UPDATE IN INTENSIVE CARE MEDICINE

Series Editor: Jean-Louis Vincent

UPDATE IN INTENSIVE CARE MEDICINE

Springer
New York
Berlin
Heidelberg
Barcelona
Hong Kong
London
Milan
Paris
Tokyo

IMMUNE RESPONSE IN THE CRITICALLY ILL

Volume Editors:

John C. Marshall, MD
Professor of Surgery
Department of Surgery
Interdepartmental Division
of Critical Care Medicine
Toronto General Hospital
University of Toronto
Toronto, Ontario, Canada

Jonathan Cohen FRCP, FRCPath,
FRCPE, FMedSci
Chairman
Department of Infectious Diseases
& Microbiology
Division of Investigative Science
Imperial College School
of Medicine
Hammersmith Hospital
London, United Kingdom

Series Editor:

Jean-Louis Vincent, MD, PhD, FCCM, FCCP
Head, Department of Intensive Care
Erasme University Hospital
Brussels, Belgium

With 46 Figures and 49 Tables

Springer

John C. Marshall, MD
Professor of Surgery
Department of Surgery
Interdepartmental Division of Critical Care Medicine
Toronto General Hospital
University of Toronto
Toronto, Ontario, Canada

Jonathan Cohen FRCP, FRCPath, FRCPE, FMedSci
Chairman
Department of Infectious Diseases & Microbiology
Division of Investigative Science
Imperial College School of Medicine
Hammersmith Hospital
London, United Kingdom

Series Editor:
Jean-Louis Vincent, MD, PhD, FCCM, FCCP
Head, Department of Intensive Care
Erasme University Hospital
Route de Lennik 808
B-1070 Brussels, Belgium

Library of Congress Cataloging-in-Publication Data applied for.

Printed on acid-free paper.

Production managed by PRO EDIT GmbH, Heidelberg, Germany.
Typeset by TBS, Sandhausen, Germany.
Printed and bound by Mercedes-Druck, Berlin, Germany.
Printed in Germany.

9 8 7 6 5 4 3 2 1

ISSN 0933-6788
ISBN 3-540-42037-1 SPIN 10797049

Springer-Verlag New York Berlin Heidelberg
A member of BertelsmannSpringer Science+Business Media GmbH

Contents

List of Contributors

E. Abraham
Division of Pulmonary Sciences
and Critical Care Medicine
University of Colorado Health
Sciences Center
Denver, Colorado
USA

M. Adib-Conquy
Unité d'Immuno-Allergie
Institut Pasteur
Paris
France

J. Andersson
Division of Infectious Diseases
Huddinge University Hospital
Huddinge
Sweden

U. Andersson
Department of Pediatrics
Huddinge University Hospital
Huddinge
Sweden

M. K. Angele
Department of Surgery
Ludwig Maximilians University
Munich
Germany

A. Ayala
Division of Surgical Research
Rhode Island Hospital
Brown University School of Medicine
Providence, Rhode Island
USA

T. R. Billiar
Department of Surgery
University of Pittsburgh
Pittsburgh, Pennsylvania
USA

T. Calandra
Department of Infectious Diseases
Centre Hospitalier Universitaire
Vaudois (CHUV)
Lausanne
Switzerland

S. E. Calvano
Department of Surgery
Robert Wood Johnson Medical School
New Brunswick, New Jersey
USA

J. M. Cavaillon
Unité d'Immuno-Allergie
Institut Pasteur
Paris
France

C. S. Chung
Center for Surgical Research
Rhode Island Hospital
Providence, Rhode Island
USA

J. Cohen
Department of Infectious
Diseases & Microbiology
Hammersmith Hospital
Division of Investigative Science
Imperial College School of Medicine
London
United Kingdom

A. K. De
Department of Surgery
University of Massachusetts
Medical School
Worcester, Massachusetts
USA

C. A. Dinarello
Department of Infectious Diseases
University Health Sciences Center
Denver, Colorado
USA

W. D. Döcke
Institute of Medical Immunology
Charité-Campus Mitte
Humboldt University Berlin
Berlin
Germany

Q. Dong
Clinical Sciences Division
Department of Medicine
University of Toronto
Toronto, Ontario
Canada

S. Donnelly
Department of Medicine & Therapeutics
University College Dublin
St. Vincent's Hospital
Dublin
Ireland

G. Downey
Clinical Sciences Division
University of Toronto
Department of Medicine
Toronto, Ontario
Canada

E. Faist
Department of Surgery
Ludwig Maximilians University
Munich
Germany

D. T. Golenbock
The Maxwell Finland Laboratory
for Infectious Diseases
Boston University School of Medicine
Boston, Massachusetts
USA

C. Haslett
Department of Respiratory Medicine
University of Edinburgh Medical School
Edinburgh
United Kingdom

H. Heine
The Maxwell Finland Laboratory
for Infectious Diseases
Boston University School of Medicine
Boston, Massachusetts
USA

D. Heumann
Department of Infectious Diseases
Centre Hospitalier Universitaire Vaudois
(CHUV)
Lausanne
Switzerland

N. Hirani
Rayne Laboratories
University of Edinburgh
Medical School
Edinburgh
United Kingdom

K. Kodys
Department of Surgery
University of Massachusetts Medical School
Worcester, Massachusetts
USA

J. Kruger
Clinical Sciences Division
University of Toronto
Department of Medicine
Toronto, Ontario
Canada

E. Lien
The Maxwell Finland Laboratory
for Infectious Diseases
Boston University School of Medicine
Boston, Massachusetts
USA

E. Lin
Department of Surgery
New York Hospital - Queens
Flushing, New York
USA

S. F. Lowry
Department of Surgery
Division of General Surgery
Robert Wood Johnson Medical School
New Brunswick, New Jersey
USA

J. C. Marshall
Department of Surgery
Interdepartmental Division
of Critical Care Medicine
Toronto General Hospital
Toronto, Ontario
Canada

P. Matzinger
National Institutes of Health
Bethesda, Maryland
USA

B. Merhad
Department of Internal Medicine
University of Michigan
Medical Center
Ann Arbor, Michigan
USA

C. L. Miller-Graziano
Department of Surgery
University of Massachusetts
Medical School
Worcester, Massachusetts
USA

M. Noursadeghi
Department of Infectious Diseases
Hammersmith Hospital
London
United Kingdom

S. M. Opal
Infectious Disease Division
Memorial Hospital of Rhode Island
Brown University Medical School
Pawtucket, Rhode Island
USA

M. R. Pinsky
Department of Anesthesiology
and Critical Care Medicine
University of Pittsburgh
School of Medicine
Pittsburgh, Pennsylvania
USA

H. Redl
Department of Clinical Traumatology
Ludwig Boltzmann Institute
Vienna
Austria

P. Reinke
Department of Nephrology
and Internal Intensive Care
Charité-Campus Mitte
Humboldt University Berlin
Berlin
Germany

A. J. Rosenbloom
Department of Anesthesiology
and Critical Care Medicine
University of Pittsburgh
Medical Center
Pittsburgh, Pennsylvania
USA

G. Y. Song
Department of Surgery
Division of Surgical Research
Rhode Island Hospital
Brown University
Providence, Rhode Island
USA

T. J. Standiford
Department of Internal Medicine
Pulmonary Inpatient Service
University of Michigan
Medical Center
Ann Arbor, Michigan
USA

P. Stokkers
Department of Experimental
Internal Medicine
Academic Medical Center
University of Amsterdam
Amsterdam
The Netherlands

R. Taneja
General Division
The Toronto General Hospital
Toronto, Ontario,
Canada

K. J. Tracey
Department of Microbiology and Immunology
Albert Einstein School of Medicine
North Shore University Hospital
Manhasset, New York
USA

W. C. Tsai
Department of Pediatric Pulmonology
University of Michigan
Medical Center
Ann Arbor, Michigan
USA

R. J. Ulevitch
Department of Immunology
Scripps Research Institute
La Jolla, California
USA

T. van der Poll
Department of Experimental
Internal Medicine
Academic Medical Center
University of Amsterdam
Amsterdam
The Netherlands

S. J. H. van Deventer
Department of Experimental
Internal Medicine
Academic Medical Center
University of Amsterdam
Amsterdam
The Netherlands

R. T. Villavicencio
Department of Surgery
University of Internal Medicine
Indiana University School of Medicine
Indianapolis, Indiana
USA

J. L. Vincent
Department of Intensive Care
Erasme University Hospital
Brussels
Belgium

H. D. Volk
Institute of Medical Immunology
Charité-Campus Mitte
Humboldt University Berlin
Berlin
Germany

H. Wang
Department of Emergency Surgery
North Shore University Hospital
Manhasset, New York
USA

L. Yue
The Toronto General Hospital
Toronto, Ontario
Canada

S. Zedler
Department of Surgery
Ludwig Maximilians University
Munich
Germany

Abbreviations

APC	Antigen presenting cell
ARDS	Acute respiratory distress syndrome
ATP	Adenosine triphosphate
BAL	Bronchoalveolar lavage
BPI	Bactericidal/permeability-increasing protein
CPB	Cardiopulmonary bypass
CRP	C-reactive protein
DIC	Disseminated intravascular coagulation
DNA	Desoxyribonucleic acid
FLICE	Fas-like IL-1β converting enzyme
FLIP	FLICE inhibitory protein
fMLP	n-formyl-methionyl-leucyl-phenylalanine
G-CSF	Granulocyte-colony stimulating factor
GMP	Guanosine monophosphate
HIV	Human immunodeficiency virus
ICAM	Intercellular adhesion molecule
ICU	Intensive care unit
IFN	Interferon
IL	Interleukin
IRAK	IL-1 receptor associated kinase
JNK	c-Jun N-terminal kinase
LBP	LPS binding protein
LPS	Lipopolysaccharide
MAPK	Mitogen activated protein kinase
MODS	Multiple organ dysfunction syndrome
MOF	Multiple organ failure
NAD	Nicotinamide adenine dinucleotide
NF-κB	Nuclear factor kappa-B
NK	Natural killer cells
NO	Nitric oxide
NOS	Nitric oxide synthase
PAF	Platelet activating factor
PARS	Poly (ADP-ribose) synthetase
pHi	Gastric intramucosal pH
PMN	Polymorphonuclear leukocyte

RANTES	Regulated upon activation normal T lymphocyte expressed and secreted
RNA	Ribonucleic acid
ROS	Reactive oxygen species
SIRS	Systemic inflammatory response syndrome
STAT	Signal transducer and activator of transcription
TGF-β	Transforming growth factor-β
TNF	Tumor necrosis factor
TRADD	TNF receptor-associated death domain
TRAF	TNF receptor-associated factor
TRAIL	TNF-related apoptosis-inducing ligand
VCAM	Vascular cell adhesion molecule

The Four Ds of the Danger Model: Distress, Damage, Destruction, and Death

P. Matzinger

Introduction

For three quarters of a century, immunologists have based their theories and experiments on the fundamental belief that the primary function of the immune system is to discriminate between self and non-self and that, if the system were perfect, it would attack everything that is non-self and be totally tolerant of anything that is self. I have abandoned this belief. Over the years too many immunological findings have accumulated that do not fit and too many questions have been raised that cannot be answered.

For example, if each individual's immune system learns what is 'self' at an early age, why are new antigens that appear at puberty not considered 'foreign' and destroyed? Why is a newly lactating breast not rejected when it begins to make new proteins? How can normal individuals contain both T and B cells capable of reacting to self antigens like DNA, keratin and myelin basic protein, yet not have destructive autoimmunity? Why are transplanted livers rejected less vigorously than transplanted hearts? Why is the immune system so bad at dealing with tumors, even when they demonstrably express new, 'non-self' antigens? Why do we not normally respond to all the foreign antigens in food, to our commensal intestinal bacteria, or to our fetuses or the sperm that begot them?

The answers to these questions cannot be easily found when we approach the immune system from the viewpoint of self/non-self discrimination (SNSD), however they fall easily into place when approached from a different direction, that of the Danger model, which holds that the immune system is far more concerned with danger and potential destruction than with the distinction between self and non-self. Below I will briefly describe the model and some of the answers it provides for the questions above.

The Danger Model

The Danger model does not require a radical re-thinking of the immune system. It borrows most of what we have learned in the last half century, adding a small but critical step that completely changes the viewpoint with which we explain most immunological phenomena. A quick overview of the theoretical additions that have been made to the original clonal selection model shows how this works.

The original clonal selection model [1] suggested that the cells we now call B cells carry clonally distributed, antigen specific, receptors and that the interaction of this receptor with antigen initiates a signal (now known as signal One or stimulation) that turns on the cell and initiates an immune response (Fig. 1a). Autoreactive cells are deleted early in life (or early in their ontogeny), thus immune responses are directed only against non-self.

This model lasted until 1969, when it was modified by Bretscher and Cohn who invented the helper cell and, to link the helper with its corresponding B cell, they invented a second signal, called 'help' [2]. They suggested that recognition of antigen (signal One) would lead to death of the B cell unless it was rescued by the receipt of timely and appropriate help (signal Two) from the helper (Fig. 1b).

This expanded model lasted until 1974, when Lafferty and Cunningham modified it again, adding a new cell (the antigen presenting cell, or APC) and a new signal (co-stimulation) [3]. They proposed that T helper cells, like B cells, die from receipt of signal One alone and become activated only if they receive a second, co-stimulatory, signal (Fig. 1c).

For the next 13 years, Bretscher and Cohn's second signal (help) [2] was studied while Lafferty and Cunningham's second signal (co-stimulation) [3] was ignored. Then, in 1986, Jenkins and Schwartz [4] discovered that gluteraldehyde fixed APCs were unable to stimulate T cell clones, and the immunological community began to study co-stimulation. Why had it taken so long? The main reason is that APCs cannot distinguish self from non-self, and if they are the cells that initiate immune responses, then the immune system cannot focus only on non-self antigens. APCs and co-stimulation, therefore, made people uncomfort-

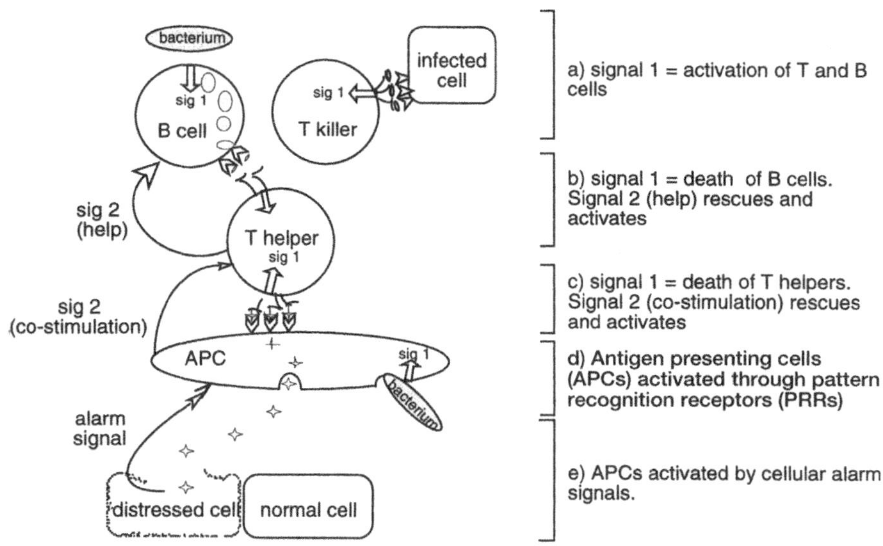

Fig. 1.1. A half century of immunological theory

able and were often dismissed or ignored until, in 1989, Charlie Janeway found an ingenious way to integrate co-stimulation into a SNSD model [5,6]. He coined the term 'pattern recognition receptors' (PRRs) for receptors on APCs that are able to recognize bacterial products, such as lipopolysaccharide (LPS), and suggested that the cells and molecules of the innate immune system have a genetically encoded memory of non-self that is specific for evolutionarily distant organisms. Starting with the hypothesis that APCs are normally at rest and must be turned on by some sort of activation signals, he suggested that binding of the PRRs activates the APCs, which only then up-regulate co-stimulatory molecules to activate T cells (Fig. 1d).

Thus, there were now two different types of non-self recognition. A genetically encoded set of PRRs relegated to the APCs and a somatically generated set of receptors expressed by T and B cells; a neat solution to the problem of how to incorporate co-stimulation into a SNSD model. However, Janeway himself pointed out that the addition of the PRRs, though explaining immune responses to bacteria and other evolutionarily distant pathogens, cannot explain the immune response to transplants or tumors, nor the dysfunction(s) that lead to many autoimmune diseases.

To solve this problem, Ephraim Fuchs and I simply followed tradition and added another set of cells and another set of signals to the current immunological family [7–9]. We suggested that all normal tissue cells, when distressed, send alarm signals that serve to activate local APCs. Cells dying normal, programmed cell deaths are usually scavenged and do not send such alarm signals, but any cell that is abnormally distressed, damaged, or destroyed necrotically, should activate its local APCs (Fig. 1e).

We do not yet know what the alarm signals might be. We presume that any molecule normally found inside cells, and that remains inside when a cell dies apoptotically but is released upon necrotic death, may serve as an alarm signal. Mitochondria, for example, might be the endogenous 'bacteria' to which the PRRs are actually directed. The internal mannose trees normally found on nascent glycoproteins might be the endogenous ligands of the mannose receptors on APCs. RNA or DNA might serve as alarm signals. Heat shock proteins might do it, especially as some of these have been shown to ferry peptides to major histocompatibility complex (MHC) molecules [10]. We presume that there will be more than one alarm signal, that some of them will be pre-packaged (for those times when a cell dies quickly) and some will be inducible (for those times when a cell is stressed, damaged, infected, or dies slowly). Whatever the alarm signals turn out to be, the Danger model suggests that it is these endogenous signals of danger, distress, damage and death, not exogenous patterns of foreignness, that are the initiators of immunity (Fig. 1e).

This simple solution turns out to have enormous explanatory and predictive power. It explains both the cases in which the immune system does the right things and many of those in which it goes wrong. In the rest of this chapter, I will very briefly show how the model deals with a number of immunological phenomena such as: 1) the need for adjuvant; 2) how the immune system deals with the appearance of new antigens as we change during life; 3) why mothers do not usually reject their fetuses; 4) why transplants are rejected; and 5) why tumors are often not rejected even though they may carry 'foreign' tumor specific antigens.

What the Model Explains

In each of the categories below I will give a brief explanation based on the two main assumptions of the Danger model, namely that primary immune responses are initiated by alarm signals from stressed or damaged tissues and that mature resting lymphocytes are rendered tolerant (deleted) by the recognition of antigen (signal One) in the absence of co-stimulation or help (signal Two). I will also deal with a couple of phenomena in each category that seem, at first sight, not to fit, showing that they can easily be fit into the model. There are many more such apparently 'non-fitting' phenomena that are actually easily explained, but will not be covered here.

The Need for Adjuvant

Janeway suggested that adjuvant works by activating APCs and here I agree. However, Janeway also suggested that the reason adjuvants activate APCs is that they mimic the bacterial products for which the APC PRRs are specific. Here I disagree, at least partly. There are many adjuvants that do not include bacterial products, such as alum, or poly I:C. Based on the Danger model, I would suggest that many adjuvants work because they either create damage or mimic the alarm signals sent by damaged cells. Complete Freund's adjuvant (CFA), the most common and effective adjuvant in experimental situations, is not allowed in humans because of the damage it does, and many biotechnology companies are trying to find effective adjuvants that do no damage. However, doing harm may be precisely what is needed.

A good candidate for an adjuvant that would do no harm comes from the efficacy of mycobacteria. There may be two reasons for its effectiveness. First, mycobacteria generate damage. Second they express many heat shock proteins. Since heat shock proteins are highly conserved throughout evolution, the heat shock proteins of mycobacteria might well mimic some of the vertebrate heat shock proteins that act as alarm signals for APCs. If we could identify these, we might be able to create adjuvants that mimic them, rather than using adjuvants that generate the damage that elicits them.

Puberty and Lactation: Maintaining Tolerance to a Changing Self

Suppose that there exists a T cell specific for a self molecule that appears late in life, for example a milk protein expressed only during pregnancy and lactation. In males, this is not a problem, but a newly lactating female risks autoimmune destruction of the lactating breast. SNSD models do not deal with this situation and I have heard several arguments suggesting that the problem does not even exist.

For example, it has been suggested that early ingestion of milk results in oral tolerance, but there are two reasons why this argument does not hold. First, oral tolerance, like all other known forms of tolerance, does not last long in the absence of antigen. Soon after weaning, it will wane. Second, there are a large number of western human females that, for social reasons, were not raised on human milk (we drank Nestle's, Carnation, Pet milk, etc.) and could not have developed oral tolerance. Yet, most do not generate autoimmunity when they themselves begin to lactate. Another argument has been that milk proteins are immunologically privileged because they do not enter the body but are secreted directly to the outside. This argument is also wrong for two reasons. First, there is no known mechanism by which cells can choose to segregate specific intermittently expressed proteins from the MHC loading system. Therefore, except in rare circumstances, the cell producing milk proteins cannot prevent milk peptides from getting to the surface on MHC molecules and becoming a target for cytotoxic T-lymphocytes (CTL). Second, though milk proteins are indeed secreted to the outside of the body, they can also be found in the circulation of lactating individuals [11, 12] and are thus available to B cells and various populations of APCs. One cannot solve the problem of the newly lactating breast (or any other organ that changes during life) by simply stating that the problem does not exist.

Why then, are newly lactating breasts not rejected? What allows us to change as we live, reach puberty, reproduce and age? The answer is that these changes are normal, that any concomitant cell death is programmed, usually apoptotic, and that these deaths do not release alarm signals to activate the immune system. If a T cell specific for a milk protein circulates into the newly lactating breast, it encounters a set of perfectly healthy tissues producing milk and expressing milk peptides on the surface in MHC grooves. The T cell binds, receives signal One without Two and dies. Suppose now that the breast becomes infected, a situation well known to sheep and dairy farmers. The infection elicits alarm signals that activate APCs, which take up the antigens in their environment (picking up milk proteins along with those of the pathogen) and present them, along with co-stimulatory molecules, to initiate an immune response. Like the pathogen specific T cells, the milk-specific T cell is stimulated, responds, kills some of the cells producing milk (sometimes also circulating to and generating an inflammation in the uninfected breast) and rests again. This cycle of stimulation and resting down continues until the infection is cleared. There are two important features that now allow the autoreactive milk-specific T cell to stop responding and become susceptible to tolerance induction. First, the immune system does not throw fuel on the fire. CTL kill by inducing apoptosis in their targets [13], ensuring that the damage done by the killers themselves does not cause activation of APCs and does not maintain the response. Second, once activated, APCs do not remain activated forever. Although it is not clear why they disappear, they do not seem to last longer than a few days. Thus the response stops when the pathogen-caused damage stops, at which time, the APCs are no longer activated to offer co-stimulatory signals. At this point, the killer becomes a resting memory cell, susceptible to signal-One-without-Two induced death. The next time it travels through the healed and normal breast tissue, it will be deleted.

Reactions against self molecules may thus be a frequent part of every immune response. However, because of the healthy tissues' ability to tolerize, the autoimmune components are short lived and tolerance is established each time. The frequency of autoreactive T cells is thus kept quite low, though it will vary with the number and concentration of expressed tissue specific antigens, the amount of traffic through the organ, and the frequency of infections and other traumas.

Why Mothers Do Not Reject Their Fetuses

Soon after Medawar did the experiment that put the SNSD model of immunity on the map, he pointed out that pregnancy was a problem [14]. After all, if the immune system should reject anything foreign, then pregnant females should reject their fetuses. However, instead of considering that the model might be wrong, he suggested that fetuses should have evolved methods to deal with their mothers' immune responses. The methods suggested over the years have been rather astonishing. For example, students are often taught that there is an immunologically and physically impermeable barrier between mother and fetus. First, this would be an unsound strategy. If the fetus were to become infected, the mother should be able to do something about it, otherwise both she and her fetus are likely to die. Even if a maternal immune response against an infected fetus results in fetal death, it is a better choice than to do nothing. Better to kill off an infected fetus and live to have another one than to die from the infection. Second, we need not worry that such an evolutionarily unsound strategy might exist. It does not; there is evidence of cellular traffic in both directions across the placenta [15].

Another suggestion has been that the fetus immunosuppresses its mother. Again this would be an evolutionarily stupid strategy. We want the individuals carrying the next generation to be as healthy as possible, not immunosuppressed! And again, it is not true. Pregnant women, for example, do not become ill with any greater frequency than non-pregnant ones.

Rather than continue through the list of possible ways in which SNSD models have dealt with pregnancy, let me offer my own solution. The Danger model suggests that pregnant females do not reject their fetuses because the fetuses do not look dangerous. The death that goes on in fetal life is programmed, apoptotic cell death, and cells dying this way do not send alarm signals to alert APCs to initiate an immune response. It does not matter that many of the fetal antigens are 'foreign' to the mother. Without alarm signals to activate her APCs, she will not initiate a response. Should the fetus become infected, however, the damage done will alert a response to clear the infection. From this viewpoint, it is not surprising that spontaneous abortion is a common concomitant of infection.

There are two situations that are commonly brought up as evidence against this view. The first is that pregnant women do worse with malaria than non-pregnant ones. This has been thought to be the result of the 'immunosuppressed' state of pregnant females. However, recent evidence shows that the reason most probably lies with the parasites, not the mother. The fetus and the malaria are fighting for the same maternal resource, blood. The fetus has had evolutionary time to generate a complex organ with which to obtain that blood, and the malaria has had evolutionary time to find a way to take advantage of that. It induces, on red cells, a receptor for a glycocalyx expressed by the placenta [16]. Thus it is not a mother's 'immunosuppressed' state that endangers her during a malaria infection, but the infectious strategy of the parasite.

The second situation is the case of Rhesus (Rh) disease, in which pregnant women that are themselves Rh negative, make antibody responses to an Rh positive fetus. Again the Danger model has no problem explaining this, mainly because it is the second pregnancy that is usually the problem, not the first. Most women become immunized at birth, and birth is dangerous. There is bleeding (and blood mixing between mother and fetus), ripping, (and surgeons with knives) causing a great deal of non-programmed cell death. At this time, an immune response may easily occur.

Thus, during healthy pregnancies, there is no danger to initiate an immune response and the fetus survives, regardless of its 'foreignness' to its mother.

Why are Transplants Rejected?

Although transplantation is meant to help, not injure, a patient, the process of transplanting a tissue involves surgical procedures that result in tissue damage and ischemic cell death. Such damage will generate alarm signals that activate both donor and host APCs, which will then home to recipient lymph nodes and present both their own antigens and any others that are captured from the damaged cells in the graft.

I have often been asked why, in that case, are grafts not rejected between identical twins, or from one part of a body to another? Or why do we not all reject our own skin when we damage it in the process of living? The answer, of course, is that it takes two things to achieve graft rejection: Alarm signals to wake up the APCs, and a sufficient frequency of reactive T cells to reject the graft. Since our own tissues are constantly in the process of tolerizing for themselves, by allowing circulating autoreactive T cells to die from the receipt of signal One without Two, the frequency of autoreactive cells to our own skin should be rather low. There will only be those that have left the thymus recently, and have not yet circulated through the skin to become tolerant. These might very well become activated after a cut, burn, or scrape causes the elaboration of alarm signals, but their frequency is too low to do much damage. Furthermore, after the skin heals (remember that killers kill by inducing apoptosis, which does not perpetuate an immune response) these autoreactive T cells will rest, become memory cells, and as they circulate, will become tolerized by signal One without Two. Thus there may be a small component of autoreactive destruction every time we damage ourselves, either physically, or by an infection, but the autoreactivity will stop when the damage stops, and the autoreactive T cells will again be deleted.

Perhaps this is why we sometimes see transient autoantibodies after a heart infarction [17]?

The best evidence that mere foreignness is not sufficient to initiate graft rejection came from a series of experiments done by Lafferty and colleagues in which they removed the APCs from thyroid or pancreatic islet grafts [18,19]. These grafts were invariably accepted, even if they differed by both major and minor histocompatibility antigens. They were not impervious to rejection, but could be rejected by recipients immunized with donor type APCs at the time of, or soon after, the transplant. This showed that the foreign antigens on the grafted tissues were available as targets for an immune response but could not elicit one. Furthermore, the grafts did not sit idly in their new hosts but, given enough time (one year in the case of thyroids) the thyroid antigens induced tolerance to themselves such that the recipients would now accept a second graft, replete with APCs. Such tolerance is all the more remarkable, considering that these are very small organs and they need to deal with a very high frequency of reactive cells.

If transplanted organs can tolerize for themselves, then why must we continue to give immunosuppressive drugs, such as cyclosporine, for the life of a transplant patient? A patient that has held on to a transplanted kidney for 15–20 years, who then tires of the side effects of the drug and stops taking it, often goes on to reject the kidney [20]. How can the Danger model cope with this? It predicts that these long standing kidneys should have had plenty of time to induce tolerance to themselves. If a grafted allogeneic thyroid can induce tolerance to itself in a year [18], why does the kidney not do it in 15 or 20 years?

The problem, it turns out, is the drug, not the model. By blocking the calcium flux that follows stimulation of the T cell receptor, cyclosporin blocks signal One [21] and, though this stops the rejection, it has the nasty side effect of suppressing the transplanted organ's natural ability to induce tolerance. If peripheral tolerance normally occurs because T cells receive signal One without Two, it cannot occur under cyclosporine blockade. The focus is beginning to shift to drugs that block signal Two, such as CTLA4-Ig and anti-CD40 ligand, which are beginning to have some measure of success in experimental transplantation [22,23]. A drug that blocks signal Two should enhance an organ's ability to induce tolerance, rather than prevent it.

Tumors

I firmly believe that we have the ability to cure a substantial percentage of tumor patients through immunization but that the current protocols do not work simply because they are performed within the wrong paradigm and are therefore performed incorrectly.

To explain why a tumor is able to grow in the face of an immune system able to recognize its mutated, or overexpressed, tumor antigens, the old SNSD models suggest that most tumors are immunosuppressive or able to somehow 'escape' from immune surveillance. The Danger model suggests instead that tumors grow simply because they are healthy cells that have lost growth control. They do not normally die necrotically and they do not put out alarm signals to alert APCs. Thus, in spite of their 'foreign' antigens, they do not elicit an immune response.

However, under experimental conditions, a tumor can sometimes be inhibited by strong immunization. In a sense, these tumors behave like Lafferty's APC depleted transplants [18,19]. They cannot initiate an immune response, but they can be destroyed by a response that is initiated in other ways. In fact, as they grow, tumors will induce tolerance to themselves in the same way that normal tissues do, by offering signal One without Two. Perhaps this is why there are no tumors of dendritic cells. A dendritic cell tumor would be able to co-stimulate for the immune response that would destroy it.

The trick would be to find ways to immunize against tumor antigens before the tumor grows large enough to tolerize the relevant T cells. This is not a new idea. First done at the turn of the century by Bill Coley [24], there has recently been renewed interest, as laboratories around the world accumulate lists of 'tumor antigens'. Many different vaccines have been tried, including tumors transfected with cytokine genes, dendritic cells fed with tumor RNA, fibroblasts, viruses, or salmonella transduced with tumor DNA, tumor DNA itself, etc. [25–29]. These vaccines have generally succeeded and failed in the same way. They protect against a tumor injected a few days later (as long as the dose of tumor is not too large), but they do not eliminate established tumors. So the search for more effective vaccines continues, as does the search for reasons why the established tumors can escape or suppress the immune response. I believe that both of these searches are misguided. The vaccines are not ineffective. They are simply used incorrectly because immuno-oncologists still adhere to models of self/non-self.

In order to clear a tumor, we need to initiate an immune response and then maintain it until the tumor is gone. It is not enough to induce a response and then stop. Under the old SNSD models, an immune response, once initiated, should continue until the target antigen is gone. However, the Danger model predicts that this is not so. The vaccinated response will wane as soon as the damage from the vaccine heals. It will not matter if tumor cells still exist in the body. They are healthy and, unlike cells damaged by a pathogen, do not send signals to maintain the response (remember that killers induce apoptotic, not necrotic death). Thus, if a tumor vaccine is given in a standard vaccination protocol (meaning a primary immunization and a boost or two) any remaining tumor cells will grow, not because they have escaped the immune system but because the immune response stops when the damage from the last boost heals. Without continuous, or repeated, damage (along with more antigen for the APCs to capture), the APCs cannot maintain the response. Following from this reasoning, the Danger model has a very simple prescription for anyone using tumor vaccines: If you have a vaccine that makes a tumor get smaller, ... DON'T STOP! Keep injecting, once every few weeks (or to coincide with the waning of the response), until the last tumor cell is gone.

Necrotic tumors: There are some tumors where necrotic death occurs. Though a quick look at the Danger model suggests that these should be eliminated, a deeper look gives a different picture. Tumors that die necrotically are usually large, solid, poorly vascularized tumors that begin to starve in the center. Starvation death is apoptotic, not necrotic and thus elicits no immune response. Eventually, however, the death rate may overload the local scavenging capacity and the dead cells then fall apart, releasing alarm signals and initiating an immune response. However, by this time the tumor is very large and has had a long time to grow and to induce tolerance in any tumor-specific T cells. Therefore the few remaining tumor-specific killers have lost the race before it starts. Each one that is activated in a local lymph node can kill a small number of tumor cells before it needs to be reactivated. In the mean time, the tumor continues to grow. I am, therefore, no longer surprised that tumor infiltrating lymphocytes (TILs) contain active killers [30]. It is a case of too little, too late. Expanding them *in vitro* is a step in the right direction, but they will not stay active forever and must be continually restimulated. This is why TIL therapy so often fails. The killers are expanded and re-injected into the patient, where they kill a number of tumor cells. The tumors become visibly smaller, and in a few cases they disappear. However, in most cases, the initial onslaught by the activated TILs is not enough to clear the tumor and, without re-stimulation, the response wanes, and any remaining tumor cells then grow again.

I believe that TIL therapy can cure tumors. We just have to let go of the old fashioned idea that the immune system, once turned on, continues to fight until the antigen is gone: It will not. It will continue to fight until the danger is gone, and it does not recognize most tumors as dangerous because the cells do not send alarm signals. We have to boost them and keep boosting.

Conclusion

In this chapter, I have discussed just a few of the areas covered by the Danger model. I hope that the principles and examples outlined in this chapter will suffice to provide a general idea of the power of the model, and will perhaps serve as a springboard for new ideas, new criticisms and new tests.

References

1. Burnet FM (1959) The clonal selection theory of acquired immunity, Vanderbilt University Press, Nashville
2. Bretscher P, Cohn M (1970) A theory of self-nonself discrimination. Science 169:1042–1049
3. Lafferty KJ, Cunningham A (1975) A new analysis of allogenic interactions. Aust J Exp Biol Med Sci 53:27–42
4. Jenkins MK, Schwartz RH (1987) Antigen presentation by chemically modified splenocytes induces antigen-specific T cell unresponsiveness in vitro and in vivo. J Exp Med 165: 302–319
5. Janeway CA Jr (1989) Approaching the asymptote? Evolution and revolution in immunology. Cold Spring Harb Symp Quant Biol 54:11–13
6. Janeway CA Jr (1992) The immune system evolved to discriminate infectious nonself from noninfectious self. Immunol Today 13:11–16
7. Matzinger P (1994) Tolerance, danger, and the extended family. Annu Rev Immunol 12: 991–1045
8. Matzinger P, Fuchs EJ (1996) Beyond "Self" and "Non- Self": Immunity is a conversation, not a war. J NIH Res 8:35–39

9. Matzinger P (1998) An innate sense of danger. Semin Immunol 10:399–415
10. Srivastava PK, Menoret A, Basu S, Binder RJ, McQuade KL (1998) Heat shock proteins come of age: primitive functions acquire new roles in an adaptive world. Immunity 8:657–665
11. Prosser CG, Eichler SJ, Farr VC, Davis SR (1992) Effect of colostrum intake on alpha-lactalbumin concentrations in serum of calves. Res Vet Sci 53:219–222
12. Stelwagen K, Farr VC, McFadden HA, Prosser CG, Davis SR (1997) Time course of milk accumulation-induced opening of mammary tight junctions, and blood clearance of milk components. Am J Physiol 273:R379–R386
13. Duke RC, Chervanak R, Cohen JJ (1983) Endogenous endonuclease-induced DNA fragmentation: an early event in cell-mediated cytolysis. Proc Natl Acad Sci USA 80:6361–6365
14. Medawar PB (1954) Some immunological and endocrinological problems raised by the evolution of viviparity in vertebrates. Symp Soc Exp Biol 7:320
15. Bonney EA (1997)The maternal immune system's interaction with circulating fetal cells. J Immunol 158:40–47
16. Fried M, Duffy PE (1996) Adherence of Plasmodium falciparum to chondroitin sulfate A in the human placenta. Science 272:1502–1504
17. Melguizo C, Prados J, Velez C, Aranega AE, Marchal JA, Aranega A (1997) Clinical significance of antiheart antibodies after myocardial infarction. Jpn Heart J 38:779–786
18. Donohoe JA, Andrus L, Bowen KM, Simeonovic C, Prowse SJ, Lafferty KJ (1983) Cultured thyroid allografts induce a state of partial tolerance in adult recipient mice. Transplantation 35:62–67
19. Bowen KM, Prowse SJ, Lafferty KJ (1981) The reversal of diabetes by islet transplantation: vulnerability of the established allograft. Science 213:1261–1262
20. Newstead CG, Johnston PA, Will EJ, Davison AM (1998)The case for withdrawal of cyclosporin after renal transplantation. Nephrol Dial Transplant 13:28–31
21. Schreiber SL, Crabtree GR (1992) The mechanism of action of cyclosporin A and FK506. Immunol Today 13:136–142
22. Larsen CP, Pearson TC (1997)The CD40 pathway in allograft rejection, acceptance, and tolerance. Curr Opin Immunol 9:641–647
23. Kirk AL, Burkly LC, Batty DS, Baumgartner RE, Berning JD, Buchanan K (1999) Treatment with humanized monoclonal antibody against CD154 prevents acute renal allograft rejection in nonhuman primates. Nature Med 5:6686–6693
24. Coley WB (1898) The treatment of inoperable sarcoma with the mixed toxins of erysipelas and bacillus prodigiosus. JAMA 389–395
25. Boczkowski D, Nair SK, Snyder D, Gilboa E (1996) Dendritic cells pulsed with RNA are potent antigen-presenting cells in vitro and in vivo. J Exp Med 184:465–472
26. Dranoff G, Jaffee E, Lazenby A, et al (1993) Vaccination with irradiated tumor cells engineered to secrete murine granulocyte-macrophage colony-stimulating factor stimulates potent, specific, and long-lasting anti-tumor immunity. Proc Natl Acad Sci USA 90:3539–3543
27. Restifo NP (1996) The new vaccines: building viruses that elicit antitumor immunity. Curr Opin Immunol 8:658–663
28. Fernandez N, Duffour MT, Perricaudet M, Lotze MT, Tursz T, Zitvogel L (1998) Active specific T-cell-based immunotherapy for cancer: nucleic acids, peptides, whole native proteins, recombinant viruses, with dendritic cell adjuvants or whole tumor cell-based vaccines. Principles and future prospects. Cytokines Cell Mol Ther 4:53–65
29. Ertl HC, Xiang Z (1996) Novel vaccine approaches. J Immunol 156:3579–3582
30. Rosenberg SA, Yannelli JR, Yang JC, et al (1994) Treatment of patients with metastatic melanoma with autologous tumor-infiltrating lymphocytes and interleukin 2. J Natl Cancer Inst 86:1159–1166

The Immune Response in Critical Illness: Excessive, Inadequate or Dysregulated

J. L. Vincent

Introduction

There have been significant advances in our understanding of the immune response in critical illness in recent years. Sepsis and its sequelae of organ dysfunction, multiple organ failure (MOF) and death, are commonly seen among the critically ill population. Newly developed therapies initially worked on the hypothesis that sepsis was the result of an overwhelming, excessive immune response, and focused on aggressive inhibition of pro-inflammatory mediators. However, although often thought of as an enemy, the septic response is, in fact, as much a friend, a normal and necessary reaction to the threat of infection. The early emphasis on the pro-inflammatory mediators involved in propagating this response, has gradually been replaced by a realization that sepsis involves both pro- and anti-inflammatory mediators acting together to create the final septic response which can be different at different times in the disease process and in different patients. In addition, mediators initially identified as anti- or pro-inflammatory may in fact exert both anti- and pro-inflammatory properties.

The inflammatory response seen in severe infections is virtually indistinguishable from that seen in other conditions including heat stroke [1,2], cardiopulmonary bypass [3], trauma [4], pancreatitis [5,6], and even in heart failure [7] and myocardial infarction [8]. In these conditions, the inflammatory response may be the result of bacterial translocation from the gut [9-11], and thus the initial triggers may, in fact, be the same as in sepsis, i.e., endotoxin or other bacterial products. Recent developments in identifying the factors involved in the body's response to lipopolysaccharide (LPS) may, in the future, present a means of distinguishing between these conditions [12].

In the immune response, whether of septic, or non-septic origin, pro- and anti-inflammatory mediators have beneficial roles to play, but both can also potentially be detrimental. For example, while high levels of the pro-inflammatory cytokine tumor necrosis factor (TNF) have been associated with the development of MOF and increased mortality in septic patients [13], and TNF is known to be involved in the development of septic shock complications such as acute respiratory distress syndrome (ARDS) [14] and renal failure, van Dissel et al. [15] reported that, in fact, the ratio of interleukin (IL)-10 to TNF, was higher in non-survivors from septic shock, i.e., they had an anti-inflammatory cytokine profile, implying that TNF is also an essential and beneficial part of host defense. Van der

Poll et al. [16] showed that induction of pneumococcal pneumonia in mice was associated, as expected, with an increase in lung TNF activity. Treatment with anti-TNF antibodies prior to intranasal inoculation with *S. pneumoniae* resulted in a fourfold increase in bacteria isolated from the lungs and blood, compared to control mice, again suggesting that TNF is an essential component of host defense. Similarly, the anti-inflammatory mediator IL-10, is released with pro-inflammatory cytokines and is believed to be important in limiting the immune response [17, 18]. Again in a mouse model, Van der Poll et al. [19] showed that the administration of IL-10 with intranasal inoculation with *S. pneumoniae*, reduced the lung concentrations of TNF, as expected, but when anti-IL-10 antibodies were administered prior to inoculation, bacterial counts fell and survival increased, suggesting that IL-10 may also hamper the immune response. In patients also, it has been suggested that IL-10 is implicated in the development of postoperative immunodepression [20].

The immune response is clearly complex; it can be excessive in terms of mediator release, but may also be inadequate. It may also be dysregulated as the cellular response to activating stimuli may be down-graded in the critically ill. In this chapter we will review current understanding about the roles of pro- and anti-inflammatory mediators in the immune response, and highlight the important implications that this understanding brings to the development and use of potential new therapies aimed at modulating the immune response in conditions such as sepsis.

Evolution of the Immune Response

An invading organism, whether bacterial, fungal, or viral, is met by the local release of pro-inflammatory mediators as the body mounts a regional defense in an attempt to eliminate the threat of infection, and promote restoration of damaged tissues. Anti-inflammatory mediators are then released to control the inflammation and restore the anti-/pro-inflammatory balance. The degree and duration of immune response varies, and some patients appear less able to restore balance, or immune homeostasis, than others, with the potential risk of organ damage, dysfunction and death; not all patients faced with an infectious insult will develop septic shock or organ failure. Why some patients do develop an excessive, persistent systemic response and others do not is uncertain, but may be due to underlying disease processes, genetic factors affecting immune status [21], immune-regulatory mechanisms such as endotoxin tolerance [22], or the size or number of infectious insults. Ongoing release of pro- and anti-inflammatory mediators continues as the body fights to restore balance.

First (Pro-Inflammatory) Phase

TNF is released early in sepsis [23] and is considered to be a key pro-inflammatory mediator for several reasons. First, TNF levels are known to be raised in patients with sepsis and increased TNF levels have been associated with increased mortality [13, 24, 25]. Second, TNF administration to healthy volunteers reproduces many of the signs of sepsis [26, 27]. Third, anti-TNF antibodies have been shown to protect animals from the harmful effects of septic shock due to endotoxin or bacteria [28, 29]. However, in the clinical situation, no anti-TNF strategy has shown similar positive results [30, 31]. One possible suggestion for this is that, unlike the experimental situation where treatments are given very soon after, or at the same time as, the septic challenge, in patients the time factor between onset of sepsis and treatment is often much greater; it may perhaps be too late to intervene when pro-inflammatory cytokine levels are already raised. Indeed, in patients with louse-borne relapsing fever, the Jarisch-Herxheimer reaction, associated with raised TNF levels [32], develops after treatment with penicillin. In these patients, administration of anti-TNF antibodies prior to the antibiotic, results in a reduced immune reaction [33]. In one anti-TNF antibody trial, treatment was administered within 12 hours of diagnosis, an inclusion criteria, but the authors commented that even at this early stage, overwhelming cytokine activation will have occurred and anti-cytokine treatment may be too late to be effective [34].

Second (Pro- and Anti-Inflammatory) Phase

The continued release of pro-inflammatory mediators triggers the release of anti-inflammatory mediators [35]. The presence of various endogenous anti-inflammatory mediators, including soluble TNF receptors, interleukin-1 receptor antagonist (IL-1ra), and IL-10, have been correlated with mortality and organ failure in patients with sepsis [18, 22, 36]. These anti-inflammatory mediators may be responsible for a down-regulation of the cellular response mechanism, with impaired production of pro-inflammatory cytokines [22, 37, 38]. The inability of cells to recover their capacity to produce cytokines, a state termed 'immunoparalysis', has been associated with increased mortality [37, 39].

Viewing the immune response as a simple pro-inflammatory phase followed by an anti-inflammatory phase with anti-inflammatory mediators released to mop up excessive pro-inflammatory mediators, is, thus, too simplistic. It has, indeed, proved impossible to find evidence of a response that is uniquely pro- or anti-inflammatory in humans. For example, patients with a worse outcome from septic shock have high levels of TNF and IL-6 as well as of IL-10 [18]. In addition, while excessive release of pro-inflammatory mediators has been generally considered deleterious, a reduced release of these factors, or excessive release of anti-inflammatory mediators, may in fact lead to an immunosuppressed state [40]. For example, in animals, TNF production is necessary in the defense against leishmaniasis [41], and similarly in some models of peritonitis [42]. Similarly, in febrile patients, those with a high IL-10 to TNF ratio, i.e., an anti-inflammatory cytokine profile, have a higher mortality [15]. Hence, excessive anti-inflammatory treatment strategies may have detrimental consequences.

Clinical Trials

Identification of many of the mediators involved in the inflammatory response to sepsis has led to the development of potential new therapies aimed at various aspects of the immune response. Such agents have been aimed either at inhibiting the release or activity of pro-inflammatory mediators, or, more recently, at augmenting the response. However, despite promising results from experimental studies in animals, both anti-inflammatory strategies [31, 43–45] and immune augmenting strategies [46] have failed to improve outcome in clinical trials of sepsis, although some of these agents have been effective in other inflammatory conditions such as Crohn's disease and rheumatoid arthritis [47–49].

The main reason for the apparent failure of these agents to influence outcome is that treatments are focused on the clinically developed syndrome rather than the underlying pathophysiological event. As we have seen the sepsis response is a necessary part of host defense and treatments aimed at modulating it must be approached with great caution. Rather than treating 'sepsis' *per se*, the underlying defect needs to be better characterized. A better definition of the immune status could, in theory, be achieved by several mechanisms, including cellular stimulation techniques and analysis of circulating mediators or inflammatory markers, but, as discussed below, in practice none of these techniques has yet been shown to be adequate.

Methods to Better Define the Immune Status

1. Cellular stimulation: The ability of monocytes to produce pro-inflammatory cytokines such as TNF, IL-1, IL-6 and IL-8, is down-regulated after stimulation with endotoxin or lipopolysaccharide in patients with severe sepsis or septic shock, and such patients have been said to be in a state of 'immunoparalysis' [39]. Identification of this reduced activity, by monitoring the degree of HLA-DR expression, has been proposed as a means of characterizing these patients and following response to treatment [40, 50].
2. Circulating cytokines: Several cytokines have been proposed as markers of the sepsis response. TNF was the first pro-inflammatory cytokine to be identified in the blood of septic patients [51], and raised levels have been correlated with poor outcome [24, 51–53]. However, not all studies have confirmed the prognostic value of TNF [54]. Interleukin-6 (IL-6) has been reported most consistently in the serum of patients with sepsis, and is generally thought to be the best cytokine marker of the severity of sepsis [55, 56]. Indeed, one clinical trial of an anti-sepsis therapy used raised IL-6 levels as an enrollment criterion [43]. The anti-inflammatory cytokine IL-10 has also been correlated with the severity of sepsis [18]. However, none of these cytokines are specific for sepsis, many being raised in other inflammatory conditions.
3. Other markers: The most commonly employed marker of infection is C-reactive protein (CRP). CRP levels increase in the presence of infection, and it has been suggested that CRP levels can be useful in predicting infection and in

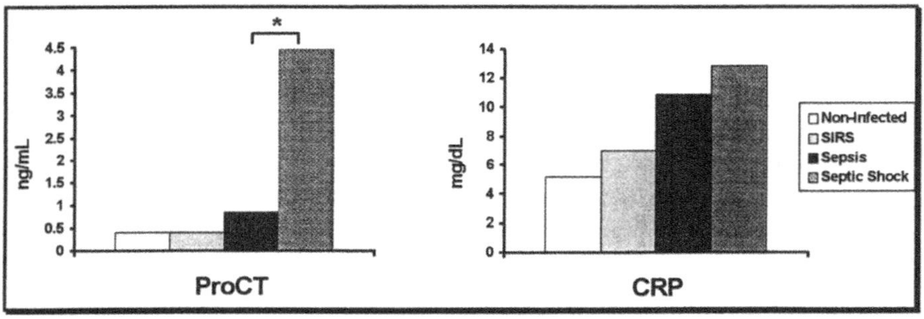

Fig. 1. Bar graph of median procalcitonin (ProCT) and C-reactive protein (CRP) levels in 205 critically ill patients during the first 96 hours following admission to the intensive care unit, divided according to severity of infection. SIRS: systemic inflammatory response syndrome; *$p < 0.05$ between groups. ProCT may be a more reliable indicator of the severity of infection that CRP. (From [60] with permission)

monitoring the effectiveness of therapy [57, 58]. The peptide procalcitonin is virtually undetectable in healthy humans, but levels are raised in patients with sepsis [59]. While probably not superior to CRP in its ability to identify the presence of infection, it may be a more useful marker of the severity of infection [60] (Fig. 1). Recent animal studies have suggested that procalcitonin may not be just an innocent bystander but may itself play an important role in the inflammatory process, as administration of procalcitonin to animals increased *E. coli*-induced mortality, and prophylactic blockade of procalcitonin offered protection [61]. Other potential candidates for sepsis markers include elastase, a marker of polymorphonuclear activation, and neopterin, a marker of macrophage activation, both of which have been shown to rise in patients with sepsis [62–64].

The Future: To Block or to Enhance ?

Whilst increased knowledge has resulted in a switch of emphasis from believing the immune response to be essentially an excessive pro-inflammatory reaction, to realizing that it has equally important anti-inflammatory components, there has not been a similar change in focus from anti-inflammatory to pro-inflammatory treatments. The pro-inflammatory cytokines remain important targets; TNF is still toxic with overwhelming evidence supporting its role in the pathogenesis and complications of sepsis. But, anti-inflammatory mediators are perhaps of equal importance; IL-10 has been shown to reduce mortality rates and the development of acute lung injury when administered to rabbits with pancreatitis [65], and to be protective against endotoxemia in mice [66].

We have been perhaps a bit blinkered in our approach to anti-sepsis treatments; too 'either/or' in our thinking. Both anti- and pro-inflammatory strategies may be effective if given to the right patient at the right time. For example, patients with a predominantly pro-inflammatory response as indicated by high IL-6 levels, may benefit from anti-inflammatory treatment [67], while patients with insufficient activation of their innate immune system may benefit from immunostimulatory therapy [40].

Experimental sepsis models usually have a clear onset and pattern with a bolus initiating dose of endotoxin or bacteria, and employ previously healthy animals of similar age and characteristics. These models have well-defined phases and treatments are given accordingly. The clinical situation is very different. Patients present at different times in the course of their disease with many other confounding factors including underlying disease processes, and non-immunologic health status. The initiating insult is rarely identifiable and may consist of repeated small insults rather than any single episode. In the clinical situation, it is therefore important not to be tempted to label patients as merely 'septic', further immune characterization is necessary. A few patients may indeed fit the classical early pro-inflammatory, late anti-inflammatory cytokine pattern, but many may have a more prolonged pro-inflammatory phase, and others may be immunosuppressed from excessive anti-inflammatory activity virtually from the beginning (Fig. 2). The ability to identify the immune status of an individual at any time, perhaps using cellular stimulation techniques as discussed above, might enable us to more appropriately target immunomodulatory therapy, for example, an anti-inflammatory agent if a pro-inflammatory phase predominates, or a pro-inflammatory agent if an anti-inflammatory phase predominates. Further monitoring of the pro/anti-inflammatory balance would then allow treatment to be ad-

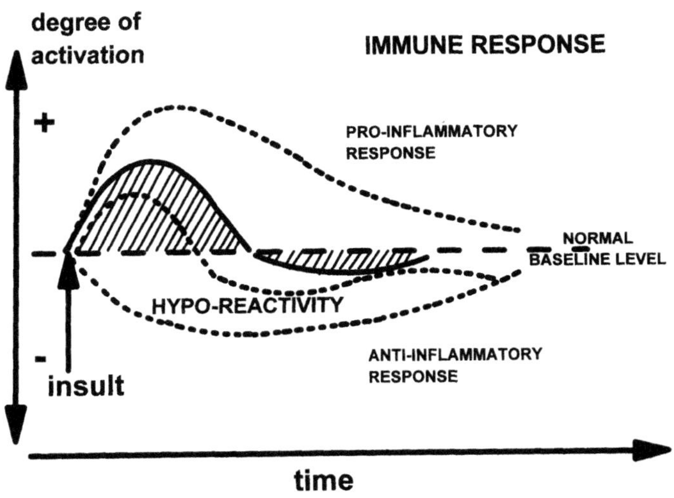

Fig. 2. Schematic representation of the possible variations in immune response. Following an infectious insult, pro- and anti-inflammatory responses develop, and return to baseline levels with time. The balance of these responses with time, in most patients, is represented by the shaded area, although some patients present a hypo-reactive response, perhaps related to previous infectious insults and cytokine down-regulation

justed according to the changing immune status. More research is clearly needed to identify the most effective techniques to define and characterize the immune response in individual patients, and to determine whether this approach, which appears clear and simple on paper, will prove to be of use in the continued search for an effective treatment in sepsis.

Conclusion

Our understanding of the inflammatory response in the critically ill has undergone rapid growth and development, from the initial identification of pro-inflammatory mediators, to a realization that it has both anti- and pro-inflammatory phases and that characterization of the balance between these two sides of the response is essential if our patients are to benefit from new anti-sepsis therapies. An immune response that is either excessive or inadequate can be detrimental. The future for clinical sepsis trials lies in more selective enrolment of individuals, perhaps based on effective identification of the degree of immune response. This will enable treatment to be based on individual disease characteristics and thus be more appropriately targeted, than the global, heterogeneous anti-sepsis approach employed in many clinical trials to date.

References

1. Bouchama A, al-Sedairy S, Siddiqui S, Shail E, Rezeig M (1993) Elevated pyrogenic cytokines in heatstroke. Chest 104: 1498–1502
2. Nylen ES, Al Arifi A, Becker KL, Snider RH Jr, Alzeer A (1997) Effect of classic heatstroke on serum procalcitonin. Crit Care Med 25: 1362–1365
3. Wan S, Marchant A, DeSmet JM, et al (1996) Human cytokine responses to cardiac transplantation and coronary artery bypass grafting. J Thorac Cardiovasc Surg 111: 469–477
4. Mimoz O, Benoist JF, Edouard AR, Assicot M, Bohoun C, Samii K (1998) Procalcitonin and C-reactive protein during the early posttraumatic systemic inflammatory response syndrome. Intensive Care Med 24: 185–188
5. de Beaux AC, Goldie AS, Ross JA, Carter DC, Fearon KC (1996) Serum concentrations of inflammatory mediators related to organ failure in patients with acute pancreatitis. Br J Surg 83: 349–353
6. Rau B, Steinbach G, Gansauge F, Mayer JM, Grunert A, Beger HG (1997) The potential role of procalcitonin and interleukin 8 in the prediction of infected necrosis in acute pancreatitis. Gut 41: 832–840
7. Testa M, Yeh M, Lee P, et al (1996) Circulating levels of cytokines and their endogenous modulators in patients with severe congestive heart failure due to coronary artery disease or heart failure. J Am Coll Cardiol 28: 964–971
8. Neumann FJ, Ott I, Gawaz M, et al (1995) Cardiac release of cytokines and inflammatory responses in acute myocardial infarction. Circulation 92: 748–755
9. Ford EG, Baisden CE, Matteson ML, Picone AL (1991) Sepsis after coronary bypass grafting: evidence for loss of the gut mucosal barrier. Ann Thorac Surg 52: 514–517
10. Brathwaite CE, Ross SE, Nagele R, Mure AJ, O'Malley KF, Garcia-Perez FA (1993) Bacterial translocation occurs in humans after traumatic injury: evidence using immunofluorescence. J Trauma 34: 586–589
11. Reed LL, Martin M, Manglano R, Newson B, Kocka F, Barrett J (1994) Bacterial translocation following abdominal trauma in humans. Circ Shock 42: 1–6

12. Ulevitch RJ (1999) Endotoxin opens the *Toll*gates to innate immunity. Nature Med 5: 144–145
13. Pinsky MR, Vincent JL, Deviere J (1993) Serum cytokine levels in human septic shock : Relation to multiple-systems organ failure and mortality. Chest 103:565–575
14. Hyers TM, Tricomi SM, Dettenmeier PA, Fowler AA (1991) Tumor necrosis factor levels in serum and bronchoalveolar lavage fluid of patients with the adult respiratory distress syndrome. Am Rev Respir Dis 144:268–271
15. van Dissel JT, van Langevelde P, Westendorp RG, Kwappenberg K, Frolich M (1998) Anti-inflammatory cytokine profile and mortality in febrile patients. Lancet 351:950–953
16. Van der Poll T, Keogh CV, Buurman WA, Lowry SF (1997) Passive immunization against tumor necrosis factor-alpha impairs host defense during pneumococcal pneumonia in mice. Am J Respir Crit Care Med 155:603–608
17. Marchant A, Devière J, Byl B, De Groote D, Vincent JL, Goldman M (1994) Interleukin-10 production during septicaemia. Lancet 344:707–708
18. Friedman G, Jankowski S, Marchant A, Goldman M, Kahn RJ, Vincent JL (1997) Blood interleukin-10 levels parallel the severity of septic shock. J Crit Care 12:183–187
19. Van der Poll T, Marchant A, Keogh CV, Goldman M, Lowry SF (1996) Interleukin-10 impairs host defense in murine pneumococcal pneumonia. J Infect Dis 174:994–1000
20. Klava A, Windsor ACJ, Farmery SM, et al (1997) Interleukin-10: A role in the development of postoperative immunosuppression. Arch Surg 132:425–429
21. Stuber F, Petersen M, Bokelmann F, Schade U (1996) A genomic polymorphism within the tumor necrosis factor locus influences plasma tumor necrosis factor-alpha concentrations and outcome of patients with severe sepsis. Crit Care Med 24:381–384
22. Van Deuren M, Van der Ven-Jongekrijk J, Demacker PN, et al (1994) Differential expression of proinflammatory cytokines and their inhibitors during the course of meningococcal infections. J Infect Dis 169:157–161
23. Hesse DG, Tracey KJ, Fong Y, et al (1988) Cytokine appearance in human endotoxemia and primate bacteremia. Surg Gynecol Obstet 166:147–153
24. Debets JM, Kampmeijer R, Van der Linden MP, Buurman WA, Van der Linden CJ (1989) Plasma tumor necrosis factor and mortality in critically ill septic patients. Crit Care Med 17:489–494
25. Borrelli E, Roux Lombard P, Grau GE, et al (1996) Plasma concentrations of cytokines, their soluble receptors, and antioxidant vitamins can predict the development of multiple organ failure in patients at risk. Crit Care Med 24:392–397
26. Michie HR, Spriggs DR, Manogue KR, et al (1988) Tumor necrosis factor and endotoxin induce similar metabolic responses in human beings. Surgery 104:280–286
27. Van der Poll T, Bueller HR, ten Cate H, et al (1990) Activation of coagulation after administration of tumor necrosis factor to normal subjects. N Engl J Med 3222:1622–1626
28. Opal SM, Cross AS, Kelly NM, et al (1990) Efficacy of a monoclonal antibody directed against tumor necrosis factor in protecting neutropenic rats from lethal infection with Pseudomonas aeruginosa. J Infect Dis 161:1148–1152
29. Fiedler VB, Loof I, Sander E, Voehringer V, Galanos C, Fournel MA (1992) Monoclonal antibody to tumor necrosis factor-alpha prevents lethal endotoxin sepsis in adult rhesus monkeys. J Lab Clin Med 120:574–588
30. Cohen J, Carlet J, INTERSEPT Study Group (1996) INTERSEPT: An international, multicenter, placebo-controlled trial of monoclonal antibody to human tumor necrosis factor-α in patients with sepsis. Crit Care Med 24:1431–1440
31. Abraham E, Anzueto A, Gutierrez G, et al (1998) Double-blind randomised controlled trial of monoclonal antibody to human tumor necrosis factor in treatment of septic shock. Lancet 351:929–933
32. Negussie Y, Remick DG, DeForge LE, Kunkel SL, Eynon A, Griffin GE (1992) Detection of plasma tumor necrosis factor, interleukins 6 and 8 during the Jarisch-Herxheimer reaction of relapsing fever. J Exp Med 175:1207–1212
33. Fekade D, Knox K, Hussein K, et al (1996) Prevention of Jarisch-Herxheimer reactions by treatment with antibodies against tumor necrosis factor α. N Engl J Med 335:311–315
34. Clark MA, Plank LD, Connolly AB, et al (1998) Effect of a chimeric antibody to tumor necrosis factor-α on cytokine and physiologic responses in patients with severe sepsis – a randomized, clinical trial. Crit Care Med 26:1650–1659

35. Granowitz EV, Santos AA, Poutsiaka DD, et al (1991) Production of interleukin-1-receptor antagonist during experimental endotoxaemia. Lancet 338:1423–1424
36. Goldie AS, Fearon KC, Ross JA, et al (1995) Natural cytokine antagonists and endogenous antiendotoxin core antibodies in sepsis syndrome. The Sepsis Intervention Group. JAMA 274:172–177
37. Munoz C, Carlet J, Fitting C, Misset B, Blérot JP, Cavaillon JM (1991) Dysregulation of in vitro cytokine production by monocytes during sepsis. J Clin Invest 88:1747–1754
38. de Waal Malefyt R, Abrams J, Bennett B, Figdor CG, de Vries JE (1991) Interleukin-10 (IL-10) inhibits cytokine synthesis by human monocytes: an autoregulatory role of IL-10 produced by monocytes. J Exp Med 174:1209–1220
39. Volk HD, Reinke P, Krausch D, et al (1996) Monocyte deactivation – rationale for a new therapeutic strategy in sepsis. Intensive Care Med 22:S474–S481
40. Döcke WD, Randow F, Syrbe HP, et al (1997) Monocyte deactivation in septic patients: restoration by IFN-γ treatment. Nature Med 3:678–681
41. Titus RG, Sherry B, Cerami A (1989) Tumor necrosis factor plays a protective role in experimental murine cutaneous leishmaniasis. J Exp Med 170:2097–2104
42. Bagby GJ, Plessala KJ, Wilson LA, Thompson JJ, Nelson S (1991) Divergent efficacy of antibody to tumor necrosis factor-α in intravascular and peritonitis models of sepsis. J Infect Dis 163:83–88
43. Reinhart K, RAMSES Study Group (1998) Treatment of severe sepsis in patients with highly elevated IL-6 levels with anti-TNF monoclonal antibody MAK 195F: The RAMSES study. Crit Care 2:P18 (Abst)
44. Opal SM, Fisher CJ, Jr., Dhainaut JF, et al (1997) Confirmatory interleukin-1 receptor antagonist trial in severe sepsis: A phase III, randomized, double-blind, placebo-controlled, multicenter trial. Crit Care Med 25:1115–1124
45. Dhainaut JF, Tenaillon A, Hemmer M, et al (1998) Confirmatory platelet-activating factor receptor antagonist trial in patients with severe gram-negative bacterial sepsis: a phase III, randomized, double-blind, placebo-controlled, multicenter trial. BN 52021 sepsis investigator group. Crit Care Med 26:1963–1971
46. Wasserman D, Ioannovich JD, Hinzmann RD, Deichsel G, Steinmann GG (1998) Interferon-gamma in the prevention of severe burn-related infections: a European phase III multicenter trial. Crit Care Med 26:434–439
47. Targan SR, Hanauer SB, Van Deventer SJ, et al (1997) A short-term study of chimeric monoclonal antibody cA2 to tumor necrosis factor alpha for Crohn's disease. N Engl J Med 337: 1029–1035
48. Stack WA, Mann SD, Roy AJ, et al (1997) Randomised controlled trial of CDP571 antibody to tumour necrosis factor-alpha in Crohn's disease. Lancet 349:521–524
49. Rankin EC, Choy EH, Kassimos D, et al (1995) The therapeutic effects of an engineered human anti-tumor necrosis factor alpha antibody (CDP571) in rheumatoid arthritis. Br J Rheumatol 34:334–342
50. Ertel W, Kremer JP, Kenney J, et al (1995) Downregulation of proinflammatory cytokine release in whole blood from septic patients. Blood 85:1341–1347
51. Waage A, Halstensen A, Espevik T (1987) Association between tumour necrosis factor in serum and fatal outcome in patients with meningococcal disease. Lancet i:355–357
52. Marks JD, Marks CB, Luce JM, et al (1990) Plasma tumor necrosis factor in patients with septic shock. Am Rev Respir Dis 141:94–97
53. Martin C, Boisson C, Haccoun M, Thomachot L, Mege JL (1997) Patterns of cytokine evolution (tumor necrosis factor-alpha and interleukin-6) after septic shock, hemorrhagic shock, and severe trauma. Crit Care Med 25:1771–1773
54. Casey LC, Balk RA, Bone RC (1993) Plasma cytokine and endotoxin levels correlate with survival in patients with the sepsis syndrome. Ann Intern Med 119:771–778
55. Damas P, Ledoux D, Nys M, et al (1992) Cytokine serum level during severe sepsis in human: IL-6 as a marker of severity. Ann Surg 215:356–362
56. Blackwell TS, Christman JW (1996) Sepsis and cytokines: Current status. Br J Anaesth 77: 110–117
57. Santolaya ME, Cofre J, Sheldon J (1994) C-reactive protein: a valuable aid for the management of febrile children with cancer and neutropenia. Clin Infect Dis 18:589–595

58. Yentis SM, Soni N, Sheldon J (1995) C-reactive protein as an indicator of resolution of sepsis in the intensive care unit. Intensive Care Med 21:602–605
59. Assicot M, Gendrel D, Carsin H, Raymond J, Guilbaud J, Bohoun C (1993) High serum procalcitonin concentration in patients with sepsis and infection. Lancet 341:515–518
60. Ugarte H, Silva E, Mercan D, de Mendonça A, Vincent JL (1999) Procalcitonin as a marker of infection in the intensive care unit. Crit Care Med 27:498–504
61. Nylen ES, Whang KT, Snider RHJr, Steinwald PM, White JC, Becker KL (1998) Mortality is increased by procalcitonin and decreased by an antiserum reactive to procalcitonin in experimental sepsis. Crit Care Med 26:1001–1006
62. Pacher P, Redl H, Frass M, Petzl DH, Schuster E, Woloszczuk W (1989) Relationship between neopterin and granulocyte elastase plasma levels and the severity of multiple organ failure. Crit Care Med 17:221–226
63. Suter PM, Suter S, Girardin E, Roux Lombard P, Grau GE, Dayer JM (1992) High bronchoalveolar levels of tumor necrosis factor and its inhibitors, interleukin-1, interferon, and elastase, in patients with adult respiratory distress syndrome after trauma, shock, or sepsis. Am Rev Respir Dis 145:1016–1022
64. Yao YM, Yu Y, Wang YP, Tian HM, Sheng ZY (1996) Elevated serum neopterin level: its relation to endotoxemia and sepsis in patients with major burns. Eur J Clin Invest 26:224–230
65. Osman MO, Jacobsen NO, Kristensen JU, et al (1998) IT 9302, a synthetic interleukin-10 agonist, diminishes acute lung injury in rabbits with acute necrotizing pancreatitis. Surgery 124:584–592
66. Hickey MJ, Issekutz AC, Reinhardt PH, Fedorak RN, Kubes P (1998) Endogenous interleukin-10 regulates hemodynamic parameters, leukocyte-endothelial cell interactions, and microvascular permeability during endotoxemia. Circ Res 83:1124–1131
67. Reinhart K, Wiegand-Löhnert C, Grimminger F, et al (1996) Assessment of the safety and efficacy of the monoclonal anti-tumor necrosis factor antibody fragment, MAK195F, in patients with sepsis and septic shock: A multicenter, randomized, placebo-controlled, dose ranging study. Crit Care Med 24:733–742

Genomics of the Sepsis Syndrome

S. J. H. van Deventer and P. Stokkers

Introduction

The mortality of patients who suffer from systemic infections is dependent on exogenous and endogenous factors. Exogenous factors include the type of microbial pathogen, the expression of virulence factors and appropriateness of medical therapy, whereas age, nutritional status, and immune deficiency are endogenous factors. It is well known that the mortality of bacterial infection markedly differs amongst genetically distinct inbred mouse strains and it has been suggested that the genetic background may also be a determinant of outcome from septic shock. Indeed, at least one study has investigated polymorphisms within the tumor necrosis factor (TNF) locus in relation to mortality from sepsis. For several reasons such studies are difficult to interpret. First, the cause of mortality in sepsis is not known, and indeed may differ among patients. From a genomics point of view it would be most important to be able to distinguish between patients that die because of overwhelming (bacterial) infection, versus those that succumb due to hypotension and ischemia/reperfusion damage, because these respective processes are controlled by different genes. Secondly, studies on disease genomics are critically dependent on the availability of an appropriate control population, or family members that express the disease. Because of the heterogeneous nature of sepsis, its occurrence at the extremes of age, the absence of families with sepsis syndrome, and the importance of underlying diseases, at present any search for the genomics of the sepsis syndrome is cumbersome and in most cases futile. On the other hand, progress has been made in the genetics of infectious disease in humans, and it has been recently reported that mutations in cytokine receptor genes (that lead to functional inactivation) pose a high risk for severe infections in humans. In mice the important Th1/Th2 cytokine switch is known to be genetically controlled, and careful studies in mice have lead to the identification of candidate susceptibility genes for mycobacterial infections. Finally, new techniques have made genetic studies of polygenic and complex diseases feasible. In this chapter, we briefly review these findings and speculate on the potential future clinical importance of (infection) genomics in the sepsis syndrome. We will not discuss associations of infectious disease with polymorphisms in the human leukocyte antigen (HLA)-, Fc receptor-, or mannose binding receptor genes, nor discuss the importance of chemokine receptors in human immunodeficiency virus (HIV) infection; the reader is referred to excellent recent reviews on these subjects [1–6].

Genetic Polymorphisms

The human genome contains more than 100 000 genes, which are molecularly defined as regions of desoxyribonucleic acid (DNA), that comprise all nucleic acid sequences necessary to produce a functional protein or ribonucleic acid (RNA). Most human genes are organized in 'exons' and 'introns' both of which are transcribed into pre-mRNA. Downstream from the last exon is the so-called 3′ untranslated region (3′UTR) that is transcribed into mRNA, and may contain certain elements that determine mRNA half-life. For example, many cytokine genes contain so-called 'Kamen and Shaw' regions that render cytokine mRNAs targets for RNAses, and thereby importantly reduce translation into protein. The 3′UTR is terminated by a motif (AATAA) that is called the polyadenylation site, which is cut by a small nuclear ribonucleoprotein particle (SNRP) and subsequently polyadenylated. Introns are rapidly excised from the pre-mRNA by various SNRPs, resulting in mRNA that contains only the exon sequences and the 3′UTR. The control of gene transcription is complex, and will not be discussed in detail. However, it is important to know that control elements for gene transcription consist of specific DNA motifs that enable binding of transcription factors, which are proteins that translocate from the cytoplasm into the nucleus upon activation of (cell)-specific receptors and signal transduction pathways. These control elements are found upstream from the first exon and together form the gene 'promoter'. Other important regulatory elements are 'enhancers' that are defined as DNA elements that can boost gene transcription regardless of the orientation, and sometimes are found at great distances from the target gene.

Two types of DNA markers are frequently used in genetic studies. Single nucleotide polymorphisms (SNPs, pronounced as 'snip') are single DNA base variations that are frequently encountered in human DNA (the frequency has been estimated at one SNP per 1000 bases in the three billion base human genome). SNPs are usually detected by differences in digestion patterns (restriction fragment length polymorphism [RFLP]) after exposure to restriction enzymes that recognize and cut specific DNA sequences (Fig. 1). In order to be informative in genetic studies, a SNP must have an allele frequency of at least 5%.

Microsatellites, also known as variable number of tandem repeat (VNTR), are a form of repetitive DNA with a unit length of 2–10 basepairs, for example (CA)n, that demonstrate extensive variations in the repeat number. Hence, the microsatellite length can be used as a genetic marker. Large parts of human DNA consist of stretches of repetitive noncoding sequences, of 'pseudogenes' (non-functional genes that arose from gene duplication) of inserted retroviral elements or of 'junk' DNA: In fact, only about 5% of human DNA consists of coding regions. Therefore, it is important to realize that many of the markers used in genetic studies are not located in parts of the gene that are transcribed (i.e., in exons) or even within elements that control gene transcription (promoters or enhancers) or translation (3′UTR of many cytokine genes). Although such markers are not directly related to gene expression, and do not explain phenotypic differences, they are frequently used for genetic fingerprinting, and in 'gene hunting'. Furthermore, genetic markers may be co-inherited with the genes of interest, which

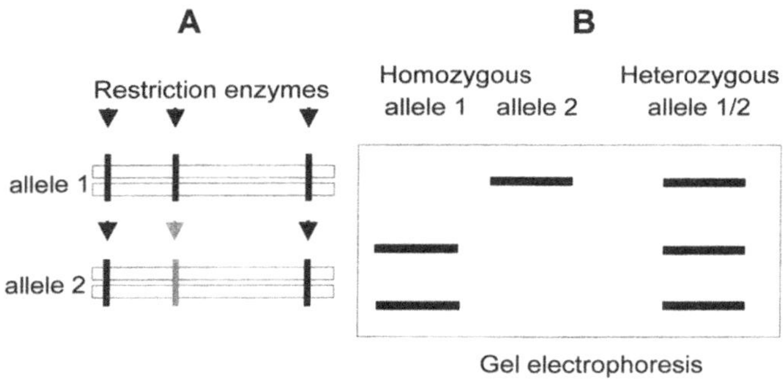

Fig. 1. Restriction fragment length polymorphisms. **A** Polymorphic differences in two alleles result in the absence of a recognition site for a specific restriction enzyme on allele 2. Consequently, the gel electrophoresis pattern of the two alleles differs and can be easily recognized (**B**)

is known as 'linkage disequilibrium'. Conversely, the mere location of a specific marker within (the vicinity of) a certain gene, does not allow any conclusion concerning its importance for gene transcription. For example, several studies have suggested that associations of a certain SNP within the TNF-α promoter with certain immune-mediated diseases were a consequence of differences in TNF-α transcription rates. Although such polymorphisms may be related to TNF-α blood levels in certain diseases, it is now known that this is a result of linkage disequilibrium with certain HLA genes that are located in the vicinity of the TNF-α gene on chromosome 6, rather than a consequence of a direct effect on transcription efficacy. In other words, the polymorphism within the TNF-α promoter region is in fact a genetic HLA marker.

Linkage and Association [7]

Genetic studies aim to correlate a genotype with a certain disease (phenotype), and even in diseases that are caused by dysfunction of single genes such correlations may be complicated by environmental effects. Many genes control the immune system, and analysis of the genetics of infectious disease (or even worse, sepsis) is further complicated by the interactions of these genes and by genetic heterogeneity. These complexities necessitate the use of sophisticated tools, including linkage analysis, allele sharing methods, association studies and transmission disequilibrium tests (TDT). Linkage analysis provides an estimation of the distance of a certain genetic marker to the disease-causing gene, based on measurement of the 'recombination fraction'. If a marker is close to the gene of interest, it will virtually always be inherited together with that gene, but if it is located far away (or on a different chromosome), crossover events during meiosis will make co-inheritance less likely. Consequently, the recombination fraction (expressed as θ) can vary between 0 and 0.5. The distance of two markers on the

DNA is expressed as Morgan, where 1 centimorgan corresponds with $\theta = 0.01$. The likelihood that the observed inheritance of the marker and the disease gene are related is expressed as the LOD (logarithm of the odds) score, and a LOD score higher than three is generally accepted as evidence for linkage [8]. Calculation of LOD scores requires construction of a model of the inheritance pattern of a disease, taking allele frequencies and disease penetrance into account [9]. For many polygenic diseases such models cannot be reliably constructed, and other techniques have to be applied. Several techniques are based on assessment of 'allele sharing' [10]. The aim of these techniques is to prove that the inheritance pattern of a genetic marker allele is not random (i.e., inherited according to Mendelian predictions), but that affected pedigree members inherit the marker allele more frequently. In many conditions (i.e., when the disease studied is rapidly fatal, or occurs at the extremes of age, conditions that are common in sepsis and many infectious diseases) no pedigree can be constructed, and the aforementioned techniques cannot be applied. In these circumstances, it is possible to apply population-based techniques. Association studies assess the frequency of marker alleles that are located near the candidate disease genes in a group of patients, and compare the outcome with the results in a matched control group. A positive result may indicate that the genetic marker indeed is the cause of the disease, or is located in the vicinity of the disease-causing gene, but association studies are prone to report false positive results [11], frequently as a consequence of inadequate matching of cases and controls. Hence, the criteria for statistical significance in association studies should be defined rather conservatively and final proof of an association usually requires evidence for linkage. Clearly, the rapidly fatal nature of many (infectious) diseases precludes application of linkage studies. In these circumstances, it is possible to estimate linkage by assessment of the transmission of marker alleles from parents to affected patients as compared to transmission of an alternative (unrelated) marker allele [12].

Lessons from Mice

Th1/Th2 Switch

Following antigenic stimulation, $CD4^+$ T lymphocytes differentiate in subpopulations that are phenotypically characterized by differences in cytokine production [13–15]. Th1 lymphocytes produce interleukin-2 (IL-2), interferon-γ (IFN-γ) and lymphotoxin, whereas Th2 lymphocytes produce IL-4, IL-5 and IL-10. The Th1/Th2 switch is controlled by the type and concentration of antigen, the route of administration, by cytokines (IL-12 and IFN-γ induce Th1 responses, IL-4, IL-6 and IL-10 Th2 responses) and by genetic factors. Inbred mouse strains are known to preferentially mount Th1 (C57/BL6) or Th2 responses (BALB/C), but although the signal transduction pathways involved in the Th1/Th2 switch have been partially characterized [16–18], the genes involved in the Th1/Th2 decision remain unknown. Still, genetic background is critically important in mouse models of disease, as is well illustrated by the important phenotypic differences of inactivation of the IL-10 gene in 129/SvEv, BALB/c (severe disease), 129 × C57BL/6J outbreds (intermediate disease), and C57BL/6J mice (mild disease) [19].

Certain disease in humans are also characterized by skewed Th1/Th2 cytokine responses. For example, Crohn's disease and rheumatoid arthritis are considered 'Th1' diseases, whereas asthma is a 'Th2' disease. As yet, the genes that control these reactions remain unknown, and cytokine responses may be differentially regulated in different body compartment (some patients with Crohn's disease have asthma). Recent genome wide scans in patients with multiple sclerosis, Crohn's disease, familial psoriasis, asthma, and type-I diabetes, have uncovered associations with several non-HLA loci, that in part overlap, and these loci contain several candidate genes that are involved in the immune response [20]. Hence it is possible that a certain genetic background may predispose for 'Th1' diseases in general (i.e., rheumatoid arthritis and Crohn's disease), whereas the expression of disease depends on non-shared genes.

It should be noted that the interaction with pathogenic microorganisms adds further complexity, because the outcome of infectious disease depends both on effective clearance of the pathogenic microorganism, and on the amplitude of the pro-inflammatory response. In most models, host immune cells need to be activated by cytokines (in particular IL-12, IFN-γ and TNF-α) to effectively kill pathogenic microorganisms. On the other hand, systemically released pro-inflammatory cytokines may kill the host by inducing systemic inflammatory responses. Therefore, survival is dependent on well-balanced pro- and anti-inflammatory responses. This point is well illustrated by the complex results of cytokine modulation in a murine model of Chagas' disease. Natural resistance of mice against infection with *Trypanosoma cruzi* is known to be associated with high levels of IFN-γ and a low production rate of IL-10 [21]. Indeed, IL-10-deficient macrophages have a defect in intracellular killing of *T. cruzi* because of insufficient induction of nitrous oxide, which can be corrected by IL-10 supplementation [22]. Infection of IL-$10^{-/-}$ mice with *T. cruzi* resulted in a higher production of TNF-α, IFN-γ and IL-12 that was associated with a lower parasite burden. Somewhat unexpectedly, in this model, the result was an earlier mortality of IL-$10^{-/-}$ mice that could be reversed by administration of anti-CD4 antibodies [23]. Therefore, it seemed that the early mortality due to *T. cruzi* infection was a result of IL-12-induced IFN-γ production by $CD4^+$ lymphocytes, which by itself is a necessary protective response. This example illustrates the point that Th1 or Th2 cytokine responses in severe infectious diseases are not 'good' or 'bad', and that the final outcome is a result of complex interactions of the host immune system with the invading microorganism. It is for this reason that it is unlikely that any genetic Th1/Th2 marker in the heterogeneous population of sepsis patients will predict outcome.

From Mouse to Man

A potentially more useful approach is the extrapolation of differences of host responses towards a single infectious agent in well-defined mouse models to the clinical setting and there is a recent example of the efficacy of such a strategy. In mice, the resistance to infection with certain mycobacteria (*M. lepraemurium*, *M. bovis*, and *M. intracellulare*) is genetically determined, and controlled by a single gene on chromosome 1 [24–26]. This gene, named natural resistance-associated macrophage protein-1 (NRAMP-1), was found to be identical to the gene that conferred resistance to *Salmonella typhymurium* and *Leishmania donovani*. Mice that are susceptible to *M. bovis* infection have a non-conservative glycine to aspartic acid substitution at position 169, and the mutant protein is not expressed [26]. Further proof for the functional importance of NRAMP-1 was provided by the demonstration that functional inactivation of the gene in mice, rendered resistant mice susceptible to mycobacterial infections [27]. The mouse and human NRAMP-1 genes encode a 60 kDa protein that is expressed in macrophages (mice) and in monocytes and granulocytes (humans). The protein has 12 putative transmembrane sites, is located in late endosomes/lysosomes and is thought to transport divalent cations such as Mn^{2+}, Mg^{2+}, Cu^{2+} and Zn^{2+} out of lysosomes [28, 29]. Because intracellular pathogens are dependent on divalent cations for intracellular survival, NRAMP-1 functions as an important mechanism of innate resistance. Others have reported that the major effect of NRAMP-1 in mouse macrophage lysosomes is acidification [30]. In West Africans, several polymorphisms have indeed been associated with a diagnosis of smear-positive tuberculosis, and infected subjects with polymorphisms in intron 4 or in the 3′UTR were particularly over-represented [31]. Recently, NRAMP-1 has also been identified as a leprosy susceptibility gene [32]. It has been reported that rheumatoid arthritis might also be linked to the NRAMP-1 gene, but the association is weak, and we have been unable to link NRAMP-1 to ulcerative colitis or Crohn's disease [33, Stokkers et al., unpublished data]. The NRAMP-1 story is an excellent example of human infection genomics that originated in mouse models. It should be appreciated that conventional linkage or association studies in humans would require study of many more patients (and their families) than the 827 subjects that were enrolled in the West African study. Hence, identification of candidate genes in animal models may importantly boost studies on infection genomics.

Cytokine and Cytokine Receptors

TNF-α

Multiple polymorphisms have been detected in the TNF-α, IL-1β, and IL-1 receptor antagonist (IL-1ra) genes, and these have been studied in relation to occurrence and severity of infectious disease. Because TNF-α has an important role in the host defense against many pathogens, and monocytes of healthy individuals show large (more than 10-fold) differences in TNF-α production after standardized stimulation [34,35] it should come as no surprise that polymorphisms in the TNF-α gene have been most extensively studied. The TNF-α gene is located on the short arm of chromosome 6, between the class I and class III histocompatibility loci [36–39]. Table 1 summarizes the ten polymorphisms that have been de-

Table 1. Polymorphisms within the TNF locus

Name	Type	Location	Number of alleles
TNFa [75, 76]	AC/GT repeat	TNF-β gene upstream region	13
TNFb [75, 76]	TC/GA repeat	TNF-β gene upstream region	5
TNFc [75, 76]	TC/GA repeat	TNF-β gene intron 1	2
TNFd [75, 76]	TC/GA repeat	LST gene	unknown
TNFe [75, 76]	TC/GA repeat	LST gene	unknown
TNFn [77, 78]	RFLP, Nco1	TNF-β gene intron 1	2
TNFr [79]	RFLP, Eco Ri	TNF-β gene exon 4	2
−308 [80]	G to A transition	TNF-α promoter region	2
−238 [81]	G to A transition	TNF-α promoter region	2
+70 [82]	C insertion position +70	TNF-α gene	2

scribed in the TNF locus, five of which are microsatellites, none of which is located within gene regulatory regions (Fig. 2). The TNFn polymorphism (a Nco1 RFLP) is in fact located in the TNF-β gene and has two alleles, known as TNFB1 and TNFB2. Although associations of certain polymorphisms with TNF production rates have been reported [40, 41] none of the polymorphisms in the TNF promoter (including the −238 and the −308 polymorphism in the TNF promoter) has a direct effect on the TNF-α transcription rate [42]. In other words, the as-

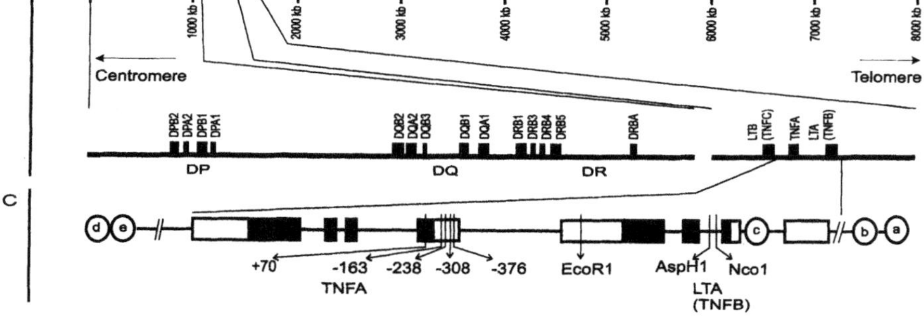

Fig. 2. Location of the TNF locus on chromosome 6 between the HLA class I and III loci. The VNTRs (a–e) are encircled and, with the exception of the TNFc VNTR, located outside the coding regions of TNF-α and TNF-β (lymphotoxin). The Nco1 'TNF' polymorphism is in fact located in an intron of the lymphotoxin gene

sociations of certain polymorphisms with TNF-α production are indirect effects, and probably result from a linkage disequilibrium with other genes on chromosome 6. It should be noted that as a consequence of their location, TNF-α alleles have a high chance to be in linkage disequilibrium with HLA genes. For example, the −308 RFLP is in tight linkage disequilibrium with the HLA A1, B8, DR3 haplotype, and may thus be linked to immune function (and eventually TNF-α production) [43, 44]. It is likely that this linkage, rather than a direct effect on TNF-α production, explains the correlation of certain TNF-α alleles with outcome of malaria, mucocutaneous Leishmania and sepsis.

The TNF-α −308 polymorphism and the TNFn RFLP (both are biallelic) have been studied in relation to outcome of infectious disease. A study in Gambia, including 376 children, reported that homozygosity for the TNF2 allele of the TNFn RFLP, which is associated with higher TNF-α production, had a relative risk of cerebral malaria of 4.0 and 7.7 for death or permanent neurological damage [45]. These effects were independent of HLA class I and class II variations. The TNF2 allele was also more frequently found in patients with mucocutaneous Leishmaniasis as compared to endemic controls, but it remains uncertain whether this association is caused by differences in TNF production [46]. In 80 patients with severe sepsis the −308 allele frequency did not differ from controls, but in a second study in 40 critically ill patients, homozygosity for the TNF2 allele was associated with higher MOF scores, increased TNF-α serum levels, and higher mortality [47, 48]. Similar findings have been reported in children with meningococcal disease [49]. In contrast, none of the polymorphisms within the TNF-α promoter is associated with the outcome of HIV infections [50]. It should be noted that the latter two studies are association studies in rather small populations, and that no further evidence for an association by linkage methods has been provided. Furthermore, as has been mentioned before, it is unlikely that these associations were a result of a direct effect on the transcription rate of TNF-α.

IL-1 Gene Family

The genes of IL-1β, IL-1α and IL-1ra are closely located on the short arm of chromosome 2, and several (restriction fragment length) polymorphisms have been identified in these genes (Fig. 3 and Table 2) [51–54]. Because IL-1ra is a natural antagonist of IL-1β, it has been suggested that an imbalance in the production of both cytokines may be a pathogenic mechanism in immune-mediated diseases. Allele 2 of a Taq1 RFLP in IL-1β is associated with higher IL-1β production, and the infrequent allele of the Mwo1 RFLP in the IL-1ra gene with lower IL-1ra production [55, 56]. Indeed, we have demonstrated that in whole blood stimulated by lipopolysaccharide (LPS), the IL-1β/IL-1L-1ra ratio was lower in carriers of both infrequent alleles, although this failed to reach statistical significance [57]. To date the (multiple) polymorphisms in the IL-1 gene family have not been studied in relation to infectious diseases, but in view of the correlations that have been found in (auto)immune disease, it is not unlikely that such associations exist.

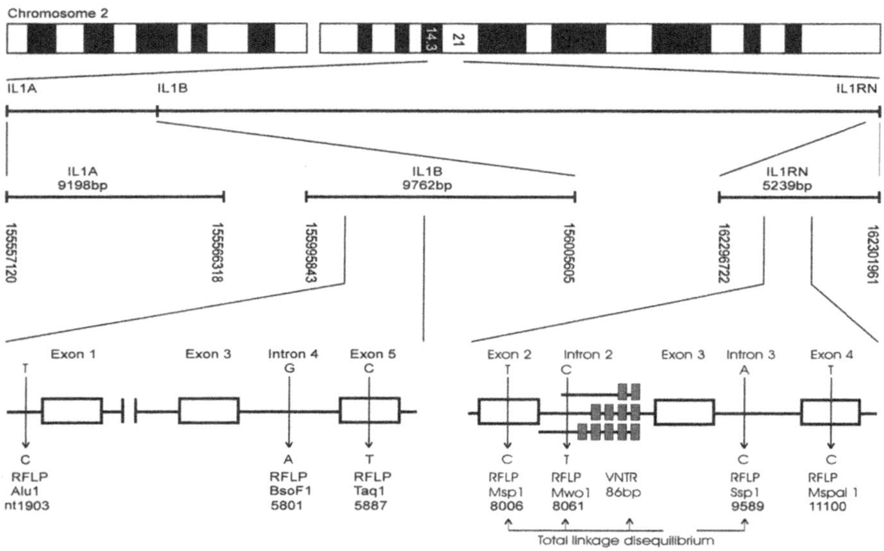

Fig. 3. The IL-1 gene family is located on chromosome 2. Several polymorphisms within the IL-1RN gene (that encodes IL-1ra) are in total linkage disequilibrium

Table 2. Polymorphisms within the IL-1 locus

Gene	Type	Location	Number of alleles
IL-1A [83]	VNTR 46 bp	intron 6	7
IL-1A [84]	RFLP	exon 5	2
IL-1A [85]	VNTR (CA repeat)		6
IL-1A [86]	C to G transition	promoter region −889	2
IL-1B [87]	C to G transition	promoter region −511	2
IL-1B [88, 89]	C to G transition	exon 5	2
IL-1B [89]	G to A transition	intron 4	2
IL-1B [89]	G to A transition	promoter region	2
IL-1RN [90, 91]	VNTR 86 bp	intron 2	5
IL-1RN [89]	T to C transition	exon 2	2
IL-1RN [89]	C to T transition	intron 2	2
IL-1RN [89]	A to C transition	intron 3	2
IL-1RN [89]	T to C transition	exon 4	2

IL-10

IL-10 is considered a prototype anti-inflammatory cytokine that down-regulates the production of a wide range of pro-inflammatory cytokines and interferes with T-lymphocyte activation, in part by reducing the expression of HLA class II molecules on antigen-presenting cells. In septic patients, blood IL-10 concentrations correlate with disease severity, and very high IL-10 concentrations have been reported in meningococcal septic shock [58]. Because patients with meningococcal septic shock are known to have very high circulating endotoxin and TNF-α concentrations, the increased IL-10 levels are considered to represent a counter-regulatory response. In a recent study, the amount of IL-10 produced in *ex vivo* stimulated blood was found to be inherited, and patients with family members with a high IL-10 production had a 20-fold increased risk for fatal outcome [59]. In febrile patients, usually due to bacterial infection, a high IL-10/TNF-α ratio on admission was also associated with increased mortality [60]. We recently confirmed this finding in a study in consecutive Thai patients with melioidosis (an infection caused by *Burkholderia pseudomallei*, that is associated with a high mortality). However, when other data, in particular the APACHE II score and IL-6 levels, were also added in a regression model, the IL-10/TNF-α ratio no longer predicted mortality (Prins and Van Deventer, unpublished data). Hence, it remains uncertain whether the IL-10/TNF-α ratio is an independent predictor of mortality in sepsis. On the other hand, the rate of IL-10 production seems to be genetically determined, although the genetic basis remains to be determined. Of interest, several polymorphisms have been located in the human IL-10 gene [61–63].

Cytokine Receptors

IFN-γ is of critical importance for successful clearance of a wide variety of (intracellular) pathogens. The IFN-γ receptor-1 gene, encoding the α-chain, is located on the long arm of chromosome 6. The α chain is expressed on most cells, and is responsible for binding IFN-γ, whereas the expression of the β chain that transduces the IFN-γ signal is cell-specific and regulated by external stimuli. Mice that are deficient for the IFN-γ receptor 1 gene (encoding the α chain) suffer from severe mycobacterial infections [64, 65]. Recently, in children suffering from severe disseminated atypical infections, homozygous mutations in the gene encoding the IFN-γ receptor α chain (IFNGR1) have been reported [66–69]. These children came from consanguinous families, and in view of the severe and often fatal phenotype, it is unlikely that such mutations occur frequently in the general population. A similar phenotype, characterized by severe infections by mycobacteria and *Salmonella* species, is caused by a mutation in the gene encoding the IL-12 receptor β chain [70]. The mutation renders cells unresponsive to IL-12, resulting in a severe deficiency of IFN-γ production.

Conclusion

Genetic factors influence the outcome of severe infectious diseases, and genetically determined differences in TNF-α and IL-10 production have been implied in the outcome of (meningococcal) septic shock. The genetic determinants of these findings have been incompletely characterized. Polymorphisms in the TNF locus do not directly affect the production rate of TNF-α, and some TNF-α polymorphisms are in linkage disequilibrium with HLA haplotypes. No cytokine deficiency syndromes are known to be involved in sepsis, but mutations that lead to inactive IFN-γ and IL-12 receptors are associated with severe infections caused by mycobacteria and *Salmonella* species. The study of the genetics of sepsis is highly complicated as a result of the heterogeneity of the sepsis syndrome, the genetic heterogeneity of patients with sepsis, and the difficulties in performing family studies. In view of these problems, how should we proceed with studies on the genetics of sepsis? One possible solution is to concentrate on well-characterized 'candidate' genes that are identified in inbred mouse strains (i.e., NRAMP-1) or in homogenous patients that suffer from a single disease (i.e., malaria or tuberculosis). The effect of polymorphisms within such genes can be assessed in association studies, but should be confirmed using linkage techniques. Therefore, not only DNA from patients, but also from their first-degree relatives should be collected.

Novel techniques enable analysis of large numbers of polymorphisms in a single test, and such assays may be applied in studies on the genomics of infectious diseases [71]. One potential application of such information would be the prediction of response to certain therapies. In view of the spectacular progress in miniaturization of molecular biology techniques, such as sequencing and PCR machines in credit card format [72–74], it is not unreasonable to expect these techniques to be applied in the clinical setting within a foreseeable period of time.

References

1. Hill AV (1998) The immunogenetics of human infectious diseases. Ann Rev Immunol 16:593–617
2. Heijnen IA, van de Winkel JG (1997) Human IgG Fc receptors. Int Rev Immunol 16:29-55
3. van der Pol W, van de Winkel JG (1998) IgG receptor polymorphisms: risk factors for disease. Immunogenetics 48:222–232
4. Abel L, Dessein AJ (1997) The impact of host genetics on susceptibility to human infectious diseases. Curr Opin Immunol 9:509–516
5. Broder CC, Collman RG (1997) Chemokine receptors and HIV. J Leukoc Biol 62:20–29
6. Kaslow RA (1997) Host genes and HIV infection: implications and applications. Emerg Infect Dis 3:401–402
7. Vogel F, Motulsky AG (1996) Human Genetics. Springer-Verlag, Berlin
8. Ott J (1991) Analysis of human genetic linkage. The Johns Hopkins University Press, Baltimore
9. Cooper DN, Schmidtke J (1992) Molecular genetic approaches to the analysis and diagnosis of human inherited disease: an overview. Ann Med 24:29–42
10. Lander ES, Schork NJ (1994) Genetic dissection of complex traits. Science 265:2037–2048
11. Lander E, Kruglyak L (1995) Genetic dissection of complex traits: guidelines for interpreting and reporting linkage results. Nat Genet 11:241–247
12. Ewens WJ, Spielman RS (1995) The transmission/disequilibrium test: history, subdivision, and admixture. Am J Hum Genet 57:455–464
13. Mosmann TR, Sad S (1996) The expanding universe of T-cell subsets: Th1, Th2 and more. Immunol Today 17:138–146
14. Nakamura T, Kamogawa Y, Bottomly K, Flavell RA (1997) Polarization of IL-4- and IFN-gamma-producing CD4+ T cells following activation of naive CD4+ T cells. J Immunol 158:1085–1094

15. Nakamura T, Lee RK, Nam SY, Podack ER, Bottomly K, Flavell RA (1997) Roles of IL-4 and IFN-gamma in stabilizing the T helper cell type 1 and 2 phenotype. J Immunol 158:2648–2653
16. Rincon M, Flavell RA (1997) T-cell subsets: transcriptional control in the Th1/Th2 decision. Curr Biol 7:R729–732
17. Rincon M, Flavell RA (1997) Transcription mediated by NFAT is highly inducible in effector CD4+ T helper 2 (Th2) cells but not in Th1 cells. Mol Cell Biol 17:1522–1534
18. Zheng W, Flavell RA (1997) The transcription factor GATA-3 is necessary and sufficient for Th2 cytokine gene expression in CD4 T cells. Cell 89:587–596
19. Berg DJ, Davidson N, Kuhn R, et al (1996) Enterocolitis and colon cancer in interleukin-10-deficient mice are associated with aberrant cytokine production and CD4(+) TH1-like responses. J Clin Invest 98:1010–1020
20. Becker KG, Simon RM, Bailey-Wilson JE, et al (1998) Clustering of non-major histocompatibility complex susceptibility candidate loci in human autoimmune diseases. Proc Natl Acad Sci USA 95:9979–9984
21. Minoprio P, el Cheikh MC, Murphy E, et al (1993) Xid-associated resistance to experimental Chagas' disease is IFN-gamma dependent. J Immunol 151:4200–4208
22. Jacobs F, Chaussabel D, Truyens C, et al (1998) IL-10 up-regulates nitric oxide (NO) synthesis by lipopolysaccharide (LPS)-activated macrophages: improved control of Trypanosoma cruzi infection. Clin Exp Immunol 113:59–64
23. Hunter CA, Ellis-Neyes LA, Slifer T, et al (1997) IL-10 is required to prevent immune hyperactivity during infection with Trypanosoma cruzi. J Immunol 158:3311–3316
24. Vidal SM, Malo D, Vogan K, Skamene E, Gros P (1993) Natural resistance to infection with intracellular parasites: isolation of a candidate for Bcg. Cell 73:469–485
25. Cellier M, Govoni G, Vidal S, et al (1994) Human natural resistance-associated macrophage protein: cDNA cloning, chromosomal mapping, genomic organization, and tissue-specific expression. J Exp Med 180:1741–1752
26. Vidal S, Gros P, Skamene E (1995) Natural resistance to infection with intracellular parasites: molecular genetics identifies Nramp1 as the Bcg/Ity/Lsh locus. J Leukoc Biol 58:382–390
27. Vidal S, Tremblay ML, Govoni G, et al (1995) The Ity/Lsh/Bcg locus: natural resistance to infection with intracellular parasites is abrogated by disruption of the Nramp1 gene. J Exp Med 182:655–666
28. Atkinson PG, Blackwell JM, Barton CH (1997) Nramp1 locus encodes a 65 kDa interferon-gamma-inducible protein in murine macrophages. Biochem J 325:779–786
29. Skamene E, Schurr E, Gros P (1998) Infection genomics: Nramp1 as a major determinant of natural resistance to intracellular infections. Ann Rev Med 49:275–287
30. Hackam DJ, Rotstein OD, Zhang W, Gruenheid S, Gros P, Grinstein S (1998) Host resistance to intracellular infection: mutation of natural resistance-associated macrophage protein 1 (Nramp1) impairs phagosomal acidification. J Exp Med 188:351–364
31. Bellamy R, Ruwende C, Corrah T, McAdam KP, Whittle HC, Hill AV (1998) Variations in the NRAMP1 gene and susceptibility to tuberculosis in West Africans. N Engl J Med 338:640–644
32. Abel L, Sanchez FO, Oberti J, et al (1998) Susceptibility to leprosy is linked to the human NRAMP1 gene. J Infect Dis 177:133–145
33. Shaw MA, Clayton D, Blackwell JM (1997) Analysis of the candidate gene NRAMP1 in the first 61 ARC National Repository families for rheumatoid arthritis. J Rheumatol 24:212–214
34. Jacob CO, Fronek Z, Lewis GD, Koo M, Hansen JA, McDevitt HO (1990) Heritable major histocompatibility complex class II-associated differences in production of tumor necrosis factor alpha: relevance to genetic predisposition to systemic lupus erythematosus. Proc Natl Acad Sci USA 87:1233–1237
35. Jacob CO, Lewis GD, McDevitt HO (1991) MHC class II-associated variation in the production of tumor necrosis factor in mice and humans: relevance to the pathogenesis of autoimmune diseases. Immunol Res 10:156–168
36. Carroll MC, Katzman P, Alicot EM, et al (1987) Linkage map of the human major histocompatibility complex including the tumor necrosis factor genes. Proc Natl Acad Sci USA 84:8535–8539

37. Dunham I, Sargent CA, Trowsdale J, Campbell RD (1987) Molecular mapping of the human major histocompatibility complex by pulsed-field gel electrophoresis. Proc Natl Acad Sci USA 84:7237–7241
38. Spies T, Morton CC, Nedospasov SA, Fiers W, Pious D, Strominger JL (1986) Genes for the tumor necrosis factors alpha and beta are linked to the human major histocompatibility complex. Proc Natl Acad Sci USA 83:8699–8702
39. Nedospasov SA, Shakhov AN, Turetskaya RL, et al (1986) Tandem arrangement of genes coding for tumor necrosis factor (TNF-alpha) and lymphotoxin (TNF-beta) in the human genome. Cold Spring Harbor Symp Quant Biol 51 Pt 1:611–624
40. Pociot F, D'Alfonso S, Compasso S, Scorza R, Richiardi PM (1995) Functional analysis of a new polymorphism in the human TNF alpha gene promoter. Scand J Immunol 42:501–504
41. Bouma G, Crusius JB, Oudkerk Pool M, et al (1996) Secretion of tumour necrosis factor alpha and lymphotoxin alpha in relation to polymorphisms in the TNF genes and HLA-DR alleles. Relevance for inflammatory bowel disease. Scand J Immunol 43:456–463
42. Brinkman BM, Zuijdeest D, Kaijzel EL, Breedveld FC, Verweij CL (1995) Relevance of the tumor necrosis factor alpha (TNF alpha) −308 promoter polymorphism in TNF alpha gene regulation. J Inflamm 46:32–41
43. Wilson AG, de Vries N, Pociot F, di Giovine FS, van der Putte LB, Duff GW (1993) An allelic polymorphism within the human tumor necrosis factor alpha promoter region is strongly associated with HLA A1, B8, and DR3 alleles. J Exp Med 177:557–560
44. Kroeger KM, Carville KS, Abraham LJ (1997) The −308 tumor necrosis factor-alpha promoter polymorphism effects transcription. Mol Immunol 34:391–399
45. McGuire W, Hill AV, Allsopp CE, Greenwood BM, Kwiatkowski D (1994) Variation in the TNF-alpha promoter region associated with susceptibility to cerebral malaria. Nature 371: 508–510
46. Cabrera M, Shaw MA, Sharples C, et al (1995) Polymorphism in tumor necrosis factor genes associated with mucocutaneous leishmaniasis. J Exp Med 182:1259–1264
47. Stuber F, Petersen M, Bokelmann F, Schade U (1996) A genomic polymorphism within the tumor necrosis factor locus influences plasma tumor necrosis factor-alpha concentrations and outcome of patients with severe sepsis. Crit Care Med 24:381–384
48. Stuber F, Udalova IA, Book M, et al (1995) −308 tumor necrosis factor (TNF) polymorphism is not associated with survival in severe sepsis and is unrelated to lipopolysaccharide inducibility of the human TNF promoter. J Inflamm 46:42–50
49. Nadel S, Newport MJ, Booy R, Levin M (1996) Variation in the tumor necrosis factor-alpha gene promoter region may be associated with death from meningococcal disease. J Infect Dis 174:878–880
50. Brinkman BM, Keet IP, Miedema F, Verweij CL, Klein MR (1997) Polymorphisms within the human tumor necrosis factor-alpha promoter region in human immunodeficiency virus type 1-seropositive persons. J Infect Dis 175:188–190
51. Webb AC, Collins KL, Auron PE, et al (1986) Interleukin-1 gene (IL1) assigned to long arm of human chromosome 2. Lymphokine Res 5:77–85
52. Furutani Y, Notake M, Fukui T, et al (1986) Complete nucleotide sequence of the gene for human interleukin 1 alpha. Nucleic Acids Res 14:3167–3179
53. Modi WS, Masuda A, Yamada M, Oppenheim JJ, Matsushima K, O'Brien SJ (1988) Chromosomal localization of the human interleukin 1 alpha (IL-1 alpha) gene. Genomics 2:310–314
54. Lafage M, Maroc N, Dubreuil P, et al (1989) The human interleukin-1 alpha gene is located on the long arm of chromosome 2 at band q13. Blood 73:104–107
55. Danis VA, Millington M, Hyland VJ, Grennan D (1995) Cytokine production by normal human monocytes: inter-subject variation and relationship to an IL-1 receptor antagonist (IL-1Ra) gene polymorphism. Clin Exp Immunol 99:303–310
56. Pociot F, Molvig J, Wogensen L, Worsaae H, Nerup J (1992) A TaqI polymorphism in the human interleukin-1 beta (IL-1 beta) gene correlates with IL-1 beta secretion in vitro. Eur J Clin Invest 22:396–402
57. Stokkers PC, van Aken BE, Basoski N, Reitsma PH, Tytgat GN, van Deventer SJ (1998) Five genetic markers in the interleukin 1 family in relation to inflammatory bowel disease. Gut 43:33–39

58. Derkx B, Marchant A, Goldman M, Bijlmer R, van Deventer S (1995) High levels of interleukin-10 during the initial phase of fulminant meningococcal septic shock. J Infect Dis 171:229–232
59. Westendorp RG, Langermans JA, Huizinga TW, et al (1997) Genetic influence on cytokine production and fatal meningococcal disease. Lancet 349:170–173
60. van Dissel JT, van Langevelde P, Westendorp RG, Kwappenberg K, Frolich M (1988) Anti-inflammatory cytokine profile and mortality in febrile patients. Lancet 351:950–953
61. Aithal PG, Grove J, Daly AK, et al (1998) Polymorphism in the interleukin-10 (IL-10) gene in patients with inflammatory bowel disease. Gastroenterology 114:a918 (Abst)
62. Turner DM, Williams DM, Sankaran D, Lazarus M, Sinnott PJ, Hutchinson IV (1997) An investigation of polymorphism in the interleukin-10 gene promoter. Eur J Immunogenet 24:1–8
63. Hajeer AH, Lazarus M, Turner D, et al (1998) IL-10 gene promoter polymorphisms in rheumatoid arthritis. Scand J Rheumatol 27:142–145
64. Huang S, Hendriks W, Althage A, et al (1993) Immune response in mice that lack the interferon-gamma receptor. Science 259:1742–1745
65. Kamijo R, Le J, Shapiro D, et al (1993) Mice that lack the interferon-gamma receptor have profoundly altered responses to infection with Bacillus Calmette-Guerin and subsequent challenge with lipopolysaccharide. J Exp Med 178:1435–1440
66. Newport MJ, Huxley CM, Huston S, et al (1996) A mutation in the interferon-gamma-receptor gene and susceptibility to mycobacterial infection. N Engl J Med 335:1941–1949
67. Jouanguy E, Altare F, Lamhamedi S, et al (1996) Interferon-gamma-receptor deficiency in an infant with fatal bacille Calmette-Guerin infection. N Engl J Med 335:1956–1961
68. Jouanguy E, Altare F, Lamhamedi-Cherradi S, Casanova JL (1997) Infections in IFNGR-1-deficient children. J Interferon Cytokine Res 17:583–587
69. Pierre-Audigier C, Jouanguy E, Lamhamedi S, et al (1997) Fatal disseminated Mycobacterium smegmatis infection in a child with inherited interferon gamma receptor deficiency. Clin Infect Dis 24:982–984
70. de Jong R, Altare F, Haagen IA, et al (1998) Severe mycobacterial and Salmonella infections in interleukin-12 receptor-deficient patients. Science 280:1435–1438
71. Wang DG, Fan JB, Siao CJ, et al (1998) Large-scale identification, mapping, and genotyping of single-nucleotide polymorphisms in the human genome. Science 280:1077–1082
72. Service RF (1998) Microchip arrays put DNA on the spot. Science 282:396–399
73. Service RF (1998) Future chips – labs on a chip – coming soon – the pocket DNA sequencer. Science 282:399–401
74. Amato I (1998) Future chips – micromachines – fomenting a revolution, in miniature. Science 282:402
75. Nedospasov SA, Udalova IA, Kuprash DV, Turetskaya RL (1991) DNA sequence polymorphism at the human tumor necrosis factor (TNF) locus. Numerous TNF/lymphotoxin alleles tagged by two closely linked microsatellites in the upstream region of the lymphotoxin (TNF-beta) gene. J Immunol 147:1053–1059
76. Jongeneel CV, Briant L, Udalova IA, Sevin A, Nedospasov SA, Cambon-Thomsen A (1991) Extensive genetic polymorphism in the human tumor necrosis factor region and relation to extended HLA haplotypes. Proc Natl Acad Sci USA 88:9717–9721
77. Webb GC, Chaplin DD (1990) Genetic variability at the human tumor necrosis factor loci. J Immunol 145:1278–1285
78. Fugger L, Morling N, Ryder LP, et al (1989) NcoI restriction fragment length polymorphism (RFLP) of the tumour necrosis factor (TNF alpha) region in primary biliary cirrhosis and in healthy Danes. Scand J Immunol 30:185–189
79. Partanen J, Koskimies S (1988) Low degree of DNA polymorphism in the HLA-linked lymphotoxin (tumour necrosis factor beta) gene. Scand J Immunol 28:313–316
80. Wilson AG, di Giovine FS, Blakemore AI, Duff GW (1992) Single base polymorphism in the human tumour necrosis factor alpha (TNF alpha) gene detectable by NcoI restriction of PCR product. Hum Mol Genet 1:353
81. D'Alfonso S, Colombo G, Della Bella S, Scorza R, Momigliano-Richiardi P (1996) Association between polymorphisms in the TNF region and systemic lupus erythematosus in the Italian population. Tissue Antigens 47:551–555

82. Brinkman BM, Kaijzel EL, Huizinga TW, Giphart MJ, Breedveld FC, Verweij CL (1995) Detection of a C-insertion polymorphism within the human tumor necrosis factor alpha (TNFA) gene. Hum Genet 96:493
83. Bailly S, di Giovine FS, Duff GW (1993) Polymorphic tandem repeat region in interleukin-1 alpha intron 6. Hum Genet 91:85–86
84. van den Velden PA, Reitsma PH (1993) Amino acid dimorphism in IL1A is detectable by PCR amplification. Hum Mol Genet 2:1753
85. Todd S, Naylor SL (1991) Dinucleotide repeat polymorphism in the human interleukin 1, alpha gene (IL1A). Nucleic Acids Res 19:3756
86. McDowell TL, Symons JA, Ploski R, Forre O, Duff GW (1995) A genetic association between juvenile rheumatoid arthritis and a novel interleukin-1 alpha polymorphism. Arthritis Rheum 38:221–228
87. di Giovine FS, Takhsh E, Blakemore AI, Duff GW (1992) Single base polymorphism at −511 in the human interleukin-1 beta gene (IL1 beta). Hum Mol Genet 1:450
88. Clay FE, Tarlow JK, Cork MJ, Cox A, Nicklin MJ, Duff GW (1996) Novel interleukin-1 receptor antagonist exon polymorphisms and their use in allele-specific mRNA assessment. Hum Genet 97:723–726
89. Guasch JF, Bertina RM, Reitsma PH (1996) Five novel intragenic dimorphisms in the human interleukin-1 genes combine to high informativity. Cytokine 8:598–602
90. Tarlow JK, Blakemore AI, Lennard A, et al (1993) Polymorphism in human IL-1 receptor antagonist gene intron 2 is caused by variable numbers of an 86-bp tandem repeat. Hum Genet 91:403–404
91. Steinkasserer A, Koelble K, Sim RB (1991) Length variation within intron 2 of the human IL-1 receptor antagonist protein gene (IL1RN). Nucleic Acids Res 19:5095

The Pro-Inflammatory Cytokine Cascade

J.-M. Cavaillon and M. Adib-Conquy

Introduction

The production of pro-inflammatory cytokines is a prerequisite for initiating the anti-infectious process, whereas their exacerbated production during severe inflammation may contribute to deleterious consequences. The capacity of interleukin (IL)-1 and tumor necrosis factor-alpha (TNF-α) to induce inflammatory mediators contributes to their pro-inflammatory properties. Phospholipase, cyclooxygenase and lipoxygenase are activated by IL-1 and TNF-α leading to the release of prostaglandins, thromboxane, leukotrienes, and platelet activating factor (PAF). Free radicals (superoxide [O_2^-], nitric oxide [NO]), and proteolytic enzymes are other mediators produced by target cells in response to IL-1 and TNF-α. Other cytokines, including chemokines such as IL-8 or some T-cell derived cytokines, such as lymphotoxin-α are also involved in the cytokine cascade (Fig. 1). Different experimental approaches have demonstrated the contribution of the pro-inflammatory cytokines to the harmful effects observed in sepsis, trauma, burns, hemorrhage, severe surgery and other pathophysiological situations leading to systemic inflammatory response syndrome (SIRS). The injection of recombinant pro-inflammatory cytokines mimics some of the clinical parameters observed in SIRS patients and the use of anti-cytokine antibodies prevents most of the deleterious effects observed in animal models of SIRS.

Nature of the Stimuli Which Initiate the Cascade

When inflammation is initiated by an infectious process, the presence of microorganisms and their derived products (membrane compounds, released toxins, intra-cellular constituents following lysis) are potent activators of cytokine production. Macrophages are probably one of the major sources of cytokines. Among Gram-negative bacterial derived compounds, endotoxin or lipopolysaccharide (LPS) is a potent inducer of cytokines. During Gram-positive bacterial infection, membrane compounds such as peptidoglycan or lipoteichoic acid are strong inducers of macrophage-derived cytokines. In addition, exotoxins behave as superantigens and trigger the release of T-cell-derived cytokines. Other cells can contribute to the release of cytokines. For example, the beneficial TNF-α observed in experimental peritonitis has been demonstrated to be released by mast

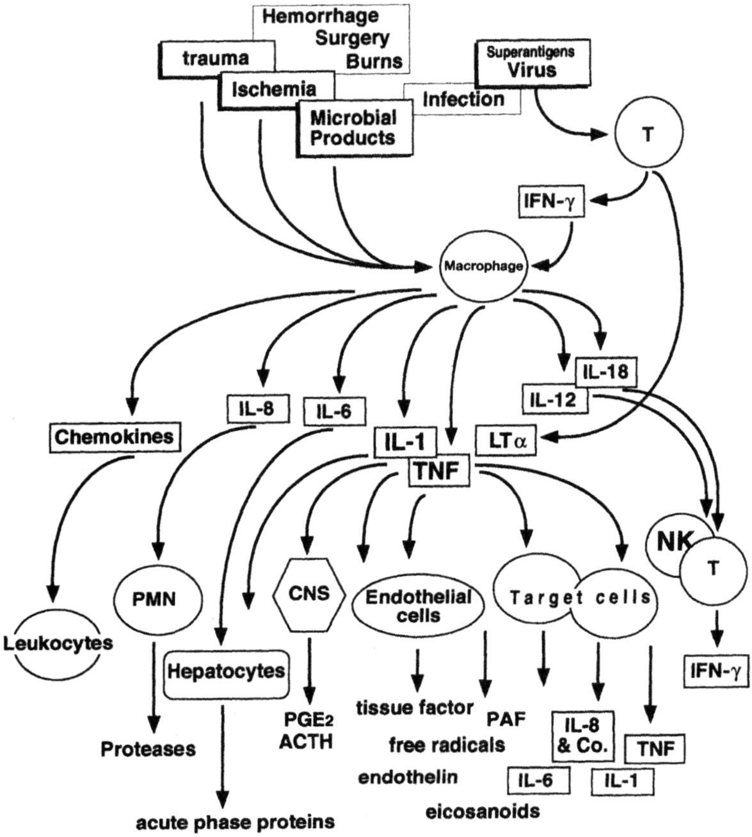

Fig. 1. Schematic representation of the pro-inflammatory cytokine cascade

cells [1]. So, in addition to the well known contribution of mast cells to inflammation observed in acquired immunity via the specific IgE antibodies, these cells play a central role during natural immunity by their capacity to release pro-inflammatory mediators in response to bacteria. Obviously, when the host is facing a stressful condition, many defense systems are activated, leading to the generation of newly synthesized or neo-generated compounds, as well as the release of pre-formed mediators. These factors have the capacity to modulate the generation of cytokines. Activation of the complement system and activation of the coagulation cascade lead to the appearance of factors (anaphylatoxins, thrombin, factor Xa) which can further enhance release of pro-inflammatory cytokines by activated macrophages. Once generated, cytokines possess the capacity of perpetuating their own production. In addition certain cytokines such as those generated by T lymphocytes (e.g., IL-3, granulocyte/macrophage colony-stimulating factor [GM-CSF]) and particularly Th1 cells (i.e., IL-2, IFN-γ) can amplify the release of the pro-inflammatory cytokines.

Bacterial derived products can also be triggering signals in pathophysiological situations that involve bacterial or endotoxin translocation. Hemorrhagic shock, burns or trauma can induce such translocation [2–4]. We have shown that in patients undergoing abdominal aortic surgery, which might be associated with mild gut ischemia, aortic clamping resulted in measurable amounts of circulating LPS and high levels of portal TNF-α suggesting local production by gut associated macrophages [5]. In an animal model, hemorrhage was also associated with local intestinal IL-6 production [6]. Other sites of production have been demonstrated during experimental models of hemorrhage, such as the lungs [7] and the peritoneum [8] where mononuclear phagocytes are a source of IL-1 and TNF-α. Very interestingly, it has been shown that resident mast cells within the tissue exposed to ischemia/reperfusion can degranulate and release pre-formed TNF-α [9]. In experimental liver ischemia and reperfusion experiments, reducing the production of IL-1 and TNF-α resulted in the reduction of polymorphonuclear leukocyte (PMN) infiltration and hepatic injury [10]. Ischemia is also associated with the local production of chemokines that contribute to the recruitment of inflammatory leukocytes [11]. *In vitro* experiments have demonstrated that hypoxia *per se* was capable of inducing the production of IL-1 and TNF-α by mononuclear cells [12]. Similarly, hypoxia induces the release of inflammatory cytokines by endothelial cells [13, 14]. Cardiopulmonary bypass (CPB) represents another inflammatory situation where the production of inflammatory cytokines occurs in various sites including peripheral blood as demonstrated by the presence of increased levels of cell-associated IL-1 in circulating monocytes [15]. The presence of cytokine transcripts in the skeletal muscle or the myocardium, and higher levels of TNF-α and IL-6 in coronary sinus blood than in arterial blood illustrates the various sites of production during CPB [16, 17]. Local production has been demonstrated within the site directly exposed to inflammation during acute pancreatitis [18], brain injury [19, 20], chest trauma [21] or laparotomy [22]. The compartmentalization of cytokine production was elegantly demonstrated in human unilateral pneumonia [23]. Bronchoalveolar lavage (BAL) levels of TNF, IL-1 and IL-6 and spontaneous production by alveolar macrophages were higher in the involved lung as compared to the non-involved lung.

Involvement of Pro-Inflammatory Cytokines in Inflammation

Activation of Endothelial Cells and Leukocyte Adherence to Endothelium

Endothelial cells are important target cells and actors during the inflammatory response. They constitute the interface between the injured tissues and the circulating leukocytes that need to be recruited. Endothelial cells are active producers of inflammatory mediators. In response to IL-1 and TNF-α, endothelial cells synthesize phospholipase and cyclooxygenase leading to the production of prostaglandins, express tissue factor enhancing the coagulation process, and release PAF, free radicals and a large panel of cytokines including IL-6 and IL-8. In addition, these cells express on their surface enhanced levels of adhesion molecules.

L- and P-selectins favor the capture of circulating leukocytes. The rolling of the cells onto the endothelium is mainly mediated by the E-selectins which together with the integrins lead to the firm adhesion of the leukocytes. Finally, integrins are involved in margination towards the tissues. Upon activation of endothelial cells by IL-1 or TNF-α, the expression of the E-selectin ELAM-1 (endothelial leukocyte adhesion molecule-1) is observed within one hour. Monocytes and neutrophils, harboring the counter-ligand Lewis X antigen, bind to the endothelium. The expression of vascular cell adhesion molecule-1 (VCAM-1) and intercellular adhesion molecule-1 (ICAM-1) occurs 4 h following IL-1 or TNF-α activation. *In vivo*, enhanced expression of these adhesion molecules has been demonstrated in various inflammatory processes. For example, augmented expression of ELAM-1 and ICAM-1 has been reported in the skin biopsies from atopic patients challenged locally with the corresponding allergen [24]. The counter-ligand for VCAM-1 is the VLA-4 molecule expressed on the surface of monocytes and lymphocytes. The counter-ligands for ICAM-1 are the LFA-1 (CD11a/CD18) and CR3 (CD11b/CD18) molecules found on the surface of monocytes and neutrophils. The activation of circulating cells leads to conformational changes of the LFA-1 and CR3 molecules that are necessary to favor a strong interaction with their ligands. Once leukocytes have adhered to endothelium, they migrate in response to chemoattractant signals locally delivered by chemokines. Blocking the chemokines by specific antibodies is associated with a lower recruitment of circulating cells and reduced inflammation [25]. Consequently, in infectious models, blocking chemokines is associated with impaired control of infection [26].

Cytokines and Coagulation

IL-1 and TNF are able to induce pro-coagulant activity on endothelial cells. Similar observations are reported with monocytes. This activity is a result of the induction of the membrane expression of tissue factor. Tissue factor combines with factor VII and initiates the coagulation cascade, activating factors X and IX. Injection of TNF in humans is associated with enhanced detection of factor X activated peptide and fragments 1 + 2 of thrombin [27]. In fact, TNF-α and IL-1 first activate fibrinolysis as assessed by enhanced levels of tissue plasminogen activator. An enhanced level of the inhibitor of tissue plasminogen activator occurs later and only then does thrombin become apparent. TNF-α and IL-1 activate coagulation via the induction of tissue factor, whereas IL-6 can also induce coagulation, independent of the induction of tissue factor. In contrast to IL-1 and TNF-α, IL-6 cannot induce fibrinolysis.

Induction of Lipid Mediators and Free Radicals

Many cells, in response to activation by IL-1 or TNF-α, release mediators derived from the metabolism of arachidonic acid either via the cyclooxygenase pathway, leading to the release of prostaglandins and thromboxanes, or via the lipoxygenase pathway leading to the release of leukotrienes. Arachidonic acid itself is generated from membrane phospholipids following the action of phospholipase A2. Neosynthesis of phospholipase A2 and inducible cyclooxygenase (COX2) occurs following the action of IL-1 or TNF-α. Prostaglandins are involved in smooth muscle contraction, mucosal edema, increased vascular permeability, cellular infiltration and mucus secretion. In addition, eicosanoids can modulate the production of pro-inflammatory cytokines: For example, prostaglandin E2 (PGE2) inhibits TNF-α production, but has no significant effect on IL-1, and enhances IL-6 production, while thromboxane A2 favors TNF-α and IL-1β production. Many activities generated by IL-1 and TNF can be suppressed by the use of cyclooxygenase inhibitors such as aspirin or ibuprofen, illustrating the contribution of PGE2 to the activities initiated by IL-1 and/or TNF-α. The action of phospholipase A2 on phosphatidylcholine generates arachidonic acid and lyso-PAF. The latter will be transformed by acetyltransferase to PAF. This factor, known to activate and aggregate platelets, is also responsible for the release of vaso-active mediators, resulting in increased permeability, vasoconstriction and bronchoconstriction.

Among the mediators induced by IL-1 and/or TNF, endothelin also acts on endothelial cells leading to vasoconstriction and increased blood pressure. Four different endothelins have been described. They are short 21 amino acid peptides derived from a 39 amino acid precursor. Endothelin acts via a 7 transmembrane domain receptor coupled to G protein.

Free radicals are also induced upon activation of the oxidative burst by IL-1 and TNF-α. Superoxide anion (O_2^-) generated upon the action of a membrane enzyme NADPH oxidase, has an anti-microbial activity but can also be toxic to local cells. It induces the peroxidation of unsaturated fatty acids leading to an alteration of membrane fluidity and permeability, as well as to the oxidation of amino acids resulting in an alteration of the proteins. Activation of the manganese superoxide dismutase by IL-1 and TNF-α generates hydrogen peroxide (H_2O_2). NO is generated from L-arginine through the action of NO synthase (NOS). Three NOS have been described – two are constitutive (NOS-1 involved in neuronal transmission and NOS-3 which contributes to the vasodilatation at homeostasis) and one is inducible (NOS-2) and produced by many cell types upon activation by IL-1 and TNF-α as well as by interferon-γ (IFN-γ) and migration inhibitory factor (MIF). The toxicity of NO is a result of its ability to inhibit glycolysis, the Krebs cycle, mitochondrial respiration, and DNA synthesis. Very unstable, NO is rapidly transformed to nitrite (NO_2^-) in the presence of H_2O and to nitrate (NO_3^-) by the effect of oxyhemoglobin.

Cytokines and Catabolism

IL-1 was previously known as catabolin and as osteoclast activating factor, a reflection of its ability to generate degradation of cartilage and to induce bone resorption. IL-6 is another cytokine which has been shown to be involved in osteolysis, particularly during the post-menopausal period. Muscle proteolysis is also observed during inflammation. The release of amino acids from muscle further enhances the pool of free amino acids available for the neosynthesis of inflammatory proteins. TNF and to a lesser extent IL-1, have this capacity when acting on muscles. Furthermore, the activation of neutrophils leads to the degranulation of these cells and thus to the release of proteases such as cathepsin and collagenase which can degrade the extracellular matrix, as well as other cellular constituents.

The Main Pro-Inflammatory Cytokines

Interleukin-1

Injection of IL-1 into animals results in hypotension, increased cardiac output and heart rate, leukopenia, thrombocytopenia, hemorrhage, pulmonary edema [28] associated with pulmonary vascular endothelial injury [29], lacticacidemia, hypoaminoacidemia and histopathological lesions in the adrenal cortex [30]. Cyclooxygenase inhibition greatly prevents these effects. IL-1 receptor antagonist (IL-1ra) is a natural IL-1 inhibitor. Early treatment with IL-1ra reduced mortality from endotoxic shock [31, 32], prevented *Staphylococcus epidermidis*-induced hypotension [33], improved survival and hemodynamic performance in *Escherichia coli* septic shock [34] and, depending on the dosage, either reduced or enhanced lethality in a model of *Klebsiella pneumoniae* infection of new born rats [35]. In agreement with these observations, IL-1ra-deficient mice are more susceptible than controls to lethal endotoxemia [36]. IL-1 converting enzyme (ICE), or caspase-1, is an enzyme required for the maturation of the 30 kDa biologically inactive IL-1β precursor to the mature 17 kDa active form of IL-1β. Survival to a lethal dose of endotoxin reached 70% among ICE-deficient animals [37] and these ICE-deficient animals showed a 50% decrease in cellular infiltrate during zymosan-induced peritonitis [38]. On the other hand IL-1β deficient mice were normally sensitive to the lethal effect of LPS [39]. The latter result suggests that, in mice, IL-1α can fulfill the role of IL-1β.

Tumor Necrosis Factor-α

TNF-α toxicity includes hemodynamic instability, fever, diarrhea, metabolic acidosis, capillary leak syndrome, activation of disseminated intravascular coagulation (DIC), late hypoglycemia, induction of a catabolic state, neurotoxicity, cachexia, organ edema, renal and hematological disorders, and acute pulmonary dysfunction, all phenomena associated with sepsis syndrome, systemic inflammatory response syndrome and the genesis of multiple organ failure (MOF) [40–44]. In a cancer patient receiving a high dose of recombinant TNF-α, a systemic inflammatory response syndrome was reported with marked hypotension, extreme generalized capillary leak syndrome and pulmonary function deterioration [45] while hepatic toxicity had been previously reported [46]. In addition, together with IL-1, TNF-α efficiently induced on endothelial cells the expression of adhesion molecules, an event which favors organ infiltration by leukocytes. Its lethal effect was synergistically enhanced by IL-1 [28], IFN-γ [47] and LPS itself [48]. Furthermore, its toxicity was influenced by circadian rhythms [49] and the route of infusion: Portal infusion of TNF-α led to high mortality, renal necrosis, and gut mucosal destruction, an effect not observed after systemic injection [50]. Anti-TNF treatments have been shown for more than a decade to be highly effective in protecting animals against endotoxic shock [51] and lethal bacteremia [52]. Such treatments also protect against pulmonary microvascular injury after intestinal ischemia injury that is associated with endotoxin translocation [53]. The soluble forms of the TNF-α receptors are natural inhibitors capable of limiting TNF-α bioactivity. Their injection into ammal models of sepsis has also been shown to be essentially protective [54–56]. Mice rendered deficient for the p55 TNF-α receptor were resistant to endotoxin in the galactosamine model, whereas high doses of LPS in the absence of galactosamine led to a lethality similar to that observed in wild-type animals; similar findings were obtained with p75 TNF receptor deficient mice [57, 58] and TNF-α/lymphotoxin-α deficient mice [59]. In contrast, over-expression of TNF in transgenic animals is associated with a severe inflammatory process localized in the over-expressing tissues, ending in cardiac failure [60], degeneration of the central nervous system [61] or erosive arthritis [62].

Interleukin-12

Among the adverse effects of IL-12, hepato- and splenomegaly, leukopenia, anemia and myelodepression have been reported [63]. These phenomena are largely IFN-γ-dependent since they have not been reported to occur in IFN-γ receptor deficient mice. Hepatomegaly is associated with infiltration of activated macrophages and natural killer (NK) cells, and single-cell necrosis. In contrast, pulmonary edema and interstitial macrophage infiltration generated by IL-12 injection has been shown to be IFN-γ-independent. In a bacillus Calmette-Guérin (BCG)-primed model of LPS-induced shock and lethality, anti-IL-12 antibodies were shown to protect mice if injected before endotoxin [64]. The protection was associated with decreased IFN-γ production.

Interferon-γ

Side-effects of IFN-γ include tachychardia, myalgia, malaise, leukopenia, and weakness. Furthermore, its synergy with the detrimental activities of LPS have been clearly established: IFN-γ enhanced LPS-induced mortality and increased levels of LPS-induced circulating TNF-α [65]. Consequently, anti-IFN-γ antibodies protected against LPS- and *E. coli*-induced mortality [65, 66]. In addition, IFN-γ was shown to be a mediator of TNF-α-induced lethality. Sublethal doses of TNF-α and IFN-γ, when injected together, led to 100% lethality in mice, and anti-

IFN-γ antibodies protected against one to four LD100 of TNF-α [47]. Mice lacking IFN-γ receptors have been shown to be resistant to LPS challenge after priming with BCG [67] or treatment with galactosamine [68].

Leukemia Inhibitory Factor (LIF) and Oncostatin M (OSM)

LIF and OSM belong to the IL-6 superfamily, sharing the gp130 chain of the receptor. However, while IL-6 and IL-11 possess certain anti-inflammatory properties (see below), LIF and OSM can be considered as pro-inflammatory cytokines. Indeed, LIF is involved in the pathogenesis of inflammation and sepsis syndrome [69]. Produced upon activation by LPS and TNF, LIF can itself induce the release of other cytokines, including IL-1, IL-6 and IL-8, by various cell types. Passive immunization against LIF in mice challenged with intraperitoneal administration of endotoxin protects them from the lethal effects and blocked increases in serum levels of IL-1 and IL-6 [70]. Levels of plasma LIF, ciliary neurotrophic factor (CNTF, another member of the IL-6 family), and OSM are elevated in septic patients [71]. Subcutaneous injection of OSM in mice causes an acute inflammatory reaction [72]. OSM favors PMN adhesion to endothelial cells and transmigration via its capacity to enhance the expression of P- and E-selectin, ICAM-1 and VCAM-1. Furthermore, OSM induces the release of IL-6 and ENA78 (an α-chemokine), but not that of IL-8.

Macrophage Migration Inhibitory Factor

Recent investigations on pituitary-derived factors resulted in the rediscovery of an old cytokine named MIF. Bernhagen et al. [73] reported that injection of MIF together with one LD40 of LPS greatly potentiated lethality, and anti-MIF antibodies fully protected against one LD50 of LPS. As previously mentioned, MIF acts to counter-regulate the inhibitory effects of glucocorticoids on inflammatory cytokine production (Fig. 2). Interestingly, it was recently shown that MIF is expressed constitutively in many tissues including lung, liver, kidney, spleen, adrenal gland, and skin. MIF exists as a preformed cytokine which is rapidly released following LPS injection [74].

Interleukin-8 and the Chemokines

Sepsis and SIRS are often associated with organ dysfunction, a reflection of the inflammatory process occurring in the tissues. One of the major features of this phenomenon is the recruitment of inflammatory leukocytes, the adherence of circulating cells to the endothelium and their response to the locally produced chemokines. Endothelial cells are highly responsive to IL-1 and TNF, in terms of adhesion molecule and tissue factor expression, as well as cytokine production.

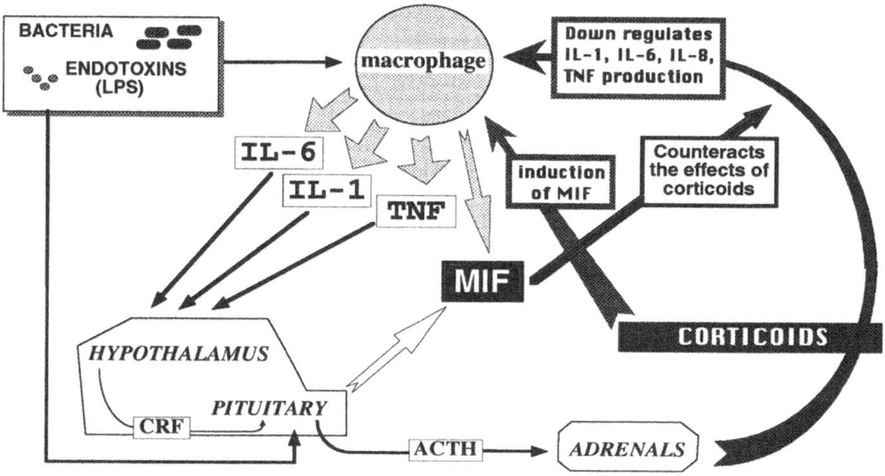

Fig. 2. Schematic representation of the regulatory loop involving down-regulation of pro-inflammatory cytokine production by glucocorticoids and its regulation by macrophage migration inhibitory factor (MIF) which behaves as a pro-inflammatory cytokine

Endothelial cell wall integrity is also perturbed by these cytokines as illustrated by the absence of endothelial damage in IL-1 receptor type I deficient mice [75]. Mice have been developed lacking molecules normally expressed on circulating leukocytes (e.g., L-selectin, CD62L) or on endothelial cells (e.g., ICAM-1). These adherence molecules are involved in the attachment of neutrophils, lymphocytes or monocytes to the endothelium [76, 77]. These deficient mice are significantly resistant to LPS-induced toxic shock lethality. Once immobilized on endothelium, leukocytes will migrate towards the tissues in response to IL-8 and the other chemokines. Thus, these chemokines favor the inflammatory cell infiltrate which contributes to the loss of tissue integrity. For example, it has been reported that neutralization of IL-8 profoundly inhibits neutrophil recruitment in an endotoxin-induced rabbit model of pleurisy, indicating that IL-8 is a major chemotactic factor in this model of acute inflammation [78]. During sepsis a large amount of IL-8 is detectable within the blood compartment, not only as a free cytokine [79] but also as a cell-associated form [80]. This first encounter of neutrophils with IL-8 led to their desensitization to further signals delivered locally by IL-8. Thus, the presence of IL-8 in the vascular space may well be a mechanism for limiting neutrophil accumulation at extracellular sites as illustrated by the defect in neutrophil migration during sepsis or endotoxemia [81–83]. Similarly, while monocyte-chemoattractant protein-1 (MCP-1) contributes to the recruitment of inflammatory macrophages within the tissues, neutralization of MCP-1 by specific antibodies before LPS administration resulted in a striking increase in mortality and injection of MCP-1 was protective [84].

The Beneficial Effects of IL-6 and IL-11

Many investigators have demonstrated that levels of circulating IL-6 correlate with severity of sepsis and may predict outcome [85–88]. Although IL-6 is often considered to be an inflammatory cytokine, most of its activities are associated with a negative control of inflammation. For example, IL-6 induces the release of IL-1ra and soluble TNF receptors [89]. Its most potent anti-inflammatory activity is linked to its capacity to induce the release of acute-phase proteins. In this context, it is interesting to note that IL-1ra has recently been identified as a product of hepatocytes, and regulated by pro-inflammatory cytokines like acute-phase proteins [90]. Furthermore, some acute-phase proteins such as the C-reactive protein (CRP), α1-anti-trypsin, and α1-acid glycoprotein, induce IL-1ra [91]. Reports have demonstrated that these acute-phase proteins can limit the inflammatory process [92], protect against meningococcal endotoxin [93], or even inhibit a lethal response to TNF [94, 95]. These results may explain why IL-6 has been shown to be protective in infectious and in septic shock models [96–98]. Nevertheless, IL-6 does possess some deleterious and pro-inflammatory effects which will be detailed below [99–102].

IL-11 belongs to the IL-6 superfamily, sharing the gp130 chain of the receptors. Although IL-11 stimulated the production of several major acute phase proteins by hepatoma cells, circulating IL-11 did not significantly participate in the production of acute-phase proteins by the liver [103]. One of the major beneficial effects of IL-11 is related to its healing activity on the intestinal tract. For example, chemotherapy and radiation both damage the small intestine mucosal barrier and lead to the entry of gastrointestinal organisms into the blood. In this lethal model, IL-11 was able to protect 80% of the animals [104]. Beneficial properties of IL-11 have also been demonstrated in a rat neonatal infectious model with group B streptococci. Prophylactic use of IL-11 enhanced the survival in this model in association with an increased number of platelets [105].

Are IL-1 and TNF the Main Directors of the Cascade?

In many pathophysiological situations, it has been reported that the production and the presence of pro-inflammatory cytokines correlates with the severity of the disease. For example, during cardiac surgery and in patients undergoing CPB, it was shown that TNF-α levels correlated with the duration of bypass and were associated with clinical complications which led to the development of SIRS/multiple organ dysfunction syndrome (MODS) [106]. More convincing is the direct demonstration that blockade of pro-inflammatory cytokines ameliorates the pathophysiological aftermath and improves survival in acute inflammatory diseases. Antibodies against TNF-α illustrate its role as a main mediator involved in the progression from local inflammation to a host-wide syndrome of organ injury. Thus anti-TNF-α antibodies were beneficial in various animal models of acute pancreatitis [107, 108], splanchnic artery occlusion [109], allograft rejection [110] or IL-2 toxicity [111]. Anti-TNF treatments reduced pulmonary injury following lower torso [112], hepatic [113], or intestinal [53] ischemia/reperfusion as assessed by reduced hemorrhage, edema, PMN sequestration, capillary leak and rise of leukotriene levels in BAL. Similarly, in hemorrhagic shock models, the use of anti-TNF-α demonstrated the contribution of this cytokine to the hemodynamic alterations, organ injury and mortality [114, 115]. In a model of zymosan-induced MODS Goris' group showed that treatment with a monoclonal antibody against TNF-α improved survival [116]. However, in humans, the therapeutic use of various anti-TNF-α approaches in sepsis has so far proven ineffective. In contrast, the use of anti-TNF-α antibodies has been shown to be particularly effective in the treatment of two chronic inflammatory diseases – rheumatoid arthritis [117] and Crohn's disease [118].

While these data indicate that TNF-α plays a major role in various acute inflammatory diseases, none fully demonstrate whether TNF is necessary for the deleterious effects associated with severe diseases. The use of TNF-deficient animals can help to answer this question. Interestingly, we demonstrated that in TNF-α/lymphotoxin-α deficient animals, LPS-induced lethality was similar to that of control animals [59], suggesting that death following endotoxin-induced shock could occur in the absence of TNF. Furthermore, we showed that 90 minutes after LPS injection the levels of circulating IL-6 in control and knock-out animals were similar, while after 3 hours, higher levels were observed in normal mice. These results indicate that TNF is not necessary for IL-6 production although its presence further enhances it. These results contrast with experiments performed with anti-TNF-α treatments which led to a significant decrease of IL-1, IL-6 and IL-8 at any time after bacterial injection [119]. On the other hand, survival can occur even with the presence of abundant circulating levels of TNF-α. In a rabbit model of endotoxin shock we have shown that hemofiltration coupled with resin adsorption significantly protected the animals from death while the levels of circulating bioactive TNF-α remained unchanged (Tetta et al., unpublished data).

Using IL-1ra to counteract the effects of IL-1, the contribution of IL-1 to various acute inflammatory diseases including pancreatitis [120], acute respiratory distress syndrome (ARDS) [121], and immune complex-induced colitis [122] or lung injury [123] has been similarly demonstrated. IL-1ra is capable of preventing LPS-induced lethality and most of the endotoxin-induced injury. The inhibition of inflammation by IL-1ra is associated with a decrease in detectable IL-1 and TNF-α as shown in the lungs of mice following hemorrhage and resuscitation [124]. While the decrease of inflammatory cytokines reflects reduction of the inflammatory process, it is also the direct consequence of a reduced production of IL-1 and TNF-α by activated phagocytes [125]. These observations further illustrate the auto-regulatory loops between IL-1 and TNF-α; each can induce the other, as well as itself.

Signaling by Pro-Inflammatory Cytokine

The Nuclear Factor-κB (NF-κB) Pathway

The inducible transcription factor NF-κB plays a major role in intracellular signaling, during inflammatory processes induced by stress, mitogens or cytokines. Indeed, this is one of the main nuclear factors that regulates the transcription of numerous genes, including cytokines and growth factors (especially pro-inflammatory cytokines such as TNF-α, IL-1β, IL-6 and IL-8), cytokine receptors, stress proteins and leukocyte adhesion molecules [126, 127]. The NF-κB family is composed of various members, p50 (NF-κB1), p52 (NF-κB2), p65 (RelA), RelB and c-Rel, which can form homo- and heterodimers [128]. In most cells, the complex that is commonly found is the p50p65 heterodimer which is a potent transactivator, while it is generally believed that the p50p50 homodimer is not [129]. NF-κB is regulated by a cytoplasmic inhibitor: IκB. This protein also is member of a large family that includes IκBα, IκBβ, IκBγ, IκBε and Bcl-3. All possess multiple regions of homology known as the ankyrin-repeat motifs. These motifs are also present in the precursors of p50 and p52, p105 and p100 respectively, which also behave as NF-κB inhibitors. In unstimulated cells, NF-κB is retained in the cytoplasm by IκB as an inactive complex. Upon stimulation, IκB is phosphorylated on serines 32 and 36, leading to its subsequent ubiquitination and its degradation by the 26S proteasome pathway. TNF-α and IL-1 are potent activators of NF-κB. As represented in Figure 3, the binding of TNF-α or IL-1 to their receptors recruits adaptator molecules which lead to the activation of an NF-κB-inducing kinase (NIK) [130]. The signaling by the TNFR1 involves a TNF receptor-associated death domain protein (TRADD) [131]. Death domains mediate protein-protein

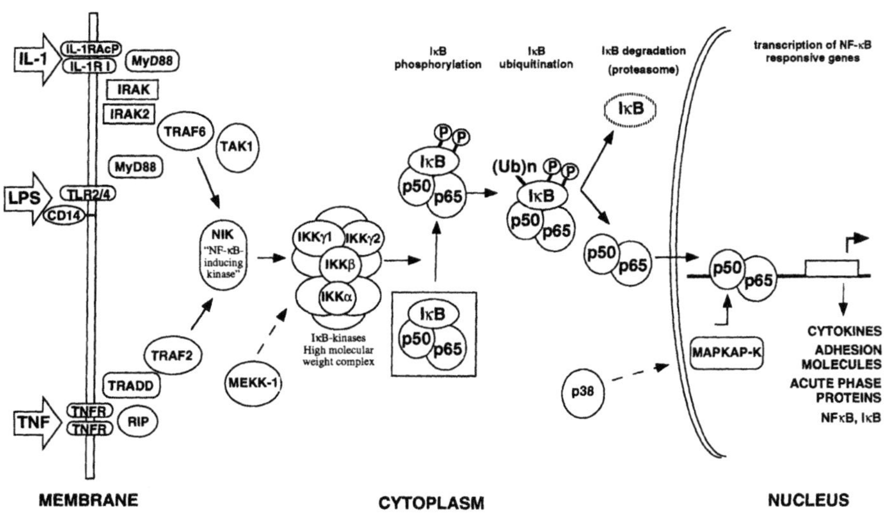

Fig. 3. Schematic cascade of NF-κB activation by TNF-α and IL-1. See text for abbreviations

interactions; TRADD can bind to the TNF receptor-associated factor-2 (TRAF2) and to receptor interacting protein (RIP), another death domain-containing kinase [132, 133]. IL-1 signaling also uses many receptor-associated proteins. The IL-1 receptor I associates with the IL-1 receptor accessory protein (IL-1RAcP) [134], and MyD88 a death domain-containing protein. MyD88 can interact with IL-1 receptor associated kinase (IRAK) that, via TRAF6, activates NIK, a MEKK-1 related kinase [135]. MEKK-1 is a mitogen-activated protein kinase (MAPK) kinase kinase implicated in one of the MAPK cascades (see the next section). The data about the contribution of this cascade to NF-κB activation remains controversial. Indeed, recombinant MEKK-1 has been shown to phosphorylate IκB *in vitro* [136] and its over expression in a fibroblastic cell line could induce NF-κB activation during TNF stimulation through the degradation of IκB [137]. However, another study showed that overexpression of inactive MEKK-1 has no inhibitory effect on NF-κB activation via TRAF2, suggesting that it does not play a role in the activation of this transcription factor [138]. Thus, it would appear that NIK, rather than MEKK-1 itself, takes part in NF-κB activation. Furthermore, NIK seems to be the convergence point of the TNF-α and IL-1-mediated NF-κB activation, since mutant forms of NIK block the signaling from the receptors of these cytokines [130]. The final step of the kinase cascade leads to the activation of protein kinases that phosphorylate IκB. These IκB kinases (IKK) are associated with a high-molecular weight cytoplasmic complex [139–141]. Overexpression of NIK, but also MEKK-1 has been shown to phosphorylate and activate IKKα and β. Finally, after the degradation of IκB, the NF-κB dimer can translocate into the nucleus, bind to DNA and activate the transcription of target genes.

The Mitogen-Activated Protein Kinases

The MAPK cascades are the other intracellular signaling pathway activated during the inflammatory process and they also lead to the activation of numerous transcription factors. Three MAPK cascades have been described to date – the extracellular signal-regulated kinases (ERK), the c-jun N terminal kinase/stress-activated protein kinase (JNK/SAPK) and the p38 pathways (Fig. 4). The first identified cascade was that of ERK. The activation of ERK1 and 2, also known as p44 and p42, is triggered by mitogens and growth factors, while the two other cascades are strongly activated by IL-1, TNF-α, LPS and cell stress [142, 143]. c-jun is a component of the activator protein(AP)-1 transcription factor and the JNK cascade leads to its phosphorylation and an enhancement of its capacity to activate transcription. The JNK pathway contains a MAPK kinase kinase, MEKK-1, which has been shown in some experiments to take part in the activation of NF-κB (see above). The p38 kinase is the last MAPK described to date and it has been implicated in the activation of various transcription factors and some reports suggest that it can play a role in the activation of NF-κB. Indeed, it has been shown that a specific inhibitor of p38 (SB203580) prevented the expression of a reporter gene under the control of NF-κB [144]. However, this was not due to an inhibition of the binding of NF-κB to DNA. Thus, p38 does not seem to regulate IκB phosphor-

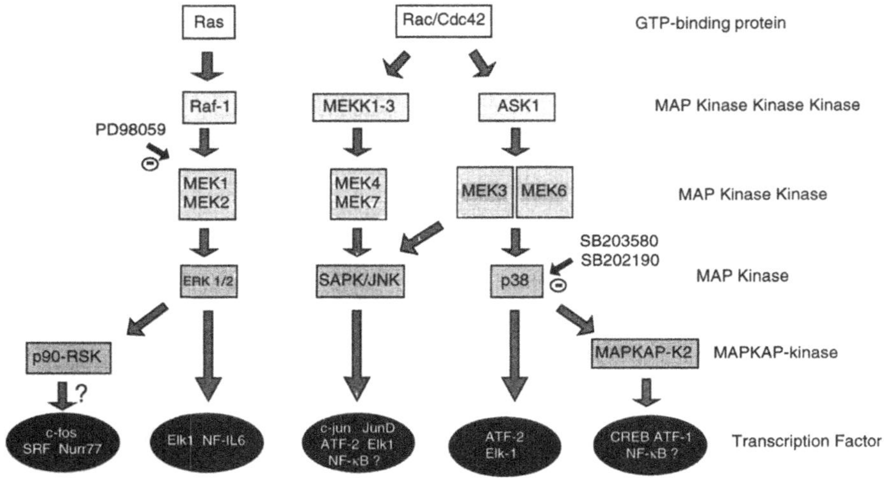

Fig. 4. Schematic representation of the three MAP kinase pathways (ERK, SAPK/JNK and p38). The ERK pathway is triggered by mitogens and growth factors while SAPK/JNK and p38 are strongly activated by endotoxin and also by cytokines such as TNF or IL-1

ylation, but most probably modulates the transactivation capacity of NF-κB via MAPKAP-kinases that in turn phosphorylate the p65 subunit. TNF and IL-1 contribute to the activation of JNK and p38 MAPK, but the molecular mechanisms between the receptors and these kinases are not completely understood. For TNF, it has been shown that TRADD, TRAF2 and RIP are implicated in the signaling leading to JNK and p38 activation [138, 145]. Furthermore, another kinase, the germinal center kinase (GCK), has been shown to interact with TRAF2 and MEKK-1 and thus could be the link between the events taking place at the receptor level and the MAPK kinase kinase [145]. For IL-1, MyD88 and IRAK are also needed for the signaling. IRAK-deficient mice showed reduced IL-1-mediated JNK and p38 activation [146]. Similarly, overexpression of MyD88 induced the activation of JNK and NF-κB while mutant forms of MyD88 inhibited their activation [135].

Inflammatory Stimuli-Induced Immune Suppression Limits the Pro-Inflammatory Cytokine Cascade

Immune depression is associated with numerous stressful conditions. Many immune responses such as delayed-type hypersensitivity, lymphoproliferative responses, NK activity, and cytokine production are diminished. Immunosuppression has often been associated with increased production of IL-10 and transforming growth factor-β (TGF-β) and levels of circulating IL-10 [147] and TGF-β [148] are increased in septic patients. Plasma IL-10 may contribute to the cell deactivation observed in septic and trauma patients [149, 150]. A similar hypothesis has been proposed for TGF-β [151–153]. In addition, in humans, the use of many drugs may further modify cell reactivity [154–156].

Reduced *ex Vivo* Cytokine Production in Critically Ill Patients

Sepsis syndrome, surgery, trauma, hemorrhage and thermal injury are associated with an augmented *in vivo* production of pro- and anti-inflammatory cytokines as assessed by their increased levels in the blood stream. Paradoxically, the capacity of circulating leukocytes from these patients to produce cytokines is reduced when compared to cells from healthy controls. Although the hyporeactivity of the cells observed in septic patients has been associated with endotoxin tolerance [157], this phenomenon is specific neither for endotoxin [158] nor for septic patients. Hyporesponsiveness of circulating leukocytes and low cytokine production have been associated with immune depression observed in these patients.

Monocyte reactivity to LPS stimulation has been particularly studied in isolated monocytes and in whole-blood assays. Monocytes from septic patients show a diminished capacity to release TNF-α, IL-1α, IL-1β, IL-6, IL-10 and IL-12 [159–165] whereas this was not the case for IL-1ra [162]. Reduced cytokine production has also been observed with other stimuli such as silica, staphylococcal enterotoxin B (SEB), killed *Streptococcus* and *Staphylococcus* [165–168]. Similarly, in patients undergoing abdominal aortic surgery [169], cardiac surgery associated with CPB [170], or trauma [171], monocyte-derived cytokine production was significantly altered.

Similar hyporeactivity has been reported when studying neutrophils. In septic patients the production of IL-1β, soluble IL-1ra and IL-8 by LPS-activated neutrophils is lower than in healthy controls [157, 172].

Indeed, the very first observation of the hyporeactivity of circulating leukocytes was demonstrated with peripheral blood lymphocytes. In this initial study, Wood et al. [173] reported decreased IL-2 production upon phytohemaglutinin (PHA) stimulation in major burn patients, with a more severe depression during the septic episodes. In patients undergoing surgery with or without CPB, hemorrhage and in trauma patients, reduced mitogen-induced IL-2 has been documented [171, 174–177]. The defect in IL-2 production was previously shown not to be related to a different $CD4^+/CD8^+$ ratio [174]. However, the different results obtained when different cell activators are used suggests that either the proportion of certain T-cell subsets may be modified in critically ill patients, or an alteration in cell reactivity may only occur among certain T-cell subsets [176]. Furthermore, certain monocyte subsets, particularly the human leukocyte antigen (HLA) DR^+ cells, have a modified frequency in injured or septic patients [178], and may, as accessory cells, contribute to the different observed T cell reactivity. IL-2 production varies depending on the animal experimental models. Concanavalin (ConA)-induced IL-2 production by spleen cells was unaffected in endotoxemia [179] and reduced in trauma, hemorrhage, peritonitis, and thermal injury models [177, 180–183]. However, one should be very careful in extrapolating these data obtained from animal models to the human situation. Mouse studies use spleen cells whereas human studies usually involve peripheral blood leukocytes. Circulating cells and cells within tissues are likely not affected similarly by the various stressful situations. IFN-γ *ex vivo* production was also reported to be altered in burns [183], trauma [171], hemorrhage [177], CPB [184] and in sepsis [165].

IL-2 and IFN-γ are both Th1 cytokines, therefore, it was of interest to know whether the production of Th2 cytokines was also modified during stressful situations. In sepsis, ConA-induced IL-2, IL-5, and IL-10 production by peripheral blood mononuclear cells was diminished, whereas this was not the case when PHA and anti-CD3 were employed as activation stimuli (Muret et al., unpublished data). In contrast, Miller-Graziano et al. [185] reported that PHA- and (anti-CD3 + anti-CD4)-induced IL-10 production were depressed in trauma patients. In animal models, the results depend on the insult and on the study. In experimental peritonitis following cecal ligature and puncture (CLP), ConA-induced IL-10 production by splenocytes was either enhanced [181] or reduced [186], and in models of hemorrhage, therma injury, and trauma, ConA-induced IL-10 production was enhanced [149, 177, 182, 183, 186].

In a mouse model of severe injury (fracture + hemorrhage) it was reported that splenocytes produce more IL-5 upon stimulation by ConA, together with an increase in IL-4 and IL-10, wheareas IL-2 production is decreased [182]. This animal model led Mack et al. [182] to postulate that there was a shift to a Th2-type splenocyte cytokine response after injury.

Reversibility of Immune Depression

The enhanced susceptibility of injured patients to infection is well known and associated with a depressed immune system. Attempts to restore immune cell reactivity have been made using IFN-γ. In mice, IFN-γ attenuated hemorrhage-induced suppression of macrophage and splenocyte function and decreased susceptibility to sepsis [187]. In humans, while the results did not show definite beneficial effects in severe surgery patients [188], IFN-γ restored monocyte reactivity and enhanced HLA DR^+ frequency [189]. Other cytokines such as IL-2, IL-12, and GM-CSF could be considered to restore immune cell activity. IL-2 enhances the survival of mice in a burn and sepsis model and its activity was enhanced by the addition of lymphokine-activated killer cells [190]. IL-12 and GM-CSF were capable of reversing the LPS-induced desensitization *in vitro* as well as *in vivo* [191, 192]. Interestingly, other natural mediators, notably growth hormone [193] and prolactin [194] are capable of abrogating the immune defects associated with stressful conditions and of protecting against sepsis.

A Too Simplistic Dichotomy

The events occurring during inflammation are not as simplistic as just an interplay between pro- and anti-inflammatory actors. Indeed, the situation is far more complex. First, the genetic background contributes to the heterogeneity of the inflammatory response in humans. Genetic polymorphisms have been reported for many pro- as well as anti-inflammatory cytokines [195–198], and, in addition, another polymorphism exists in terms of target cell reactivity in response to cytokine signaling [199]. While an excess of pro-inflammatory cytokines may be deleterious and even kill when used in animal models, these same cytokines are essential in the initiation of the anti-infectious response. More recently, their anti-inflammatory potential has even been outlined. For example, in response to an injection of myelin oligodendrocyte glycoprotein, a model which mimics human systemic sclerosis, TNF deficient mice display a more severe auto-immune mediated demyelination than their wild type counterparts [200]. In *in vitro* models, when delivered early enough to the cells, TNF can prevent the INF-γ-primed production of NO [201] or IL-12 [202]. The amount of the delivered cytokine may also influence its property. For example, while low concentrations of IL-12 exacerbated the disease in an experimental model of arthritis, IL-12 behaved as an anti-inflammatory cytokine when delivered at higher concentrations [203]. Surprisingly, INF-γ could inhibit the production of LPS-induced chemokines MIP-1α and MIP-1β to the same extent as IL-10 and TGF-β [204].

IL-4, IL-10, IL-13, IFN-α and TGF-β are considered as anti-inflammatory cytokines because of their capacity to inhibit the release of pro-inflammatory cytokines, to induce the production of IL-1ra and the release of soluble TNF receptor, and to limit some of the pro-inflammatory activities of IL-1 and TNF. However, many available examples illustrate that the pro- or anti-inflammatory properties of these cytokines may depend on the nature of the target cell, the nature of the stimuli the cell has encountered, the sequence of the events and the nature of the environmental factors.

While IL-4 inhibits the IL-1- or TNF-induced expression of ICAM-1 and ELAM-1 on the surface of endothelial cells, it favors the expression of VCAM-1, allowing the adherence of basophils and eosinophils [205]. Also, IL-4 inhibits the LPS-induced production of IL-8 by macrophages, but amplifies that of endothelial cells [206]. Similarly, while IL-13 diminishes chemokine production in activated macrophages, it induces the synthesis of MCP-1 in endothelial cells [207]. Whether a mediator exerts an inhibiting or, on the contrary, an enhancing property may also be linked to the timing of its exposure to the target cells. For example, IL-4 and IL-13 inhibit IL-6, IL-12, MCP-1 and TNF production when added simultaneously to activated monocytes whereas they enhance the production of these cytokines when they are delivered before the activating signals [208–210]. IL-4, which can block TNF production by LPS-activated freshly isolated monocytes, is unable to inhibit the TNF production by 7-day cultured monocytes stimulated by LPS but can block the IL-1 production [211]. The nature of the activator results in a different profile; IL-4 was shown not to interfere with the production of RANTES (regulated on activation, normal T expressed and secreted) by human monocytes activated by IFN-γ whereas it amplified it when the cells were activated by TNF [212]. Similarly, IL-13 inhibits TNF and IL-8 production in human whole blood assays in the presence of LPS while it does not modify the TNF production when heat killed streptococci are used as activators [213].

The nature of the responding cell may also influence the quality of the modulation of the response by TGF-β. While TGF-β1 limited the production of IL-1α and IL-8 in macrophages, it induced their production in epithelial cells [214].

IL-10 which is undoubtely an anti-inflammatory cytokine, has been shown in various models to behave differently. IL-10 may well have some pro-inflammatory properties. Evidence from *in vivo* work (graft rejection [215], ocular inflammation [216], auto-immune diseases [217], anti-tumor activity [218]) suggests that in some circumstances, IL-10 may also behave as an immunostimulatory and/or pro-inflammatory cytokine. Injection of an adenocarcinoma expressing IL-10 gene results in a far more severe local inflammation than the non-transfected adenocarcinoma, as evaluated in terms of the presence of MCP-1 and inducible NOS, of leukocyte infiltrate and expression of adherence molecules [219]. Some *in vitro* reports have shown that IL-10 could also favor certain aspects of the inflammatory response. Thus, IL-10 induced E-selectin expression on small and large blood-vessel endothelial cells [220]. IL-10 may behave differently depending on the nature of the target cells. For example, a consistent, or even enhanced, production of IL-8 has been reported by dendritic cells [221] and endothelial cells [206]. While IL-10 could perfectly repress the production of IL-8 by LPS-activated blood neutrophils, such inhibition could not be obtained when neutrophils were derived from the sputum of patients with chronic bronchial sepsis [222]. While IL-10 repressed the production of NO by macrophages or keratinocytes [223, 224], it did not modify its release by mesangial cells [225] and even enhanced the production of NO by bone marrow derived macrophages and osteoclasts [226, 227]. The inhibitory capacity of IL-10 may also depend on the nature of the triggering agent. For example, the modulatory activity of IL-10 on the proliferation or the cytotoxic activity of $CD8^+$ T lymphocytes was different when cells were activated with allogenic monocytes, anti-CD3 antibodies or IL-2 [228]. IL-10 repressed the LPS-induced IL-8 production by neutrophils but not TNF-α-induced IL-8 production [229]. We have shown in *in vitro* experimental studies that IL-10 primed leukocytes and led to enhanced production of TNF and IL-6 upon further stimulation by LPS. The prevention of monocyte adherence by red cells in the whole-blood assays or by cultures of peripheral blood mononuclear cells on teflon, contributed to this observation [230]. Altogether, these results indicate that IL-10-induced modulation of cytokine production depends on the *in vitro* experimental procedures used and on the *in vivo* localization of the event. A similar effect has been reported concerning the pre-treatment with IL-10 of human cell clones which then produced higher levels of IL-2, IL-4, IFN-γ, and TNF [231]. This observation was shown to be associated with the anti-apoptotic property of IL-10 on T cells. On T lymphocytes infected with human immunodeficiency virus (HIV), IL-10 was shown to act synergistically with TNF to favor viral replication and even to induce the production of TNF [232]. On other cells such as mast cells, IL-10 can behave differently. IL-10 can inhibit cytokine generation by mast cells [233] but can act synergistically with c-Kit ligand to increase cyclooxygenase-2 expression and PGD2 production [234].

IL-6 is also considered as an anti-inflammatory cytokine, mainly for its action on hepatocytes and its capacity to induce the production of acute phase proteins which are essentially anti-inflammatory. However, in contrast, IL-6 can induce bone resorption [235], muscle atrophy [236], anemia [237] and can prime neutrophils for the production of PAF and superoxide anion [99, 100]. While IL-6 does not activate endothelial cells, it induces MCP-1, MCP-3, and IL-8 production, signal transducer and activator of transcription (STAT)-3 activation, and ICAM-1 expression, in the presence of its soluble receptor which is naturally found in plasma [102].

Another fascinating example of discordance between dogma and reality is given by the effect of cortisol infusion in human volunteers. While an injection of LPS at the end of the cortisol infusion did not lead to detectable circulating TNF, the same injection 14 to 144 h after the infusion led to far higher levels of TNF and IL-6 as compared with the same volunteers who did not receive the cortisol treatment [238]. Other examples will almost certainly appear in the next few months, illustrating, if necessary, that we still have a lot to understand and should be very careful when analyzing the inflammatory response during SIRS.

Conclusion

The generation of pro-inflammatory cytokines and the capacity of some of them to further induce the production of others within self-amplifying loops plays a major role in the perpetuation of the inflammatory process. However, most inflammatory mediators can be induced by other signals, such as microbial derived products or ischemia, activating the coagulation cascade and the complement system. The capacity of the pro-inflammatory cytokines to further induce a wide type of inflammatory mediator is characteristic of their activities. Of course natural counter-regulation occurs through the generation of acute phase proteins, anti-inflammatory cytokines, endogenous corticoids and heat shock proteins. These later events, together with the reduced capacity of circulating leukocytes to further produce cytokines, may reflect what Louis Pasteur called "Natura medicatrix". When this natural negative regulation appears insufficient, in many animal model of severe inflammation, the therapeutical blocking of the induction or the activities of the major pro-inflammatory cytokines has been demonstrated to be helpful. In human, such approaches have so far been rather disappointing in patients with acute inflammation and systemic inflammatory response syndrome but appear highly promising in some chronic inflammatory diseases such as rheumatoid arthritis or Crohn's disease.

References

1. Echtenacher B, Männel D, Hültner L (1996) Critical protective role of mast cells in a model of acute septic peritonitis. Nature 381:75–77
2. Rush B, Sori A, Murphy T, Smith S, Flanagan J, Machiedo G (1988) Endotoxemia and bacteremia during hemorrhagic shock. The link between trauma and sepsis. Ann Surg 207:549–554
3. Bahrami S, Schlag G, Yao YM, Redl H (1995) Significance of translocation/endotoxin in the development of systemic sepsis following trauma and/or haemorrhage. Prog Clin Biol Res 392:197–208

4. Yao YM, Bahrami S, Leichtfried G, Redl H, Schlag G (1995) Pathogenesis of hemorrhage-induced bacteria/endotoxin translocation in rats. Effects of recombinant bactericidal/permeability-increasing protein. Ann Surg 221:398–405
5. Cabié A, Farkas J-C, Fitting C, et al (1993) High levels of portal TNF-α during abdominal aortic surgery in man. Cytokine 5:448–453
6. Wang W, Smail N, Wang P, Chaudry IH (1998) Increased gut permeability after hemorrhage is associated with upregulation of local and systemic IL-6. J Surg Res 79:39–46
7. Le Tulzo Y, Shenkar R, Kaneko D, et al (1997) Hemorrhage increase cytokine expression in lung mononuclear cells in mice. J Clin Invest 99:1516–1524
8. Zhu XL, Ayala A, Zellweger R, Morrison MH, Chaudry IH (1994) Peritoneal macrophages show increased cytokine gene expression following haemorrhagic shock. Immunology 83: 378–383
9. Frangogiannis NG, Lindsey ML, Michael LH, et al (1998) Resident cardiac mast cells degranulate and release preformed TNF, initiating the cytokine cascade in experimental canine myocardial ischemia/reperfusion. Circulation 98:699–710
10. Suzuki S, Toledo-Peryera LH (1994) Interleukin-1 and tumor necrosis factor production as the initial stimulants of liver ischemia and reperfusion. J Surg Res 57:253–258
11. Safirstein R, Megyesi J, Saggi SJ, et al (1991) Expression of cytokine-like genes JE and KC is increased during renal ischemia. Am J Physiol 261:F1095–F1101
12. Ghezzi P, Dinarello CA, Bianchi M, Rosandich ME, Repine JE, White CW (1991) Hypoxia increases production of interleukin-1 and tumor necrosis factor by human mononuclear cells. Cytokine 3:189–194
13. Shreeniwas R, Koga S, Karakurum M, et al (1992) Hypoxia-mediated induction of endothelial cell interleukin-1α. J Clin Invest 90:2333–2339
14. Karakurum M, Shreeniwas R, Chen J, et al (1994) Hypoxic induction of interleukin-8 gene expression in human endothelial cells. J Clin Invest 93:1564–1570
15. Haeffner-Cavaillo N, Rousselier N, Pnozio O, et al (1989) Induction of IL-1 production in patients undergoing cardiopulmonary bypass. J Thorac Cardiovasc Surg 98:1100–1106
16. Burns S, Newburger J, Xiao M, Mayer J, Walsh A, Neufeld E (1995) Induction of interleukin-8 messenger RNA in heart and skeletal muscle during pediatric cardiopulmonary bypass. Circulation 92 :II-315–II-321
17. Wan S, Desmet JM, Barvais L, Goldstein M, Vincent JL, Leclerc JL (1996) Myocardium is a major source of proinflammatory cytokines in patients undergoing cardiopulmonary bypass. J Thorac Cardiovasc Surg 112:806–811
18. Gross V, Andreesen R, Leser H-G, et al (1992) Interleukin-8 and neutrophil activation in acute pancreatitis. Eur J Clin Invest 22:200–203
19. Giulian D, Lachman LB (1985) Interleukin-1 stimulation of astroglial proliferation after brain injury. Science 228:497–499
20. Holmin S, Schalling M, Höjeberg B, Nordqvist AC, Skeftruna AK, Mathiesen T (1997) Delayed cytokine expression in rat brain following experimental contusion. J Neurosurg 86: 493–504
21. Keel M, Ecknauer E, Stocker R, et al (1996) Different pattern of local and systemic release of proinflammatory and anti-inflammatory mediators in severely injured patients with chest trauma. J Trauma 40:907–914
22. Badia JM, Whawell SA, Scott-Coombes DM, Abel PD, Williamson RCN, Thompson JN (1996) Peritoneal and systemic cytokine response to laparotomy. Br J Surg 83:347–348
23. Dehoux MS, Boutten A, Ostinelli J, et al (1994) Compartmentalized cytokine production within the human lung in unilateral pneumonia. Am J Respir Crit Care Med 150:710–716
24. Kyan-Aung U, Haskard DO, Poston RN, Thornhill MH, Lee TH (1991) ELAM-1 and ICAM-1 mediate the adhesion of eosinophils to endothelial cells in vitro and are expressed by endothelium in allergic cutaneous inflammation in vivo. J Immunol 146:521–528
25. Mulligan MS, Jones ML, Bolanowski MA, et al (1993) Inhibition of lung inflammatory reactions in rats by an anti-human IL-8 antibody. J Immunol 150:5585–5595
26. Huffnagle GB, Strieter RM, Standiford TJ, et al (1995) The role of monocyte chemotactic protein-1 in the recruitment of monocytes and CD4+ T cells during a pulmonary *Cryptococcus neoformans* infection. J Immunol 155:4790–4797

27. van der Poll T, Buller HR, ten Cate H, et al (1990) Activation of coagulation after administration of tumor necrosis factor to normal subjects. N Engl J Med 322:1622–1627
28. Okusawa S, Gelfand J, Lkejima T, Connolly R, Dinarello C (1988) Interleukin 1 induces a shock like state in rabbit. Synergism with tumor necrosis factor and the effect of cyclooxygenase inhibition. J Clin Invest 81:1162–1172
29. Goldblum SE, Yoneda K, Cohen DA, McClain CJ (1988) Provocation of pulmonary vascular endothelial injury in rabbits by human recombinant IL-1 beta. Infect Immun 56:2255–2263
30. Fischer E, Marano MA, Barber AE, et al (1991) Comparison between effects of interleukin-1 administration and sublethal endotoxemia in primates. Am J Physiol 261:R442–R452
31. Ohlsson K, Bjökk P, Bergenfield M, Hageman R, Thompson R (1990) Interleukin-1 receptor antagonist reduces mortality from endotoxin shock. Nature 348:550–552
32. Alexander HR, Doherty GM, Buresh CM, Venzon DJ, Norton JA (1991) A recombinant human receptor antagonist to interleukin-1 improves survival after lethal endotoxemia in mice. J Exp Med 173:1029–1032
33. Aiura K, Gelgand J, Burke J, Thompson R, Dinarello C (1993) Interleukin-1 receptor antagonist prevents S. epidermidis hypotension and reduces circulating levels of TNF and IL-1β in rabbits. Infect Immun 61:3342–3350
34. Fischer E, Marano MA, Van Zee KJ, et al (1992) Interleukin-1 receptor blockade improves survival and hemodynamic performance in Escherichia coli septic shock, but fails to alter host responses to sublethal endotoxemia. J Clin Invest 89:1551–1557
35. Mancilla J, Garcia P, Dinarello CA (1993) The IL-1 receptor antagonist can either reduce or enhance the lethality of *Klebsiella pneumoniae* sepsis in newborn rats. Infect Immun 61: 926–932
36. Hirsch E, Irikura VM, Paul SM, Hirsh D (1996) Functions of interleukin 1 receptor antagonist in gene knockout and overproducing mice. Proc Natl Acad Sci USA 93:11008–11013
37. Li P, Allen H, Banerjee S, et al (1995) Mice deficient in IL-1β converting enzyme are defective in production of mature IL-1β and resistant to endotoxic shock. Cell 80:401–411
38. Fantuzzi G, Ku G, Harding MW, et al (1997) Response to local inflammation of IL-1-beta-converting enzyme-deficient mice. J Immunol 158:1818–1824
39. Fantuzzi G, Hui Z, Faggioni R, et al (1996) Effect of endotoxin in IL-1β deficient mice. J Immunol 157:291–296
40. Natanson C, Eichenholz PW, Danner RL, et al (1989) Endotoxin and TNF challenges in dogs simulate the cardiovascular profile of human septic shock. J Exp Med 169:823–832
41. Van der Poll T, Romijn JA, Endert E, Borm JJ, Buller HR, Sauerwein HP (1991) TNF mimics the metabolic response to acute infection in healthy humans. Am J Physiol 261:E457–E465
42. Ciancio MJ, Hunt J, Jones SB, Filkins JP (1991) Comparative and interactive in vivo effects of tumor necrosis factor alpha and endotoxin. Circ Shock 33:108–120
43. Eichacker PQ, Hoffman WD, Farese A, et al (1991) TNF but not IL-1 in dogs causes lethal lung injury and multiple organ dysfunction similar to human sepsis. J Appl Physiol 71:1979–1989
44. Edwards MJ, Heniford BT, Miller FN (1993) Tumor necrosis factor mediates disseminated intravascular inflammation in the genesis of multiple organ edema. J Surg Res 54:140–144
45. Oldhafer KJ, Kuse ER (1998) High dose tumor necrosis factor alpha leads to the systemic inflammatory response syndrome. Am J Med 105:346–347
46. Schilling PJ, Murray JL, Markowitz AB (1992) Novel tumor necrosis factor toxic effects. Pulmonary hemorrhage and severe hepatic dysfunction. Cancer 69:256–260
47. Doherty GM, Lange JR, Langstein HN, Alexander HR, Buresh CM, Norton JA (1992) Evidence for IFN-gamma as a mediator of the lethality of endotoxin and tumor necrosis factor-alpha. J Immunol 149:1666–1670
48. Rothstein JL, Schreiber H (1988) Synergy between TNF and bacterial products causes hemorrhagic necrosis and lethal shock in normal mice. Proc Natl Acad Sci USA 85:607–611
49. Hrushesky WJM, Langevin T, Kim YJ, Wood PA (1994) Circadian dynamics of tumor necrosis factor alpha lethality. J Exp Med 180:1059–1065
50. Kahky MP, Daniel CO, Cruz AB, Gaskill HV (1990) Portal infusion of tumor necrosis factor increases mortality in rats. J Surg Res 49:138–145
51. Beutler B, Milsark IW, Cerami AC (1985) Passive immunization against cachectin/tumor necrosis factor protects mice from lethal effect of endotoxin. Science 229:869–871

52. Tracey KJ, Fong Y, Hesse DG, et al (1987) Anti-cachectin/TNF monoclonal antibodies prevent septic shock during lethal bacteraemia. Nature 330:662–664
53. Caty MG, Guice KS, Oldham KT, Remick DG, Kunkel SI (1990) Evidence for tumor necrosis factor-induced pulmonary microvascular injury after intestinal ischemia-reperfusion injury. Ann Surg 212:694–700
54. Van Zee K, Kohno T, Fisher E, Rock C, Moldawer L, Lowry S (1992) TNF soluble receptors circulate during experimental and clinical inflammation and can protect against excessive tumor necrosis factor α *in vitro* and *in vivo*. Proc Natl Acad Sci USA 89:4845–4849
55. Lesslauer W, Tabuchi H, Gentz R, et al (1991) Recombinant soluble tumor necrosis factor receptor proteins protect mice from LPS-induced lethality. Eur J Immunol 21:2883–2886
56. Ashkenazi A, Marsters S, Capon D, et al (1991) Protection against endotoxic shock by a tumor necrosis factor receptor immunoadhesin. Proc Natl Acad Sci USA 88:10535–10539
57. Pfeffer K, Matsuyama T, Kundig TM, et al (1993) Mice deficient for the 55 kd tumor necrosis factor receptor are resistant to endotoxic shock, yet succumb to L. monocytogenes infection. Cell 73:457–467
58. Erickson SL, de Sauvage F, Kikly K, et al (1994) Decreased sensitivity to tumour-necrosis factor but normal T-cell development in TNF receptor-2-deficient mice. Nature 372: 560–563
59. Amiot F, Fitting C, Tracey KJ, Cavaillon J-M, Dautry F (1997) LPS-induced cytokine cascade and lethality in LTα/TNF-α deficient mice. Mol Med 3:864–875
60. Bryant D, Becker L, Richardson J, et al (1998) Cardiac failure in transgenic mice with myocardial expression of tumor necrosis factor. Circulation 97:1375–1381
61. Probert L, Akassoglou K, Kassiotis G, Pasparakis M, Alexopoulou L, Kollias G (1997) TNF-alpha transgenic and knockout models of CNS inflammation and degeneration. J Neuroimmunol 72:137–141
62. Butler DM, Malfait AM, Mason LJ, et al (1997) DBA/1 mice expressing the human TNF transgen develop a severe erosive arthritis. J Immunol 159:2867–2876
63. Ryffel B (1997) Interleukin-12: role of interferon-γ in IL-12 adverses effects. Clin Immunol Immunopath 83:18–20
64. Wysocka M, Kubin M, Vieira LQ, et al (1995) IL-12 is required for interferon-gamma production and lethality in lipopolysaccharide-induced shock in mice. Eur J Immunol 25: 672–676
65. Heinzel FP (1990) The role of interferon-gamma in the pathology of experimental endotoxemia. J Immunol 145:2920–2924
66. Silva AT, Cohen J (1992) Role of interferon-gamma in experimental Gram-negative sepsis. J Infect Dis 166:331–335
67. Kamijo R, Le J, Shapiro D, et al (1993) Mice that lack the interferon-gamma receptor have profoundly altered responses to infection with Bacillus Calmette-Guerin and subsequent challenge with lipopolysaccharide. J Exp Med 178:1435–1440
68. Car BD, Eng VM, Schnyder B, et al (1994) Interferon-gamma receptor deficient mice are resistant to endotoxic shock. J Exp Med 179:1437–1444
69. Waring P, Wycherley K, Cary D, Nicola N, Metcalf D (1992) Leukemia inhibitory factor levels are elevated in septic shock and various inflammatory body fluids. J Clin Invest 90: 2031–2037
70. Block MI, Berg M, McNamara MJ, Norton JA, Fraker DL, Alexander HR (1993) Passive immunization of mice against D factor blocks lethality and cytokine release during endotoxemia. J Exp Med 178:1085–1090
71. Guillet C, Fourcin M, Chevalier S, Pouplard A, Gascan H (1995) ELISA detection of circulating levels of LIF, OSM and CNTF in septic shock. Ann NY Acad Sci 762:407–412
72. Modur V, Feldhaus MJ, Weyrich AS, et al (1997) Oncostanin M is a proinflammatory mediator. In vivo effects correlates with endothelial cell expression of inflammatory cytokines and adhesion molecules. J Clin Invest 100:158–168
73. Bernhagen J, Calandra T, Mitchell RA, et al (1993) MIF is a pituitary-derived cytokine that potentiates lethal endotoxaemia. Nature 365:756–759
74. Bacher M, Meinhardt A, Lan HY, et al (1997) Migration inhibitory factor expression in experimentally induced endotoxemia. Am J Pathol 150:235–246

75. Sutton ET, Norman JG, Newton CA, Hellermann GR, Richards IS (1997) Endothelial structural integrity is maintained during endotoxic shock in an interleukin-1 type 1 receptor knockout mouse. Shock 7:105–110
76. Tedder TF, Steeber DA, Pizcueta P (1995) L-selectin-deficient mice have impaired leukocyte recruitment into inflammatory sites. J Exp Med 181:2259–2264
77. Xu H, Gonzalo J, St Pierre Y, et al (1994) Leucocytosis and resistance to septic shock in intercellular adhesion molecule 1-deficient mice. J Exp Med 180:95–109
78. Broaddus VC, Boylan AM, Hoeffel JM, Kim KJ, Sadick M, Chuntharapai A (1994) Neutralization of IL-8 inhibits neutrophils influx in a rabbit model of endotoxin-induced pleurisy. J Immunol 152:2960–2967
79. Marty C, Misset B, Tamion F, Fitting C, Carlet J, Cavaillon J-M (1994) Circulating interleukin-8 concentrations in patients with multiple organ failure of septic and nonseptic origin. Crit Care Med 22:673–679
80. Marie C, Fitting C, Cheval C, et al (1997) Presence of high levels of leukocyte-associated IL-8 upon cell activation and in patients with sepsis syndrome. Infect Immun 65:865–871
81. Gimbrone MA, Obin MS, Brock AF, et al (1989) Endothelial interleukin-8: a novel inhibitor of leukocyte-endothelial interactions. Science 246:1601–1603
82. Solomkin JS, Bass RC, Bjornson HS, Tindal CJ, Babcock GF (1994) Alterations of neutrophil responses to TNF-α and IL-8 following human endotoxemia. Infect Immun 62:943–947
83. Cunha FQ, Cunha Tamashiro WMS (1992) Tumour necrosis factor-alpha and interleukin-8 inhibit neutrophil migration in vitro and in vivo. Mediators Inflamm 1:397–401
84. Zisman DA, Kunkel SL, Strieter RM, et al (1997) MCP-1 protects mice in lethal endotoxemia. J Clin Invest 99:2832–2836
85. Waage A, Brandtzaeg P, Halstensen A, Kierulf P, Espevik T (1989) The complex pattern of cytokines in serum from patients with meningococcal septic shock. Association between interleukin-6, interleukin-1, and fatal outcome. J Exp Med 169:333–338
86. Hack C, de Groot E, Felt-Bersma R, et al (1989) Increased plasma levels of interleukin-6 in sepsis. Blood 74:1704–1710
87. Muñoz C, Misset B, Fitting C, Bleriot JP, Carlet J, Cavaillon J-M (1991) Dissociation between plasma and monocyte-associated cytokines during sepsis. Eur J Immunol 21:2177–2184
88. Calandra T, Gerain J, Heumann D, Baumgartner JD, Glauser MP (1991) High circulating levels of interleukin-6 in patients with septic shock: evolution during sepsis, prognostic value, and interplay with other cytokines. Am J Med 91:23–29
89. Tilg H, Trehu E, Atkins MB, Dinarello CA, Mier JW (1994) Interleukin-6 (IL-6) as an anti-inflammatory cytokine: induction of circulating IL-1 receptor antagonist and soluble tumor necrosis factor receptor p55. Blood 83:113–118
90. Gabay C, Smith MF, Eidlen D, Arend WP (1997) Interleukin-1 receptor antagonist is an acute phase protein. J Clin Invest 99:2930–2940
91. Tilg H, Vannier E, Vachino G, Dinarello CA, Mier JW (1993) Antiinflammatory properties of hepatic acute phase proteins: preferential induction of interleukin 1 (IL-1) receptor antagonist over IL-1 beta synthesis by human peripheral blood mononuclear cells. J Exp Med 178:1629–1636
92. Heuertz RM, Piquette CA, Webster RO (1993) Rabbits with elevated serum C-reactive protein exhibit diminished neutrophil infiltration and vascular permeability in C5a-induced alveolitis. Am J Pathol 142:319–328
93. Moore DF, Rosenfeld MR, Gribbon PM, Winlove CP, Tsai CM (1997) Alpha-1 acid glycoprotein (orosomucoid): interaction with bacterial lipopolysaccharide and protection from sepsis. Inflammation 21:69–82
94. Libert C, Vanmolle W, Brouckaert P, Fiers W (1996) Alpha1-antitrypsin inhibits the lethal response to TNF in mice. J Immunol 157:5126–5129
95. Libert C, Brouckaert P, Fiers W (1994) Protection by alpha 1-acid glycoprotein against tumor necrosis factor-induced lethality. J Exp Med 180:1571–1575
96. Mancuso G, Tomasello F, Migliardo M, et al (1994) Beneficial effects of interleukin-6 in neonatal mouse models of group B streptococcal disease. Infect Immun 62:4997–5002
97. Barton BE, Jackson JV (1993) Protective role of interleukin 6 in the lipopolysaccharide-galactosamine septic shock model. Infect Immun 61:1496–1499

98. Yoshizawa KI, Naruto M, Ida N (1996) Injection time of interleukin-6 determines fatal outcome in experimental endotoxin shock. J Interferon Cytokine Res 16:995–1000
99. Borish L, Rosenbaum R, Albury L, Clark S (1989) Activation of neutrophils by recombinant interleukin-6. Cell Immunol 121:280–289
100. Biffl WL, Moore EE, Moore FA, Barnett CC, Silliman CC, Peterson VM (1996) Interleukin-6 stimulates neutrophil production of platelet activating factor. J Leuk Biol 59:569–574
101. Denis M (1992) Interleukin-6 in mouse hypersensitivity pneumonitis: changes in lung free cells following depletion of endogenous IL-6 or direct administration of IL-6. J Leuk Biol 52:197–201
102. Romano M, Sironi M, Toniatti C, et al (1997) Role of IL-6 and its soluble receptor in induction of chemokines and leukocyte recruitment. Immunity 6:315–325
103. Gabay C, Singwe M, Genin B, et al (1996) Circulating levels of IL-11 and leukaemia inhibitory factor (LIF) do not significantly participate in the production of acute-phase proteins by the liver. Clin Exp Immunol 105:260–265
104. Du XX, Doerschuk CM, Orazi A, Williams DA (1994) A bone marrow stromal-derived growth factor, interleukin-11, stimulates recovery of small intestinal mucosal cells after cytoablative therapy. Blood 83:33–37
105. Chang M, Williams A, Ishizawa L, Knoppel A, van de Ven C, Cairo MS (1996) Endogenous interleukin-11 (IL-11) expression is increased and prophylactic use of exogenous IL-11 enhances platelet recovery and improves survival during thrombocytopenia associated with experimental group B streptococcal sepsis in neonatal rats. Blood Cells Mol Dis 22:57–67
106. Khabar KSA, ElBarbary MA, Khouqeer F, Devol E, Al-Gain S, Al-Halees Z (1997) Circulating endotoxin and cytokines after cardiopulmonary bypass: differential correlation with duration of bypass and systemic response/multiple organ dysfunction syndromes. Clin Immunol Immunopathol 85:97–103
107. Grewal HP, Mohey el Din A, Gaber L, Kotb M, Gaber AO (1994) Amelioration of the physiologic and biochemical changes of acute pancreatitis using an anti-TNF polyclonal antibody. Am J Surg 167:214–219
108. Hughes CB, Grewal HP, Gaber LW, et al (1996) Anti-TNF therapy improves survival and ameliorates the pathophysiological sequelae in acute pancreatitis in the rat. Am J Surg 171: 274–280
109. Squadrito F, Altavilla D, Ioculano M, et al (1992) Passive immunization with antibodies against tumor necrosis factor protects from the lethality of splanchnic occlusion shock. Circ Shock 37:236–244
110. Imagawa DK, Millis JM, Seu P, et al (1991) The role of tumor necrosis factor in allograft rejection. III. Evidence that anti-TNF antibody therapy prolongs allograft survival in rats with acute rejection. Transplantation 51:57–62
111. Fraker DJ, Langstein HN, Norton JA (1989) Passive immunization against tumor necrosis factor partially abrogates interleukin-2 toxicity. J Exp Med 170:1015–1020
112. Welbourn R, Goldman G, O'Riordain M, et al (1991) Role of tumor necrosis factor as mediator of lung injury following lower torso ischemia. J Appl Physiol 70:2645–2649
113. Collettti LM, Remick DG, Burtch GD, Kunkel SL, Strieter RM, Campbell DA (1990) Role of tumor necrosis factor in the pathophysiologic alterations after hepatic ischemia/reperfusion injury in the rat. J Clin Invest 85:1936–1943
114. Zingarelli B, Squadrito F, Altavilla D, Calapai G, Di Rosa M, Caputi AP (1994) Role of TNF in acute hypovolemic hemorrhagic shock in rats. Am J Physiol 266:H1512–H1515
115. Bahrami S, Yao YM, Leichtfried G, Redl H, Marzi I, Schlag G (1997) Significance of TNF in hemorrhage-related hemodynamic alteration, organ injury and mortality in rats. Am J Physiol 272:H2219–H2226
116. Jansen MJJM, Hendriks H, Hermsen R, van der Meer JWM, Goris RJA (1998) A monoclonal antibody against tumour necrosis factor improves survival in experimental multiple organ dysfunction syndrome. Cytokine 10:904–910
117. Elliot MJ, Maini RN, Feldmann M, et al (1994) Randomised double-blind comparison of chimeric monoclonal antibody to tumor necrosis factor versus placebo in rheumatoid arthritis. Lancet 344:1105–1110

118. van Dullemen HM, van Deventer SJ, Hommes DW, et al (1995) Treatment of Crohn's disease with anti-TNF chimeric monoclonal antibody (cA2). Gastroenterology 109:129–135
119. Fong Y, Tracey KJ, Moldawer LL, et al (1989) Antibodies to cachectin/tumor necrosis factor reduce IL-1β and IL-6 appearance during lethal bacteremia. J Exp Med 170:1627–1633
120. Norman JG, Franz MG, Fink GS, et al (1995) Decreased mortality of severe acute pancreatitis after proximal cytokine blockade. Ann Surg 221:625–634
121. Pugin J, Ricou B, Steinberg KP, Suter PM, Martin TR (1996) Proinflammatory activity in bronchoalveolar lavage fluids from patients with ARDS, a prominent role for interleukin-1. Am J Respir Crit Care Med 153:1850–1856
122. Cominelli F, Nast CC, Clark BD, et al (1990) IL-1 gene expression, synthesis, and effect of specific IL-1 receptor blockade in rabbit immune complex colitis. J Clin Invest 86:972–980
123. Shanley TP, Peters JL, Jones ML, Chensue SW, Kunkel SL, Ward PA (1996) Regulatory effects of endogenous interleukin-1 receptor antagonist protein in immunoglobulin G immune complex-induced lung injury. J Clin Invest 97:963–970
124. Abraham E, Allbee J (1994) Effects of therapy with IL-1ra on pulmonary cytokine expression following hemorrhage and resuscitation. Lymphokine Cytokine Res 13:343–347
125. Marsh CB, Moore SA, Pope MHA, Wewers MD (1994) IL-1ra supresses endotoxin-induced IL-1 and TNF release from mononuclear phagocytes. Am J Physiol 267:L39–L45
126. Wulczyn FG, Krappmann D, Scheidereit C (1996) The NF-κB/Rel and IκB families: mediators of immune response and inflammation. J Mol Med 74:749–769
127. Baldwin AS, Jr (1996) The NF-κB and IκB proteins: new discoveries and insights. Ann Rev Immunol 14:649–683
128. Ghosh S, May MJ, Kopp EB (1998) NF-κB and Rel proteins: evolutionarily conserved mediators of immune responses. Ann Rev Immunol 16:225–260
129. Schmitz ML, Baeuerle PA (1991) The p65 subunit is responsible for the strong transcription activating potential of NF-κB. EMBO J 10:3805–3817
130. Malinin NL, Boldin MP, Kovalenko AV, Wallach D (1997) MAP3K-related kinase involved in NF-κB induction by TNF, CD95 and IL-1. Nature 385:540–544
131. Hsu H, Xiong J, Goeddel DV (1995) The TNF receptor 1–associated protein TRADD signals cell death and NF-activation. Cell 81:495–504
132. Rothe M, Wong SC, Henzel WJ, Goeddel DV (1994) A novel family of putative signal transducers associated with the cytoplasmic domain of the 75 KDa tumor necrosis factor receptor. Cell 78:681–692
133. Hsu H, Huang J, Shu HB, Baichwal V, Goeddel DV (1996) TNF-dependent recruitment of the protein kinase RIP to the TNF receptor-signaling complex. Immunity 4:387–396
134. Greenfeder SA, Nunes P, Kwee L, Labow M, Chizzonite RA, Ju G (1995) Molecular cloning and characterization of a second subunit of the interleukin-1 receptor complex. J Biol Chem 270:13757–13765
135. Burns K, Martinon F, Esslinger C, et al (1998) MyD88, an adapter protein involved in interleukin-1 signaling. J Biol Chem 273:12203–12209
136. Lee FS, Hagler J, Chen J, Maniatis T (1997) Activation of the IκBα kinase complex by MEKK1, a kinase of the JNK pathway. Cell 88:213–222
137. Hirano M, Osada S-I, Aoki T, et al (1996) MEK kinase is involved in tumor necrosis factor α-induced NF-κB activation and degradation of IκB-α. J Biol Chem 271:13234–13238
138. Liu Z, Hsu H, Goeddel DV, Karin M (1996) Dissection of the TNF receptor 1 effector functions: JNK activation is not linked to apoptosis while NF-κB activation prevents cell death. Cell 87:565–576
139. Di Donato JA, Hayakawa M, Rothwarf DM, Zandi E, Karin M (1997) A cytokine-responsive IκB kinase that activates the transcription factor NF-κB. Nature 388:548–554
140. Zandi E, Rothwarf DM, Delhase M, Hayakawa M, Karin M (1997) The IκB kinase complex (IKK) contains two kinase subunits, IKKα and IKKβ, necessary for IκB phosphorylation and NF-κB activation. Cell 91:243–252
141. Rothwarf DM, Zandi E, Natoli G, Karin M (1998) IKK-γ is an essential regulatory subunit of the IκB kinase complex. Nature 395:297–300
142. Westwick JK, Weitzel C, Minden A, Karin M, Brenner DA (1994) TNF-α stimulates AP-1 activity through prolonged activation of the c-jun kinase. J Biol Chem 269:26396–26401

143. Raingeaud J, Gupta S, Rogers JS, et al (1995) Pro-inflammatory cytokines and environmental stress cause p38 mitogen-activated protein kinase activation by dual phosphorylation on tyrosine and threonine. J Biol Chem 270:7420–7426
144. Wesselborg S, Bauer MKA, Vogt M, Schmitz ML, Schulze-Osthoff K (1997) Activation of transcription factor NF-κB and p38 mitogen-activated protein kinase is mediated by distinct and separate stress effector pathways. J Biol Chem 272:12422–12429
145. Yuasa T, Ohno S, Kehrl JH, Kyriakis JM (1998) TNF signaling to stress-activated protein kinase (SAPK)/Jun NH2-terminal kinase (JNK) and p38. J Biol Chem 273:22681–22692
146. Kanakaraj P, Schafer PH, Cavender DE, et al (1998) IL-1 receptor-associated kinase (IRAK) requirement for optimal induction of multiple IL-1 signaling pathways and IL-6 production. J Exp Med 187:2073–2079
147. Marchant A, Devière J, Byl B, De Groote D, Vincent J, Goldman M (1994) Interleukin-10 production during septicaemia. Lancet 343:707–708
148. Marie C, Cavaillon J-M, Losser M-R (1996) Elevated levels of circulating transforming growth factor-β1 in patients with the sepsis syndrome. Ann Intern Med 125:520–521
149. Ayala A, Lehman DL, Herdon CD, Chaudry IH (1994) Mechanism of enhanced susceptibility to sepsis following hemorrhage. Interleukin-10 suppression of T-cell response is mediated by eicosanoid-induced interleukin-4 release. Arch Surg 129:1172–1178
150. Brandtzaeg P, Osnes L, Øvstebø R, Joø GB, Westwik AB, Kierulf P (1996) Net inflammatory capacity of human septic shock plasma evaluated by a monocyte-based target cell assay: identification of IL-10 as a major functional deactivator of human monocytes. J Exp Med 184:51–60
151. Miller-Graziano CL, Szabo G, Griffey K, Mehta B, Kodys K, Catalano D (1991) Role of elevated monocyte TGFβ production in post-trauma immunosuppression. J Clin Immunol 11:95–102
152. Ayala A, Meldrum DR, Perrin MM, Chaudry IH (1993) The release of transforming growth factor-beta following haemorrhage: its role as a mediator of host immunosuppression. Immunology 79:479–484
153. Ayala A, Knotts JB, Ertel W, Perrin MM, Morrison MH, Chaudry IH (1993) Role of interleukin 6 and transforming growth factor-beta in the induction of depressed splenocyte responses following sepsis. Arch Surg 128:89–94
154. Sheeran P, Hall GM (1997) Cytokines in anaesthesia. Br J Anaesth 78:201–219
155. Bencsics A, Elenkov IJ, Vizi ES (1997) Effect of morphine on lipopolysaccharide-induced tumor necrosis factor-alpha production in vivo: Involvement of the sympathetic nervous system. J Neuroimmunol 73:1–6
156. Hill GE, Pohorecki R, Alonso A, Rennard SI, Robbins RA (1996) Aprotinin reduces interleukin-8 production and lung neutrophil accumulation after cardiopulmonary bypass. Anesth Analg 83:696–700
157. McCall CE, Grosso-Wilmoth LM, LaRue K, Guzman RN, Cousart SL (1993) Tolerance to endotoxin-induced expression of the interleukin-1β gene in blood neutrophils of humans with the sepsis syndrome. J Clin Invest 91:853–861
158. Cavaillon JM (1995) The nonspecific nature of endotoxin tolerance. Trends Microbiol 3: 320–324
159. Helminen M (1991) Interleukin-1 production from peripheral blood monocytes in septic infections in children. Scand J Infect Dis 23:607–611
160. Muñoz C, Carlet J, Fitting C, Misset B, Bleriot JP, Cavaillon JM (1991) Dysregulation of in vitro cytokine production by monocytes during sepsis. J Clin Invest 88:1747–1754
161. Sekatrian JC, Yee J, Christou NV (1994) Reduced tumor necrosis factor-α production in lipopolysaccharide-treated whole blood from patients in the intensive care unit. Arch Surg 129:187–192
162. Van Deuren M, Van Der Ven-Jongekrijg H, Demacker PNM, et al (1994) Differential expression of proinflammatory cytokines and their inhibitors during the course of meningococcal infections. J Infect Dis 169:157–161
163. Marchant A, Alegre M, Hakim A, et al (1995) Clinical and biological significance of interleukin-10 plasma levels in patients with septic shock. J Clin Immunol 15:265–272
164. Randow F, Syrbe U, Meisel C, et al (1995) Mechanism of endotoxin desensitization: involvement of interleukin 10 and transforming growth factor β. J Exp Med 181:1887–1892

165. Ertel W, Keel M, Neidhardt R, et al (1997) Inhibition of the defense system stimulating interleukin-12 interferon-γ pathway during critical illness. Blood 89:1612–1620
166. Luger A, Graf H, Schwarz HP, Stummvoll HK, Luger TA (1986) Decreased serum IL-1 activity and monocyte IL-1 production in patients with fatal sepsis. Crit Care Med 14:458–461
167. Cavaillon J-M, Muñoz C, Marty C, et al (1993) Cytokine production by monocytes from patients with sepsis syndrome and by endotoxin-tolerant monocytes. In: Levin J, Alving CR, Munford RS, Stütz PL (eds) Bacterial endotoxin: recognition and effector mechanisms. Elsevier Sc. Publ., New York, pp 275–284
168. Astiz M, Saha D, Lustbader D, Lin R, Rackow E (1996) Monocyte response to bacterial toxins, expression of cell surface receptors, and release of anti-inflammatory cytokines during sepsis. J Lab Clin Med 128:597–600
169. Cabié A, Fitting C, Farkas J-C, et al (1992) Influence of surgery on in-vitro cytokine production by human monocytes. Cytokine 4:576–580
170. Kleinschmidt S, Wanner GA, Buβmann D, et al (1998) Proinflammatory cytokine gene expression in whole blood from patients undergoing coronary artery bypass surgery and its modulation by pentoxifylline. Shock 9:12–20
171. Faist E, Mewes A, Strasser T, et al (1988) Alteration of monocyte function following major injury. Arch Surg 123:287–292
172. Marie C, Muret J, Fitting C, Losser M-R, Payen D, Cavaillon J-M (1998) Reduced ex vivo interleukin-8 production by neutrophils in septic and non-septic systemic inflammatory response syndrome. Blood 91:3439–3446
173. Wood J, Rodrick M, O'Mahony J, et al (1984) Inadequate interleukin 2 production. A fundamental immunological deficiency in patients with major burns. Ann Surg 200:311–320
174. Rodrick MM, Wood JJ, O'Mahony JB, et al (1986) Mechanisms of immunosupression associated with severe nonthermal traumatic injuries in man: production of interleukin-1 and 2. J Clin Immunol 6:310–318
175. Grzelak I, Olszewski WL, Rowinski W (1989) Blood mononuclear cell production of IL-1 and IL-2 following moderate surgical trauma. Eur Surg Res 21:114–122
176. Hisatomi K, Isomura T, Kawara T, et al (1989) Changes in lymphocyte subsets, mitogen responsiveness, and interleukin-2 production after cardiac operations. J Thorac Cardiovasc Surg 98:580–591
177. Abraham E, Chang YH (1992) Haemorrhage-induced alteration in function and cytokine production of T cells and T cell subpopulations. Clin Exp Immunol 90:497–502
178. Hershman MJ, Cheadle WG, Wellhausen SR, Davidon P, Polk HC (1990) Monocyte HLA-DR antigen expression characterizes clinical outcome in the trauma patient. Br J Surg 77: 204–207
179. Ertel W, Keel M, Steckholzer U, Ungethüm U, Trentz O (1996) IL-10 attenuates the release of pro-inflammatory cytokines but depresses splenocyte function in murine endotoxemia. Arch Surg 131:51–56
180. Meldrum DR, Ayala A, Perrin MM, Ertel W, Chaudry IH (1991) Diltiazem restores IL-2, IL-3, IL-6 and IFN-gamma synthesis and decreases host suceptibility to sepsis following hemorrhage. J Surg Res 51:158–164
181. Ayala A, Deol ZK, Lehman DL, Herdon CD, Chaudry IH (1994) Polymicrobial sepsis but not low-dose endotoxin infusion causes decreased splenocyte IL-2/IFN-gamma release while increasing IL-4/IL-10 production. J Surg Res 56:579–585
182. Mack VE, McCarter MD, Naama HA, Calvano SE, Daly JM (1996) Dominance of T-helper 2-type cytokine after severe injury. Arch Surg 131:1303–1309
183. O'Sullivan ST, Lederer JA, Horgan AF, Chin DHL, Mannick JA, Rodrick ML (1995) Major injury leads to predominance of the T helper-2 lymphocyte phenotype and diminished interleukin-12 production associated with decreased resistance to infection. Ann Surg 222: 482–492
184. Naldini A, Borrelli E, Cesari S, Giomarelli P, Toscano M (1995) In vitro cytokine production and T-cell proliferation in patients undergoing cardiopulmonary by-pass. Cytokine 7: 165–170
185. Miller-Graziano CL, De AK, Kodys K (1995) Altered IL-10 levels in trauma patients monocytes and T lymphocytes. J Clin Immunol 15:93–104

186. Napolitano L, Campbell C (1995) Polymicrobial sepsis following trauma inhibits interleukin-10 secretion and lymphocyte proliferation. J Trauma 39: 104–111
187. Ertel W, Morrison MH, Ayala A, Dean R, Chaudry IH (1992) Interferon-γ attenuates hemorrhage-induced suppression of macrophage and splenocyte functions and decreases susceptibility to sepsis. Surgery 111: 177–187
188. Dries DJ, Jurkovich GJ, Maier RV, et al (1994) Effect of interferon-gamma on infection-related death in patients with severe injuries. A randomized, double-blind, placebo-controlled trial. Arch Surg 129: 1031–1041
189. Döcke WD, Randow F, Syrbe U, et al (1997) Monocyte deactivation in septic patients: restoration by IFNγ treatment. Nature Med 3: 678–681
190. Mendez M, Molloy R, O'Rioirdain D, et al (1993) Lymphokine activated killer cells enhance IL-2 prevention of sepsis-related death in a murine model of thermal injury. J Surg Res 54: 565–570
191. Bundschuh DS, Barsig J, Hartung T, et al (1997) Granulocyte-macrophage colony-stimulating factor and IFN-gamma restore the systemic TNF-alpha response to endotoxin in lipopolysaccharide-desensitized mice. J Immunol 158: 2862–2871
192. Randow F, Docke WD, Bundschuh DS, Hartung T, Wendel A, Volk HD (1997) In vitro prevention and reversal of lipopolysaccharide desensitization by IFN-gamma, IL-12, and granulocyte-macrophage colony-stimulating factor. J Immunol 158: 2911–2918
193. Inoue T, Saito H, Fukushima R, et al (1995) Growth hormone and insulin like growth factor I enhance host defense in a murine sepsis model. Arch Surg 130: 1115–1122
194. Zellweger R, Zhu XH, Wichmann MW, Ayala A, DeMaso CM, Chaudry IH (1996) Prolactin administration following hemorrhagic shock improves macrophage cytokine release capacity and decreases mortality from subsequent sepsis. J Immunol 157: 5748–5754
195. Pociot F, Briant L, Jongeneel CV, et al (1993) Association of tumor necrosis factor (TNF) and class II major histocompatibility complex alleles with the secretion of TNFα and TNFβ by human mononuclear cells: a possible link to insulin-dependent diabetes mellitus. Eur J Immunol 23: 224–231
196. Danis VA, Millington M, Hyland VJ, Grennan D (1995) Cytokine production by normal human monocytes: inter-subject variation and relationship to an IL-1 receptor antagonist (IL-1Ra) gene polymorphism. Clin Exp Immunol 99: 303–310
197. Turner DM, Williams DM, Sankaran D, Lazarus M, Sinnott PJ, Hutchinson IV (1997) An investigation of polymorphism in the interleukin-10 gene promoter. Eur J Immunogenet 24: 1–8
198. Walley AJ, Cookson W (1996) Investigation of an interleukin-4 promoter polymorphism for associations with asthma and atopy. J Med Genet 33: 689–692
199. Bender JR, Sadeghi MM, Watson C, Pfau S, Pardi R (1994) Heterogeneous activation thresholds to cytokines in genetically distinct endothelial cells: evidence for diverse transcriptional responses. Proc Natl Acad Sci USA 91: 3994–3998
200. Liu J, Marino MW, Wong G, et al (1998) TNF is a potent anti-inflammatory cytokine in auto-immune-mediated demyelination. Nature Med 4: 78–83
201. Erwig L-P, Kluth DC, Walsh GM, Rees AJ (1998) Initial cytokine exposure determines function of macrophages and renders them unresponsive to other cytokines. J Immunol 161: 1983–1988
202. Hodge-Dufour J, Marino MW, Horton ME, et al (1998) Inhibition of interferon-γ induced interleukin-12 production: a potential mechanism for the anti-inflammatory activities of tumor necrosis factor. Proc Natl Acad Sci USA 95: 13 806–13 811
203. Kasama T, Yamazaki J, Hanaoka R, et al (1999) Biphasic regulation of the development of murine type II collagen-induced arthritis by interleukin-12: Possible involvement of endogenous interleukin-10 and tumor necrosis factor alpha. Arthritis Rheum 42: 100–109
204. Sherry B, Espinoza M, Manogue KR, Cerami A (1998) Induction of the chemokine β peptides, MIP-1α and MIP-1β by lipopolysaccharide is differentially regulated by immunomodulatory cytokines γ-IFN, IL-10, IL-4 and TGFβ. Mol Med 4: 654–657
205. Schleimer RP, Sterbinsky SA, Kaiser J, et al (1992) IL-4 induces adherence of human eosinophils and basophils but not neutrophils to endothelium. Association with expression of VCAM-1. J Immunol 148: 1086–1092

206. De Beaux AC, Maingay JP, Ross JA, Fearon KC, Carter DC (1995) Interleukin-4 and interleukin-10 increase endotoxin-stimulated human umbilical vein endothelial cell interleukin-8 release. J Interferon Cytokine Res 15:441–445
207. Goebeler M, Schnarr B, Toksoy A, et al (1997) Interleukin-13 selectively induces monocyte chemoattractant protein-1 synthesis and secretion by human endothelial cells. Involvement of IL-1Rα and Stat-6 phosphorylation. Immunology 91:450–457
208. Kambayashi T, Jacob CO, Strassmann G (1996) IL-4 and IL-13 modulate IL-10 release in endotoxin-stimulated murine peritoneal mononuclear phagocytes. Cell Immunol 171:153–158
209. D'Andrea A, Ma X, Aste-Amezaga M, Paganin C, Trinchieri G (1995) Stimulatory and inhibitory effects of interleukin (IL)-4 and IL-13 on the production of cytokines by human peripheral blood mononuclear cells: priming for IL-12 and tumor necrosis factor alpha production. J Exp Med 181:537–546
210. Minty A, Ferrara P, Caput D (1997) Interleukin-13 effects on activated monocytes lead to novel cytokine secretion profiles intermediate between those induced by interleukin-10 and by γ-interferon. Eur Cytokine Netw 8:189–201
211. Hart PH, Jones CA, Finlay-Jones JJ (1995) Monocytes cultured in cytokine-defined environments differ from freshly isolated monocytes in their responses to IL-4 and IL-10. J Leukoc Biol 57:909–918
212. Marfaing-Koka A, Maravic M, Humbert M, Galanaud P, Emilie D (1996) Contrasting effects of IL-4, IL-10 and corticosteroids on RANTES production by human monocytes. Int Immunol 8:1587–1594
213. Marie C, Fitting C, Muret J, Payen D, Cavaillon J-M (1999) Interleukin-8 production in whole blood assays: is interleukin-10 responsible for the downregulation observed in sepsis? Cytokine (in press)
214. Kumar NM, Rabadi NH, Sigurdson LS, Schunemann HJ, Lwebuga-Mukasa JS (1996) Induction of interleukin-1 and interleukin-8 mRNAs and proteins by TGF beta(1) in rat lung alveolar epithelial cells. J Cell Physiol 169:186–199
215. Qian SG, Li W, Li YP, et al (1996) Systemic administration of cellular interleukin-10 can exacerbate cardiac allograft rejection in mice. Transplantation 62:1709–1714
216. Rosenbaum JT, Angell E (1995) Paradoxical effects of IL-10 in endotoxin-induced uveitis. J Immunol 155:4090–4094
217. Moritani M, Yoshimoto K, Tashiro F, et al (1994) Transgenic expression of IL-10 in pancreatic islet A cells accelerates autoimmune insulitis and diabetes in non-obese diabetic mice. Intern Immunol 6:1927–1936
218. Berman RM, Suzuki T, Tahara H, Robbins PD, Narula SK, Lotze MT (1996) Systemic administration of cellular IL-10 induces an effective specific and long-lived immune response against established tumor in mice. J Immunol 157:231–238
219. Di Carlo E, Coletti A, Modesti A, Giovarelli M, Forni G, Musiani P (1998) Local release of interleukin-10 by transfected mouse adenocarcinoma cells exhibits pro- and anti-inflammatory activity and results in a delayed tumor rejection. Eur Cytokine Netw 9:61–68
220. Vora M, Romero LI, Karasek MA (1996) Interleukin-10 induces E-selectin on small and large blood vessel endothelial cells. J Exp Med 184:821–829
221. Buelens C, De Groote D, Goldman M, Willems F (1996) Differential effects of interleukin-10 on the production of interleukin-12 and interleukin-8 by human dendritic cells generated from peripheral blood. Transplant Proc 28:3255–3256
222. Pang G, Ortega M, Zighang R, Reeves G, Clancy R (1997) Autocrine modulation of IL-8 production by sputum neutrophils in chronic bronchial sepsis. Am J Respir Crit Care Med 155:726–731
223. Becherel PA, Le Goff L, Ktorza S, et al (1995) Interleukin-10 inhibits IgE-mediated nitric oxide synthase induction and cytokine synthesis in normal human keratinocytes. Eur J Immunol 25:2992–2995
224. Cunha FQ, Moncada S, Liew FY (1992) Interleukin-10 inhibits the induction of nitric oxide synthase by interferon-gamma in murine macrophages. Biochem Biophys Res Commun 182:1155–1159
225. Fouqueray B, Boutard V, Philippe C, et al (1995) Mesangial cell-derived interleukin-10 modulates mesangial cell response to lipopolysaccharide. Am J Pathol 147:176–182

226. Betz-Corradin SB, Fasel N, Buchmuller-Rouiller Y, Ransijn A, Smith J, Mauel J (1993) Induction of macrophage nitric oxide production by interferon-gamma and tumor necrosis factor-alpha is enhanced by interleukin-10. Eur J Immunol 23:2045–2048
227. Sunyer T, Rothe L, Jiang X, Osdoby P, Collin-Osdoby P (1996) Proinflammatory agents, IL-8 and IL-10, upregulate inducible nitric oxide synthase expression and nitric oxide production in avian osteoclast-like cells. J Cell Biochem 60:469–483
228. Groux H, Bigler M, de Vries JE, Roncarolo MG (1998) Inhibitory and stimulatory effects of IL-10 on human CD8+ T cells. J Immunol 160:3188–3193
229. Marie C, Pitton C, Fitting C, Cavaillon J-M (1996) Regulation by anti-inflammatory cytokines (IL-4, IL-10, IL-13, TGFβ) of interleukin-8 production by LPS- and/or TNFα-activated human polymorphonuclear cells. Mediators Inflamm 5:334–340
230. Adib-Conquy M, Petit A-F, Marie C, Fitting C, Cavaillon J-M (1999) Paradoxical priming effects of interleukin-10 on cytokine production. Int Immunol 11:689–698
231. Lelievre E, Sarrhouilhe D, Morel F, Preud'homme JL, Wijdenes J, Lecron JC (1998) Preincubation of human resting T cell clones with interleukin-10 strongly enhances their ability to produce cytokine after stimulation. Cytokine 10:831–840
232. Rabbi MF, Finnegan A, Al-Harthi L, Song S, Roebuck KA (1998) Interleukin-10 enhances tumor necrosis factor-activation of HIV-1 transcription in latently infected T cells. J AIDS Hum Retrovirol 19:321–331
233. Arock M, Zuany-Amorim C, Singer M, Benhamou M, Pretolani M (1996) Interleukin-10 inhibits cytokine generation from mast cells. Eur J Immunol 26:166–170
234. Moon TC, Murakami M, Ashraf M, Kudo I, Chang HW (1998) Regulation of cyclooxygenase-2 and endogenous cytokine expression by bacterial lipopolysaccharide that acts in synergy with c-kit ligand and Fce receptor I crosslinking in cultured mast cells. Cell Immunol 185:146–152
235. Ishimi Y, Miyaura C, Jin CH, et al (1990) IL-6 is produced by osteoblasts and induces bone resorption. J Immunol 145:3297–3303
236. Tsujinaka T, Fujita J, Ebisui C, et al (1996) Interleukin-6 receptor antibody inhibits muscle atrophy and modulates proteolytic systems in interleukin-6 transgenic mice. J Clin Invest 97:244–249
237. Jongen-Lavrencic M, Peeters HRM, Rozemuller H, et al (1996) IL-6 induced anaemia in rats: possible pathogenic implications for anaemia observed in chronic inflammations. Clin Exp Immunol 103:328–334
238. Barber AE, Coyle SM, Marano MA, et al (1993) Glucocorticoid therapy alters hormonal and cytokine responses to endotoxin in man. J Immunol 150:1999–2006

Inhibitory Cytokines

T. Calandra and D. Heumann

Introduction

Over the last 15 years our understanding of the pathophysiology of inflammation and sepsis has progressed considerably [1]. Microbial constituents, such as the lipopolysaccharide (LPS, endotoxin) of Gram-negative bacteria and the exotoxins or cell-wall fragments of Gram-positive bacteria, have been shown to be potent activators of a wide range of cells, including monocytes/macrophages, neutrophils and endothelial cells. On stimulation, these cells release mediators that play a critical role in the host response to invasion by microorganisms, and serve to orchestrate the cellular and humoral components contributing to the development of inflammatory and immune reactions. Inflammation is an essential feature of host defenses and should thus be kept in check. Indeed, severe sepsis and septic shock are manifestations of an overwhelming, dysregulated inflammatory host response characterized by a massive activation of several systems leading to multiple organ dysfunction and death in a high proportion of cases.

A large body of evidence derived from studies performed in animals and in humans supports the concept that sepsis is caused by an uncontrolled pro-inflammatory response. Systemic injection of bacterial toxins such as LPS, toxic shock syndrome toxin-1 (TSST-1) or streptococcal pyrogenic exotoxin A (SPEA), or of bacteria, or the presence of a bacterial infection, stimulates the production of pro-inflammatory mediators, including the cytokines tumor necrosis factor (TNF)-α and interleukin (IL)-1 [2]. Neutralization of these cytokines has been associated with protection from death in selected animal models. During the last decade, over twenty Phase II and Phase III clinical trials of non glucocorticoid anti-inflammatory agents have been conducted. Studies of adjunctive therapies with monoclonal antibodies against TNF, soluble TNF receptors, antagonists of the IL-1 receptor, bradykinin, and platelet-activating factor (PAF), and prostaglandins, have so far yielded disappointing results [3]. While there are many possible explanations for these negative results, including the lack of activity of the agents used, inappropriate trial design or timing of intervention, or the fact that targeting one single molecule may not be sufficient, some investigators have questioned the 'pro-inflammatory only' theory.

During the course of sepsis patients also develop an anti-inflammatory response, sometimes designated as the compensatory anti-inflammatory response syndrome (CARS). Several studies have shown that monocytes of septic patients become hyporesponsive in the post-acute phase of septic shock [4–6]. These observations lend support to the concept that this anti-inflammatory response may deactivate the monocytes and lead to a state of 'immunoparalysis'. However, it is unclear whether the hyporesponsiveness of monocytes and macrophages is the result of an active process of down-regulation or simply reflects a state of post-battle cellular exhaustion of these professional 'warriors'. In this chapter we will review our current knowledge about cytokines with anti-inflammatory properties that are likely to be involved in the pathophysiology of severe infections. We also will discuss the mechanisms by which they may contribute to limit the magnitude of the septic shock syndrome.

Biological Characteristics of Anti-Inflammatory Mediators

Cytokines are often classified into two main categories depending upon whether they exert pro-inflammatory or anti-inflammatory activities. Yet, the pro-inflammatory versus anti-inflammatory dichotomy is an oversimplification, as several cytokines may exert both pro-inflammatory and anti-inflammatory effects depending on the target cells. Cytokines and soluble cytokine receptors with anti-inflammatory properties are listed in Table 1. All these molecules inhibit the production of the pro-inflammatory cytokines TNF and IL-1 and as such are considered to be anti-inflammatory mediators.

In 1986, Mosmann and collaborators first reported that clones of murine helper T (Th) cells could be divided into two subsets based on the type of cytokines that they produced. Th1 clones produced interferon (IFN)-γ, IL-2 and other cytokines, but not IL-4, IL-5 and IL-10, whereas Th2 clones produced IL-4, IL-5, IL-10 and other cytokines, but not IFN-γ and IL-2 [7]. Th1 cells play a central role in cell-mediated immunity (delayed-type hypersensitivity reactions and activation

Table 1. Cytokines and soluble cytokine receptors with anti-inflammatory properties

Cytokines	**Activity**
IL-10	Suppression of lymphocyte and monocyte/macrophage functions
IL-4	Reduction of LPS-induced cytokine synthesis by monocytes and macrophages
IL-13	Down-regulation of monocyte and macrophage functions
IL-6	Inhibition of TNF and IL-1 production
TGF-β	Deactivation of monocytes and macrophages (decreased expression of MHC class II, inhibition of TNF and IL-1 synthesis)
IL-1ra	Inhibition of IL-1-mediated cell activation by blocking IL-1 binding to its receptor
Soluble receptors	
TNFR p55, p75	Binding of TNF and prevention of ligand-receptor interaction
IL-6R	Prolongation of the half-life of IL-6

of macrophages), whereas Th2 cells are critical for the development of humoral immunity (antibody production and IgE-mediated immune responses). Each subset also exerts inhibitory functions on its counterpart. IFN-γ released by Th1 cells and IL-12 produced by phagocytic cells inhibit the growth of antigen-stimulated Th2 cells and the production of IL-4 by these cells, while IL-4 and IL-10 released by Th2 cells inhibit cellular responses and cytokine production by Th1 cells. Since this landmark observation, it has become apparent that Th1 and Th2 clones represent two extremes and that most T-cell clones express mixed cytokine patterns [8]. It is likely that sepsis triggers the activation and proliferation of both Th1 and Th2 cells, but the mechanisms by which the expansion of Th1 and Th2 clones is regulated during sepsis and septic shock is essentially unknown.

Interleukin-10 (IL-10) (Table 2)

IL-10 was originally identified as a product of murine Th2 clones that inhibited the production of Th1 cytokines, including IL-2 and IFN-γ [7], hence its initial designation as cytokine synthesis inhibition factor (CSIF). IL-10 is also produced by monocytes/macrophages and B-cells. IL-10 exhibits profound immunosuppressive properties, but also some immunostimulatory effects on B-cells, as it upregulates major histocompatibility complex (MHC) class II expression and augments the proliferation and differentiation of activated B cells [9]. IL-10 is a potent anti-inflammatory molecule that suppresses cell-mediated immune responses and inhibits macrophage-dependent T-cell proliferation and cytokine production by activated macrophages, neutrophils, Th1 and natural killer (NK) cells. IL-10 inhibits most of the cytokines involved in inflammatory and immune responses, including TNF-α, IL-1, IL-6, IL-8, IL-12, granulocyte/macrophage-colony stimulating factor (GM-CSF), granulocyte-colony stimulating factor

Table 2. Effects of IL-10 in various mouse models of shock or infection

Model	Effect	References
LPS (endotoxemia)	Beneficial	[63–66]
Staphylococcal enterotoxin B	Beneficial	[67]
Staphylococcal enterotoxin B	Beneficial	[67]
Group B streptococci (s.c.)	Beneficial	[68]
Pseudomonas aeruginosa (pneumonia)	Beneficial	[69]
Cecal ligation and puncture (CLP)	Beneficial	[74]
Klebsiella pneumoniae (pneumonia)	Harmful	[70]
Streptococcus pneumoniae (pneumonia)	Harmful	[71]
Listeria monocytogenes (i.v.)	Harmful	[72]
Candida albicans (i.v.)	Harmful	[73]
Cecal ligation and puncture (CLP)	No effect	[74]

Studies were performed in mice given either anti-IL-10 antibodies or exogenous recombinant IL-10 or in IL-10-deficient mice.

(G-CSF), macrophage inflammatory protein (MIP)-1α, MIP-1β, IL-2, IL-3 and IFN-γ, and is therefore the prototype of an anti-inflammatory molecule. The precise mechanism of the inhibitory effects of IL-10 is still unclear. Both transcriptional and post-transcriptional mechanisms have been proposed to explain the mode of action of IL-10 [10-12]. On the one hand, IL-10 has been shown to inhibit nuclear localization of nuclear factor-kappa B (NF-κB) in monocytes stimulated by LPS or TNF [13]. On the other hand, IL-10 was found to promote degradation of TNF, IL-1α and IL-1β mRNA [14]. In addition, IL-10 down-regulates surface expression of TNF receptors and up-regulates shedding of p75 and p55 soluble TNF receptors [15, 16].

Targeted disruption of the IL-10 gene confirms the anti-inflammatory properties of IL-10. IL-10-deficient mice suffer from chronic enterocolitis characterized by mucosal hyperplasia, inflammatory reactions and aberrant expression of MHC class II molecules on epithelia [17]. Studies performed with IL-10 knockout mice reveal the presence of high levels of TNF-α in colonic sections and of IFN-γ in supernatants of explanted intestinal tissue. No spontaneous cytokine production is observed in other tissues, but post-stimulation tissue expression of pro-inflammatory cytokines is up-regulated in IL-10 deficient mice compared to wild-type animals [18].

Interleukin-4 (IL-4)

IL-4 is an18 kDa cytokine produced by activated T cells of the Th2 subset, by $CD4^+$ $NK1.1^+$ T cells, and by mast cells and basophils. The IL-4 gene is located on the human chromosome 5 and on mouse chromosome 11, mapping to regions also containing the IL-3, IL-5, IL-13 and GM-CSF genes. The mature proteins are made of 129 and 120 amino acids, respectively. Like most cytokines, IL-4 acts on a variety of cells expressing the high-affinity IL-4 type I receptor (IL-4Rα). The IL-4Rα is a heterodimer consisting of a 140 kDa IL-4 specific ligand binding chain (α chain) and the signaling chain (γ chain), also called the common γ chain (γ_c), that is shared with several other cytokines such as IL-2 and IL-7 [19]. A number of non T cells express an alternate form of the IL-4R, the type II receptor, consisting of the IL-4Rα and IL-13Rα and thus can also transduce the IL-4 signal. IL-4 was originally discovered as a B-cell growth factor. Subsequent studies showed that IL-4 is essential for immunoglobulin class switch, augmenting the production and release of IgG1 and IgE. It also induces the expression of cell surface molecules on B cells, such as the class II MHC molecules and the low affinity Fcε receptor II (FcεRII or CD23). IL-4 is critical in the development of the Th2 subtype of $CD4^+$ T helper cell and also can affect the development of $CD8^+$ effector cells. Moreover, IL-4 plays an important role in hematopoiesis, stimulating precursor cells, and in allergic responses, and exerts stimulatory effects on cells that contribute to inflammation, including macrophages, endothelial cells, stromal cells and fibroblasts (for a review see [20]). Therefore, in many ways IL-4 is an essential component of late-phase inflammatory reactions.

Like IL-10, IL-4 exhibits anti-inflammatory properties. IL-4 suppresses the production of several pro-inflammatory molecules, including the monocyte/macrophage cytokine TNF-α, and IL-1 and metalloproteinases [21-24]. Yet, in contrast to IL-10, IL-4 suppresses the release of p75 TNF receptors [16].

Interleukin-13 (IL-13)

IL-13 is a recently described IL-4-like cytokine produced mainly by activated T cells ($CD4^+$ and $CD8^+$ cells) that acts on B cells and on monocytes, but not on T cells [25]. Primarily expressed by Th2 cells, human IL-13 is also released by Th1 and Th0 clones. The IL-13 gene maps to a cytokine gene cluster on human chromosome 5 and mouse chromosome 11, suggesting that these cytokines (IL-3, IL-4, IL-5, GM-CSF) may have evolved by gene duplication events. IL-13 shares many biological activities with IL-4, but the IL-13 mediated effects are more restricted and IL-13 is generally less potent than IL-4. This is partly due to the fact that IL-4 and IL-13 interact and compete for the high-affinity IL-4Rα. The structure of the IL-13 receptor is complex. IL-13, but not IL-4, clearly binds to the IL-13Rα1 and IL-13Rα2 chains. Different combinations of the α-chains (IL-13Rα1, IL-13Rα2), the IL-4Rα and the IL-2Rγ_c chains have been detected on various cells [26]. However, the exact composition of the receptor complexes engaging each individual cytokine has not been completely elucidated. IL-13 exerts growth promoting effects on B cells and induces immunoglobulin class switching (IgG4 and IgE). Like IL-4, IL-13 enhances B cell expression of MHC class II, the low affinity Fcε receptor II (FcεRII or CD23), soluble IgM and of CD71 and CD72. IL-13 directly stimulates IFN-γ production by NK cells, but also exerts synergistic effects with IL-4. In contrast to IL-4, human IL-13 does not activate human T cells. It does not inhibit T cell proliferation induced by IL-4.

IL-13 is a very potent modulator of monocyte/macrophage functions, affecting cell morphology, expression of surface molecules, and production of cytokines. Interestingly, IL-13 exhibits dual effects on monocytes, both stimulatory and inhibitory. IL-13 has been found to up-regulate the expression of several integrins (CD11b, CD11c, CD18, CD29 and CD29) and of MHC class II, CD13 and CD23, on the one hand, but also to down-regulate the expression of CD14, CD64 (FcγRI), CD32(FcγRII) and CD16(FcγRIII) on the other hand. Like IL-10 and IL-4, IL-13 inhibits the production of pro-inflammatory cytokines (TNF-α, IL-1α, IL-1β, IL-6, IL-10), chemokines (IL-8 and MIP-1α) and hematopoietic growth factors (G-CSF and GM-CSF) by LPS-stimulated monocytes and macrophages. Of note, IL-4 and IL-13 inhibitory activities occur even in the presence of anti-IL-10 antibodies, indicating that their effects are not mediated by IL-10.

Both transcriptional and post-transcriptional regulatory mechanisms account for the inhibitory effects of IL-13. IL-4 and IL-13 have little effect on TNF mRNA accumulation but inhibit mRNA translational activation in LPS-induced mouse macrophages [27]. IL-13, like IL-10, suppresses TNF-induced activation of NF-κB [28]. The precise mechanism of inhibition provided by IL-4 and IL-13 is still not defined, but evidence suggests the involvement of a repressive transcription factor (STAT6) that antagonizes NF-κB activity [29, 30]. Interestingly, IL-13 potentiates the production of IL-6 following LPS exposure in mice, while inhibiting that of TNF at the same time [31].

Transforming Growth Factors-Beta (TGF-β)

The TGF-β family of cytokines is composed of five isoforms, of which three, TGF-β1, TGF-β2 and TGF-β3, are expressed in mammals. Macrophages, T and B lymphocytes, endothelial cells, platelets, fibroblasts, astrocytes, osteoblasts and osteoclasts are important cellular sources of TGF-β. In contrast to most cytokines, TGF-β is expressed constitutively by many cells and tissues and is up-regulated upon stimulation. TGF-β regulates the growth and differentiation of several cell types (TGF-β2 and TGF-β3) and plays an important role in inflammation, immune responses and tissue repair (TGF-β1) [32]. For an extensive review of the molecular biology of the TGF-βs genes, the biochemical characteristics and biological activities of the various isoforms of TGF-β proteins, and of the TGF-β receptors and signaling pathways, the reader should refer to a recent chapter on this subject [33].

TGF-β has been shown to exhibit both pro-inflammatory and immunosuppressive activities, promoting inflammatory and immune responses at the tissue level, while acting as a suppressor of the immune system at the systemic level. TGF-β released in response to tissue injury and inflammation stimulates chemotaxis of leukocytes (neutrophils, monocytes, lymphocytes), mast cells and fibroblasts and induces the production of pro-inflammatory mediators (TNF-α, IL-1 and IL-6). TGF-β was one of the first cytokines reported to deactivate monocytes and macrophages, and evidence supporting this function was clearly established by targeted disruption of the TGF-β1 gene. Indeed, TGF-β1-deficient mice develop multiple foci of inflammation, characterized by extensive leukocyte infiltration, and overexpress molecules such as MHC class I and II and the cytokines TNF-α, MIP-1α and IFN-γ, causing the death of the animals [34]. TGF-β suppresses the proliferation and differentiation of T cells and B cells and inhibits the synthesis of cytokines (IL-2, IFN-γ, IL-3, GM-CSF, TNF-α) induced by mitogens. Deactivation of macrophages by TGF-β results in the inhibition of TNF-α and IL-1 production and in a reduced expression of MHC class II. TGF-β1 and IL-10 use different mechanisms to inhibit TNF and IL-1 synthesis by LPS-stimulated macrophages. They do not suppress transcription of the TNF and IL-1 genes, but act at a post-transcriptional level. IL-10 degrades preformed mRNA, whereas TGF-β1 interferes with protein translation [14]. IL-10 is 25-fold more potent than TGF-β1 in inhibiting TNF. Moreover, IL-1 production is blocked by IL-10, but not by TGF-β1 [14]. Like IL-10, IL-4 and IL-13, TGF-β up-regulates IL-1ra production by LPS-stimulated monocytes and down-regulates the expression of the IL-1 receptor type 1 [35–38].

IL-1 Receptor Antagonist (IL-1ra)

IL-1ra is the third member of the IL-1 gene family. IL-1α and IL-1β are agonists, whereas IL-1ra is a naturally occurring, specific receptor antagonist. IL-1ra exists in different forms: Soluble IL-1ra, intracellular IL-1raI, and intracellular IL-1raII, that are either soluble or cytoplasmic, constitutive or inducible [2]. Like IL-1β, IL-1ra is induced by viruses, bacteria, yeasts, soluble microbial products and the pro-inflammatory cytokines IL-1 and TNF. The production of IL-1ra is up-regulated by IL-4, IL-10, IL-13 and TGF-β [35-38]. IL-1ra competes with IL-1 for binding to IL-1 receptors, resulting in a strong inhibition of IL-1-mediated cell stimulation. The formation of a heterodimer consisting of IL-1 receptor 1 and IL-1 accessory protein (IL-1R-AcP) is believed to play a key role in cell activation by IL-1. It is postulated that IL-1ra binds to the IL-1 type I receptor, but cannot bind to IL-1R-AcP, providing the basis for the inhibitory effect of IL-1ra [2]. IL-1ra does not trigger a signal and thus is devoid of any agonist activity, even when injected intravenously into humans at concentrations 10^6-fold greater than those of IL-1α or IL-1β. It is beyond the scope of this chapter to review all the existing data on the biological activities of IL-1ra in healthy volunteers and in models of inflammation, infection, autoimmune and malignant diseases. The reader should refer to an excellent review article published recently by Dinarello [39] and to the chapter written by the same author in this book. IL-1ra has been given to a large number of patients with septic shock and rheumatoid arthritis, and to patients with steroid resistant graft versus host disease and with acute or chronic myelogenous leukemia. Unfortunately, two large Phase III clinical trials of IL-1ra conducted in patients with septic shock have not confirmed the dose-dependent reduction of mortality that was observed in the initial open-label, 99-patient Phase II study. By contrast, the results obtained with IL-1ra in patients with rheumatoid arthritis look promising [39].

Interleukin-6 (IL-6)

IL-6 has long been viewed as a pro-inflammatory cytokine. This assumption was derived primarily from the observation that IL-6 was secreted in copious amounts together with TNF-α and IL-1 after LPS challenge or during acute infections and that these three cytokines were involved in the initiation of the acute phase response [40]. IL-6 was reported to play a detrimental role in endotoxemia based on the results obtained with neutralizing anti-IL-6 antibodies [41], but this paper was subsequently retracted [42]. Recent experiments have demonstrated that sub-neutralizing amounts of anti-IL-6 antibodies increase, rather than decrease, the half-life of IL-6. IL-6 inhibits the synthesis of LPS-induced IL-1 and TNF production and IL-6 is the major inducer of the acute phase response with anti-inflammatory potential [40]. Experiments performed in IL-6-deficient mice, or in mice treated either with anti-IL-6 antibodies or with recombinant IL-6, have shown that IL-6 is required to cure infections caused by *Escherichia coli, Streptococcus pneumoniae, Listeria monocytogenes* or *Mycobacterium tuberculosis* and

Table 3. Effects of IL-6 in various mouse models of shock or infection

Model	Effect	References
TNF-induced shock	No effect	[75]
Endotoxemia	No effect	[76]
Endotoxemia	Beneficial	[76]
S. aureus enterotoxin B-induced shock	Beneficial	[77]
Escherichia coli (i.p.)	Beneficial	[76]
Streptococcus pneumoniae (pneumonia)	Beneficial	[78]
Listeria monocytogenes (i.v.)	Beneficial	[79]
Ischemia/reperfusion injury	Beneficial	[80]
Mycobacterium tuberculosis (i.v.)	Beneficial	[81]

Studies were performed in IL-6-deficient mice or in mice given either anti-IL-6 antibodies or exogenous recombinant IL-6.

to reduce the mortality of *S. aureus* enterotoxin B-induced shock, but does not seem to play a critical role in shock induced by LPS or TNF (Table 3). Thus, IL-6 should perhaps be regarded as an anti-inflammatory, rather than a pro-inflammatory molecule.

Soluble Receptors

TNF is an important component of the cytokine network that is activated during sepsis. The biological activity of TNF is effected through two TNF receptors present on target cells, the TNFR1 (or TNFR-p55) and the TNFR2 (or TNFR-p75). These receptors are shed from the membrane upon cell activation and circulate as soluble molecules. The soluble TNFR-p55 and TNFR-p75 are naturally occurring inhibitors of TNF activity that serve two functions [43, 44]. First, the shedding of the TNF receptors in response to inflammatory stimuli results in a transient desensitization of the cell, thereby providing a mechanism for inhibition of TNF activity. Second, soluble TNF receptors also bind TNF and may thus inhibit TNF bioactivity by preventing its binding to the membrane-bound receptor. Conversely, these soluble receptors may exert a detrimental effect, especially at low concentrations, by prolonging TNF activity, allowing the complex to dissociate later in the course of the disease [45]. This is known to occur with the soluble p75 TNF receptor [46–48]. Our current understanding of the *in vivo* interactions between TNF and the soluble TNF receptors is far from complete. In addition to inhibiting the effects of their ligands, soluble receptors can also facilitate ligand-mediated signaling. This mechanism is common among the IL-6 family of soluble receptors, for which both agonistic and antagonistic effects have been observed [49]. Similar to what has been seen with TNF, complexes of IL-6 and soluble IL-6 receptor were found to markedly prolong the IL-6 plasma half-life [50].

Anti-inflammatory Molecules in Experimental Animal Models of Septic Shock

Although LPS undoubtedly plays an important role in the pathophysiology of Gram-negative infections, the administration of LPS does not completely mimic the complex host-pathogen interactions that take place during sepsis and septic shock. Furthermore, many infections are now caused by Gram-positive organisms, whose cell walls are devoid of LPS. To get a more complete picture of the role of inhibitory cytokines, one should study their effect in experimental models of sepsis induced by toxins (endotoxin and exotoxins), by Gram-negative and Gram-positive bacteria, and by intracellular pathogens. Anti-inflammatory mediators, such as IL-10, IL-13, IL-1ra or soluble TNF receptors have all been shown to protect galactosamine-sensitized mice from lethal endotoxemia (Table 2, Table 4). Protection was associated with reduced levels of circulating TNF-α, which is a critical determinant of death in this model. IL-6 plays a beneficial role in the resolution of experimental bacterial infections, but does not appear to be a major determinant for outcome in experimental endotoxemia or TNF-induced shock (Table 3). By contrast, administration of anti-inflammatory mediators (IL-4, IL-10, IL-13, IL-1ra and the soluble TNF receptors) actually aggravate the infection, especially when caused by Gram-positive bacteria or intracellular pathogens (Table 2, Table 4) [51]. The bacterial species used to trigger infection and the size of the inoculum (i.e., the severity of the infection) are critical factors to be taken into account. For a given pathogen and a given experimental model it is often not possible to predict whether an anti-inflammatory strategy will be beneficial or detrimental. Furthermore, inhibitory cytokines do not always exert comparable effects in a given infectious model. These results illustrate the difficulty of modulating the immune response in sepsis. The fact that a molecule suppresses LPS-induced TNF or IL-1 production by monocytes *in vitro*, does not mean that this

Table 4. Effects of IL-13 or of IL-4 in various mouse models of shock or infection

Model	Effect	References
IL-13		
LPS (endotoxemia)	Beneficial	[82, 83]
Listeria monocytogenes (i.v.)	Harmful	[84]
IL-4		
Borrelia burgdorferi (s.c.)	Beneficial	[85]
Pseudomonas aeruginosa (pneumonia)	Beneficial	[86]
Staphylococcus aureus (arthritis)	Harmful	[87]
Listeria monocytogenes (i.v.)	Harmful	[88]
Salmonella typhimurium (i.v.)	Harmful	[89]
Candida albicans (i.p.)	No effect	[90]

Studies were performed in mice given either anti-IL-13 or anti-IL-4 antibodies, or exogenous recombinant IL-13 or IL-4 or in IL-13- or IL-4-deficient mice.

anti-inflammatory effect is the main function of that mediator. Indeed, as mentioned previously, cytokines such as IL-4, IL-6, IL-13 and TGF-β also exhibit critical pro-inflammatory and immunostimulatory functions within the immune system.

Anti-inflammatory Molecules in Human Septic Shock

Pro-inflammatory cytokines and anti-inflammatory mediators have been detected in the blood and body fluids of septic shock patients. However, several problems related to the timing and processing of samples and to the cytokine assays, complicate the interpretation of these data. These problems are further confounded by the fact that we do not completely understand how mediator networks are regulated, nor the role of individual cytokines in the pathogenesis of sepsis and septic shock. Moreover, cytokines are measured in the blood in the presence of their natural inhibitors and very little information is available on cell-associated cytokines in the tissues.

In most of the studies presented in Table 5, there was a correlation between the amount of circulating mediator and the severity of the disease. Generally, blood levels were higher in non-survivors than in survivors. In fulminant meningococcal septic shock, mediators are released in larger amounts than during the course of sepsis caused by other bacteria. This could be related to high circulating levels of endotoxin [52]. From the data in Table 5, it appears that levels of soluble TNFR-p55 range between 5 and 20 ng/ml, levels of soluble TNFR-p75 between 20 and 100 ng/ml. Levels of IL-10 are especially elevated in patients with meningococcemia (10–20 ng/ml, but sometimes up to 100 ng/ml), but usually do not exceed 1 ng/ml in patients with septic shock caused by other organisms. Among cytokines, IL-6 was found to be the best predictor of disease severity and outcome. Levels as high as 500 ng/ml were observed in severe cases. Levels of IL-1ra do not exceed 20 ng/ml. IL-4 has rarely been detected in the circulation of septic patients, and if so in small amounts, usually below 1 ng/ml [53–55]. Similarly, IL-13 is undetectable in most patients with sepsis [56]. Few data have been published

Table 5. Studies of serum concentrations of anti-inflammatory mediators in patients with septic shock

Mediators	Type of Disease	References
Soluble TNF receptors	Meningoccemia	[54, 91, 92]
	Sepsis	[53, 55, 57, 93-96]
IL-10	Meningococcemia	[52, 97]
	Sepsis	[55, 56, 98, 99]
IL-6	Sepsis	[57, 93, 98, 100–103]
IL-4/IL-13	Sepsis	[53–56]
IL-1ra	Sepsis	[55–57, 93]
TGF-β	Sepsis	[57]

for TGF-β [57]. For convenience, cytokine levels are usually measured in the bloodstream. However, they may play a more important autocrine or paracrine role at the primary site of infection or tissue injury, but there is little information on that topic.

A 30 molar excess of soluble TNFR-p55 and a 300 molar excess of soluble TNFR-p75 are necessary to achieve >50% of inhibition of TNF toxicity *in vitro* [43]. The serum concentrations of soluble TNFR-p55 detected in critically ill patients are in the range of 5 to 10 ng/ml and thus appear to be capable of partially inhibiting TNF, which usually circulates at concentrations below 500 pg/ml [46, 47, 58]. In contrast to the soluble TNFR, extremely high (i.e., non physiological) concentrations of IL-1ra are needed to completely inhibit the binding of IL-1 to target cells [2]. With regard to IL-10, IL-4 and IL-13, high concentrations of these cytokines are required to partially suppress LPS-induced TNF production by monocytes *in vitro* [11, 27, 59]. However, they are in the range of the levels of IL-4 and of IL-10 measured in patients with septic shock patients (1–10 ng/ml). Overall, studies performed in septic patients suggest that the anti-inflammatory mediators circulate at concentrations in the range of those shown to inhibit cytokine production by mononuclear cells activated by LPS. It is therefore possible that they modulate the magnitude of the pro-inflammatory response *in vivo*. Yet, the pathogenesis of septic shock is very complex and it is unclear whether the results obtained *in vitro* with isolated cells stimulated with bacterial toxins can be extrapolated to the situation of a patient with septic shock caused by live bacteria. Moreover, many of the so-called anti-inflammatory or inhibitory mediators are multifunctional molecules with pro-inflammatory properties that are essential for host defenses. Thus, the fact that one of these molecules can be measured in the bloodstream does not necessarily mean that the host response is anti-inflammatory.

Role of Anti-Inflammatory Mediators in Monocyte Deactivation in Septic Shock

It is well documented that monocytes presensitized with LPS have a strongly reduced capacity to produce pro-inflammatory cytokines (especially TNF) in response to a second LPS stimulus (for a review see [60]). This phenomenon also occurs *in vivo* and has been called tolerance, adaptation, or hyporesponsiveness. Several mechanisms have been proposed to explain how monocytes from healthy donors become tolerant to LPS. Among these are the down-regulation of LPS receptors, the induction of inhibitory molecules or the production of anti-inflammatory mediators, such as anti-inflammatory cytokines or glucocorticoid hormones. Similar to what happens during tolerance, monocytes or whole blood from septic patients release minimal amount of cytokines (such as TNF) following LPS stimulation [4–6]. Although similarities exist between LPS-tolerant monocytes and monocytes isolated from critically-ill or septic patients, there are important differences as well (see [61] for a review).

IL-10, IL-4, IL-13, and TGF-β all decrease, or may even completely suppress, the synthesis of pro-inflammatory cytokines *in vitro*. Kinetic studies of cytokine production have shown that the release of anti-inflammatory cytokines is delayed compared to that of the pro-inflammatory ones. There is now ample evidence that these cytokines, especially IL-10 and TGF-β, are essential effector molecules of LPS tolerance and that they may themselves replace LPS to induce monocyte hyporesponsiveness [62]. In whole blood assays, the presence of anti-inflammatory molecules may inhibit pro-inflammatory events triggered by LPS. Brandtzaeg and co-workers [6] observed that circulating anti-inflammatory cytokines exert profound inhibitory effects. The IL-10 present in the plasma of patients with meningococcal sepsis was found to suppress the cytokine response of LPS-stimulated monocytes of healthy donors [6]. Plasma levels of IL-10 may be as high as 40 ng/ml in patients with meningococcal septic shock, but they usually do not exceed 1 ng/ml in other septic conditions and might therefore only partly inhibit the production of pro-inflammatory molecules. Thus, this observation may not be relevant when septic shock is caused by other microorganisms. Similar considerations also apply for the other anti-inflammatory molecules TGF-β, IL-1ra or the soluble forms of the TNF receptors.

Conclusion

In vitro studies have shown that the cytokines IL-1ra, IL-10, IL-4, IL-13, TGF-β, IL-6 and the soluble TNF receptors exert suppressive effects on immune cells (lymphocytes, monocytes, macrophages), inhibiting or down-modulating a wide range of pro-inflammatory mediators, hence their designation as anti-inflammatory mediators. However, these inhibitory functions represent only one facet of the complex biological activities of these molecules, that also exhibit critical immunostimulatory functions within the immune system. *In vivo*, IL-1ra, IL-10, IL-4, IL-13, TGF-β, IL-6, soluble TNFR-p55 and TNFR-p75 have been detected in the circulation of patients with sepsis, severe sepsis or septic shock. Similar to what has been observed for the pro-inflammatory cytokines, the serum concentrations of the anti-inflammatory mediators often correlate with the severity of the disease, and often with the clinical outcome. Whether septic shock patients die because the anti-inflammatory response is insufficient to control a superabundant inflammatory response, or because it induces a state of relative immunosuppression that impairs host defense mechanisms, is difficult to establish. In fact, except for IL-1ra, TNFR-p55, TNFR-p75 and possibly IL-10, it is difficult to determine whether the anti-inflammatory properties of these mediators exceed the pro-inflammatory features that are likely to be put into action during sepsis. Further work is needed to improve our understanding of the very complex pathophysiology of sepsis and septic shock.

References

1. Heumann D, Glauser MP (1994) Pathogenesis of septic shock. Sci Am 1/5:28–37
2. Dinarello CA (1996) Biologic basis for interleukin-1 in disease. Blood 87:2095–2147

3. Bone RC (1996) Why sepsis trials fail. JAMA 276:565–566
4. Munoz C, Carlet J, Fitting C, Misset B, Blériot JP, Cavaillon JM (1991) Dysregulation of in vitro cytokine production by monocytes during sepsis. J Clin Invest 88:1747–1754
5. Ertel W, Kremer JP, Kenney J, et al (1995) Downregulation of proinflammatory cytokine release in whole blood from septic shock patients. Blood 85:1341–1347
6. Brandtzaeg P, Osnes L, Ovstebo R, Joo GB, Westwik AB, Kierulf P (1996) Net inflammatory capacity of human septic shock plasma evaluated by a monocyte-based target cell assay: identification of interleukin-10 as a major functional deactivator of human monocytes. J Exp Med 184:51–60
7. Mosmann TR, Cherwinski H, Bond MW, Giedlin MA, Coffman RL (1986) Two types of murine helper T-cell clone. I. Definition according to profiles of lymphokine activities and secreted proteins. J Immunol 136:2348–2357
8. Kelso A (1995) Th1 and Th2 subsets: paradigms lost? Immunol Today 16:374–379
9. Moore KW, O'Garra A, de Waal Malefyt R, Vieira P, Mosmann TR (1993) Interleukin 10. Annu Rev Immunol 11:165–190
10. de Waal Malefyt R, Abrams J, Bennett B, Figdor CG, de Vries JE (1991) Interleukin 10 (IL-10) inhibits cytokine synthesis by human monocytes: an autoregulatory role of IL-10 produced by monocytes. J Exp Med 174:1209–1220
11. Clarke CJ, Hales A, Hunt A, Foxwell BMJ (1998) IL-10 mediated suppression of TNF-α production is independent of its ability to inhibit NFκB activity. Eur J Immunol 28:1719–1726
12. Takeshita S, Gage RG, Kishimoto T, Vredevoe DL, Martinez- Maza D (1996) Differential regulation of IL-6 gene transcription and expression by IL-4 and IL-10 in human monocytic cell lines. J Immunol 156:2591–2598
13. Wang P, Wu P, Siegel ML, Egan RW, Billah MM (1995) Interleukin (IL)-10 inhibits nuclear factor κB (NFκB) activation in human monocytes. IL-10 and IL-4 suppress cytokine synthesis by different mechanisms. J Biol Chem 270:9558–9563
14. Bogdan C, Paik J, Vodovotz Y, Nathan C (1992) Contrasting mechanisms for suppression of macrophage cytokine release by transforming growth factor-β and interleukin-10. J Biol Chem 267:23301–23308
15. Dickensheets HL, Freeman SL, Smith MF, Donnelly RP (1997) Interleukin-10 upregulates tumor necrosis factor receptor type II (p75) gene expression in endotoxin-stimulated human monocytes. Blood 90:4162–4171
16. Joyce DA, Gibbons DP, Geen P, Steer JH, Feldmann M, Brennan FM (1994) Two inhibitors of pro-inflammatory cytokine release, interleukin-10 and interleukin-4, have contrasting effects on release of soluble p75 tumor necrosis factor receptor by cultured monocytes. Eur J Immunol 24:2699–2705
17. Kühn R, Löhler J, Rennick D, Rajewsky K, Müller W (1993) Interleukin-10-deficient mice develop chronic enterocolitis. Cell 75:263–274
18. Rennick D, Davidson N, Berg D (1995) Interleukin-10 gene knock-out mice: a model of chronic inflammation. Clin Immunol Immunopathol 76:S174–S178
19. Callard RE, Matthews DJ, Hibbert L (1996) IL-4 and IL-13 receptors: are they one and the same ? Immunol Today 17:108–110
20. Brown MA, Hural J (1997) Functions of IL-4 and control of its expression. Crit Rev Immunol 17 :1–32
21. te Velde AA, Huijbens RJF, de Vries JE, Figdor CG (1990) Interleukin-4 (IL-4) inhibits secretion of IL-1β, tumor necrosis factor α, and human IL-6 by human monocytes. Blood 76: 1392–1397
22. Essner R, Rhoades K, McBride WH, Morton DL, Economou JS (1989) IL-4 down-regulates IL-1 and TNF gene expression in human monocytes. J Immunol 142:3857–3861
23. de Waal Malefyt R, Figdor CG, Huijbens R, et al (1993) Effects of IL-13 on phenotype, cytokine production, and cytotoxic function of human monocytes. J Immunol 151:6370–6381
24. Lacraz S, Nicod L, Galve-de Rochemonteix B, Baumberger C, Dayer JM, Welgus HG (1992) Suppression of metalloproteinase biosynthesis in human alveolar macrophages by interleukin-4. J Clin Invest 90:382–388
25. Zurawski G, de Vries JE (1994) Interleukin 13, and interleukin 4-like cytokine that acts on monocytes and B cells, but not on T cells. Immunol Today 15:19–26

26. Murata T, Obiri NI, Debinski W, Puri RK (1997) Structure of the IL-13 receptor: analysis of subunit composition in cancer and immune cells. Biochem Biophys Res Commun 238: 90–94
27. Mijatovic T, Kruys V, Caput D, Defrance P, Huez G (1997) Interleukin-4 and -13 inhibit tumor necrosis factor-α mRNA translational activation in lipopolysaccharide-induced mouse macrophages. J Biol Chem 272 : 14394–14398
28. Manna SK, Aggarwal BB (1998) IL-13 suppresses TNF-induced activation of nuclear factor-κB, activation protein-1, and apoptosis. J Immunol 161:2863–2872
29. Bennett BL, Cruz R, Lacson RG, Manning AM (1997) Interleukin-4 suppression of tumor necrosis factor α-stimulated E-selectin gene transcription is mediated by STAT6 antagonism of NF-κB. J Biol Chem 272:10212–10219
30. Shen CH, Stavnezer J (1998) Interaction of Stat6 and NF-κB: direct association and synergistic activation of interleukin-4 induced transcription. Mol Cell Biol 18:3395–3404
31. Di Santo E, Meazza C, Sironi M, et al (1997) IL-13 inhibits TNF production but potentiates that of IL-6 in vivo and ex vivo in mice. J Immunol 159:379–382
32. Letterio JJ, Roberts AB (1997) TGF-β: a critical modulator of immune cell function. Clin Immunol Immunopathol 84:244–250
33. Krakauer T, Vilcek J, Oppenheim JJ (1999) Proinflammatory cytokines. TNF and IL-1 families, chemokines, TGF-β, and others. In: Paul WE (ed) Fundamental Immunology. Lippincott-Raven, Philadelphia, pp 775–811
34. Shull MM, Ormsby I, Kier AB, et al (1992) Targeted disruption of the mouse transforming growth factor-β1 gene results in multifocal inflammatory disease. Nature 359:693–699
35. Kline JN, Fisher PA, Monick MM, Hunninghake GW (1995) Regulation of interleukin-1 receptor antagonist by Th1 and Th2 cytokines. Am J Physiol 269:L92–L98
36. Vannier E, Miller MC, Dinarello CA (1992) Coordinated antiinflammatory effects of interleukin 4: interleukin 4 suppresses interleukin 1 production but up-regulates gene expression and synthesis of interleukin 1 receptor antagonist. Proc Natl Acad Sci USA 89: 4076–4080
37. Muzio M, Re F, Sironi M, et al (1994) Interleukin-13 induces the production of interleukin-1 receptor antagonist (IL-1ra) and the expression of the mRNA for the intracellular (keratinocyte) form of IL-1ra in human myelomonocytic cells. Blood 83:1738–1743
38. Cassatella MA, Meda L, Gasperini S, Calzetti F, Bonora S (1994) Interleukin 10 (IL-10) upregulates IL-1 receptor antagonist production from lipopolysaccharide-stimulated human polymorphonuclear leukocytes by delaying mRNA degradation. J Exp Med 179:1695–1699
39. Dinarello CA (1998) Interleukin-1, interleukin-1 receptors and interleukin-1 receptor antagonist. Intern Rev Immunol 16:457–499
40. Barton BE (1997) IL-6: insights into novel biological activities. Clin Immunol Immunopathol 85:16–20
41. Starnes HF, Pearce MK, Tewari A, Yim JH, Zou JC, Abrams JS (1990) Anti-IL-6 monoclonal antibodies protect against lethal Escherichia coli infection and lethal tumor necrosis factor-alpha challenge in mice. J Immunol 145:4185–4191
42. Starnes HF, Pearce MK, Tewari A, Yim JH, Zou JC, Abrams JS (1992) Anti-IL-6 monoclonal antibodies protect against lethal Escherichia coli infection and lethal tumor necrosis factor-alpha challenge in mice. J Immunol 148:1968
43. VanZee KJ, Kohno T, Fischer E, Rock CS, Moldawer LL, Lowry SF (1992) Tumor necrosis factor soluble receptors circulate during experimental and clinical inflammation and can protect against excessive tumor necrosis factor α in vitro and in vivo. Proc Natl Acad Sci USA 89:4845–4849
44. Spinas GA, Keller U, Brockhaus M (1992) Release of soluble receptors for tumor necrosis factor (TNF) in relation to circulating TNF during experimental endotoxinemia. J Clin Invest 90:533–536
45. Aderka D, Engelmann H, Maor YBC, Wallach D (1992) Stabilization of the bioactivity of tumor necrosis factor by its soluble receptors. J Exp Med 175:323–329
46. Moller B, Ellermann-Eriksen S, Storgaard M, Obel N, Bendtzen K, Petersen CM (1996) Soluble tumor necrosis factor (TNF) receptors conserve TNF bioactivity in meningitis patient spinal fluid. J Infect Dis 174:557–563

47. Evans TJ, Moyes D, Carpenter A, et al (1994) Protective effect of 55- but not 75-kD soluble tumor necrosis factor receptor-immunoglobulin G fusion proteins in an animal model of Gram-negative sepsis. J Exp Med 180:2173–2179
48. Mohler KM, Torrance DS, Smith CA, et al (1993) Soluble tumor necrosis factor (TNF) receptors are effective therapeutic agents in lethal endotoxemia and function simultaneously as both TNF carriers and TNF antagonists. J Immunol 151:1548–1561
49. Heaney ML, Golde DW (1996) Soluble cytokine receptors. Blood 87:847–857
50. Peters M, Jacobs S, Ehlers M, et al (1996) The function of the soluble interleukin-6 (IL-6) receptor in vivo: sensitization of human soluble IL-6 receptor transgenic mice towards IL-6 and prolongation of the plasma half-life of IL-6. J Exp Med 183:1399–1406
51. Heumann D, Glauser MP (1996) Anticytokine strategies for the treatment of septic shock: relevance of animal models. Curr Top Microbiol Immunol 216:299–311
52. Derkx B, Marchant A, Goldman M, Bijlmer R, van Deventer S (1995) High levels of interleukin-10 during the initial phase of fulminant meningococcal septic shock. J Infect Dis 171: 229–232
53. Zeni F, Vindimian M, Pain P, Gery P, Tardy B, Bertrand J.C. (1995) Antiinflammatory and proinflammatory cyokines in patients with severe sepsis. J Infect Dis 172:1171–1172
54. van Deuren M, van der Ven-Jongekrijk J, Bartelink AKM, van Dalen R, Sauerwein RW, Van der Meer JWM (1995) Correlation between proinflammatory cytokines and antiinflammatory mediators and the severity of disease in meningococcal infections. J Infect Dis 172: 433–439
55. Kasai T, Inada K, Takakuwa T, et al (1997) Anti-inflammatory cytokine levels in patients with septic shock. Res Commun Mol Pathol Pharmacol 98:34–42
56. van der Poll T, de Waal Malefyt R, Coyle SM, Lowry SF (1997) Antiinflammatory cytokine responses during clinical sepsis and experimental endotoxemia: sequential measurements of plasma soluble interleukin (IL)-1 receptor type II, IL-10, and IL-13. J Infect Dis 175: 118–122
57. Marie C, Losser MR, Fitting C, Kermarrec N, Payen D, Cavaillon JM (1997) Cytokines and soluble cytokine receptors in pleural effusions from septic and nonseptic patients. Am J Resp Crit Care Med 156:1515–1522
58. Aiura K, Gelfand JA, Burke JF, Thompson RC, Dinarello CA (1993) Interleukin-1 (IL-1) receptor antagonist prevents Staphylococcus epidermidis-induced hypotension and reduces circulating levels of tumor necrosis factor and IL-1 beta in rabbits. Infect Immun 61: 3342–3350
59. Wang P, Wu P, Siegel MI, Egan RW, Billah MM (1994) IL-10 inhibits transcription of cytokine genes in human peripheral blood mononuclear cells. J Immunol 153:811–816
60. Ziegler-Heitbrock HWL (1995) Molecular mechanism in tolerance to lipopolysaccharide. J Inflamm 45:13–26
61. Heumann D, Glauser MP, Calandra T (1998) Monocyte deactivation in septic shock. Curr Opin Infect Dis 11:279–283
62. Randow F, Syrbe U, Meisel C, Krausch D, Zuckermann H, Platzer C, Volk HD (1995) Mechanism of endotoxin desensitization: involvement of interleukin-10 and transforming growth factor β. J Exp Med 181:1887–1892
63. Standiford TJ, Strieter RM, Lukacs NW, Kunkel SL (1995) Neutralization of IL-10 increases lethality in endotoxemia. Cooperative effects of macrophage inflammatory protein-2 and tumor necrosis factor. J Immunol 155:2222–2229
64. Howard M, Muchamuel T, Andrade S, Menon S (1993) Interleukin 10 protects mice from lethal endotoxemia. J Exp Med 177:1205–1208
65. Gérard C, Bruyns C, Marchant A, et al (1993) Interleukin 10 reduces the release of tumor necrosis factor and prevents lethality in experimental endotoxemia. J Exp Med 177:547–550
66. Marchant A, Bruyns C, Vandenabeele P, et al (1994) Interleukin-10 controls interferon-γ and tumor necrosis factor production during experimental endotoxemia. Eur J Immunol 24: 1167–1171
67. Florquin S, Amraoui Z, Abramowicz D, Goldman M (1998) Systemic release and protective role of IL-10 in staphylococcal enterotoxin B-induced shock in mice. J Immunol 153: 2618–2623

68. Cusumano V, Genovese F, Mancuso G, Carbone M, Fera MT, Teti G (1996) Interleukin-10 protects neonatal mice from lethal Group B streptococcal infection. Infect Immun 64: 2850–2852
69. Sawa T, Corry DB, Gropper MA, Ohara M, Kurahashi K, Wiener-Kronisch JP (1997) IL-10 improves lung injury and survival in *Pseudomonas aeruginosa* pneumonia. J Immunol 159:2858–2866
70. Greenberger MJ, Strieter RM, Kunkel SL, Danforth JM, Goodman RE, Standiford TJ (1995) Neutralization of IL-10 increases survival in a murine model of *Klebsiella* pneumonia. J Immunol 155:722–729
71. van der Poll T, Marchant A, Keogh Cv, Goldman M, Lowry SF (1996) Interleukin-10 impairs host defense in murine pneumococcal pneumonia. J Infect Dis 174:994–1000
72. Dai W, Köhler G, Brombacher F (1997) Both innate and acquired immunity to *Listeria monocytogenes* infections are increased in IL-10-deficient mice. J Immunol 158:2259–2267
73. Tonnetti L, Spaccapelo R, Cenci E, et al (1995) Interleukin-4 and -10 exacerbate candidiasis in mice. Eur J Immunol 25:1559–1565
74. Remick DG, Garg SJ, Newcomb DE, Wollenberg G, Huie TK, Bolgos GL (1998) Endogenous IL-10 fails to decrease the mortality of morbidity of sepsis. Crit Care Med 26:895–904
75. Libert C, Takahashi N, Cauwels A, Brouckaert P, Bluethmann H, Fiers W (1994) Response of interleukin-6-deficient mice to tumor necrosis factor-induced metabolic changes and lethality. Eur J Immunol 24:2237–2242
76. Dalrymple SA, Slattery R, Aud DM, Krishna M, Lucian LA, Murray R (1996) Interleukin-6 is required for a protective immune response to systemic *Escherichia coli* infection. Infect Immun 64:3231–3235
77. Barton BE, Shortall J, Jackson JV (1996) Interleukins 6 and 11 protect mice from mortality in a staphylococcal enterotoxin-induced toxic shock model. Infect Immun 64:714–718
78. van der Poll T, Keogh Cv, Guirao X, Buurman WA, Lowry SF (1997) Interleukin-6 gene-deficient mice show impaited defense against pneumococcal pneumonia. J Infect Dis 176: 439–444
79. Kopf M, Baumann H, Freer G, et al (1994) Impaired immune and acute-phase responses in interleukin-6-deficient mice. Nature 368:339–342
80. Camargo CA, Madden JF, Gao W, Selvan RS, Clavien PA (1997) Interleukin-6 protects liver against warm ischemia/reperfusion injury and promotes hepatocyte proliferation in the rodent. Hepatology 26:1513–1520
81. Ladel CH, Blum C, Dreher A, Reifenberg K, Kopf M, Kaufmann SHE (1997) Lethal tuberculosis in interleukin-6-deficient mutant mice. Infect Immun 65:4843–4849
82. Muchamuel T, Menon S, Pisacane P, Howard MC, Cockayne DA (1997) IL-13 protects mice from lipopolysaccharide-induced lethal endotoxemia. correlation with down-modulation of TNF-α, IFN-γ, and IL-12 production. J Immunol 158:2898–2903
83. Nicoletti F, Mancuso G, Cusumano V, et al (1997) Prevention of endotoxin-induced lethality in neonatal mice by interleukin-13. Eur J Immunol 27:1580–1583
84. Flesch IE, Wandersee A, Kaufmann SH (1997) Effects of IL-13 on murine listeriosis. Intern Immunol 9:467–474
85. Keane-Myers A, Maliszewski CR, Finkelman FD, Nickell SP (1996) Recombinant IL-4 augments resistance to *Borrelia burgdorferi* infections in both normal susceptible and antibody-deficient susceptible mice. J Immunol 156:2448–2494
86. Jain-Vora S, LeVine AM, Chroneos Z, Ross GF, Hull WM, Whitsett JA (1998) Interleukin-4 enhances pulmonary clearance of *Pseudomonas aeruginosa*. Infect Immun 66:4229–4236
87. Hultgren O, Kopf M, Tarkowski A (1998) *Staphylococcus aureus*-induced septic arthritis and septic death is decreased in IL-4-deficient mice: role of IL-4 as promoter for bacterial growth. J Immunol 160:5082–5087
88. Szalay G, Ladel CH, Blum C, Kaufmann SHE (1996) IL-4 neutralization or TNF-α treatment ameliorate disease by an intracellular pathogen in IFN-γ receptor-deficient mice. J Immunol 157:4746–4750
89. Everest P, Allen J, Papakonstantinopoulou A, Mastroeni P, Roberts M, Dougan G (1997) *Salmonella typhimurium* infections in mice deficient in interlukin-4 production. Role of IL-4 in infection-associated pathology. J Immunol 159:1820–1827

90. Kaposzta R, Tree P, Marodi L, Gordon S (1998) Characteristics of invasive candidiasis in gamma interferon- and interleukin-4-deficient mice: role of macrophages in host defense against *Candida albicans*. Infect Immun 66:1708–1717
91. van Deuren M, Frieling TM, van der Ven-Jongekrijg J, et al (1998) Plasma patterns of tumor necrosis factor-α and TNF soluble receptors during acute meningococcal infections and the effect of plasma exchange. Clin Infect Dis 26:918–923
92. Girardin E, Roux-Lombard P, Grau GE, Suter P, Galatti H, the J5 study group (1992) Imbalance between tumour necrosis factor-alpha and soluble TNF receptor concentrations in severe meningococcaemia. Immunology 76:20–23
93. Goldie AS, Fearon CH, Ross JA, et al (1995) Natural cytokine antagonists and endogenous antiendotoxin core antibodies in sepsis syndrome. JAMA 274:172–177
94. van der Poll T, Jansen J, van Leenen D, et al (1993) Release of soluble receptors for tumor necrosis factor in clinical sepsis and experimental endotoxemia. J Infect Dis 168:955–960
95. Ertel W, Scholl FA, Galatti H, Bonaccio M, Schildberg FW, Trentz O (1994) Increased release of soluble tumor necrosis factor receptors into blood during clinical sepsis. Arch Surg 129: 1330–1337
96. Froon AHM, Bemelmans MHA, Greve JW, Van der Linden CJ, Buurman WA (1994) Increased plasma concentrations of soluble tumor necrosis factor receptors in sepsis syndrome: correlation with plasma creatinine values. Crit Care Med 22:803–809
97. Lehmann AK, Halstensen A, Sornes S, Rokke O, Waage A (1998) High levels of interleukin 10 in serum are associated with fatality in meningococcal disease. Infect Immun 63:2109–2112
98. Gomez-Jimenez J, Martin MC, Sauri R, et al (1995) Interleukin-10 and the monocyte/macrophage-induced inflammatory response in septic shock. J Infect Dis 171:472–475
99. Marchant A, Alegre ML, Hakim A, et al (1998) Clinical and biological significance of interleukin-10 plasma levels in patients with septic shock. J Clin Immunol 15:266–273
100. Hack CE, De Groot ER, Felt-Bersma RJF, et al (1989) Increased plasma levels of interleukin-6 in sepsis. Blood 74:1704–1710
101. Calandra T, Gerain J, Heumann D, Baumgartner JD, Glauser MP, the Swiss-Dutch J5 Immunoglobulin Study Group (1991) High circulating levels of interleukin-6 in patients with septic shock: Evolution during sepsis, prognostic value and interplay with other cytokines. Am J Med 91:23–29
102. Damas P, Ledoux D, Nys M, et al (1992) Cytokine serum level during severe sepsis in human IL-6 as a marker of severity. Ann Surg 215:356–362
103. Frieling JTM, van Deuren M, Wijdenes J, et al (1995) Circulating interleukin-6 receptor in patients with sepsis syndrome. J Infect Dis 171:469–472
104. Bean AGD, Freiberg RA, Andrade S, Menon S, Zlotnik A (1993) Interleukin-10 protects mice against staphylococcal enterotoxin B-induced lethal shock. Infect Immun 61:4937–4939
105. van der Poll T, Marchant A, Buurman WA, et al (1995) Endogenous IL-10 protects mice from death during septic peritonitis. J Immunol 155:5397–5401
106. Barton BE, Jackson JV (1993) Protective role of interleukin 6 in the lipopolysaccharide-galactosamine septic shock model. Infect Immun 61:1496–1499
107. Marie C, Cavaillon JM, Losser MR (1996) Elevated levels of circulating transforming growth factor-beta 1 in patients with the sepsis syndrome Ann Intern Med 125:520–521

Interleukin-1β and Interleukin-18: Two Cytokine Precursors for Interleukin-1β Converting Enzyme (Caspase-1)

C. A. Dinarello

Introduction

During the analysis of the human interleukin (IL)-1β precursor cDNA [1], the open reading frame resulted in a protein with a molecular weight of 31 000 Daltons but lacking a signal peptide. The interpretation of this leaderless precursor of IL-1β was rather difficult since it was not clear how the mature form was cleaved naturally. We had expressed an intermediate form of recombinant IL-1β with a molecular weight of 21 000 Daltons. This species of IL-1β was biologically weak. Upon cleavage with elastase, an 18 000 IL-1β form resulted, which possessed a 100-fold increase in biological activity [2]. The elastase N-terminus was not that of the natural IL-1β reported in 1985 by the Belgians which had an N-terminus at alanine 117 [3]. That N-terminus indicated no specific cleavage protease and therefore, it remained unclear for several years exactly how and what protease cleaved precursor IL-1β into a mature peptide with an N-terminus at alanine 117. The discovery of the IL-1β converting enzyme (ICE) as a unique intracellular protease opened a door on an entirely new area of cytokine biology and inflammation in that there are intracellular proteases which function to cleave proteins which lack a classic signal peptide. ICE was the first enzyme of this class described for cutting the precursor for IL-1β; other members of the ICE family were clearly involved in other intracellular biological processes.

Cleavage of Precursor IL-1β by ICE

The precursor of IL-1β requires cleavage by ICE before the mature form is secreted. The 45-kDa precursor of ICE requires two internal cleavages before becoming the enzymatically active heterodimer comprised of a 10 and 20-kDa chain. The active site cysteine is located on the 20-kDa chain. ICE itself contributes to autoprocessing of the ICE precursor by undergoing oligomerization with itself or homologs of ICE [4, 5]. ICE is a member of a family of intracellular cysteine proteases called caspases, a term used to connote a cysteine protease cleaving after an aspartic acid residue [6]. ICE is caspase-1.

Two molecules of the ICE heterodimer form a tetramer with two molecules of precursor IL-1β for cleavage [4, 7]. The aspartic acid at position 116 of the precursor IL-1β is the recognition amino acid for ICE cleavage. ICE does not cleave the IL-1α precursor. Enzymes such as elastase [2] and granzyme A [8] cleave precursor IL-1β at amino acid 112 and 120 respectively yielding biologically active IL-1β. The propiece of IL-1β can be found both inside and outside the cell [9]. In addition, the propiece exhibits biological activity as a chemoattractant for fibroblasts via an IL-1 receptor (IL-1R)-mediated event [10].

In the presence of a tetrapeptide competitive substrate inhibitor of ICE, the generation and secretion of mature IL-1β is reduced and precursor IL-1β accumulates mostly inside but also outside the cell [11]. This latter finding supports the concept that precursor IL-1β can be released from a cell independent of processing by ICE. Similar to that of thioredoxin [12] and basic fibroblast growth factor (FGF) [13], exocytosis has been proposed as a possible mechanism of precursor IL-1β release. A putative membrane 'channel' where active ICE is localized has also been proposed. In this model, mature IL-1β is released through this channel [14]. When ICE activity is blocked by a reversible competitive substrate inhibitor, greater amounts of precursor IL-1β are found in the supernatants [11, 14] and thus, the putative channel may provide a passive secretory pathway for both precursor IL-1β and mature IL-1β. Macrophages from ICE deficient mice do not release mature IL-1β upon stimulation *in vitro* [15, 16]. Although neutrophil enzymes such as elastase and granzyme A [8] can cleave precursor IL-1β at sites close to alanine 117, precursor IL-1β accumulates in cells from ICE-deficient mice. Interestingly, IL-1α production in macrophages from ICE deficient mice is reduced. This remains an unexplored area.

ICE Also Cleaves Precursor IL-18

Unlike IL-1β deficient mice [17], ICE-deficient mice are resistant to lethal endotoxemia [15, 16]. Although IL-1β and ICE deficient mice do not have circulating mature IL-1β following endotoxin, ICE deficient mice lack inferferon-γ (IFN-γ) in the circulation following endotoxin [18, 19]. The role of IFN-γ in rodent models of endotoxin shock was shown in IFN-γ receptor deficient mice which are resistant to lethal endotoxemia [20]. However, in humans, a role for IFN-γ in septic shock patients, including those with Gram-negative bacteremia, appears to be beneficial rather than harmful [21]. Therefore, the resistance of ICE-deficient mice to endotoxemia is due to the lack of a factor, not IL-1β, which induces IFN-γ. This factor was originally identified as IFN-γ inducing factor (IGIF) [22]. IGIF is now called IL-18 (see below). Because IL-18, like IL-1β, lacks a signal peptide, the precursor of IL-18 requires a specific cleavage and ICE is the intracellular enzyme that cleaves precursor IL-18. This was shown in two reports in which precursor IL-18 was expressed and then cleaved by recombinant ICE [18, 19].

IL-18 Is a New Member of the IL-1 Family

Discovery of IFN-γ Inducing Factor

In 1989, an endotoxin-induced serum activity that induced IFN-γ from mouse spleen cells was described by Nakamura and co-workers [22]. This serum activity functioned not as a direct inducer of IFN-γ but rather as a co-stimulant together with IL-2 or mitogens. An attempt to purify the activity from post-endotoxin mouse serum revealed an apparently homogeneous 50–55 kDa protein [23]. Since other cytokines can act as co-stimulants for IFN-γ production, the failure of neutralizing antibodies to IL-1, IL-4, IL-5, IL-6, or tumor necrosis factor (TNF) to neutralize the serum activity suggested that it was a distinct factor. In 1995, a third report was published from the same scientists demonstrating that the endotoxin-induced co-stimulant for IFN-γ production was present in extracts of livers from mice preconditioned with *P. acnes* [24]. In this model, the hepatic macrophage population (Kupffer cells) expands dramatically, and in these mice, a low dose of bacterial lipopolysaccharide (LPS), which in non-preconditioned mice is not lethal, becomes lethal. The factor, named IGIF, was purified to homogeneity from 1200 grams of *P. acnes*-treated mouse livers. Its molecular weight was 18–19 kDa and a N-terminal amino acid sequence was reported [24]. Similar to the endotoxin-induced serum activity, IGIF purified from liver homogenates did not induce IFN-γ by itself but functioned primarily as a co-stimulant with mitogens or IL-2.

Neutralizing antibodies to mouse IGIF were shown to prevent liver damage induced by LPS in *P. acnes* pre-conditioned mice [25]. Others had previously reported the importance of IFN-γ as a mediator of LPS-induced toxicity in pre-conditioned mice. For example, neutralizing anti-IFN-γ antibodies protected mice against Shwartzman-like shock [26] and galactosamine-treated mice deficient in the IFN-γ receptor were resistant to LPS-induced death [20]. Hence, it was not unexpected that neutralizing antibodies to murine IGIF protected *P. acnes*-preconditioned mice against LPS-induced liver toxicity [25].

Molecular Cloning of IGIF

Degenerate oligonucleotides derived from amino acid sequences of IGIF purified from liver homogenates were used to clone a murine IGIF cDNA [25]. Recombinant murine IGIF did not induce IFN-γ by itself but only in the presence of a mitogen or IL-2. However, most importantly, the co-induction of IFN-γ was independent of IL-12 induction of IFN-γ. After the murine form was cloned [25], the human cDNA sequence for IGIF was reported in 1996 [27]. Recombinant human IGIF exhibited IGIF activity reported for the naturally occurring molecule [27]. For example, human recombinant IGIF was without direct IFN-γ-inducing activity on human T-cells but acted as a co-stimulant for production of IFN-γ and other T-helper cell-1 (Th1) cytokines [27]. IGIF induced T-cell and natural killer (NK) cell IFN-γ production independently of IL-12 (and *vice versa*) [24, 25]. Hence, IGIF has been thought of primarily as a co-stimulant for Th1 cytokine production by acting as a co-stimulant for IFN-γ production with IL-12, IL-2, microbial agents or mitogens, particularly in NK cells [28–30]. The cytokine also acts as a co-stimulant for Fas ligand-mediated cytotoxicity of murine T cells and NK cell clones [31, 32]. In the human myelomonocytic cell line KG-1, IL-18 directly induces Fas ligand and apoptosis [33]. *In vivo*, endogenous IGIF activity appears to account for IFN-γ production in *P. acnes*-preconditioned mice injected with LPS [24]. This has been demonstrated using neutralizing anti-mouse IL-18 as well as the ICE-deficient mouse [18, 19].

IGIF and IL-1β and the Naming of IL-18

Scientists at the DNAX Research Institute analyzed the computer generated protein folding pattern of murine IGIF and compared its pattern to those of other cytokines. Using a compatibility relatedness program, mature murine IGIF had the highest score with mature human IL-1β; furthermore, the IGIF amino acid sequence matched best with amino acids which form the all-β pleated sheet folding pattern of human IL-1β [34]. A high degree of alignment was present in the sequences that comprise the twelve β-sheets of the mature IL-1β structure. Using this alignment of conserved amino acids, there is a 19% positional identity of mature murine IGIF to mature human IL-1β and a 12% identity to human IL-1α. Using this same positional alignment, the identity of IL-1β to IL-1α is 23%. It was suggested that the name IGIF be changed to IL-1γ [34]. Does IGIF bind to IL-1 type I receptors? This would be an essential criterion for assigning the name IL-1γ since the type I IL-1 receptor is the ligand receptor and an essential chain of the IL-1 receptor signaling complex for the biological activity of IL-1. In the absence of evidence that IGIF binds to the IL-1 receptor type I [35], IL-18 rather than IL-1γ is a more appropriate name [27].

IL-18 and IL-1 Share the Same Receptor Family

The IL-18 Receptor Complex

Torigoe et al. described the purification and characterization of a human IL-18 receptor [36]. The purified protein had a molecular weight between 60–100 kDa and its amino acid sequence revealed 100% identity to a previously known member of the IL-1 receptor family which had been termed the IL-1 receptor related protein (IL-1Rrp) [37]. IL-1Rrp had remained an orphan receptor until recently. When the IL-1Rrp was first reported, it was clear that it was indeed a member of the IL-1 receptor family, although it did not bind IL-1α, IL-1β or IL-1 receptor antagonist (IL-1ra) [37]. This was an unexpected finding because the IL-1Rrp was isolated from a library using degenerate oligonucleotides from conserved amino acids in the extracellular domains of the IL-1 type I receptor.

Until the studies by Torigoe et al., the ligand for IL-1Rrp was unknown but it would be likely that the ligand was structurally related to members of the IL-1 family. However, despite its relatedness, neither IL-1α nor IL-1β bind to IL-1Rrp [37]. When the extracellular domain of the IL-1Rrp was expressed as a fusion protein linked to the Fc domain of IgG, the IL-1Rrp did not bind IL-1 on a Biacore chip [37]. However, a chimeric molecule was constructed comprised of the extracellular domains of the IL-1 type I receptor linked to the transmembrane and cytosolic domain of the IL-1 Rrp. When transfected into COS cells, this chimeric receptor did exhibit IL-1 functional activity upon binding of IL-1. Therefore, although the IL-1 Rrp is a member of the IL-1 receptor family and its extracellular domains do not bind IL-1 itself, IL-1Rrp transmits a signal similar to that of the IL-1R.

IL-1Rrp is the Binding Component of the IL-18 Receptor Complex

Torigoe et al. reported that IL-1Rrp is the functional component of the IL-18 receptor primarily based on the observation that antibodies to IL-1 Rrp prevent IL-18 activity [36]. Yet, in terms of other cytokine receptors, IL-18 binding to the L428 cell line used in the purification process was low (Kd of 18.5 nM). Thomassen reported a Kd of 25 nM for IL-18 [38]. The Kd for IL-18 binding to IL-1Rrp expressed transiently on COS cells was 45 nM [36]. These are unusually low affinities for a cytokine with a biological activity in the pM range. Nevertheless, IL-1Rrp is unquestionably essential for IL-18 activity and an integral part of the IL-18 signaling complex. Therefore, the term IL-18Rα replaces the term IL-1Rrp. But, a second binding chain in a putative IL-18 receptor complex likely exists in order to form a high affinity complex which characterizes all cytokine receptor signaling.

Nakanishi's group have reported that there are both high (0.4 nM) and low (40 nM) affinity binding sites for IL-18 in murine primary T-cells [39]. Clearly the IL-18Rα could account for the low affinity IL-18 binding sites. Thus, a second chain resulting in a greater affinity would explain the higher affinity. This 'other' receptor chain has been identified as the 'accessory' protein-like (AcPL) receptor [40], and is related to the IL-1 accessory protein identified by Greenfeder et al. [41]. Similar to the IL-1 accessory protein, the IL-18 AcPL does not bind to its ligand but rather binds to the complex formed by IL-18 with the IL-18Rα chain [40]. This heterodimeric is likely the high affinity complex.

There is a comparable finding in the identification of the IL-1 receptor complex. For nearly 9 years, IL-1 activity was thought to be due to a single chain receptor, the 80 kDa IL-1R type I [42]. The second chain was discovered in 1995; it was termed the IL-1R accessory protein (IL-1R-AcP) [41]. This latter receptor is essential to IL-1 signaling, although IL-1R-AcP does not bind to any IL-1 ligand. Similar to many cytokine receptors, the receptor consists of a heterocomplex of a ligand binding chain (often termed the α chain of the receptor) plus an accessory chain (often termed the β chain) which transmits the signal. The importance of the IL-1R-AcP for IL-1 activity was shown using antibodies to IL-1R-AcP which is an essential part of the heterodimeric IL-1R complex.

Therefore, the IL-18Rα is unlikely to be the sole component of the IL-18 receptor signaling apparatus and is certainly not the high affinity ligand binding receptor chain. It is likely that the IL-18 receptor complex is comprised of a ligand binding chain of IL-1Rrp (IL-18Rα), with the second chain being the non-IL-18 binding AcPL (IL-18Rα) [40]. As described below [43], an IL-18 binding protein (IL-18BP) has been purified from human urine and would likely be the soluble (extracellular) form of the IL-18Rα chain. But a transmembrane form of the IL-18BP has not been isolated to date despite murine cDNA cloning and human genomic analyses [43]. Thus, the IL-18BP is a third gene product and appears to be the 'decoy' receptor of IL-18, similar to the IL-1R type II which is the decoy receptor for IL-1.

Isolation and Purification of an IL-18 Binding Protein from Human Urine

Using methods established for the purification and characterization of ligand binding cytokine receptors in human urine (44–47), a 38 kDa IL-18BP was purified to homogeneity from urine using ligand affinity chromatography and the N-terminal amino acids determined [43]. The amino acid sequence of the IL-18BP is not that of a known cytokine receptor presently listed in the data banks. Although this binding protein likely represents the extracellular domain of the ligand binding receptor chain, to date a transmembrane and cytosolic component to the IL-18BP has not been found.

Similar to neutralizing antibodies to IL-18 [48], the IL-18BP prevents LPS-induced IFN-γ production [43]. Also, similar to anti-IL-18 antibodies, IL-18BP does not affect IFN-γ production following stimulation with mitogens such as concanavalin A. However, unlike antibodies to IL-18, the IL-18BP does not exhibit species specificity and hence human IL-18BP neutralizes both human and murine IL-18 [43].

IL-18 Signal Transduction is Similar to that of IL-1

It is clear that IL-1 and IL-18 do share signaling pathways, particularly in activating the processes by which nuclear factor-kappa B (NF-κB) translocates to the nucleus. In terms of IFN-γ production, IL-1α, IL-1β and IL-18 each induce IFN-γ in the presence of IL-2 or IL-12 [29, 49]. IL-18 is 5–10 times more potent that either form of IL-1 [29] which suggests, expectedly, that signal transduction of IL-1 and IL-18 cannot be identical. However, the recruitment of IL-IR-associated kinase (IRAK) to the IL-18 receptor complex places IL-18 signaling high in the signaling cascade that it shares with IL-1. For IL-1 signaling, one of the earliest events is the formation of the heterocomplex of the ligand IL-1 with the type I IL-1R and the IL-1R-AcP [41]. This complex then recruits IRAK [50]. The topic of IL-1 signal transduction related to NF-κB activation has been reviewed in detail [51, 52]. The IL-1R-AcP is essential for the recruitment and activation of IRAK [53, 54]. In fact, deletion of specific amino acids in the IL-1R-AcP cytoplasmic domain results in loss of IRAK association [53] and these same amino acids are present in the IL-1 Rrp (IL-18Rα). In addition, an intracellular adapter molecule termed MyD88 appears to dock to the complex allowing IRAK to become phosphorylated [50, 55]. IRAK then dissociates from the IL-1R complex and associates with TNF receptor associated factor-6 (TRAF-6) [56]. TRAF-6 then phosphorylates NF-κB-inducing kinase (NIK) [57] and NIK phosphorylates the inhibitory κB kinases (IKK-1 and IKK-2) [58]. Once phosphorylated, IκB is rapidly degraded by a ubiquitin pathway liberating NF-κB which translocates to the nucleus for gene transcription.

IRAK also associates with the IL-18R complex [28, 59]. This was demonstrated using IL-12 stimulated T-cells followed by immunoprecipitation with anti-IL-18R or anti-IRAK [59]. Furthermore, IL-18 triggered cells also recruited TRAF-6 [59]. Like IL-1 signaling, myeloid differentiation (MyD)88 has a role in IL-18 signaling. MyD88-deficient mice do not produce acute phase proteins and have diminished cytokine responses. Recently, Th1-developing cells from MyD88 deficient mice were unresponsive to IL-18-induced activation of NF-κB and c-Jun N-terminal kinase (JNK) [60]. Thus, MyD88 is an essential component in the signaling cascade that follows IL-1R as well as IL-18R binding. It appears that the cascade of sequential recruitment of MyD88, IRAK and TRAF-6 followed by the activation of NIK and degradation of IKK and release of NF-κB are nearly identical for IL-1 as well as for IL-18. Indeed, in cells transfected with IL-18Rα (IL-1Rrp) and then stimulated with IL-18, translocation of NF-κB is observed using electromobility shift assay [36]. In U1 macrophages which already express the gene for IL-1Rrp,

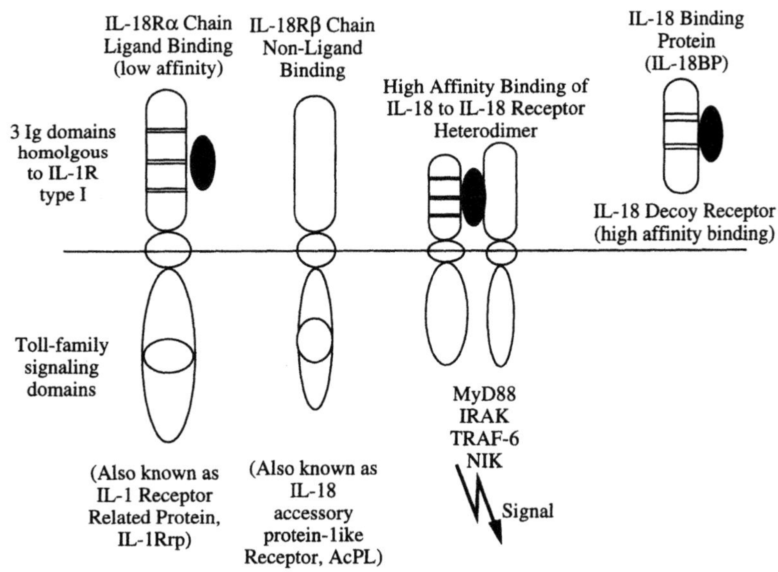

Fig. 1. Model for IL-18 signal transduction. IL-18 binds to the IL-18Rα chain (also known as IL-1Rrp) and recruits the IL-18Rβ chain (also known as AcPL). This heterodimeric complex recruits MyD88 and IL-1 receptor-associated kinase (IRAK). Phosphorylated IRAK activates TNF receptor-associated factor (TRAF)-6 and in turn nuclear factor-kappa B (NF-κB)-inducing kinase (NIK). This results in activation of inhibitory kappa B (IκB) kinase (IKK) and then phosphorylation of IκB. Phosphorylated IκB degrades and releases the p50 and p65 components of NF-κB. Free NF-κB migrates through nuclear pores and translocates to nuclear DNA for gene transcription

there is translocation of NF-κB and stimulation of the human immunodeficiency virus-type 1 (HIV-1) production [61].

Figure 1 is a working model of the proposed IL-18 signaling resulting in translocation of NF-κB to the nucleus. However, not shown is the evidence that IL-18 signaling activates p38 mitogen activated protein kinase (MAPK). In U1 cells stimulated with IL-18, IL-8 synthesis is reduced by nearly 90% in the presence of a specific p38 MAPK inhibitor [61]. In murine T-cells, IL-18 stimulated the phosphorylation of p42 MAPK and p56lck [62].

IL-18 as a Pro-Inflammatory Cytokine

IL-18 Induces Chemokines in Monocytes and NK Cells

There is no dearth of evidence for the role of chemokines in promoting inflammation. For example, the neutrophil-activating chemokine IL-8 is a primary agonist in several pathologic processes of the lung. It is presently unclear whether IL-18 has a role in the eosinophilic infiltration of asthma but the global stimulation of both CXC and CC chemokines by IL-18 [63] warrants consideration that eosinophilic chemokines are induced from cells expressing receptors for IL-18. In this regard, the macrophage cell line U1, which is derived from the histiocytic lymphoma cell U937, releases IL-8 when stimulated by IL-18 [61]. In addition, the myelomonocytic leukemia cell line KG-1 also releases IL-8 when stimulated with IL-18 [33]. This topic has recently been reviewed [64].

Is there a broader role for IL-18? Does the cytokine possess other biological activities, not only as a co-stimulant for Th1 cytokines, but as a direct acting pro-inflammatory cytokine? The ability of IL-18 to induce CC and CXC chemokines places IL-18 in a strategic role in inflammation. Using freshly obtained human peripheral blood mononuclear cells, mature, recombinant IL-18 induced IL-8 gene expression and synthesis [63]. Using IL-1ra to block IL-1 activity in these cells, IL-18-induced IL-8 production was reduced by 40%. When TNF activity was inhibited using soluble receptors for TNF, IL-18-induced IL-8 production was reduced by 80% suggesting that the primary action of IL-18 was via a TNF-dependent pathway. Although IL-8 in peripheral blood mononuclear cell cultures was derived from the $CD14^+$ cell population (and not the $CD3^+$ cells), the source of TNF was the $CD3^+$ and the NK cells. Therefore, the inflammatory cytokine cascade initiated by IL-18 in the mixed peripheral blood mononuclear cell population starts with triggering of constitutive IL-18 receptors on lymphocytes and NK cells leading to TNF production; in turn, TNF stimulates IL-1 and IL-8 from the $CD14^+$ cell. The induction of TNF can be observed at the level of gene expression within two hours following exposure to IL-18. IL-18 also stimulates the synthesis of macrophage chemoattractant protein-1 (MCP-1) in these cultures [63]. These results are consistent with the ability of IL-18 to activate the translocation of NF-κB in peripheral T-cells and fibroblasts [28, 36, 65].

Consistent with the induction of TNF in these models is the observation that IL-18 induces HIV-1 expression. At concentrations as low as 100 pM, mature IL-

18 induces p24 synthesis in a chronically infected macrophage cell line called U1 [61]. The increase in p24 is an indication of production of competent virus by these cells. Similar to the observation in peripheral blood mononuclear cells, HIV-1 p24 production by IL-18 is inhibited by blocking the activity of endogenously produced TNF [61]. Furthermore, the induction of p24 by IL-18 is reduced by inhibition of endogenous nitric oxide (NO) synthesis [66]. Again, these observations are consistent with the ability of IL-18 to activate NF-κB translocation. As discussed below, one chain of the IL-18R complex is the L-1Rrp which upon transient transfection into COS-1 cells results in NF-κB translocation [36]. In murine cloned T-cells, IL-18 stimulation results in a macromolecular complex precipitated by an antibody to IRAK [28]. In these same cells, IL-18 does not activate signal transducer and activator of transcription (STAT) 4 which characteristically occurs following IL-12 treatment [28]. Since IRAK activates a kinase cascade leading to degradation of IκB and activation of NF-κB, these findings are consistent with IL-18 induction of TNF from T-cells and IL-8 from macrophages [63].

IL-18 Up-regulates Expression of Fas Ligand

IL-18 enhances Fas ligand expression and induces apoptosis in Fas-expressing human myelomonocytic KG-1 cells [33]. KG-1 cells are monocyte like and also produce the intercellular adhesion molecule-1 (ICAM-1). IL-18 increases ICAM-1 expression in these macrophagic cells [67]. These cells also express constitutively Fas antigen (CD95) and after exposure to IL-18, KG-1 cells became apoptotic. Fas ligand is up-regulated in T-cells and NK cells following incubation with IL-18 [31]. In the liver, cytotoxic T-lymphocytes are thought to contribute to the destruction of hepatic cells, particularly when infected by viruses. Cytotoxic T-cells and NK cells isolated from the liver and then stimulated with IL-18 exhibit enhanced killing of Jurkat T-cells [68]. The IL-18-induced enhanced killing by liver-derived cytotoxic T lymphocytes was via a perforin-dependent pathway and not CD95 [68]. Liver-derived NK cells also exhibited enhanced killing of Jurkat cells following exposure to IL-18 but the mechanism was thought to be independent of TNF. However, failure to detect TNF in cell culture supernatants is not an argument that any cellular change is TNF independent since membrane forms of TNF are biologically active but often hardly measurable in supernatant. In fact, the ability of IL-18 to induce HIV-1 in U1 cells [61] and IL-8 in peripheral blood mononuclear cells [63] is TNF dependent. In both studies, the dependence on TNF was demonstrated by reducing the IL-18 effect with soluble TNFp55 receptor. Therefore, it is likely that IL-18 induced killing by liver NK cells can still be due to induction of membrane TNF.

Conclusion

The use of inhibitors of ICE provides a novel mechanism for reducing IL-1 and IL-18 mediated responses during infectious and inflammatory diseases. Unlike blocking these cytokines with specific inhibitors such as IL-1ra, soluble IL-1 receptors or the IL-18 binding protein, such inhibitors of ICE are not specific. Nevertheless, they may find a role in treatment of the critically ill patient since animal studies reveal effectiveness in models of systemic inflammation.

Acknowledgment. These studies are supported by NIH Grant AI15614.

References

1. Auron PE, Webb AC, Rosenwasser LJ, et al (1984) Nucleotide sequence of human monocyte interleukin 1 precursor cDNA. Proc Natl Acad Sci USA 81:7907–7911
2. Dinarello CA, Cannon JG, Mier JW, et al (1986) Multiple biological activities of human recombinant interleukin 1. J Clin Invest 77:1734–1739
3. Van Damme J, De Ley M, Opdenakker G, Billiau A, De Somer P (1985) Homogeneous interferon-inducing 22K factor is related to endogenous pyrogen and interleukin-1. Nature 314: 266–268
4. Wilson KP, Black JA, Thomson JA, et al (1994) Structure and mechanism of interleukin-1β converting enzyme. Nature 370:270–275
5. Gu Y, Wu J, Faucheu C, et al (1995) Interleukin-1β converting enzyme requires oligomerization for activity of processed forms in vivo. EMBO J 14:1923–1931
6. Alnemri ES, Livingston DJ, Nicholson DW, et al (1996) Human ICE/CED-3 protease nomenclature. Cell 87:171
7. Walker NP, Talanian RV, Brady KD, et al (1994) Crystal structure of the cysteine protease interleukin-1 beta-converting enzyme: a (p20/p10)2 homodimer. Cell 78:343–352
8. Irmler M, Hertig S, MacDonald HR, et al (1995) Granzyme A is an interleukin-1β-converting enzyme. J Exp Med 181:1917–1922
9. Higgins GC, Foster JL, Postlethwaite AE (1994) Interleukin-1 beta propeptide is detected intracellularly and extracellularly when human monocytes are stimulated with LPS in vitro. J Exp Med 180:607–614
10. Higgins GC, Foster JL, Postlethwaite AE (1993) Synthesis and biological activity of human interleukin-1β propiece in vitro. Arthritis Rheum 39:S153 (Abst)
11. Thornberry NA, Bull HG, Calaycay JR, et al (1992) A novel heterodimeric cysteine protease is required for interleukin-1 beta processing in monocytes. Nature 356:768–774
12. Rubartelli A, Bajetto A, Allavena G, Wollman E, Sitia R (1992) Secretion of thioredoxin by normal and neoplastic cells through a leaderless secretory pathway. J Biol Chem 267: 24161–24164
13. Mignatti P, Rifkin DB (1991) Release of basic fibroblast growth factor, an angiogenic factor devoid of secretory signal sequence: a trivial phenomenon or a novel secretion mechanism? J Cell Biochem 47:201–217
14. Singer II, Scott S, Chin J, et al (1995) The interleukin-1 beta-converting enzyme (ICE) is localized on the external cell surface membranes and in the cytoplasmic ground substance of human monocytes by immuno-electron microscopy. J Exp Med 182:1447–1459
15. Li P, Allen H, Banerjee S, et al (1995) Mice deficient in interleukin-1 converting enzyme (ICE) are defective in production of mature interleukin-1β and resistant to endotoxic shock. Cell 80:401–411
16. Kuida K, Lippke JA, Ku G, et al (1995) Altered cytokine export and apoptosis in mice deficient in interleukin-1β converting enzyme. Science 267:2000–2003
17. Fantuzzi G, Zheng H, Faggioni R, et al (1996) Effect of endotoxin in IL-1β-deficient mice. J Immunol 157:291–296
18. Gu Y, Kuida K, Tsutsui H, et al (1997) Activation of interferon-γ inducing factor mediated by interleukin-1β converting enzyme. Science 275:206–209
19. Ghayur T, Banerjee S, Hugunin M, et al (1997) Caspase-1 processes IFN-gamma-inducing factor and regulates LPS-induced IFN-gamma production. Nature 386:619–623

20. Car BD, Eng VM, Schnyder B, et al (1994) Interferon γ receptor deficient mice are resistant to endotoxic shock. J Exp Med 179:1437–1444
21. Doecke WD, Randow F, Syrbe U, et al (1997) Monocyte deactivation in septic patients: restoration by IFN-gamma treatment. Nat Med 3:678–681
22. Nakamura K, Okamura H, Wada M, Nagata K, Tamura T (1989) Endotoxin-induced serum factor that stimulates gamma interferon production. Infect Immun 57:590–595
23. Nakamura K, Okamura H, Nagata K, Komatsu T, Tamura T (1993) Purification of a factor which provides a costimulatory signal for gamma interferon production. Infect Immun 61: 64–70
24. Okamura H, Nagata K, Komatsu T, et al (1995) A novel costimulatory factor for gamma interferon induction found in the livers of mice causes endotoxic shock. Infect Immun 63: 3966–3972
25. Okamura H, Tsutsui H, Komatsu T, et al (1995) Cloning of a new cytokine that induces interferon-γ. Nature 378:88–91
26. Heremans H, van Damme J, Dillen C, Dikman R, Billiau A (1990) Interferon-γ, a mediator of lethal lipopolysaccharide-induced Shwartzman-like shock in mice. J Exp Med 171: 1853–1861
27. Ushio S, Namba M, Okura T, et al (1996) Cloning of the cDNA for human IFN-γ-inducing factor, expression in Escherichia coli, and studies on the biologic activities of the protein. J Immunol 156:4274–4279
28. Robinson D, Shibuya K, Mui A, et al (1997) IGIF does not drive Th1 development but synergizes with IL-12 for interferon-γ production and activates IRAK and NFκB. Immunity 7:571–581
29. Hunter CA, Timans J, Pisacane P, et al (1997) Comparison of the effects of interleukin-1α, interleukin-1β and interferon-γ inducing factor on the production of interferon-γ by natural killer. Eur J Immunol 27:2787–2792
30. Kohno K, Kataoka J, Ohtsuki T, et al (1997) IFN-γ-inducing factor (IGIF) is a co-stimulatory factor on the activation of Th1 but not Th2 cells and exerts its effect independently of IL-12. J Immunol 158:1541-1550
31. Dao T, Ohashi K, Kayano T, Kurimoto M, Okamura H (1997) Interferon-γ-inducing factor, a novel cytokine, enhances Fas ligand-mediated cytotoxicity of murine T helper cells. Cell Immunol 173:230–235
32. Tsutsui H, Nakanishi K, Matsui K, et al (1996) IFN-γ-inducing factor up-regulates Fas ligand-mediated cytotoxic activity of murine natural killer cell clones. J Immunol 157:3967–3973
33. Ohtsuki T, Micallef MJ, Kohno K, Tanimoto T, Ikeda M, Kurimoto M (1997) Interleukin-18 enhances Fas ligand expression and induces apoptosis in Fas-expressing human myelomonocytic KG-1 cells. Anticancer Res 17:3253–3258
34. Bazan JF, Timans JC, Kaselein RA (1996) A newly defined interleukin-1? Nature 379:591
35. Udagawa N, Horwood NJ, Elliot J, et al (1997) Interleukin-18 is produced by osteoblasts and acts via granulocyte macrophage colony-stimulating factor and not via interferon-γ to inhibit osteoclast formation. J Exp Med 185:1005–1012
36. Torigoe K, Ushio S, Okura T, et al (1997) Purification and characterization of the human interleukin-18 receptor. J Biol Chem 272:25737–25742
37. Parnet P, Garka KE, Bonnert TP, Dower SK, Sims JE (1996) IL-1Rrp is a novel receptor-like molecule similar to the type I interleukin-1 receptor and its homologues T1/ST2 and IL-1R AcP. J Biol Chem 271:3967–3970
38. Thomassen E, Bird TA, Renshaw BR, Kennedy MK, Sims JE (1998) Binding of interleukin-18 to the interleukin-1 receptor homologous receptor, IL-1Rrp1 leads to activation of signaling pathways similar to those used by interleukin-1. J Interferon Cytokine Res 18:1077–1088
39. Yoshimoto T, Takeda K, Tanaka T, et al (1998) IL-12 upregulates IL-18 receptor expression on T cells, Th1 cells and B cells: synergism with IL-18 for IFN-γ production. J Immunol 161: 3400–3407
40. Born TL, Thomassen E, Bird TA, Sims JE (1998) Cloning of a novel receptor subunit, AcPL, required for interleukin-18 signaling. J Biol Chem 273:29445–29450
41. Greenfeder SA, Nunes P, Kwee L, Labow M, Chizzonite RA, Ju G (1995) Molecular cloning and characterization of a second subunit of the interleukin-1 receptor complex. J Biol Chem 270:13757–13765

42. Sims JE, Gayle MA, Slack JL, et al (1993) Interleukin-1 signaling occurs exclusively via the type I receptor. Proc Natl Acad Sci USA 90:6155–6159
43. Novick D, Kim SH, Fantuzzi G, Reznikov L, Dinarello CA, Rubinstein M (1999) Interleukin-18 binding protein: a novel modulator of the Th1 cytokine response. Immunity 10:127–136
44. Novick D, Engelmann H, Wallach D, Rubinstein M (1989) Soluble cytokine receptors are present in normal human urine. J Exp Med 170:1409–1414
45. Engelmann H, Novick D, Wallach D (1990) Two tumor necrosis factor-binding proteins purified from human urine. Evidence for immunological cross-reactivity with cell surface tumor necrosis factor receptors. J Biol Chem 265:1531–1536
46. Novick D, Cohen B, Rubinstein M (1994) The human interferon α/β receptor: characterization and molecular cloning. Cell 77:391–400
47. Novick D, Engelmann H, Wallach D, Leitner O, Revel M, Rubinstein M (1990) Purification of soluble cytokine receptors from normal human urine by ligand-affinity and immunoaffinity chromatography. J Chromat 510:331–337
48. Fantuzzi G, Puren AJ, Harding MW, Livingston DJ, Dinarello CA (1998) IL-18 regulation of IFN-γ production and cell proliferation as revealed in interleukin-1β converting enzyme-deficient mice. Blood 91:2118–2125
49. Hunter CA, Chizzonite R, Remington JS (1995) IL-1β is required for IL-12 to induce the production of IFN-γ by NK cells. J Immunol 155:4347–4354
50. Croston GE, Cao Z, Goeddel DV (1995) NFkB activation by interleukin-1 requires an IL-1 receptor-associated protein kinase activity. J Biol Chem 270:16514–16517
51. Martin MU, Falk W (1997) The interleukin-1 receptor complex and interleukin-1 signal transduction. Eur Cytokine Netw 8:5–17
52. O'Neill LAJ, Greene C (1998) Signal transduction pathways activated by the IL-1 receptor family: ancient signaling machinery in mammals, insects, and plants. J Leukoc Biol 63:650–657
53. Wesche H, Korherr C, Kracht M, Falk W, Resch K, Martin MU (1997) The interleukin-1 receptor accessory protein is essential for IL-1-induced activation of interleukin-1 receptor-associated kinase (IRAK) and stress-activated protein kinases (SAP kinases). J Biol Chem 272:7727–7731
54. Huang J, Gao X, Li S, Cao Z (1997) Recruitment of IRAK to the interleukin 1 receptor complex requires interleukin 1 receptor accessory protein. Proc Natl Acad Sci USA 94:12829–12832
55. Cao Z (1998) Signal transduction of interleukin-1. Eur Cytokine Netw 9:378 (Abst)
56. Cao Z, Xiong J, Takeuchi M, Kurama T, Goeddel DV (1996) Interleukin-1 receptor activating kinase. Nature 383:443–446
57. Malinin NL, Boldin MP, Kovalenko AV, Wallach D (1997) MAP3K-related kinase involved in NF-kappaB induction by TNF, CD95 and IL-1. Nature 385:540–544
58. DiDonato JA, Hayakawa M, Rothwarf DM, Zandi E, Karin M (1997) A cytokine-responsive I kappaB kinase that activates the transcription factor NF-kappaB. Nature 388:548–554
59. Kojima H, Takeuchi M, Ohta T, et al (1998) Interleukin-18 activates the IRAK-TRAF6 pathway in mouse EL-4 cells. Biochem Biophys Res Commun 244:183–186
60. Adachi O, Kawai T, Takeda K, et al (1998) Targeted disruption of the MyD88 gene results in loss of IL-1- and IL-18-mediated function. Immunity 9:143–150
61. Shapiro L, Puren AJ, Barton HA, et al (1998) Interleukin-18 stimulates HIV type 1 in monocytic cells. Proc Natl Acad Sci USA 95:12550–12555
62. Tsuji-Takayama K, Matsumoto S, Koide K, et al (1997) Interleukin-18 induces activation and association of p56lck and MAPK in a murine TH1 clone. Biochem Biophys Res Commun 237:126–130
63. Puren AJ, Fantuzzi G, Gu Y, Su MSS, Dinarello CA (1998) Interleukin-18 (IFN-γ-inducing factor) induces IL-1β and IL-8 via TNFα production from non-CD14+ human blood mononuclear cells. J Clin Invest 101:711–724
64. Luster AD (1998) Chemokines – chemotactic cytokines that mediate inflammation. N Engl J Med 338:436–445
65. Matsimoto S, Tsuji-Takayama K, Aizawa Y, et al (1997) Interleukin-18 activates NFkB in murine T helper type I cells. Biochem Biophys Res Commun 234:454–457

66. Mühl H, Dinarello CA (1997) Macrophage inflammatory protein-1α production from LPS-stimulated human adherent peripheral blood mononuclear cells is inhibited by the nitric oxide synthase inhibitor N^G-monomethyl-L-arginine. J Immunol 159:5063–5069
67. Kohka H, Yoshino T, Iwagaki H, et al (1998) Interleukin-18/interferon-gamma-inducing factor, a novel cytokine, up-regulates ICAM-1 (CD54) expression in KG-1 cells. J Leukoc Biol 64:519–527
68. Dao T, Mehal WZ, Crispe IN (1998) IL-18 augments perforin-dependent cytotoxicity of liver NK-T cells. J Immunol 161:2217–2222

Bacterial Toxins Induce Selective Cytokine Patterns *In Vivo* and *In Vitro*

J. Andersson and U. Andersson

Introduction

Sepsis due to Gram-negative, Gram-positive or fungal organisms is among the most common causes of death in intensive care units (ICUs) in Western society [1]. Currently, 28-day mortality in sepsis is estimated to be 20–40% depending on the etiological agent and presence of complicating medical disorders [2–6]. An even higher mortality has been associated with septic shock, affecting approximately half of the patients with sepsis. Investigations performed in patients included in recent immunomodulatory trials have estimated that 35–60% of patients with septic shock died within 28 days following onset of disease [7, 8].

Although the pathophysiology of systemic inflammation induced by sepsis and resulting in organ dysfunction is complex, cytokines, along with abnormalities of coagulation and the complement system, are probably the major mediators of endothelial damage and life-threatening inflammation. Endogenously produced cytokines have the ability to cure, or kill, the host depending on cytokine pattern and total amounts of cytokines produced. Thus, cytokines are small proteins that regulate immune activation, inflammation, cell turnover as well as cell traffic and are probably the main regulators of endothelial function and microcirculation including organ oxygenation [9–12].

Extensive *in vitro* studies, as well as animal models, have generated information about how bacterial toxins can trigger immediate production of pro-inflammatory cytokines [13–17]. However, interleukin (IL)-1, tumor necrosis factor (TNF)-α , IL-6, IL-8 and interferon (IFN)-γ detection *in vivo* in septic patients has been difficult, and significantly increased serum and plasma concentrations have only been detected in subgroups of patients [17–20]. Even if IL-1β, TNF-α and IL-6 serum concentrations indeed have been shown to correlate with prognosis in a direct way, recent studies have questioned the results and suggested that it is actually the delicate balance between expression of pro-inflammatory cytokines and counter-regulatory cytokines including IL-1 receptor antagonist (IL-1ra), IL-10, transforming growth factor (TGF)-β [21], and cationic deactivating molecules such as spermine, that determines the prognosis [22, 23]. Thus, there is always a delicate balance between pro-inflammatory mediators and counter inflammatory regulators, in addition to immunregulatory type 1 cytokines such as IFN-γ, IL-2 and TNF-β, IL-15 and IL-18 as well as type 2 cytokines IL-4, IL-5, IL-10 and IL-13.

Endogenous Cytokine Production in Blood

In health, cytokines are produced at low constitutive levels detectable at picogr/ml serum or plasma while the great majority of human cells express huge numbers of cytokine specific cell surface receptors. Invasive bacterial infections or secreted toxins may rapidly, within minutes, induce production of pro-inflammatory cytokines which in turn induce shedding of cytokine specific receptors and production of counter-regulatory cytokines [25–27]. Immunocytochemical staining using cytokine specific antibodies with neutralizing activity enables the detection of individual cytokine producing cells in peripheral blood mononuclear cells. We have determined the frequency of cytokine producing cells in the blood in 150 healthy blood donors at the single cell level. IL-1α and β as well as TNF-α producing cells have been detected at a frequency of 1:1000 to 1:5000 cells in healthy conditions. Counter-regulatory cytokines such as IL-1ra have been detected in 1:500 cells while IL-10 producing cells were present at a level of 1:5000 to 1:10000 cells [28, 29]. Type 1 (IL-2, IFN-γ, TNF-β), as well as type 2 (IL-4, IL-5, IL-13), cytokine immunoregulatory expressing cells were normally not present above frequencies of 1:5000 to 1:10000 cells in healthy conditions [28, 39]. Serum and plasma assessments have indicated that these cytokines can be identified at picogram concentrations while soluble cytokine specific receptors are detectable at 50–500 fold higher concentrations (at nanogram levels) [27]. Thus, serum normally contains excessive levels of soluble receptors in comparison to its reciprocal cytokine and has the capacity to neutralize secreted cytokines in the vascular compartment. Induction of inflammation therefore occurs within a relatively short time frame in the range of a few hours when specific cytokine concentrations temporarily increase above the levels of soluble receptors and are able to generate systemic immune activation. This is followed by elevation in the levels of soluble receptors, neutralizing the cytokine. Assays can measure free and soluble-receptor bound cytokines in serum and plasma. In addition, cytokines function in a paracrine and autocrine fashion in cell-to-cell contact and are often difficult to detect in serum and plasma. The half-life of unbound cytokines in serum or plasma is estimated to be around 2.5 to 5 minutes; they are rapidly degraded by proteolytic activity and eliminated by the renal route. It is thus debatable how cytokines should optimally be measured in disorders associated with inflammation since there are obviously many complicating factors which limit the ability to elucidate this complex signaling system via assessments of serum/plasma or circulating blood cells.

Bacterial Cytokine Induction is Compartmentalized

Measurements performed in lymphoid sites such as the spleen, lymph nodes and liver, and even lung tissue, would probably generate useful data; however, these measurements cannot generally be obtained. There is, therefore, need for improved strategies for measuring cytokines at local sites of inflammation. Such information would help us to understand the pathogenesis of invasive bacterial and fungal disorders and improve our knowledge on how immunomodulation might be adopted in the future [26, 31, 32]. Trials in patients with sepsis using immunomodulatory approaches such as IL-1ra, TNF-blockade, soluble TNF receptors or exogenous inhibitors of nitric oxide (NO) have failed to reduce mortality and have led to these immunomodulatory approaches being abandoned [2–8].

Cytokine Patterns Induced by Bacterial Toxins

Our group has studied the cytokine patterns generated by various bacterial toxins or attenuated bacteria *in vitro* and *ex vivo*, and the cytokine pattern and compartmentalization of the site of production. We have used *Escherichia coli*, endotoxin from *E.coli* and *Shigella dysenteriae* type 1, *Staphylococcus aureus* exotoxin A and B (SEA, SEB), streptococcal group A, in an attenuated form or a few of its exotoxins, streptococcal pyrogenic exotoxin A, B, C, and F (SPEA, B, C and F) as well as bacillus Calmette-Guérin (BCG), and have compared cytokine responses between these various microbial toxins. To measure cytokine producing cells at the single cell level, a carefully selected fixation and permeabilization method was developed using formaldehyde and saponin in association with cytokine specific monoclonal antibodies selected for having cytokine neutralizing activity [28, 32]. Since the majority of cytokines are secreted through the Golgi-endoplasmatic route, producer cells show accumulation of the cytokine in the Golgi organelle. This generates a specific juxtanuclear localized staining signal which is easily separated from cytokine binding cells having only a cell surface staining pattern. Quantification of cytokine producing cells has been performed by use of an *in situ* imaging technique using software that determined positive cells by morphometric and densitometric criteria and, therefore, did not need any gating for discrimination of positive or negative cell populations [33]. This technique has been adapted both for activated cells in suspension *in vitro*, as well as for cryopreserved tissue biopsies. Cytokine producing cells were assessed in a similar manner allowing for a detection sensitivity of one positive cell per 1000 cells analyzed [34]. This technique has been used for assessment of IL-1 to IL-15, TNF-α, TNF-β, IFN-α, IFN-γ, granulocyte colony-stimulating factor (G-CSF) and granulocyte/macrophage colony stimulating factor (GM-CSF), TGF-β_{1-3} as well as chemokines such as IL-8, macrophage inflammatory protein (MIP)-1α, MIP-1β and RANTES (regulated upon activation, normal T cell expressed and secreted).

Cytokine Induction by Endotoxin and Gram-Negative Bacteria

Endotoxins derived from *E.coli* or *Shigella dysenteriae* type 1 were used to stimulate peripheral blood cells from healthy blood donors, and induced expression of IL-1α, IL-1β, and TNF-α within 1 to 3 hours, followed by IL-6 and IL-8; expression of IL-10 as well as IL-12 and TGF-β occurred 6–12 h later (Fig. 1A) [26, 29]. Endotoxin induced pro-inflammatory cytokines in macrophages and monocytes

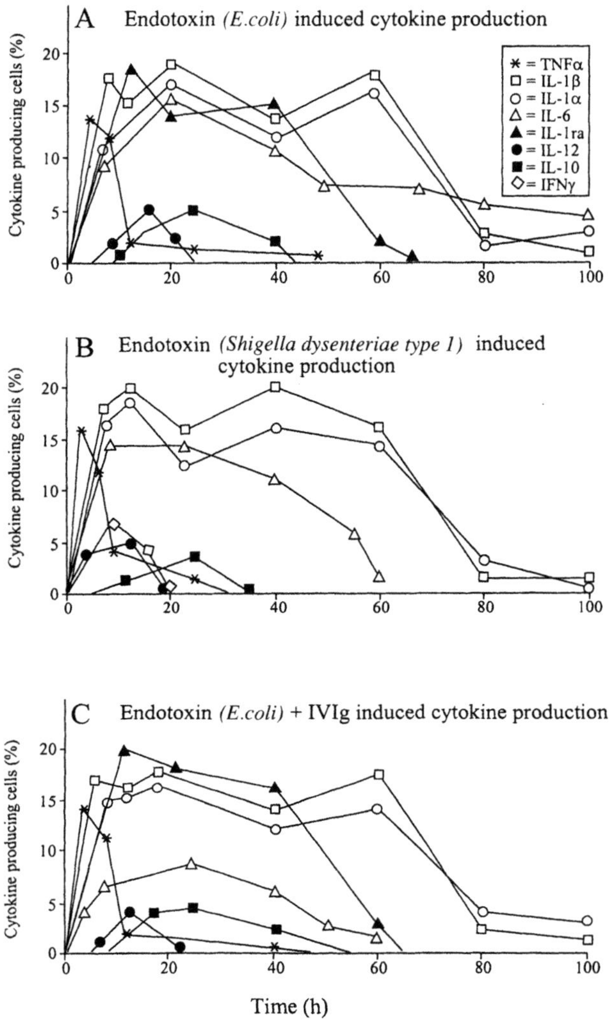

Fig. 1A–C. A kinetic study of cytokine production in peripheral blood mononuclear cells after stimulation with *E.coli*-derived LPS (**A**), or with LPS from *Shigella dysenteriae* type 1 (**B**). The cell cultures contained 15–25% monocytes and 75–85% lymphocytes. Graph A indicates that *E.coli* endotoxin induced expression of TNF-α, IL-8, IL-1α, IL-1β, IL-6, IL-12 and IL-10, in that chronological order. Unstimulated cultured peripheral blood mononuclear cells did not show increased cytokine expression for any of the studied cytokines $<0.1\%$. The cytokine pattern with *Shigella dysenteriae* type 1 endotoxin (**B**) was very similar to that induced by *E.coli*-derived LPS with the exception that IFN-γ expression in T-lymphocytes was also induced. **C** illustrates the immunomodulating effects of IVIg on LPS (*E.coli*) induced cytokine production in peripheral blood mononuclear cells. All cytokine producing cells were monocytes as judged by two color staining with a monocyte marker. The cytokine pattern overall was almost identical to that found when stimulating the peripheral blood mononuclear cells with endotoxin without IVIg, with the exception that the incidence of IL-6 expressing cells was significantly down-regulated in the IVIg treated peripheral blood mononuclear cell cultures ($p<0.01$). Each cytokine has a specific label as indicated in the box throughout the figure with the exception of lipopolysaccharide (LPS) derived from *Shigella dysenteriae* type 1 which also induced IFN-γ production in T-lymphocytes (Fig. 1B) [35]. Stimulation of epithelial cells from renal and uroepithelial mucosa with LPS resulted in excessive IL-1α, IL-1β, IL-6 and IL-8 expression while the production of TNF-α was absent or expressed at a frequency below 1% (Fig. 2) [36]. In contrast,

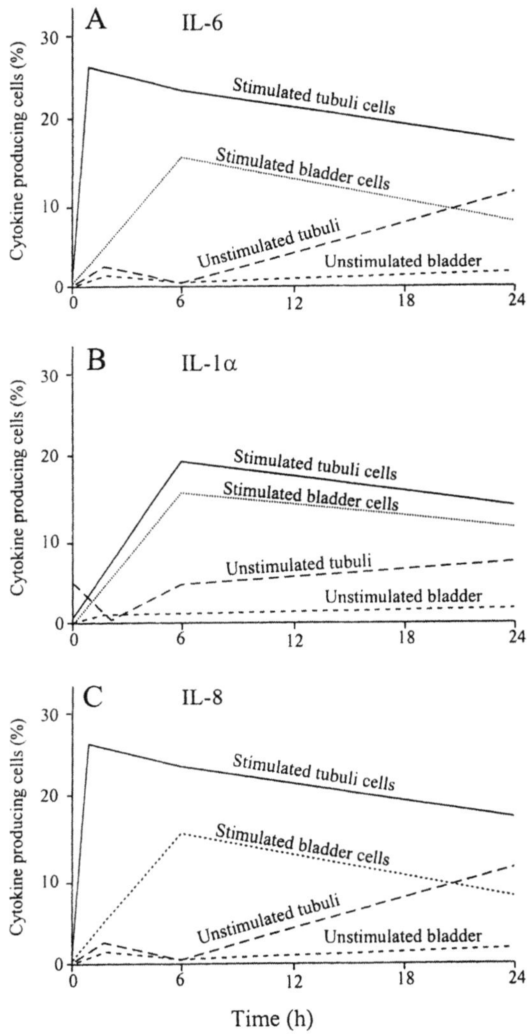

Fig. 2. Selective induction of cytokine expression, IL-6 (**A**), IL-1α (**B**) and IL-8 (**C**) after challenge with *E.coli*, Hu734, in human urinary tract epithelial cells. Assessments were performed at the single cell level by use of an indirect immunofluorescence technique and cytokine specific monoclonal antibodies. The incidence of cytokine producing cells were compared between *E.coli* challenged cells and cultured unstimulated tubuli and bladder epithelial cells. Significant induction of IL-6, IL-1α and IL-8 ($p<0.01$) were noticed for both tubuli and bladder epithelial

no cytokine expression occurred in colon epithelial cells when exposed to the same LPS. Thus, endotoxin has the ability to induce cytokine production in specific epithelial cells.

Lack of Endotoxin Neutralizing Antibodies in Serum

In order to determine whether LPS neutralizing antibodies are present in normal serum, cells were activated in the presence of 100% AB-serum by endotoxin; a similar cytokine pattern as described above was seen. In addition, we have tested lots of pooled human IgG from various commercial sources (IVIg) and have never detected any significant LPS-neutralizing efficacy even when added in Ig-concentrations from 1 up to 10 mg/ml. No inhibition of IL-1α, β, TNF or IL-8 could be identified (Fig 1C) [37]. However, we noticed a significant drop in the frequency of IL-6 producing cells [37]. These results would suggest that biological neutralizing antibodies to endotoxin derived from various *E.coli* strains do not occur in normal human IgG (Fig. 1C).

Cytokine Production *in Vivo* in Gram-Negative Infections

We have compared IL-1 and TNF-α serum or plasma levels in patients suffering from Gram-negative septicemia with those of patients with Gram-positive bacteremia, and found significantly higher levels of IL-1β and TNF-α in patients with Gram-negative sepsis ($p<0.01$) [38]. We have also analyzed cytokine patterns in 30 patients with invasive *Shigella dysenteriae* type 1 infection. IL-1β and TNF-α were detectable throughout the initial 1-4 days of disease followed by a late increase in IFN-γ (after 5 days) while most other cytokines analyzed (IL-4, IL-5, IL-12, IL-13) could not be found to be increased in serum or plasma [25]. In contrast, stool analysis revealed a different pattern with an initial 10–100 fold increase of TNF-α, IL-1β, IL-6, and IL-4. IFN-γ production again occurred at later time-points (day 7-30) than that of the pro-inflammatory cytokines [25]. In colon biopsies we found persistently increased IL-1β, IL-1α, TNF-α, IL-6, IL-2 in addition to IL-4 and IL-10 responses [26]. IFN-γ producing cells were not increased before day 7 while TGF-β was significantly elevated throughout the study period (30 days). These data indicate that the pro-inflammatory cytokines were initially shed predominantly in the mucosal site with some spill-over to serum and plasma and that the immunoregulatory cytokines were predominantly found at the local site of infection [25]. The delayed induction of IFN-γ may be a pathogenic factor contributing to the persistence and spread of the intracellular *Shigella* bacteria reducing the capacity of the macrophages to kill the invasive bacterial infection [39]. Furthermore, attenuated *Hemophilus influenzae* were incubated with mononuclear cells isolated from tonsil tissue from patients suffering from tonsillar hyperplasia. These cells could also be induced to express IL-1, TNF, IL-6, IL-8 as well as low levels of IL-2, IFN-γ and IL-4, a predominantly inflammatory and type 1 cytokine response, although IL-4 and IL-10 producing cells were also evident [40].

Cytokine Synthesis Analyzed at the Single-Cell Level Before and After Revaccination with Tetanus Toxoid

Tetanus toxoid (TT) is a potent immunogen which evokes strong antibody responses after immunization. TT was used as a model bacterial antigen to study the production of cytokines at the single cell level during an *in vitro* immune response. Peripheral blood mononuclear cells were obtained from healthy volunteers before and 9 weeks after *in vivo* TT vaccination and were cultured with antigen *in vitro*. The kinetics of cytokine synthesis as well as frequencies of cytokine-producing cells were determined at the single cell level by immunofluorescent intracellular staining of the cytokine protein. The phenotype of the producer cells was determined by concomitant staining of surface markers.

Two patterns of cytokine synthesis were induced by TT. T-lymphocytes expressed a number of lymphokines (IL-2, IL-3, IL-4, IL-19, IFN-γ and TNF-β), each with distinct kinetics of synthesis. This cytokine expression was strictly dependent on previous exposure of the donor to TT and positively correlated with the level of tetanus immunity, as judged by TT-specific antibody levels in plasma as well as antigen-driven lymphoproliferation. Cells producing IL-2, IFN-γ and particularly TNF-β, dominated this *in vitro* response. The frequencies of TT-specific cytokine producing cells (IL-2, IL-3, IL-4, TNF-β) obtained prior to re-immunization were always below 1/1000 T-cells [30]. Much higher incidences were noticed in peripheral blood mononuclear cells obtained 9 weeks after revaccination and after 96–120 hours in culture; 1.0–1.3% of the cells produced TNF-β frequencies at least 10-fold higher than for any of the other lymphokines assayed (Fig. 3). The cytokines IL-1α, IL-1β, IL-6 and TNFα were produced by monocytes. This inflammatory monokine response was independent of the TT-specific immune status of the donors, was characterized by a rapid onset and was transient.

Induction of Cytokines by Exotoxins Derived from *Staph. Aureus* or Streptococcal Group A Bacteria

Cytokine Production in Experimental Models

In experimental models, peripheral blood mononuclear cells *in vitro* stimulated by SEA or SEB, or by SPEA, B, C and F, all generated a very complex immune response [29]. In addition to a gradual onset of expression of pro-inflammatory cytokines, predominantly IL-1β but also TNF-α and IL-6, excessive IFN-γ, TNF-β and IL-2 induction was noticed with a similar pattern for all these exotoxins (Fig. 4A) [41]. All toxins also induced IL-12 production. These protein toxins thus generated a type 1 cytokine response plus a pro-inflammatory cytokine response that persisted for up to three days following one course of stimulation [42]. When these cells were re-stimulated with the same exotoxin for at least three times, we noticed a gradual decrease in the number of cells that expressed IL-2, IFN-γ and TNF-β, while IL-4 and IL-10 expressing cells emerged at an increased frequency. Most of these exotoxins have superantigenic properties and can therefore induce

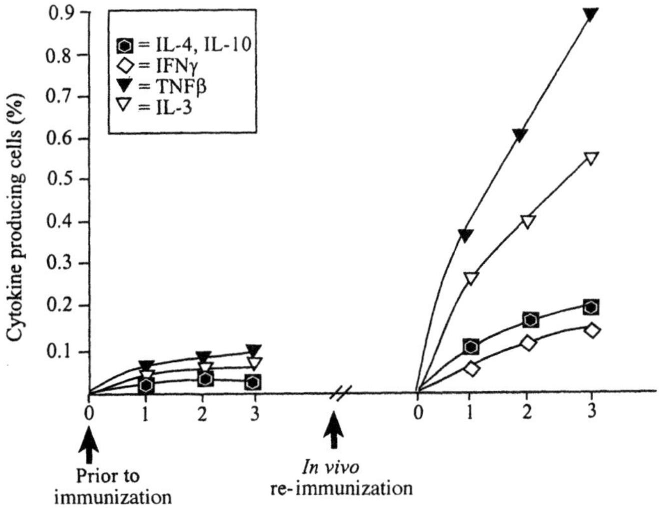

Fig. 3. A kinetic study of cytokine production at the single cell level in peripheral blood mononuclear cells stimulated with tetanus toxoid (TT). Cytokine producing cells were determined by indirect immunofluorescent staining by use of cytokine specific monclonal antibodies. Approximately 10,000 cells were counted for each single cytokine. Peripheral blood mononuclear cells were collected before (day 0) and after (week 3) vaccination *in vivo* with TT and cultured in the presence of 50 ng/ml TT. Cells were harvested after 24, 48 and 72 hours of culture and assessed for cytokine expression. Prior to TT immunization the incidence of all the studied cytokine producing cells was below 1/1000. In contrast, a significant induction of TNF-β, IL-3, IL-4, IL-10 and IFN-γ expressing cells was noticed after *in vitro* re-stimulation of peripheral blood mononuclear cells obtained after *in vivo* immunization with TT

up to 30% of all T-cells to express cytokines. It is known that these exotoxins interact with antigen presenting cells, major histocompatibility complex (MHC) class II and the Vβ part of the T-cell receptor on lymphocytes inducing cytokine production in both cell types.

Exotoxin-Induced Cytokine Production *in Vivo*

We have also injected SEA or SEB intraperitoneally in healthy mice and studied the induction of cytokine production *in vivo*. We initially found cytokine producing cells at the local inguinal lymph nodes as well as in the spleen (Fig. 4B and C). The cytokine pattern completely overlapped that found after stimulation of human peripheral blood mononuclear cells *in vitro* [31,43]. Thus, both SEA and SEB-induced IL-1, TNF-α and lymphocytes of particular $CD4^+$ and $CD8^+$ cells contributed to the cytokine cascade [31, 43]. Initially CD4 cells produced TNF-α and the type 1 cytokines, but beyond 24 hours of stimulation, $CD8^+$ cells also contributed in increasing frequencies. SPEA stimulation of epithelial cells from the urinary tract mucosa did not result in any cytokine production at all. Thus, *Staph. aureus* and streptococcal group A exotoxin induced cytokine production in immunocompetent cells, predominantly the antigen presenting cells and T-cells.

Cytokines in Invasive Streptococcal Infection: Importance of Neutralizing Antibodies

Assessments of biopsy specimens obtained from patients with invasive streptococcal group A infection, indicate that IL-1β and TNF-α are rapidly expressed at the site of infection, but are overwhelmed by excessive IFN-γ and IL-2 producing cells. Two observations suggest that locally produced toxins with superantigenic properties may have an important pathogenic role in these disorders (Fig. 4).

Cells from healthy blood donors showed large inter-individual variations in the frequency of responder cells following SPEA, SPEC as well as SEA and SEB stimulation [29, 44]. The TNF-α producing cells were predominantly $CD4^+$ and $CD8^+$ T-cells with less than 40% of the TNF producing cells being macrophages. We therefore investigated the ability of serum to neutralize the biologic activity of the superantigens. Indeed patients with invasive streptococcal group A infectious diseases were all characterized by a selective lack of neutralizing capacity against at least one of the superantigens despite the fact that enzyme-linked immunosorbent assay (ELISA) assessments of serum showed that all patients had detectable antibodies [45, 46]. In addition, supplementation of IVIg resulted in a significant decrease in IL-2, IFN-γ and TNF-β producing cells *in vitro* even if IVIg was added up to 24 hours after superantigenic stimulation of peripheral blood mononuclear cells (Fig. 5) [47]. Thus, IgG has important biological toxin neutralizing capacity and may protect individuals from severe systemic manifestations of *Staph. aureus* and streptococcal group A infections; IVIg may be of clinical benefit in life threatening invasive disorders with *Staph. aureus* or streptococcal group A [48]. We have therefore recently initiated a placebo controlled trial 'StreptIg001' of IVIg treatment in patients with invasive life threatening streptococcal group A infection.

A different cytokine pattern was evident in cryopreserved tissue from tonsil biopsies obtained from peri-tonsillitis. An extensive pro-inflammatory cytokine pattern (IL-1, TNF-α, IL-6, IL-8, GM-CSF), but no induction of IL-2, IFN-γ or TNF-β, was found (Fig. 6).

Cytokine Pattern Induced by BCG Immunization

We obtained peripheral blood mononuclear cells from healthy adult individuals vaccinated against tuberculosis by BCG during childhood. We noticed a very complex interaction between pro- and counter-regulatory cytokine responses initially characterized by pro-inflammatory cytokines such as IL-1, TNF and IL-6 followed by extensive production of IL-2, IFN-γ and TNF-β (Fig. 7). This was re-

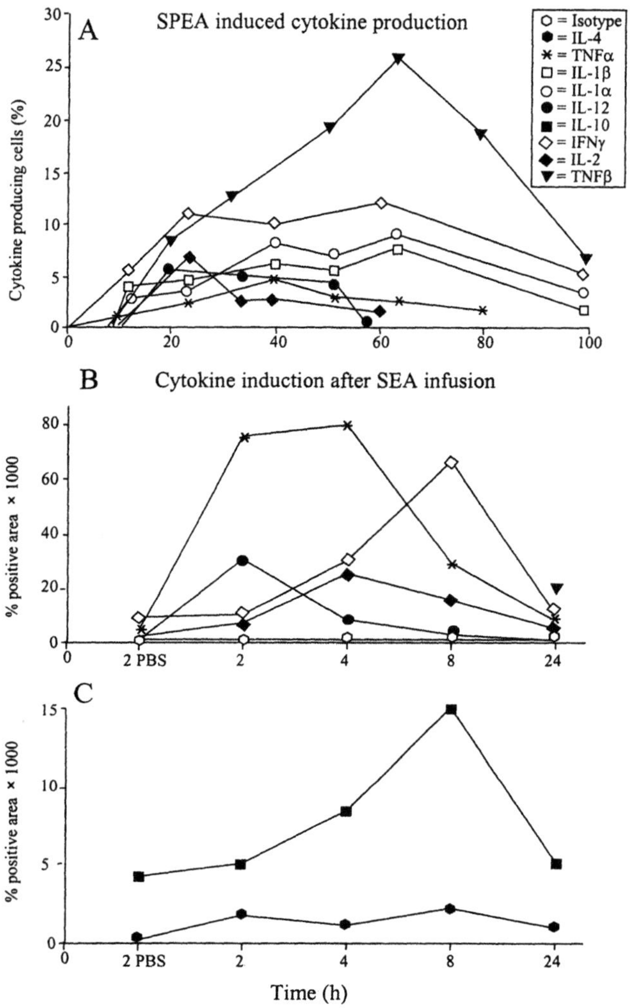

versed after the seventh day of culture, reverting to a type 2 cytokine pattern with dominance of IL-4, IL-10 and IL-13, and extensive expression of TGF-β and IL-1ra, in association with a reduction in the number of IL-1 and TNF-α expressing cells [49]. This dichotomy of type 1 and type 2 responses has not been noticed for any other microbial toxins tested so far and may indicate that the attenuated *Mycobacterium bovis* secretes various toxins or immunoregulatory proteins at different time points. It may reflect that this intracellular pathogen circumvents type 1 up-regulated macrophage killing of the bacteria via induction of IL-4 and IL-10 which may counteract a generation of oxygen radicals, and by this means inhibits immune response-mediated elimination of this intracellular pathogen. Stimulation by BCG in the presence of IVIg resulted in reduced TNF-α, IL-2, IFN-γ and

Fig. 4. A The graph illustrates a kinetic study of cytokine expression in peripheral blood mononuclear cells after stimulation with streptococcal pyrogenic exotoxin A (SPEA). The mean values of 5 separate experiments are shown. The cell culture contained 15–20% monocytes and 80–85% lymphocytes. The incidence of cytokine producing cells was determined at the single cell level by use of an indirect immunohistochemical technique and approximately 2000 cells were counted for each specific cytokine. SPEA predominantly induced TNF-β and IFN-γ expression in a huge number of T-lymphocytes as revealed by two color staining. In addition, IL-1 was extensively induced in monocytes while TNF-α was found both in T-lymphocytes as well as in monocytes. Cells were harvested at indicated time periods following stimulation with SPEA. **B** and **C** Computerized image assessments of cytokine production at the single cell level in cryopreserved spleen tissue sections obtained from mice injected with Staphyloccus enterotoxin A (SEA) in the foot pad. The graphs illustrate the cytokine expression pattern obtained within 2–24 h after immunization with SEA. Initially an extensive TNF-α expression was followed by IL-12, IFN-γ and IL-2 expression. IL-4 and IL-10 expression occurred later with a peak after 8 h of stimulation, however at significantly lower incidences when compared to pro-inflammatory and type 1 cytokines. At this time-point pro-inflammatory as well as type 1 cytokine induction was significantly down-regulated. Thus, SEA was characterized by pro-inflammatory and type 1 cytokine responses followed by a significantly less prominent type 2 cytokine pattern, and the incidence of cytokine producing cells was virtually normalized within 24 hours following primary stimulation. The incidence of cytokine expressing cells following SEA exposure was compared with animals exposed to phosphate buffered saline (PBS) which did not induce any significant cytokine expression

TNF-β expressing cells (Fig. 7B) [48]. The inhibition was not as extensive as that noticed for *Staph. aureus* and streptococcal group A exotoxins. Thus, neutralizing antibodies may affect the immune response following BCG and may have a protective importance, although not to the extent noticed for Gram-positive exotoxins. This may indicate that cellular immune mediated responses are much more important in *Mycobacterium tuberculosis* infections than the humoral response once the infection has been established (Fig. 7).

Differences in Gram-Negative and Gram-Positive Immune Responses

One may speculate about the clinical importance of various microbial toxins and how they induce various cytokine patterns and compartmentalization of cytokine producing cells. The current results indicate that endotoxin, in particular, generates a pro-inflammatory cytokine production in macrophages, monocytes, and epithelial cells, and activates granulocytes, contributing to the pro-inflammatory cytokine pool (Table 1). Gram-negative organisms predominantly multiply at mucosal sites where the ability of IgG antibodies to block endotoxin-mediated immune activation is limited. In invasive Gram-negative infection endotoxin may directly activate monocytes/macrophages and endothelial cells for rapid induction of pro-inflammatory cytokines at this site [50, 51]. This would explain why Gram-negative infections are characterized by excessive and measurable levels of IL-1β and TNF-α, the two major cytokines in the development of septic shock [1–6]. Since IgG do not seem to be of vital importance in the neutralization of the biologic activity of endotoxin, other endogenous immune modulatory

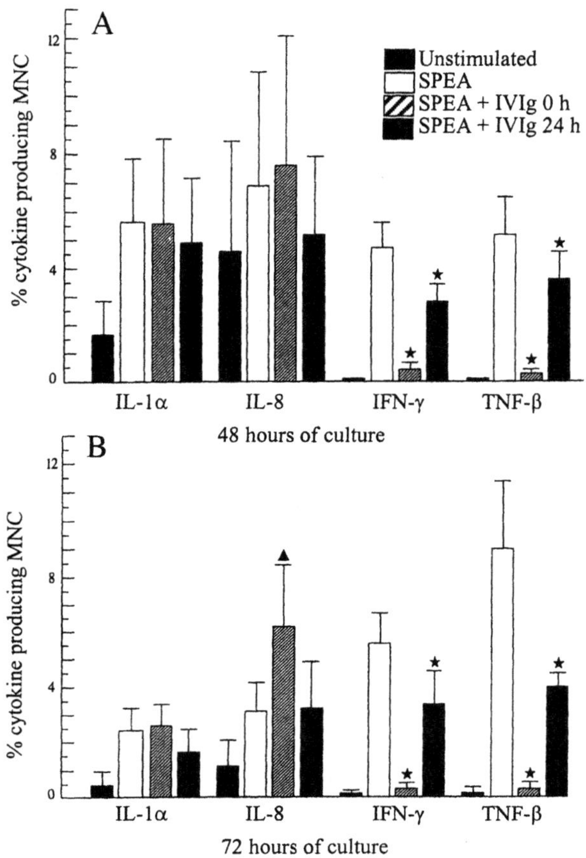

Fig. 5A, B. The frequency of cytokine producing cells after streptococcal pyrogenic exotoxin A (SPEA) stimulation alone or in the presence of IVIg (5 mg/ml). The top panel (**A**) shows the results after 48 hours of culture and the lower panel (**B**) after 72 hours of culture. IVIg was added either prior to simulation (0 h) or 24 hours after initiation of the cultures. Statistically significant inhibition of cytokine production is indicated by * ($p<0.05$, student's t-test). Data represent mean ± SD of seven experiments with different donors. The results are given as the percentage of positive cells per total number of cells counted (4000 cells for each cytokine). Unstimulated cells were used as a negative control for each time-point. The filled triangles indicate a significant induction of a specific cytokine expression by IVIg. The graph illustrates that the IVIg indeed were able to suppress cytokine expression even when added 24 hours after SPEA stimulation

mechanisms (bacterial/permeability-increasing protein [BPI], spermine, cationic deactivating proteins) are probably of greater importance [21–23]. Indeed, BPI can block LPS and LPS binding protein (LBP) complexes, preventing attachment to signaling receptors on macrophages and epithelial cells. Anti-inflammatory cytokines such as TGF-β, IL-10, IL-11 as well as prostaglandin E2 (PGE2) and spermine, may be of central importance in deactivating the macrophage and normalizing the inflammatory induction. Thus, exogenous addition of spermine,

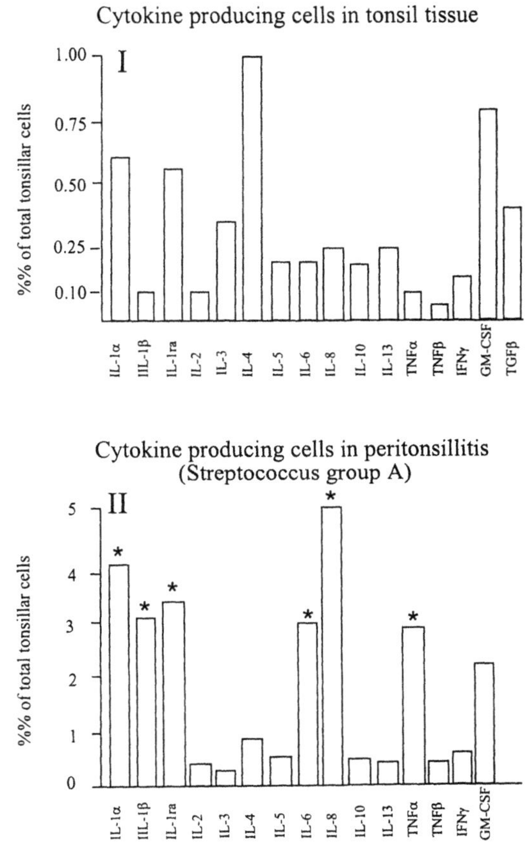

Fig. 6. The bars represent cytokine expression in cryopreserved tonsillar tissue assessed by computerized imaging of immunohistochemically stained tissue. (**I**) are mean values of four biopsies from patients with tonsillar hyperplasia and (**II**) represents assessments of three biopsies from patients with peritonsillitis. Significant induction of IL-1α, IL-1β, TNF-α, IL-6 and IL-8 was found as compared with tonsillar hyperplasia (* indicates $p < 0.01$)

PGE2 or interference with the induction of excessive NO production may be of more central clinical importance than direct inactivation of IL-1 and TNF-α in Gram-negative invasive infections [22, 23]. Previous clinical trials using IL-1ra or antibodies to human TNF-α in addition to use of soluble p55 type 1 TNF receptors have not been successful [8]. Even institution of anti-TNF antibodies within 12 hours of the onset of septic shock has not been able to provide a significant reduction in mortality rates within 28 days following the onset of disease [7]. This may be due to the extremely rapid induction of TNF-α and IL-1 production *in vivo* through the direct interaction between LPS and its target cells without requiring the contribution of other immunocompetent cells. Pooled human IgG will obviously not have the capacity to block endotoxin-mediated immune activation. It remains to be investigated whether more late-acting macrophage deactivating substances, such as the cationic macrophage deactivating factor, spermine, could actually affect prognosis in septic shock conditions. The tetravalent guanylhydrazone CNI-1493, is a synthetic molecule, with overlapping activity to that of spermine, having a significant inhibitory effect on TNF-α synthesis [52]. This molecule has the unique property of inhibiting macrophage activation even in the

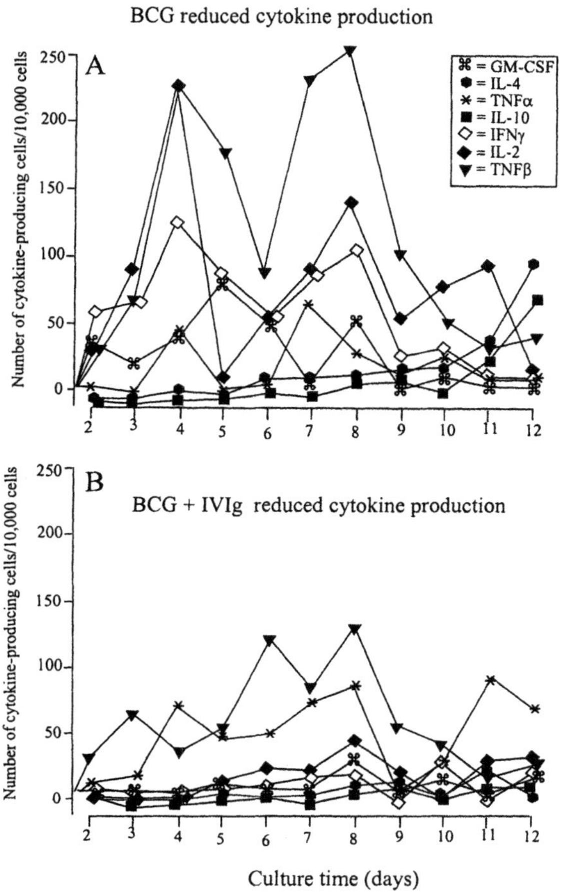

Fig. 7A, B. A kinetic study of cytokine production in peripheral blood mononuclear cells co-cultured with live attenuated *Mycobacterium bovis* (BCG). **A** The graph represents results from BCG stimulated cultures. The incidence of cytokine producing cells was determined by an indirect immunofluorescence technique and use of cytokine specific monoclonal antibodies. Approximately 2000 cells were counted for each specific cytokine. The data represents 1/7 experiments which all gave basically similar results. The cell cultures contained 10–20% monocytes and 80–90% lymphocytes. BCG initially induced type-1 cytokine responses with the biphasic kinetic response which was later followed by induction of IL-4 and IL-10. Cells were harvested daily for 12 days and assessed for incidence of cytokine expressing cells. The peripheral blood mononuclear cells were obtained from adult healthy blood donors who had experienced BCG vaccination in childhood. **B** The graph represents BCG stimulation of the same donor in the presence of IVIg 5 mg/ml. A significant inhibition of the number of cytokine expressing cells was evident for IL-2, IFN-γ, TNF-β and GM-CSF and also for IL-4 and IL-5 ($p < 0.01$). However, no suppression of TNF-α expression occurred

presence of IFN-γ induced macrophage migration inhibitory factor (MIF) production and has the capacity to override IFN-γ mediated up-regulation of macrophage activity [53]. Thus, in contrast to steroids, CNI-1493 may inhibit macrophage activation and cytokine production even in the presence of large amounts of IFN-γ and MIF [52].

The *in vitro* experiments, as well as results from animal models and the relatively limited information from clinical observations in *Staph. aureus* and streptococcal group A infection, would indicate that these bacteria have a different pathogenetic role in the induction of septic shock. These conditions seem to be associated with the production of exotoxins in susceptible individuals who lack exotoxin-neutralizing antibodies [45, 46]. The T-cell compartments in lymphoid sites and spleen may be central sites for the induction of cytokines, characterized by a gradual onset of pro-inflammatory cytokines as well as IL-2, IFN-γ and TNF-β (Table 1). In order to control the pathogenic mechanisms induced by these two bacterial agents, molecules which are actually distributed to lymphoid sites may be necessary. Since IFN-γ is induced very rapidly, and early in the clinical event, steroids may not be efficacious. However, studies using IVIg indicate that neutralizing antibodies may inhibit type 1 cytokine production even if IVIg is given up to 24 hours after the initiation of inflammatory responses [48]. Humoral immune responses seem to be of central importance in the protection and regulation of inflammatory responses indicated by streptococcal group A or *Staph. aureus* exotoxins. Even if the recently published NORASEPT II trial, using neutralizing antibodies to TNF [7], did not show that blockade of TNF was of superior clinical significance in Gram-positive versus Gram-negative infections, a prior trial (INTERSEPT) indicated that a subgroup of Gram-positive infections may have a better response to blockade of TNF as compared to Gram-negative infections [38]. This may be due to the more gradual onset of TNF-α production in Gram-positive sepsis compared to Gram-negative septicemia. Indeed, measurement of plasma nitrate in the recently finished NG-methyl-L-arginine (LNMA) study (affecting NO synthesis) showed two different kinetic curves for NO induction. Nitrate production was much more inhibited by LMNA in Gram-positive infections as compared to Gram-negative infections, highlighting how different cytokine patterns and compartmentalization may affect the net outcome in NO produc-

Table 1. Illustration of the different cytokine patterns in human monocytes and T-lymphocytes induced by lipopolysaccharide (LPS) or streptococcal pyrogenic exotoxin A (SPEA)

Cytokine	LPS#	SPEA
	% of monocytes expressing cytokines*	
IL-1β	70–90	5–10
TNF-α	60–80	10–20
IL-6	60–80	5–10
	% of T-lymphocytes expressing cytokines*	
IL-2	0	2–8
IFN-γ	0–1	10–20
TNF-β	0	10–25

* The frequencies of cytokine expressing cells were determined by *in situ* imaging at the single cell level following 72 hours of *in vitro* culture of peripheral blood mononuclear cells.
# LPS = endotoxin from *E.coli* serotype 0128.B12.

tion. Far too little scientific interest has focused on the differences in pathogenesis between Gram-negative and Gram-positive infections and we speculate that, in fact, various pathogens will have to be dealt with individually in order to affect outcome in invasive diseases.

The enormously complex cytokine pattern induced by BCG exposure to peripheral blood mononuclear cells from previously vaccinated individuals may be a reflection of attenuated bacteria secreting a vast pool of various toxins which activate various pathways of the cytokine signaling system and would indicate that the immune response is not synchronized, at least not *in vitro*, following immunization with this bacterial pathogen [49]. Thus, in addition to anti-tuberculous therapy, synchronization and induction of type 1 cytokine responses may be of central importance in generating a better cure to tuberculosis.

Conclusion

We now have available tools to study immunopathogenesis based on bacterial etiology. However, assessments of blood and serum must be combined with local tissue approaches and studies of cytokine production at the single cell level in order to understand pathogenic mechanisms. Immunomodulation likely needs to be more focused on specific pathogens; emphasizing the need for rapid diagnostic tests, perhaps based on gene detection assays or bacterial cell wall constituents (peptidoglycan and endotoxin) in order to tailor treatment to each specific agent. A great deal of work is ahead of us!

Acknowledgments. The authors would like to thank Lena Radler for excellent technical assistance. We are grateful for the donation of cytokine-specific antibodies from Drs. J. Abrams, G. Adolf, M. Ceska, and H. Towbin. This work was supported by grants from Baxter Healthcare Corporation, the National Cancer Institute (grants No. 2490 and 2766), the Medical Research Council (grants No. 09082 and 10850) and the von Kantzow Foundation.

References

1. Parrillo JE, Parker MM, Natanson C, et al (1990) Septic shock in humans. Advances in the understanding of pathogenesis, cardiovascular dysfunction, and therapy. Ann Intern Med 113:227–242
2. Bone RC, Fisher CJ Jr, Clemmer TP, Slotman GJ, Metz CA, Balk RA (1987) A controlled clinical trial of high-dose methylprednisolone in the treatment of severe sepsis and septic shock. N Engl J Med 317:653–658
3. The HA-1A Sepsis Study Group (1991) Treatment of gram negative bacteremia and septic shock with HA-1A human monoclonal antibody against endotoxin: a randomized, double-blind placebo-controlled trial. N Engl J Med 324:429–436
4. Parillo JE (1991) Management of septic shock: present and future. Ann Intern Med 115: 491–493
5. Sands KE, Bates DW, Lanken PN, et al for the Academic Medical Center Consortium Sepsis Project Working Group (1997) Epidemiology of sepsis syndrome in 8 academic medical centers. JAMA 278:234–240

6. Rangel-Frausto MS, Pitter D, Costigan M, Hwang T, Davis CS, Wenzel RP (1996) The natural history of the systemic inflammatory response syndrome (SIRS): a prospective study. JAMA 273:117–123
7. Abraham E, Anzueto A, Gutierrez G, et al (1998) Double-blind randomised controlled trial of monoclonal antibody to human tumour necrosis factor in treatment of septic shock. Lancet 351:929–933
8. Abraham E, Glauser MP, Butler T, et al for the Ro 45-2081 Study Group (1997) p55 tumor necrosis factor receptor fusion protein in the treatment of patients with severe sepsis and septic shock. A randomized controlled multicenter trial. JAMA 277:1531–1538
9. Chaves-Carballo E, Bouchama A (1998) A role for cytokines in toxic shock syndrome? J Pediatr 133:169–175
10. Myers PR, Parker JL, Tanner MA, Adams HR (1994) Effects of cytokines tumor necrosis factor alpha and interleukin 1 beta on endotoxin-mediated inhibition of endothelium-derived relaxing factor bioactivity and nitric oxide production in vascular endothelium. Shock 1:73–78
11. Griffin GE (1988) Cytokines involved in human septic shock – the model of the Jarisch-Herxheimer reaction. J Antimicrob Chemother 41 (Suppl A):25–29
12. Shapiro L, Gelfand JA (1993) Cytokines and sepsis: pathophysiology and therapy. New Horiz 1:13–22
13. Standiford TJ, Strieter RM (1992) TNF and IL-1 in sepsis: good cytokines gone bad. J Lab Clin Med 120:179–180
14. Calandra T, Gerain J, Heumann D, Baumgartner JD, Glauser MP for the Swiss-Dutch J5 Immunoglobulin Study Group (1991) High circulating levels of interleukin-6 in patients with septic shock: evolution during sepsis, prognostic value, and interplay with other cytokines. Am J Med 91:23–29
15. Dinarello CA (1991) The proinflammatory cytokines interleukin-1 and tumor necrosis factor and treatment of the septic shock syndrome. J Infect Dis 163:1177–1184
16. Waage A, Brandtzaeg P, Halstensen A, Kierulf P, Espevik T (1989) The complex pattern of cytokines in serum from patients with meningococcal septic shock. Association between interleukin 6, interleukin 1, and fatal outcome. J Exp Med 169:333–338
17. Tracey KJ, Cerami A (1989) Cachectin/tumor necrosis factor and other cytokines in infectious disease. Curr Opin Immunol 1:454–461
18. Dofferhoff AS, Bom VJ, de Vries-Hospers HG, et al (1992) Patterns of cytokines, plasma endotoxin, plasminogen activator inhibitor, and acute-phase proteins during the treatment of severe sepsis in humans. Crit Care Med 20:185–192
19. Endo S, Inada K, Inoue Y, et al (1992) Two types of septic shock classified by the plasma levels of cytokines and endotoxin. Circ Shock 38:264–274
20. Martin C, Saux P, Mege JL, Perrin G, Papazian L, Gouin F (1994) Prognostic values of serum cytokines in septic shock. Intensive Care Med 20:272–277
21. van Dissel JT, van Langervelde P, Westendorp RGJ, Kwappenberg K, Frölich M (1998) Anti-inflammatory cytokine profile and mortality in febrile patients. Lancet 351:950–953
22. Zhang M, Caragine T, Wang H et al (1997) Spermine inhibits proinflammatory cytokine synthesis in human mononuclear cells: a counterregulatory mechanism that restrains the immune response. J Exp Med 185:1759–1768
23. Wang H, Zhang M, Soda K, Sama A, Tracey KJ (1997) Fetuin protects the fetus from TNF. Lancet 350:861–862
24. Bone RC (1997) Important new findings in sepsis. JAMA 278:249–255
25. Raqib R, Wretlind B, Andersson J, Lindberg AA (1995) Cytokine secretion in acute shigellosis is correlated to disease activity and detected more in stool than in plasma. J Infect Dis 171:376–384
26. Raqib R, Lindberg AA, Wretlind B, Bardhan PK, Andersson U, Andersson J (1995) Persistence of local cytokine production in shigellosis in acute and convalescent stages. Infect Immun 63:289–296
27. Raqib R. Lindberg AA, Björk L, et al (1995) Down-regulation of gamma interferon, tumor necrosis factor type I, interleukin 1 (IL-1) type I, IL-3, IL-4, and transforming growth factor β type I receptors at the local site during the acute phase of Shigella infection. Infect Immun 63:3079–3087

28. Sander B, Andersson J, Anderson U (1991) Assessment of cytokines by immunofluorescence and the paraformaldehyde-saponin procedure. Immunol Rev 119:65–93
29. Andersson J, Nagy S, Björk L, Brams J, Holm S, Andersson U (1992) Bacterial toxin-induced cytokine production studied at the single-cell level. Immunol Rev 127:69–96
30. Fernandez V, Andersson J, Andersson U, Troye-Blomberg M (1994) Cytokine synthesis analyzed at the single-cell level before and after revaccination with tetanus toxoid. Eur J Immunol 24:1808–1815
31. Litton MJ, Dohlsten M, Lando PA, et al (1996) Antibody-targeted superantigen therapy induces tumor-infiltrating lymphocytes, excessive cytokine production, and apoptosis in human colon carcinoma. Eur J Immunol 26:1–9
32. Andersson J, Abrams J, Björk L, et al (1994) Concomitant *in vivo* production of 19 different cytokines in human tonsils. Immunology 83:16–24
33. Björk L, Fehniger T, Andersson U, Andersson J (1996) Computerized assessment of production of multiple human cytokines at the single cell level using image analysis. J Leukoc Biol 59:287–293
34. Andersson U, Litton MJ, Fehniger T, Ulfgren A-K, Andersson J (1999) Detection and quantification of cytokine-producing cells by immunostaining. In: Patterson B (ed) Molecular probes for cytokine and gene detection. CRC press, Chicago (in press)
35. Raqib R, Gustafsson A, Andersson J, Bakheit M (1997) A systemic downregulation of IFNγ production is associated with susceptibility to Shigellosis. Infect Immunity 65:5338–5341
36. Agace W, Hedges S, Andersson U, Andersson J, Ceska M, Svanborg C (1993) Selective cytokine production by epithelial cells following exposure to *Escherichia coli*. Infect Immunity 61:602–609
37. Andersson JP, Andersson UG (1990) Human intravenous immunoglobulin modulates monokine production in vitro. Immunology 71:372–376
38. Cohen J, Carlet J for the International Sepsis Trial Study Group (1996) INTERSEPT: An international multicentre placebo-controlled trial of monoclonal antibody to human tumor necrosis factor-alpha in patients with sepsis. Crit Care Med 24:1431–1440
39. Raqib R, Wretlind B, Lindberg AA, Ljungdahl Å, Andersson J (1996) Pathogenesis and immune responses in shigellosis. In: Microbial Pathogenesis and Immune Response II. Ann NY Acad Sci 797:299–302
40. Ågren K, Brauner A, Andersson J (1998) *Haemophilus influenzae* and *Streptococcus pyogenes group A* challenge induce of Th1 type of cytokine response in cells obtained from tonsillar hypertrophy and recurrent tonsillitis. ORL J Otorhinolaryngol Relat Spec 60:35–41
41. Björk L, Andersson J, Ceska M, Andersson U (1992) Endotoxin and Staphylococcus aureus enterotoxin A induce different patterns of cytokines. Cytokine 4:513–519
42. Norrby-Teglund A, Norgren M, Holm SE, Andersson U, Andersson J (1994) Similar cytokine induction profiles of a novel streptococcal exotoxin, MF, and pyrogenic exotoxin A and B. Infect Immunity 62:3731–3738
43. Litton MJ, Dohlsten M, Hansson J, et al (1997) Tumor therapy with an antibody-targeted superantigen generates a dichotomy between local and systemic immune response. Am J Pathol 150:1607–1618
44. Björk L, Andersson U, Chauvet JM, Skansén-Saphir U, Andersson J (1994) Quantification of superantigen induced IFNγ production by computerised image analysis - inhibition of cytokine production and blast transformation by pooled human IgG. J Immunol Methods 175: 201–213
45. Norrby-Teglund A, Kaul R, Low DE, et al (1996) Plasma from patients with severe invasive group A streptococcal infections treated with normal polyspecific IgG inhibits streptococcal superantigen-induced T cell proliferation and cytokine production. J Immunol 156: 3057–3064
46. Eriksson BKG, Andersson J, Holm SE, Norgren M (1998) Epidemiological and clinical aspects of invasive group A streptococcal infections and the streptococcal toxic shock syndrome. J Clin Infect 27:1428–1436
47. Skansén-Saphir U, Andersson J, Björk L, Andersson U (1994) Lymphokine production induced by streptococcal pyrogenic exotoxin-A is selectively down-regulated by pooled human IgG. Eur J Immunol 24:916–922

48. Andersson U, Björk L, Skansén-Saphir U, Andersson J (1994) Pooled human IgG modulates cytokine production in lymphocytes and monocytes. Immunol Rev 139: 21–42
49. Sander B, Skansén-Saphir U, Damm O, Håkansson L, Andersson J, Andersson U (1995) Sequential production of Th1 and Th2 cytokines in response to live bacillus Calmette-Guérin. Immunology 86:512–518
50. Ge Y, Ezzell RM, Clark BD, Loiselle PM, Amato SF, Warren HS (1997) Relationship to tissue and cellular interleukin-1 and lipopolyaccharide after endotoxemia and bacteremia. J Infect Dis 176:1313–1321
51. Sutton TE, Norman JG, Newton CA, Hellerman GR, Richards IS (1997) Endothelial structural integrity is maintained during endotoxic shock in an interleukin-1 type 1 receptor knockout mouse. Shock 7:105–110
52. Björk L, Tracey K, Ulrich P, et al (1997) Targeted suppression of cytokine production in monocytes but not in T-lymphocytes by a tetravalent guanylhydrazone (CNI-1493). J Infect Dis 176:1303–1312
53. Calandra T, Bernhagen J, Metz CN, et al (1995) MIF is a glucocorticoid-induced modulator of cytokine production. Nature 377:68–71

The Acute Phase Response and Enhancing Resistance to Bacterial Infection

M. Noursadeghi and J. Cohen

Introduction

The use of prophylactic antibiotics is commonplace prior to invasive procedures and in immunocompromised patients. For many years surgeons have argued that antibiotics suffer from the intrinsic limitation that even broad-spectrum therapy inevitably omits some microbial species [1]. Despite aseptic techniques, infections are the commonest complication of surgery. Studies in the U.S. have reported 27% infection rates in-patients undergoing major gastro-intestinal surgery, resulting in longer hospital length of stay. The extra cost per infected patient was estimated at almost $ 13 000 in 1993 [2]. Nosocomial infections similarly complicate intensive care, cancer chemotherapy, elderly and malnourished patients, severe trauma and burns, amongst others. The problem is compounded by increasing reports of microbial resistance to antibiotics resulting in therapeutic failure, an issue of worldwide concern [3–4]. Hospitals are particularly at risk because the extensive use of antibiotics produces a selection pressure for organisms which are resistant to multiple agents. Thus the development of alternative or adjunctive approaches to antibiotic therapy has become imperative. Augmentation of the host immune response would seem an obvious approach. Indeed, the manipulation of the adaptive immune system with vaccines has been very successful against specific pathogens. Manipulation of the innate immune system however has been comparatively neglected as a potential strategy to enhance non-specific resistance to infection. Over the last two decades encouraging results from work with animal models of infection have been accumulating. In parallel, our understanding of the structure and function of the host acute phase response has also improved. This constitutes the humoral component of innate host defense and may provide a target for improving non-specific resistance to bacterial infection. We first provide an overview of the acute phasc response with particular reference to its role in host defense and then discuss the evidence for the mechanisms by which non-specific resistance to bacterial infection has been enhanced in animal models.

The Acute Phase Response

The acute phase response is a cytokine-induced physiological reaction to infection and tissue injury consisting of well described quantitative and qualitative changes in plasma protein synthesis [5]. It is highly conserved in all endothermic species, suggesting it confers a survival advantage. The precise nature of this survival advantage however remains elusive. In addition to the temporal association of the acute phase response with infection, it has become clear that many of its components have important physiological roles in host defense mechanisms. As summarized schematically in Fig. 1, we will outline the signaling pathways and

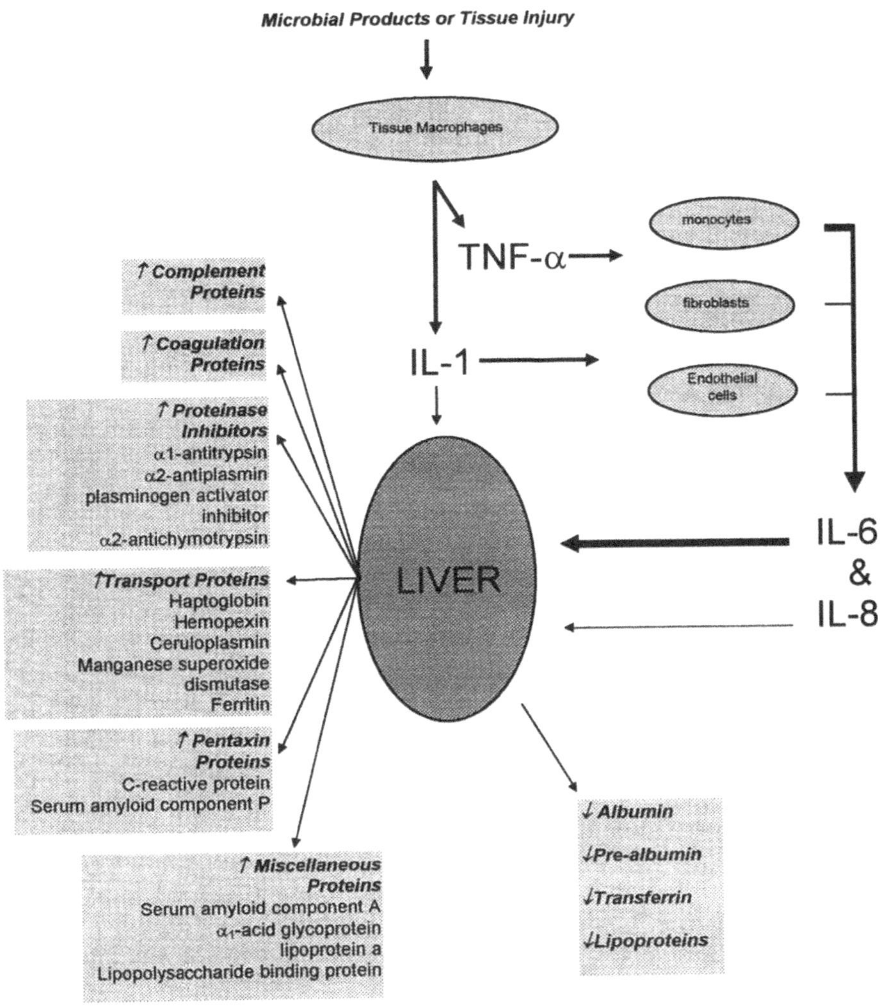

Fig. 1. Schematic outline of the acute phase response

plasma protein changes which constitute the acute phase response with particular reference to proteins which demonstrate anti-microbial effects.

Increased sedimentation rates of red blood cells in severely ill patients, reflecting greatly elevated plasma protein concentrations is well recognized [6]. Abernathy and Avery [7] first applied the term 'acute phase' to sera from acutely ill patients, containing C-reactive protein (CRP), then identified as a precipitin of pneumococcal C-polysaccharide [8]. CRP became known as the acute phase protein. As assays for specific plasma proteins were developed a multitude of changes in acute phase sera were described [9]. These consisted of increased levels of complement, coagulation and transport proteins as well as proteinase inhibitors, serum amyloid protein A (SAA), the classic acute phase pentraxin proteins, CRP and serum amyloid component P (SAP) and a number of other miscellaneous proteins. Hepatocytes were identified as the major cells responsible for the synthesis of these proteins [10]. It has become evident however that some acute phase protein can be produced in a variety of tissues by monocytes, endothelial cells and fibroblasts. The finding that changes in protein concentration were preceded by alterations in mRNA levels indicated that these changes were the result of *de-novo* protein synthesis [11].

Induction of the Acute Phase Response

Since infection or injury at a distant site produces changes in the liver, the existence of humoral or neural mediators was evident. In animal models, an acute phase response is induced experimentally by injection of substances such as turpentine, silver nitrate or casein which produce sterile tissue inflammation. Leukocytes, being the dominant population of cells at inflammatory foci, were examined as a possible source of such mediators. The supernatants of leukocyte cultures were found to stimulate the synthesis of a number of acute phase proteins in rabbit, rat and murine animal models [12–14]. When stimulated by phagocytosis or bacterial products such as endotoxin or muramyl peptides, monocyte culture supernatants were particularly effective inducers of acute phase response protein synthesis [15]. Three products of stimulated monocytes, interleukin-1 (IL-1, originally leukocytic endogenous mediator), tumour necrosis factor-α (TNF-α) and IL-6, originally hepatocyte stimulating factor, were identified by their ability to induce acute phase protein synthesis in both cultured hepatocytes and *in vivo* animal models [16–21]. All these cytokines, whilst undetectable in resting serum are elevated following an infection. Each has wide ranging multisystem effects apart from hepatocyte stimulation. These include fever, hemodynamic changes, leukocyte proliferation and activation, proteolysis and gluconeogenesis [22–24], suggesting they are key regulators of the host response to infection. TNF-α and IL-1 levels rise within 1 to 4 hours following infection and notably stimulate the synthesis of IL-6 by monocytes, fibroblasts and endothelial cells. Accordingly IL-6 levels peak at 6 to 12 hours and the acute phase proteins after 12 to 24 hours [25, 26]. The precise signaling pathways inducing the acute phase response are complex and incompletely understood. Recombinant cytokines used in hepatocyte cultures to isolate their individual effects revealed that IL-1 and TNF-α each stimulate the production of small subsets of acute phase proteins [19]. IL-6 stimulated a wider range of these proteins and enhanced the IL-1 effect. Indeed the combination of IL-1, IL-6 and dexamethasone was required to achieve maximal stimulation [27]. Although IL-6 has been considered as the dominant acute phase stimulant, *in vivo* studies with recombinant IL-6 have revealed that its effect is incomplete [21]. Recent work with genetically engineered IL-6 deficient mice has also demonstrated that whilst the acute phase response following injection of turpentine is abolished, the response to lipopolysaccharide (LPS) is preserved suggesting that there may more than one signaling pathway to acute phase response induction [28]. A number of other monocyte derived cytokines such as IL-8, interferon-γ (IFN-γ), leukemia inhibitory factor (LIH), transforming growth factor-β (TGF-β) and IL-11 have been added to the list which may be involved in this signaling pathway [29–31]. Moreover, evidence is also available to suggest that bacterial products such as LPS may stimulate hepatocyte acute phase protein synthesis directly in the absence of cytokines [32].

The Role of Acute Phase Proteins in Host Defense

Complement: Certain components of the acute phase response have clear roles in host defense. Of these the complement proteins are best understood. They act in sequential fashion to form enzyme cascades, the products of which have well documented biological effects [33]. The central event is cleavage of the most abundant component C3 and binding of its C3b fragment to microbial surfaces or immune complexes. Thereafter this fragment may act as an opsonin recognized by specific CR1 receptors on monocytes, macrophages and neutrophils promoting phagocytosis of the bound target. Alternatively it may serve as the ligand for binding of complement components C5–9 forming the membrane attack complex on microbial cell surfaces, thereby having a direct microbicidal effect. As a component of non-specific host defense, spontaneous hydrolysis of C3 leads to a sequence of interactions with factors B and D and cleavage of C3. C3b is then stabilized by binding to microbial cell wall components and complement factor P. This is known as the alternative pathway of complement activation. Its functional significance is revealed by deficiencies of factors C3, B or P which result in recurrent pyogenic infections [34]. C3a and C5a are also biologically active fragments contributing to host defense [35]. They increase recruitment of leukocytes to sites of tissue infection by receptor-mediated effects on endothelial cells and leukocytes. They increase local blood flow and capillary permeability, enhance neutrophil-endothelial cell interactions and induce production of cytokines and other inflammatory mediators from these cells. C5a in particular is a potent chemotactic factor for neutrophils. Complement is also an effector mechanism for the specific immune response by the classical pathway in which the complement component C1q binds Fc segments of immunoglobulins [36]. This leads to cleavage of factors C2 and C4 forming the C4b2a convertase enzyme which actively cleaves C3. The fragment C4a has similar pro-inflammatory properties to C3a and C5a.

Coagulation Proteins: The main function of the coagulation proteins is of course hemostasis which is a critical component of tissue repair. In addition however the clotting cascade may also potentiate host defense processes. As a result of tissue injury and activation of the contact system in the clotting cascade, high molecular weight kininogen (HMWK) is cleaved and leads to the release of kinin molecules. These have a pro-inflammatory effect, characterized by local vasodilatation and increased capillary permeability in addition to stimulation of synthesis of cytokine and eicosanoid mediators from inflammatory cells [37]. Indeed the acute phase response in rats includes proteins that are directly related to kininogens and may contribute to this effect [38].

Transport Proteins: The presence of blood, free hemoglobin or soluble iron compounds enhances the lethality of certain bacteria [39–41]. Indeed in a clinical setting, the co-existence of blood and bacteria in a wound can lead to life threatening infection [42]. Many pathogenic microorganisms require iron for growth and the availability of iron is therefore a significant limiting factor to the replication of such organisms [43–44]. The acute phase response includes increased synthesis of transport proteins such as haptoglobin which bind free hemoglobin in a stable complex, that is rapidly cleared by the reticulo-endothelial system [45]. In so doing, haptoglobin limits the availability of iron to microorganisms. *In vitro*, haptoglobin reduces bacterial replication in media containing blood and *in vivo* it suppresses hemoglobin driven bacterial peritonitis [46]. It contributes directly to non-specific host defense as a natural bacteriostat. A number of other metal binding acute phase reactants such as hemopexin, ceruloplasmin and manganese superoxide dismutase are likely to impart a similar effect by limiting essential bacterial nutrients. Many acute phase proteins are proteinase inhibitors. They are most likely to function as a mechanism for limiting the damage caused by the wide variety of degradative enzymes which are released from inflammatory cells and as a result of tissue injury [47].

Pentraxins: The acute phase proteins CRP and SAP are related molecules, referred to as pentraxins [9]. They have approximately 50–60% amino acid sequence homology (in man) and are both composed of non-covalently associated polypeptide sub-units arranged with cyclic pentameric symmetry. They also share a capacity for calcium dependent binding to specific ligands. There is little evidence however to demonstrate functional homology. They were originally identified and individually purified by their differing ligand specificities. Moreover whilst CRP levels may increase by a factor of 10^3 with the acute phase response in man, that of SAP remains relatively constant. This phenomenon is reversed in mice where SAP is the major pentraxin acute phase reactant [48]. A large body of evidence has accumulated to suggest that CRP augments anti-microbial host defenses. It enhances phagocytosis of a variety of bacteria [49–51], but the mechanism by which it does so is not clear. Phospho-choline residues are the main ligands for CRP. Their presence in some microbial organisms allows the interaction of CRP with a wide variety of pathogens, including bacteria such as *S. pneumoniae* and *H. influenzae* [52, 53]. These observations have led to the description of CRP as an opsonin. In the presence of CRP, neutrophils demonstrate enhanced phagocytosis, including phagocytosis of particles not containing phospho-choline. Concomitant treatment of these neutrophils with phorbol myristate acetate (PMA) or concanavalin A and low dose CRP led to increased super-oxide anion production, whilst higher doses of CRP surprisingly inhibited respiratory burst activity [54]. Intriguingly CRP also inhibits neutrophil chemotaxis [55]. It was postulated therefore that CRP stimulation of neutrophil function may involve a negative feedback system to limit potentially cytotoxic neutrophil activity. A CRP-specific receptor has recently been reported on leukocytes which may mediate phagocytosis of CRP-bound microbes [56, 57]. A more widely accepted explanation however is that CRP activates complement via the classical pathway by binding C1q [58]. In doing so C3b may be generated, which as already discussed, is a well-recognized opsonin. Indeed complement dependent binding of CRP-ligand complexes to complement receptors is well recognized [59]. Activation of complement is also the likely mechanism for *H. influenzae* sensitivity to serum killing mediated by CRP [53]. The *in vivo* functional importance of the interaction of CRP with pneumococci and its antimicrobial effect is further illustrated by experiments in which mice given human CRP passively demonstrate dramatically improved survival in *S. pneumoniae* models of infection [60, 61]. Similarly, mice transgenic for human CRP had reduced bacteremia by day 2 and enhanced survival by day 5, after intra-peritoneal *S. pneumoniae* infection [62]. The physiological functions of SAP are also emerging. It was originally identified by its ability to bind amyloid fibrils [11], making them resistant to proteolysis [63]. The significance of these interactions is highlighted in experiments with genetically engineered SAP deficient mice ($SAP^{-/-}$) which are more resistant to amyloidosis [64]. Like CRP, SAP also binds C1q and may activate complement by the classical pathway [65]. Intriguingly it also binds bacteria such as *S. pyogenes* and *Klebsiella rhinoscleromatis* [66]. This suggests that SAP may contribute to innate resistance to infection. Although evidence demonstrating an anti-bacterial effect is not widely published, experiments investigating the susceptibility of $SAP^{-/-}$ mice to a variety of infections are underway and may provide interesting results.

Serum Amyloid Component A: SAA is an acute phase protein which derives its name from biochemical and immunocytochemical homology to amyloid A (AA) fibrils. Indeed it is the precursor of AA protein. In acute phase serum, SAA is a component of lipoproteins, particularly high-density lipoprotein (HDL), comprising up to 50% of the total apoproteins of HDL. Acute phase SAA-rich HDL is cleared more rapidly from the circulation than its non-acute phase counterpart, but the physiological role of this interaction is not known. SAA has not been widely implicated in anti-microbial host defense [9].

Enhancing Resistance to Bacterial Infections

For many years, evidence has been accumulating suggesting the potential benefit of enhancing non-specific resistance to bacterial infections. Thus far, this research has been almost wholly confined to animal experiments. A wide variety of reagents has been used in different models of infection. These data are summarized in Table 1. All are characterized by pre-treatment of animals with a pro-inflammatory agent prior to bacterial infection. Broadly these reagents fall into two groups: Microbial products and cytokines. The evidence for the mechanisms by which they produce their effect is incomplete. Many of these reagents induce an acute phase response which may be the critical factor in enhancing non-specific resistance to bacterial infection.

Indirect Stimulation of the Acute Phase Response: Pre-Treatment with Bacterial Products

Muramyl Dipeptide: The bacterial products which have successfully enhanced non-specific host resistance are predominantly cell wall constituents such as muramyl dipeptides (MDP), glucans and LPS. Following observations that they may have lymphocyte stimulatory effects, *C. parvum* and bacillus Calmette-Guérin (BCG), were amongst the first to be evaluated. In mouse models of surgical wound infection, simulated by insertion of *E. coli* or *Staph. aureus* laden thigh sutures, both these agents, administered 7–14 days before infection, reduced bacterial counts in the infected tissue by half, compared with control animals [1]. In order to improve on these results efforts were made to identify the active constituents of these organisms.

Progressive fractionation of the mycobacterial cell wall in Freund's complete adjuvant led to the isolation of MDP and the synthesis of its analogs [67]. These are water-soluble peptidoglycans composed of 6 aminoacids. Pre-treatment of mice with MDP reduced mortality from intravenous, intramuscular or intraperitoneal *K. pneumoniae* infection [68]. MDP was effective when given intravenously, intramuscularly, sub-cutaneously or orally. This effect was observed when MDP was administered any time between 4 days before, and 1 hour after, bacterial challenge. It was most effective when given 24 hours before infection. This increased resistance to bacterial infection was subsequently demonstrated with other bacteria including *S. pneumoniae*, *P. aeruginosa* and *L. monocytogenes* [69, 70]. In addition MDP, when given by subcutaneous injection to mice 48 hours prior to inoculation with *K. pneumoniae* and *Staph. aureus* laden thigh sutures, reduced mortality and bacterial cell counts from infected tissue at 24 hours after infection [71]. The ability of MDP to enhance resistance to bacterial infection was also tested in immunocompromised hosts. Using the *K. pneumoniae* laden thigh suture model in mice, MDP pre-treatment was shown to reduce local and systemic bacterial growth and produce a six fold increased survival in mice immunosuppressed with cyclophosphamide [72]. In the same infection model, mice compromised by malnutrition resulting from a 48-hour period of acute starvation or a 2-week period of protein deprivation, demonstrated reduced mortality when pre-treated with MDP [73]. Finally this reagent also demonstrated a beneficial effect when administered after established infection.

Bacteremia and mortality were both reduced from simulated surgical wound infection in mice when a combination of MDP and antibiotics were given 6 hours after bacterial challenge, compared to antibiotic treatment only [74]. Moreover this observation was also evident when MDP was given alone, compared with no treatment. Notably however the beneficial effect was quantitatively lower when compared to MDP administration prior to infection.

These series of experiments led to the observation that MDP had systemic effects. They were characterized by fever, sleep induction and hemodynamic changes [75]. Although they were initially thought to be direct effects of MDP on neurochemicals, the observation that MDP stimulates macrophages *in vitro* to produce IL-1 led to suggestions that IL-1 mediated these effects and that they may be part of a systemic acute phase response [76]. More recently it has become evident that MDP stimulates macrophages to produce the pro-inflammatory cytokines TNF-α and IL-6, in addition to IL-1 [77]. Indeed, increased levels of the acute phase reactant α-1 glycoprotein have been reported following injection of MDP in mice [78]. Some effort has been made to uncover the mechanism by which MDP stimulates macrophages. Although cell surface binding sites for MDP have been described [79], no clear candidate for a specific MDP receptor has been identified. Interestingly MDP induced cytokine release by monocytes is not reduced by prior repeated stimulation with LPS (which results in tolerance to LPS and a diminished cytokine response) [80]. This suggests that MDP stimulation of monocytes involves cell surface receptors or intra-cellular signaling pathways which are different from that used by LPS.

MDP enhances host defenses by stimulating phagocytic cell activity. Indirect evidence for this is provided by observations from animal experiments in which a consistent characteristic of MDP is its capacity to contain bacteria at the site of inoculation [73], and its efficacy despite cyclophosphamide treatment which particularly affects lymphocytes and neutrophils but spares tissue macrophages [81]. Direct evidence however comes from *in vivo* experiments in which clearance of colloid carbon by the reticulo-endothelial system is enhanced in shocked mice by MDP pre-treatment [82]. In addition, polymorphonuclear cells from foci of infection in MDP pre-treated mice were present in greater number, showed increased viability and had more visibly phagocytosed bacteria than control animals [83]. *In vitro*, neutrophils demonstrate greater chemotaxis in the presence of MDP [84]. The synthetic derivative of MDP, murabutide, enhances phagocytic activity of neutrophils *in vitro*, associated with up-regulation of cell surface CR1 and Fc-γ receptors and the bacterial endotoxin ligand CD14 [85]. Whether enhanced activity of phagocytic cells is the result of a direct effect on cells, a contribution from the acute phase response or stimulation by cytokines is not known. The tentative observation that there are a greater number of circulating monocytes in MDP treated animals [74] is likely to be the effect of colony stimulating activity and lends support to the latter explanation.

Table 1. Summary of substances used to enhance host resistance in animal studies

Substance	Administration route	Timing	Organism	Inoculation route	Animal	Outcome	References
Muramyl dipeptides	i.v., i.m., s.c., and p.o.	4 d pre–1 hr post infection	*K. pneumoniae* *P. aeruginosa* *S. pneumoniae*	i.v., i.m., i.p. i.p.	normal mice	reduced mortality	[68] [69] [70]
	i.v., i.p., and s.c. s.c.	48 hrs pre-infection	mixed *K. pneumoniae* and *Staph. aureus*	thigh sutures	normal mice	reduced mortality and bacterial cell counts from infected tissue	[71]
	s.c.	24 hrs pre-infection	*K. pneumoniae*	thigh sutures	neutropenic or malnourished mice	reduced mortality and reduced local and systemic bacterial growth	[72, 73]
Glucans	i.v.	7–4 d pre-infection	*Staph. aureus*	i.v.	normal mice	reduced mortality	[91]
	i.v. or i.n.		*P. pseudomallei*	i.n.	normal rat	reduced mortality with i.n. glucan only	[92]
	i.v.	4–6 hrs pre-infection	*E. coli* *Staph. aureus*	i.v. i.v.	normal mice	reduced mortality	[99]
	i.m.	24 hrs pre-infection	mixed intraabdominal infection		normal rat	reduced mortality and bacterial counts	[99]
LPS	i.p. or s.c.	24 hrs pre-infection	*E. coli*	i.p.	normal mice	Reduced mortality and bacterial counts	[113]
	i.p.	24 hrs pre-infection	*S. epidermidis*	i.p.	normal mice	reduced mortality and bacterial counts	[114]
IL-1	i.v.	at same time and post-infection	*L. monocytogenes*	i. p.	mouse	reduced liver and spleen bacterial counts	[118]
	i.v.	72–24 hrs pre-infection	*P. aeruginosa* *K. pneumonia* *S. typhimurium* *Staph. aureus*	i.p. i.p. i.p. i.v.	normal and neutropenic mice	reduced mortality and local and systemic bacterial counts	[119–124]

TNF-α	i.p.	24 hrs pre-infection	*L. monocytogenes*	i.v.	normal mice	reduced mortality	[130]
	i.p.	6–12 hrs pre-infection	*S. typhimurium*	i.p.	normal mice	reduced mortality and bacterial counts in those receiving TNF-α 6–12 hrs pre-infection only	[115]
IL-6	i.v.	24 hrs pre-infection	*P. aeruginosa*	i.m.	normal mice	no survival benefit	[133]
	i.v.	24 hrs pre-infection–48 hrs post infection	*L. monocytogenes*	i.v.	normal mice	no survival benefit	[134]
IL-8	i.p.	24 hrs pre–6 hrs post-infection	*P. aeruginosa*	i.m.	normal mice	no survival benefit and no reduction in bacterial counts	[136]

i.m.: intramuscular; i.v.: intravenous; i.p.: intraperitoneal; p.o.: oral; s.c.: subcutaneous.

Glucans: Glucan is a water-insoluble β-1,3-glucopyranose polysaccharide isolated from the inner cell walls of baker's yeast (*Saccharomyces cerevisiae*) and widely referred to as β-glucan [86, 87]. It was originally identified as the active moiety of a crude insoluble yeast cell wall extract called zymosan, which was shown to be a stimulant of the reticuloendothelial system [88]. The administration of glucan to rats or mice led to an increase in weight and size of lymph nodes and the spleen as a result of greater numbers of activated macrophages [89, 90]. In view of this apparent immunostimulant property glucan was evaluated as an agent which may enhance antibacterial resistance. In a mouse model of systemic *Staph. aureus* infection, administration of intravenous glucan 7 and 4 days prior to inoculation, led to a significant reduction in mortality [91]. Pre-treatment of rats with intravenous glucan enhanced resistance to both intra-peritoneal and low dose intranasal *Francisella tularensis* challenge whilst pre-treatment with intranasal glucan reduced mortality from aerosolized *Pseudomonas pseudomallei* infection [92]. These studies revealed macrophage hyperplasia in lymphoid tissue, increased circulating levels of serum lysozyme and increased phagocytosis as determined by colloidal carbon clearance. Enhancement of non-specific cellular defense mechanisms were therefore postulated as the mechanism by which glucan confers bacterial resistance.

Particulate zymosan, from which glucan was originally purified, is able to activate the alternative pathway and may have complement mediated interaction with phagocytic cells [93]. However the observation that zymosan is also phagocytosed in the absence of complement and immunoglobulin [94], suggested that it may interact directly with monocytes and neutrophils. Indeed a number of putative cell-surface receptors for glucan have been described [95]. Not surprisingly, glucan induces IL-1 and TNF-α production by monocytes *in vitro* and the levels of these cytokines are elevated *in vivo* following the administration of glucan [96–98]. In light of its potent anti-bacterial effect, soluble synthetic derivatives of glucan were developed and explored with a view to possible clinical applications. One such derivative, called poly-(1–6)-β-glucotriosyl-(1–3)-β-glucopyranose glucan (PGG-glucan) has been effective in animal studies and provides further insight into the mechanism by which resistance to bacterial infection may be enhanced. Pre-treatment of mice with intravenous PGG-glucan 4–6 hours before bacterial challenge reduced mortality to approximately 40% from intravenous *E. coli* and *Staph. aureus* LD_{70} infections [99]. In the same report, using a rat model of mixed intra-abdominal infection including *E. coli*, *P. mirabilis*, streptococcal species, bacteroides species and *C. perfringens*, PGG-glucan was similarly effective when administered as an intramuscular injection 24 hours before bacterial challenge, reducing mortality 5–6 fold. Moreover its anti-microbial effect has also been demonstrated against antibiotic-resistant organisms in a guinea pig model of intramuscular infection inducing abscess formation with methicillin resistant strains of *Staph. aureus* and *Staph. epidermidis* [100]. Its anti-microbial effect was highlighted by quantitative bacteriology which demonstrated significantly lower bacterial counts in PGG-glucan treated animals.

Like its parent molecule, PGG-glucan interacted with cell-surface receptors on monocytes and neutrophils, but possibly different from those previously characterized as glucan-receptors [101, 102]. PGG-glucan can induce a transient rise in total leukocyte counts, and primes them to exhibit enhanced phagocytosis and respiratory burst activity following subsequent stimulation [103]. In an attempt to further characterize the anti-bacterial mechanisms, a series of passive transfer experiments were undertaken. In a rat model of mixed intra-abdominal infection spleen cell, splenic cell lysates, peripheral blood leukocytes and serum from PGG-glucan treated animals were passively transferred by intra-peritoneal injection into PGG-glucan naïve animals four hours prior to bacterial challenge [104]. Consistent with the hypothesis that cellular effector mechanisms are predominantly responsible for the effect of PGG-glucan, transfer of peripheral blood leukocytes or spleen cells reduced mortality in this model of infection from approximately 70% to 13% and 5% respectively. Surprisingly however transfer of serum also reduced mortality to 6%. This suggests that humoral effector mechanisms of host defense may also be augmented by PGG-glucan. Despite this observation other studies provide indirect evidence that such humoral effect is unlikely to be mediated by components of the acute phase response. In particular *in vitro* studies have failed to demonstrate PGG-glucan induction of pro-inflammatory cytokines [105] and although activation of nuclear factor-IL-6α does occur, PGG-glucan does not induce IL-6 mRNA synthesis [106].

Lipopolysaccharide: LPS is a highly conserved glycolipid component of Gram-negative bacterial cell walls which has long been recognized as the cause of Gram-negative septic shock [107]. The lipid A component of LPS binds to a plasma protein called LPS-binding protein (LBP), which augments interaction of LPS with leukocytes [108]. The complex binds to the cell surface protein CD14 and leads to intra-cellular signaling which stimulates the production of cytokines. Toll-like receptors (TLR) have recently been described as a transmembrane protein which may mediate intra-cellular signaling [109]. LPS is a very potent stimulator of TNF-α, IL-1 and IFN-γ production by myeloid cells and *in vivo* induces a systemic cytokine cascade, implicated in the pathogenesis of septic shock [110]. The physiological role of this cytokine cascade, which in turn induces the acute phase response must be to augment host defenses in response to detection of a highly conserved bacterial product. Indeed the ability of LPS to enhance resistance to bacterial infection was initially observed over 40 years ago [111, 112]. This effect has been re-examined more recently. In mice the administration of LPS at doses insufficient to induce septic shock, by intraperitoneal or subcutaneous routes, 24 hours prior to intraperitoneal challenge with *E. coli* led to reduced mortality [113]. This was associated with a reduction of viable bacteria recoverable from the animals only 3–4 hours after infection. A synthetic derivative of LPS, monophosphoryl lipid A (MPLA) was similarly effective against mouse models of intraperitoneal *E. coli* and *Staph. epidermidis* infection [114]. The mechanisms for LPS induced resistance to bacterial infection may be diverse. Direct leukocyte activation and the consequent cytokine cascade undoubtedly augment the cellular effector mechanisms of host defense. Interestingly LPS-induced resistance to infection can be blocked by antibodies to TNF-α [115]. LPS is also a potent stimulator of the acute phase response in human and experimental animal models, thereby also enhancing humoral components of non-specific host defense. The cytokine response to LPS is however variable and modified by genetic factors. In a line of low-responder mice, pre-treatment with LPS failed to increase resistance to a model of *K. pneumoniae* infection, in contrast to a sub-line of high-responder mice [116]. Finally, part of the protective effect of LPS may be by virtue of its ability to induce tolerance, in which the subsequent cytokine and systemic response to LPS is diminished [117].

Direct Stimulation of the Acute Phase Response: Pre-Treatment with Cytokines

Although a number of different host defense strategies have been implicated in enhancing resistance to bacterial infections, it is notable that all the bacterial products that have been discussed stimulate myeloid cells, particularly monocytes, to produce cytokines such as IL-1, TNF-α and IFN-γ, which in turn stimulate IL-6 and IL-8 synthesis. The logical progression in evaluating agents which improve non-specific host defenses and in further understanding the mechanisms which may be involved, was therefore to study the effect of individual cytokines in animal models of infection.

IL-1: IL-1 exists in two biochemically distinct forms, IL-1α and IL-1β. They are encoded by separate genes and share only 26% amino-acid homology (in humans). Both are translated as 31 kDa precursors, cleaved by serine proteases to 17.5 kD mature proteins. IL-1β production predominates following inflammatory stimuli but both bind the same receptor and have the same spectrum of biological activity with equal potency [24]. Recombinant IL-1α (rIL-1α) given intravenously to mice concomitantly receiving an intraperitoneal *L. monocytogenes* infection produced an anti-microbial effect in which fewer viable bacteria were recoverable from the liver and spleen in comparison to control animals [118]. Pre-treatment of mice with intravenous rIL-1α 72 and 24 hours prior to intraperitoneal inoculation with 2–5 times the LD_{50} of *P. aeruginosa*, *K. pneumoniae*, *S. typhimurium* and *S. pneumoniae*, or intravenous *Staph. aureus* led to an IL-1 dose dependent reduction in mortality, ranging from no protection at 0.01 μg per mouse to 75–100% survival at 10 μg per mouse [119]. In a series of reports, pretreatment with rIL-1 (α and β) was found to enhance resistance to bacterial infections in mice rendered neutropenic by cyclophosphamide [119–124]. In these studies improved survival was consistently associated with reduced viable bacteria recovered from blood or tissues of animals. This improved bacterial clearance indicated that IL-1 did have a clear anti-microbial effect. The mechanism of this effect is unknown.

IL-1 can certainly stimulate the production of other cytokines. For example following infection for example with *L. monocytogenes*, IL-1 pre-treated mice demonstrated an earlier burst of colony stimulating factor production when compared with control animals [118]. Since this cytokine increases circulating neutrophil counts, reduces apoptosis and enhances phagocytosis a significant role for neutrophils was suggested [125]. Higher peripheral neutrophil counts in normal mice and accelerated neutrophil recovery in cyclophosphamide treated mice have been reported following IL-1 pre-treatment and subsequent bacterial infection [122]. Increased accumulation of neutrophils into the peritoneal cavity of mice pre-treated with IL-1 has also been demonstrated after intraperitoneal infection with *K. pneumoniae* or *L. monocytogenes* [120]. The cellular response correlated well with increased survival. In contrast however, in mice rendered neutropenic with either repeated cyclophosphamide administration or sub-lethal total body irradiation, the protective effect of IL-1 pre-treatment remained intact [124].

In one study enhanced resistance to infection was only observed when IL-1 and the subsequent bacterial challenge were administered into the same site [123]. Based upon this observation, enhanced activity of resident macrophages was postulated as an important mechanism. Pre-treatment of neutropenic mice with low dose (8–800 ng per mouse) recombinant IL-1β by single intraperitoneal or intramuscular injection 24 hours before LD_{90} infection with intramuscular *P. aeruginosa* or *S. pneumoniae* led to 60% survival, but did not result in improved bacterial clearance. In this study respiratory burst activity by peritoneal macrophages was assessed as superoxide production, but no difference was demonstrated between IL-1 pre-treated and untreated animals [121]. The putative role of humoral inflammatory mediators, such as prostaglandins and leukotrienes was also considered; however administration of the cyclooxygenase inhibitor, ibuprofen, did not diminish IL-1 induced resistance to infection. Instead the observation that resistance to infection was maximal when IL-1 was administered 24 hours before infection, rather than immediately before or 6 hours after infection led to the suggestion that since this was consistent with the time required to achieve a maximal acute phase response, acute phase proteins may be necessary.

This possibility was addressed more directly in a similar mouse model demonstrating enhanced resistance by pre-treatment with low dose recombinant IL-1β (80–800 ng per mouse) to both *K. pneumoniae* and *P. aeruginosa* infection [126]. Mice were treated with intraperitoneal D-galactosamine (GALN). This liver specific blocker of RNA and protein synthesis acts by depleting uridine triphosphate thereby abrogating the acute phase response in response to IL-1 and subsequent infection. Its effect was verified by demonstrating failure of increases in serum levels of SAA or fibrinogen following IL-1 treatment, but increased IL-6 levels demonstrating that the cytokine cascade mediating the acute phase response was intact. GALN administration (at doses that did not cause hepatotoxicity) 30 minutes prior to IL-1 treatment and 24 hours prior to bacterial challenge totally abolished the IL-1 induced survival benefit. All mice treated with GALN alone survived and GALN pre-treatment without IL-1 did not increase mortality associated with subsequent infection. Although enhanced bacterial clearance has been consistently observed in infections following IL-1 pre-treatment, a modification of the physiological response to infection may also contribute to reduced mortality.

IL-1 pre-treated mice were found to have reduced circulating TNF-α and IL-6 levels following infection with *K. pneumoniae* and *P. aeruginosa*, and reduced

LPS-stimulated production of IL-1α and TNF-α [127]. Interestingly this was associated with down-regulation of mRNA for the type I IL-1 receptor (IL-1RI) and the type 1 TNF receptor in several organs, but up-regulation of mRNA for IL-1 receptor antagonist (IL-1ra) in these organs. IL-1 pre-treatment may therefore reduce the effects of the systemic cytokine cascade that follows infection thereby abrogating its deleterious effects. In further experiments concomitant pre-treatment of mice with IL-1ra or a neutralizing antibody to IL-RI eliminated IL-1 induced enhanced survival [128].

TNF-α: TNF-α is a 17 kDa polypeptide cytokine which, like IL-1, appears as an early mediator of the cytokine cascade in sepsis and enhances induction of the acute phase response [27]. TNF-α is also an excellent candidate for increasing non-specific host defenses through cellular mechanisms. In *in vitro* studies TNF-α increases neutrophil longevity, aggregation, chemotaxis, phagocytosis, respiratory burst activity and degranulation [125, 129]. Following an observation that LPS-induced enhanced resistance to bacterial infection was reduced by antibodies to TNF-α, this cytokine was also evaluated for its anti-microbial effects [115]. Pre-treatment of mice with intraperitoneal recombinant human TNF-α 24 hours prior to infection with 4 to 7 times LD_{50} *L. monocytogenes* by intravenous injection resulted in a dose dependent reduction in mortality [130]. The dose used to achieve maximal effect was noted to be higher than endogenous TNF levels following LPS pre-treatment which confers a similar protection. Recombinant murine TNF-α given intraperitoneally to mice receiving intraperitoneal *S. typhimurium* infection enhanced bacterial clearance only in those animals treated with TNF-α 6 or 12 hours before bacterial challenge, but not in those receiving TNF-α simultaneously or after infection [115]. An increased influx of neutrophils into the peritoneal cavity was also noted. These results were associated with a reduction in mortality in TNF-α treated animals. The dose of TNF-α required to achieve this effect did not produce a shock like state. The beneficial effect of TNF-α pre-treatment was again abolished by co-administration of anti-TNF-α antibodies.

IL-6: IL-6 is a 26 kDa polypeptide cytokine, predominantly produced by monocytes, endothelial cells and fibroblasts in response to stimulation from IL-1 and TNF-α. IL-6 is the major cytokine stimulant of the acute phase response and many of the biological effects of IL-1 and TNF-α are thought to be mediated by IL-6 [22]. The development of a genetically engineered IL-6 deficient ($IL\text{-}6^{-/-}$) mouse has provided further insight into its physiological functions. In particular $IL\text{-}6^{-/-}$ mice are reported to demonstrate increased susceptibility to a variety of bacteria. Infection with *L. monocytogenes* resulted in 10^2–10^3 higher bacterial titres in the spleen and liver as compared to control animals ($IL\text{-}6^{+/+}$) [30]. In another model of sub-lethal *L. monocytogenes* infection normal control animals were able to clear the infection but IL-6 deficient mice demonstrated uncontrolled replication of bacteria in the spleen and liver and accordingly a high mortality rate 2 to 3 days after infection [131]. Administration of exogenous recombinant murine IL-6 to $IL\text{-}6^{-/-}$ mice, 24 hours before infection, at the time of infection and 24 hours afterwards, enhanced resistance to this infection to levels greater than that of normal IL-6$^{+/+}$ control mice. During the course of these experiments it was noted that IL-6$^{-/-}$ mice did not produce a peripheral blood neutrophilia after infection. The significance of neutrophils was further highlighted by demonstrating that exogenous IL-6 did not revert the susceptibility phenotype of IL-6$^{-/-}$ mice which have been neutrophil depleted by the monoclonal antibody RB6-8C5.

More recently IL-6$^{-/-}$ mice used in a model of pneumonia produced by intranasal inoculation of *S. pneumonia*, died significantly earlier than control animals [132]. IL-6$^{-/-}$ mice had 6-fold more bacterial colonies isolated from lung homogenates at 40 hours after inoculation than IL-6$^{+/+}$ animals, confirming the significance of IL-6 in bacterial clearance. As expected IL-6$^{-/-}$ mice were noted to have a highly attenuated acute phase response in response to infection. Of interest, however, was the observation that IL-6$^{-/-}$ mice also demonstrated higher pulmonary levels of IL-1β, TNF-α and IFN-γ after induction of pneumonia. This was interpreted as evidence that the absence of the negative feed back loop of IL-6 on these pro-inflammatory cytokines may also have contributed to higher mortality. However despite the wealth of evidence that the presence of IL-6 provides a survival benefit in animal models of infection, pre-treatment of normal mice with IL-6 does not appear to enhance resistance to subsequent bacterial infection. Pre-treatment of mice with recombinant murine and human IL-6 did not provide a survival benefit from subsequent infection from *P. aeruginosa* administered by intramuscular injection nor did it enhance the IL-1 effect when both cytokines were given together 24 hours before infection [133]. Treatment with intravenous recombinant human IL-6 at the same time as intravenous inoculation with *L. monocytogenes* did not reduce subsequent viable bacterial counts from liver and spleen specimens nor was there any protective effect with repeated IL-6 treatment at 12 hourly intervals, from 24 hours before infection to 48 hours afterwards [134]. Whilst treatment with IL-1 and TNF-α individually did enhance bacterial clearance in this model, concomitant treatment with IL-6 did not synergize their effect. In a model of intramuscular *P. aeruginosa* infection in granulocytopenic mice, pre-treatment with recombinant human IL-6 24 hours before bacterial challenge, produced only a very small survival benefit when used at extremely high doses of 800 ng per mouse whereas 80 ng of recombinant human IL-1 was sufficient to produce a greater survival benefit [133].

IL-8: IL-8 is an 8 kDa polypeptide cytokine which belongs to the chemokine gene family. It is produced by monocytes, neutrophils, endothelial cells and a variety of mesothelial cell types in response to stimulation by LPS, IL-1 or TNF-α. Its primary function is to activate and chemoattract neutrophils to sites of inflammation [135]. IL-8 has also recently been proposed to be a stimulus for hepatocyte acute phase protein synthesis [33]. In light of these biological functions which putatively augment both cellular and humoral components of non-specific host defense, IL-8 was examined for its ability to enhance host resistance to bacterial infection in mouse models. Pre-treatment with intraperitoneal IL-8 24 hours or 30 minutes before, or 6 hours after, infection with intramuscular *P. aeruginosa*, did not significantly improve survival [136]. Instead, in mice receiving IL-8 30 minutes before or 6 hours after bacterial challenge, there was a higher mortality than control animals. In contrast, mice that received IL-8 30 minutes before *K. pneumoniae* infection by the same intraperitoneal route, did demonstrate improved survival. This protective effect was not apparent in neutropenic mice. Quantitative bacteriological analyses in these experiments showed no difference between IL-8 pre-treated and untreated mice in either model of infection. Although it was suggested that IL-8 may enhance resistance to bacteria by a neutrophil dependent mechanism, if given at the site of infection no difference in peripheral blood or peritoneal neutrophil number was evident. In comparison to IL-1 induced protection which was used as the positive control, pre-treatment with IL-8 was ineffective.

Future Work and Clinical Applications

Several different agents have been described that enhance non-specific host resistance to bacterial infections. The evidence for the possible mechanisms which lead to reduced mortality or improved bacterial clearance seems inconsistent, but it cumulatively highlights a number of general observations that may be useful in guiding future work. It is apparent that multiple mechanisms in host defense may contribute to resistance to bacterial infections, rather than there being a predominance of any one component. Therefore in order to achieve non-specific resistance we must aim to use non-specific stimulators of host defense. It is difficult to make comparisons of efficacy between agents because of differences in the models of infection and route, timing and dose of immunostimulants employed. Despite this it is apparent that MDP, glucans and the early cytokines IL-1 and TNF-α are the most effective in enhancing resistance to infection. These agents all have pleiotropic effects, stimulating both cellular and humoral components of innate immunity. By comparison, cytokines such as IL-6 or IL-8 which have slightly more specific actions are clearly less effective in enhancing non-specific resistance. In line with this observation a number of studies have demonstrated that pre-treatment of mice with multiple stimulants is more effective than each individual component used by itself [115, 137, 138]. The phenomenon of LPS-tolerance was echoed in the observations that pre-treatment with certain cytokines down-regulated the systemic cytokine response to subsequent infection by altering circulating levels, expression of their natural antagonists and their receptors. Therefore modifying the physiological response to sepsis may improve survival independently of improving microbial killing.

Down-regulating the cytokine cascade is the approach that has been most energetically pursued in attempts to improve the outcome of established severe sepsis in clinical studies. Unfortunately this has had minimal success [139]. Enhancing bacterial clearance by inducing the acute phase response and stimulating cellular components of non-specific host defense has not been sufficiently examined. Certainly, amplifying the pro-inflammatory cytokine cascade in established sepsis would be a diametrically opposite approach to that studied so far and intuitively unlikely to succeed. However, doing so prior to the onset of severe infection may be beneficial. Enhancing the resistance to bacterial infection has almost exclusively been studied in animal models and clinical studies are long overdue. In the past, clinical trials were impractical because agents such as MDP and glucans were toxic. In recent years, however, synthetic derivatives have been developed which are less toxic. PGG-glucan is active in numerous animal studies and has been selected as one such derivative and a randomized, double blind, placebo controlled Phase I/II clinical trial has been conducted [140]. Thirty four immunocompetent patients, undergoing elective major non-cardiac, thoracic surgery or abdominal surgery received either multiple intravenous doses of 0.5 mg/kg PGG-glucan or saline at 12–24 hours before surgery, 1–4 hours before surgery and 48 hours after surgery. There was no difference in adverse drug experiences between the two groups and the mean white blood cell counts were comparable throughout the trial period. There were significantly fewer culture positive infections in the PGG-glucan group compared with controls. More extensive trials with this agent are under-way. A derivative of LPS such as MPLA has been effective in animal studies with less toxicity than LPS. Preliminary human studies suggest that they are safe and that they may attenuate the toxic effects to subsequent challenge with bacterial endotoxin [141]. Human studies are required not only to evaluate the clinical effect of these agents, but also to further refine our understanding of host defense mechanisms in man and find other opportunities to manipulate them for therapeutic advantage. Ultimately, prevention of infection by stimulating non-specific host defense mechanisms may prove to be a more useful strategy than attempting to modify the immunological chaos of established severe sepsis.

References

1. Rouben DP, Fagelman K, McCoy MT, Polk HC Jr (1977) Enhancement of nonspecific host defenses against local bacterial challenge. Surg Forum 28:44–45
2. Shulkin DJ, Kinosian B, Glick H, Glen-Puschett C, Daly J, Eisenber JM (1993) The economic impact of infections. An analysis of hospital costs and charges in surgical patients with cancer. Arch Surg 128:449–452
3. Hart CA (1998) Antibiotic resistance: an increasing problem? It always has been, but there are things we can do. Br Med J 316:1255–1256
4. Levy SB (1998) Multidrug resistance – A sign of the times. N Engl J Med 338:1376–1378
5. Pepys MB (1996) The acute phase response and C-reactive protein. In: Weatherall DJ, Ledingham JGG, Warrell DA (eds) Oxford Textbook of Medicine, 3rd edn. Oxford University Press, Oxford, pp 1527–1533
6. Sox HC Jr, Liang MH (1986) The erythrocyte sedimentation rate. Guidelines for rational use. Ann Intern Med 104:515–523
7. Abernathy TJ, Avery OT (1941) Occurrence during acute infections of protein not normally present in patients' sera and effect of calcium floculation reaction with C-polysaccharide of pneumococcus. J Exp Immunol 73:173–182
8. Tillet WS, Francis C (1930) Serological reactions in pneumonia with non-protein somatic fraction of pneumococcus. J Exp Med 52:561–571
9. Pepys MB, Baltz ML (1983) Acute phase proteins with special reference to C-reactive protein and related proteins (pentaxins) and serum amyloid A protein. Adv Immunol 34:141–212

10. Crane LJ, Miller DL (1983) Plasma protein induction by isolated hepatocytes. Mol Cell Biochem 53–54:89–109
11. Morrow JF, Stearman RS, Peltzman CG, Potter DA (1981) Induction of hepatic synthesis of serum amyloid A protein and actin. Proc Natl Acad Sci USA 78:4718–4722
12. Zenser TV, DeRubertis FR, Beisel WR, et al (1975) A protein from polymorphonuclear leukocytes (LEM) which affects the rate of hepatic amino acid transport and synthesis of acute-phase globulins. Endocrinology 96:651–661
13. Kampschmidt RF, Upchurch HF, Eddington CL, Pulliam LA (1973) Multiple biological activities of a partially purified leukocytic endogenous mediator. Am J Physiol 224:530–533
14. Powanda MC, Cockerell GL, Pekarek RS (1973) Amino acid and zinc movement in relation to protein synthesis early in inflammation. Am J Physiol 225:399–401
15. Sipe JD, Vogel SN, Ryan JL, McAdam KP, Rosenstreich DL (1979) Detection of a mediator derived from endotoxin-stimulated macrohpages that induces the acute phase serum amyloid A response in mice. J Exp Med 150:597–606
16. Ramadori G, Sipe JD, Dinarello CA, Mizel SB, Colten HR (1985) Pretranslational modulation of acute phase hepatic protein synthesis by murine recombinant interleukin 1 (IL-1) and purified human IL-1. J Exp Med 162:930–942
17. Goldman ND, Liu TY (1987) Biosynthesis of human C-reactive protein in cultured hepatoma cells is induced by a monocyte factor(s) other than interleukin-1. J Biol Chem 262: 2363–2368
18. Darlington GJ, Wilson DR, Lachman LB (1986) Monocyte-conditioned medium, interleukin-1, and tumor necrosis factor stimulate the acute phase response in human hepatoma cells in vitro. J Cell Biol 103:787–793
19. Perlmutter DH, Dinarello CA, Punsal PI, Colten HR (1986) Cachectin/tumor necrosis factor regulates hepatic acute-phase gene expression. J Clin Invest 78:1349–1354
20. Heinrich PC, Castell JV, Andus T (1990) Interleukin-6 and the acute phase response. Biochem J 265:621–636
21. Marinkovic S, Jahreis GP, Wong GG, Baumann H (1989) IL-6 modulates the synthesis of a specific set of acute phase proteins in vivo. J Immunol 142:808–812
22. Dinarello CA (1988) Biology of interleukin 1. FASEB J 2:108–115
23. Wong GG, Clark SC (1988) Multiple actions of interleukin 6 within a cytokine network. Immunol Today 9:137–139
24. Selby P, Hobbs S, Viner C, et al (1987) Tumour necrosis factor in man: clinical and biological observations. Br J Cancer 56:803–808
25. Blackwell TS, Christman JW (1996) Sepsis and cytokines: current status. Br J Anaesth 77: 110–117
26. Nakayama T, Sonoda S, Urano T, Yamada T, Okada M (1993) Monitoring both serum amyloid protein A and C-reactive protein as inflammatory markers in infectious diseases. Clin Chem 39:293–297
27. Baumann H, Prowse KR Marinkovic S, Won KA, Jahreis GP (1989) Stimulation of hepatic acute phase response by cytokines and glucocorticoids. Ann NY Acad Sci 557:280–295
28. Kopf M, Bauman H, Freer G, et al (1994) Impaired immune and acute phase responses in interleukin-6–deficient mice. Nature 368:339–342
29. Morimoto A, Murakami N, Takada M, Teshirogi S, Watanabe T (1987) Fever and acute phase response induced in rabbits by human recombinant interferon-gamma. J Physiol (Lond) 391:209–218
30. Kishimoto T, Akira S, Narazaki M, Taga T (1995) Interleukin-6 family of cytokines and gp130. Blood 86:1243–1254
31. Wigmore SJ, Fearon KCH, Maingay JP, Lai PBS, Ross JA (1997) Interleukin-8 can mediate acute phase protein production by isolated human hepatocytes. Am J Physiol 273: E721–E726
32. Mazuski JE, Tolman K, Shapiro MJ (1997) Effects of cytokine antagonists on the hepatic acute-phase response. J Surg Res 68:161–169
33. Whaley K (1986) The complement system. In: Whaley K (ed) Complement in health and disease. MTP Press, Lancaster, pp 1–35

34. Morgan BP, Walport MJ (1991) Complement deficiency and disease. Immunol Today 12:301–306
35. Frank MM, Fries LF (1991) The role of complement in inflammation and phagocytosis. Immunol Today 12:322–326
36. Miletic VD, Frank MM (1995) Complement-immunoglobulin interactions. Curr Opin Immunol 7:41–47
37. Stewart JM (1993) The kinin system in inflammation. Agents Actions Suppl 42:145–157
38. Anderson KP, Heath EC (1985) The relationship between rat major acute phase protein and the kininogens. J Biol Chem 260:12065–12071
39. Bornside GH, Cohn I Jr (1968) Hemoglobin as a bacterial virulence-enhancing factor in fluids produced in strangulation intestinal obstruction. Am Surg 34:63–67
40. Krizek TJ, Davis JH (1966) Endogenous wound infection. J Trauma 6:239–248
41. Lee JT Jr, Ahrenholz DH, Nelson RD, Simmons RL (1979) Mechanisms of the adjuvant effect of hemoglobin in experimental peritonitis. V. The significance of the coordinated iron component. Surgery 86:41–48
42. Moss JP (1981) Historical and current perspectives on surgical drainage. Surg Gynecol Obstet 152:517–527
43. Griffiths E, Rogers HJ, Bullen JJ (1980) Iron, plasmids and infection. Nature 284:508–509
44. Weinberg ED (1974) Iron and susceptibility to infectious disease. Science 184:952–956
45. Krauss S, Sarcione EJ (1966) Role of the liver in the catabolism of serum haptoglobin. Proc Soc Exp Biol Med 122:1019–1022
46. Eaton JW, Brandt P, Mahoney JR (1982) Haptoglobin: A natural bacteriostat. Science 215: 691–693
47. Roberts RM, Mathialagan N, Duffy JY, Smith GW (1995) Regulation and regulatory role of proteinase inhibitors. Crit Rev Eukaryot Gene Expr 5:385–436
48. Pepys MB, Baltz M, Gomer K, Davies AJS, Doenhoff M (1979) Serum amyloid P-component is an acute phase reactant in the mouse. Nature 278:259–261
49. Ganrot PO, Kindmark CO (1969) C-reactive protein – A phagocytosis-promoting factor. J Clin Lab Invest 24:215–219
50. Kindmark CO (1971) Stimulating effect of C-reactive protein on phagocytosis of various species of pathogenic bacteria. Clin Exp Immunol 8:941–948
51. Nakayama S, Mold C, Gewurz H, du Clos TW (1982) Opsonic properties of C-reactive protein in vivo. J Immunol 128:2435–2438
52. Mold C, Edwards KM, Gewurz H (1982) Effect of C-reactive protein on the complement-mediated phagocytosis of human neutrophils by Streptococcus pneumoniae serotypes 3 and 6. Infect Immun 37:987–992
53. Weiser JN, Pan N, McGowan KL, Musher D, Martin A, Richards J (1998) Phosphorylcholine on the lipopolysaccharide of *Haemophilus influenzae* contributes to persistence in the respiratory tract and sensitivity to serum killing mediated by C-reactive protein. J Exp Med 187:631–640
54. Buchta R, Fridkin M, Pontet M, Contessi E, Scaggiante B, Romeo D (1987) Modulation of human neutrophil function by C-reactive protein. Eur J Biochem 163:141–146
55. Zhong W, Zen Q, Tebo J, Schlottmann K, Coggeshall M, Mortensen RF (1998) Effect of human C-reactive protein on chemokine and chemotactic factor-induced neutrophil chemotaxis and signaling. J Immunol 161:2533–2540
56. Zen Q, Zhong W, Mortensen RF (1997) Binding site on human C-reactive protein (CRP) recognized by the leukocyte CRP-receptor. J Cell Biochem 64:140–151
57. Crowell RE, Du-Clos TW, Montoya G, Heaphy E, Mold C (1991) C-reactive protein receptors on the human monocytic cell line U-937. Evidence for additional binding to Fc gamma RI. J Immunol 147:3445–3451
58. Volanakis JE, Kaplan MH (1974) Interaction of C-reactive protein complexes with the complement system. II. Consumption of guinea pig complement by CRP complexes: requirement for human C1q. J Immunol 113:9–17
59. Mold C, Gurule C, Otero D, Du Clos TW (1996) Complement-dependent binding of C-reactive protein to human erythrocyte CR1. Clin Immunol Immunopathol 81:153–160

60. Horowitz J, Volanakis JE, Briles DE (1987) Blood clearance of Streptococcus pneumoniae by C-reactive protein. J Immunol 138:2598–2603
61. Yother J, Volanakis JE, Briles DE (1982) Human C-reactive protein is protective against fatal Streptococcus pneumoniae infection in mice. J Immunol 128:2374–2376
62. Szalai AJ, Briles DE, Volanakis JE (1995) Human C-reactive protein is protective against fatal Streptococcus pneumoniae infection in transgenic mice. J Immunol 155:2557–2563
63. Tennent GA, Lovat LB, Pepys MB (1995) Serum amyloid P component prevents proteolysis of the amyloid fibrils of Alzheimer disease and systemic amyloidosis. Proc Natl Acad Sci USA 92:4299–4303
64. Botto M, Hawkins PN, Bickerstaff MC, et al (1997) Amyloid deposition is delayed in mice with targeted deletion of the serum amyloid P component gene. Nature Med 3:855–859
65. Bristow CL, Boackle RJ (1986) Evidence for the binding of human serum amyloid P component to C1q and Fab gamma. Mol Immunol 23:1045–1052
66. Hind CR, Collins PM, Baltz ML, Pepys MB (1985) Human serum amyloid P component, a circulating lectin with specificity for the cyclic 4,6-pyruvate acetal of galactose. Interactions with various bacteria. Biochem J 225:107–111
67. Parant M (1979) Biological properties of a new synthetic adjuvant, muramyl dipeptide (MDP). Springer Semin Immunopathol 2:101–118
68. Chedid L, Parant M, Parant F, Lefrancher P, Choay J, Lederer E (1977) Enhancement of nonspecific immunity to Klebsiella pneumoniae infection by a synthetic immunoadjuvant (N-acetylmuramyl-L-alanyl-D-isoglutamine). Proc Natl Acad Sci USA 74:2089–2093
69. Fraser-Smith EB, Matthews TR (1981) Protective effect of muramyl dipeptide analogs against infections of Pseudomonas aeruginosa or Candida albicans in mice. Infect Immun 34:676–683
70. Humphres RC, Henika PR, Ferraresi RW, Krahenbuhl JL (1980) Effects of treatment with muramyl dipeptide and certain of its analogs on resistance to Listeria monocytogenes in mice. Infect Immun 30:462–466
71. Ausobsky JR, Trachtenberg LS, Polk HC Jr (1982) Enhancement of non-specific host defenses against combined local bacterial challenge. Surg Forum 33:46–47
72. Galland RB, Heine KJ, Polk HC Jr (1982) Nonspecific stimulation of host defenses against bacterial challenge in immunosuppressed mice. Arch Surg 118:333–337
73. Galland RB, Polk HC (1982) Non-specific stimulation of host defenses against a bacterial challenge in malnourished hosts. Br J Surg 69:665–668
74. Polk HC Jr, Galland RB, Ausobsky JR (1982) Nonspecific enhancement of resistance to bacterial infection. Evidence of an effect supplemental to antibiotics. Ann Surg 196:436–441
75. Masek K (1986) Immunopharmacology of muramyl peptides. FASEB J 45:2549–2551
76. Dinarello CA, Krueger JM (1986) Induction of interleukin-1 by synthetic peptides and naturally occuring muramyl peptides. FASEB J 45:2545–2548
77. Darcissac ECA, Bahr GM, Pouillart PR, Riveau GJ, Parant MA (1996) Selective potentiation of cytokine expression in human whole blood by murabutide, a muramyl dipeptide analogue. Cytokine 8:658–666
78. Sedgwick AD, Hooke RE, Lees P, May SA (1987) Modulation of lymphocyte activating factor activity (interleukin-1) and acute phase proteins in pertussis-induced air pouch inflammation by muramyl dipeptide. Agents Actions 21:113–120
79. Karnovsky ML (1986) Muramyl peptides in mammalian tissues and their effects at the cellular level. FASEB J 45:2556–2560
80. Roth J, Aslan T, Storr B, Zeisberger E (1997) Lack of cross tolerance between LPS and muramyl dipeptide in induction of circulating TNF-α and IL-6 in guinea pigs. Am J Physiol 273: R1529–R1533
81. Makinodan T, Santos GW, Quinn RP (1979) Immunosuppressive drugs. Pharmacol Rev 22: 189–247
82. Ausobsky JR, Cheadle WG, Brosky BG, Polk HC Jr (1984) Muramyl dipeptide increases tolerance to shock and bacterial challenge in mice. Br J Surg 71:151–153
83. Lamont PM, Maier KG, Melton L, Polk HC Jr (1987) Stimulatory effects of muramyl dipeptide upon neutrophils isolated from a local bacterial infection. Br J Exp Path 68:655–661

84. Brown GL, Kellerman J, Lamont P, Sciutto M, Berbos E, Polk HC Jr (1985) Muramyl dipeptide and polymorphonuclear leukocyte chemotaxis *in vitro*. J Surg Res 39:128–132
85. Riveau GJ, Brunel-Riveau BG, Audibert FM, Chedid LA (1991) Influence of muramyl dipeptide on human blood leukocyte functions and their membrane antigens. Cell Immunol 134:147–156
86. Bacon JSD, Farmer VC, Jones D, Taylor IF (1969) The glucan component of the cell wall of Baker's yeast (*Saccharomyces cerevisiae*) considered in relation to its ultrastructure. Biochem J 114:556–557
87. Phaff HJ (1963) Cell wall of yeasts. Ann Rev Microbiol 17:15–30
88. Riggi SJ, Di Luzio NR (1961) Identification of a reticuloendithelial stimulating agent in zymosan. Am J Physiol 200:297–300
89. Ashworth CT, Di Luzio NR, Riggi SJ (1963) A morphological study of the effect of reticuloendothelial stimulation upon hepatic removal of minute particles from the blood of rats. Exp Mol Pathol (Suppl 1):83–103
90. Di Luzio NR, Wooles WR (1964) Effect of splenectomy and X-irradiation on antibody formation in reticuloendothelial hyperfunctional mice. J Reticuloendothel Soc 1:248–263
91. Kokoshis PL, Williams DL, Cook JA, Di Luzio NR (1978) Increased resistance to *Staphylococcus aureus* infection and enhancement of serum lysozyme activity by glucan. Science 199:1340–1342
92. Reynolds JA, Kastello MD, Harrington DG, et al (1980) Glucan-induced enhancement of host resistance to selected infectious diseases. Infect Immun 30:51–57
93. Fearon DT, Austen KF (1977) Activation of the complement pathway due to resistance zymosan bound cation convertase to endogenous regulatory mechanisms. Proc Natl Acad Sci USA 74:1683
94. Czop JK, Fearon DT, Austen KF (1978) Opsonin-independent phagocytosis of activators of the alternative complement pathway by human monocytes. J Immunol 120:1132–1138
95. Czop JK (1986) The role of beta-glucan receptors on blood and tissue leukocytes in phagocytosis and metabolic activation. Pathol Immunopathol Res 5:286–296
96. Suzuki T, Ohno N, Chiba N, Miura NN, Adachi Y, Yadomae T (1996) Immunopharmacological activity of the purified insoluble glucan, zymocel, in mice. J Pharm Pharmacol 48:1243–1248
97. Seljelid R, Figenschau Y, Bogwald J, Rasmussen LT, Austgulen R (1989) Evidence that tumor necrosis induced by aminated beta 1–3D polyglucose is mediated by a concerted action of local and systemic cytokines. Scand J Immunol 30:687–694
98. Sherwood ER, Williams DL, McNamee RB, Jones EL, Browder IW, Di-Luzio NR (1987) Enhancement of interleukin-1 and interleukin-2 production by soluble glucan. Int J Immunopharmacol 9:261–267
99. Onderdonk AB, Cisneros RL, Hinkson P, Ostroff G (1992) Anti-infective effect of poly-β-1-6-glucotrisyl-β1-3-glucopyranose glucan *in vivo*. Infect Immun 60:1642–1647
100. Kernodle DS, Gates H, Kaiser AB (1998) Prophylactic anti-infective activity of poly-[1–6]-β-D-glucopyranosyl-[1–3]-β-D-glucopyranose glucan in a guinea pig model of staphylococcal wound infection. Antimicrob Agents Chemother 42:545–549
101. Zimmerman JW, Lindermuth J, Fish PA, Palace GP, Stevenson TT, DeMong DE (1998) A novel carbohydrate-glycosphingolipid interaction between a β-(1–3)-glucan immunomodulator, PGG-glucan, and lactosylceramide of human leukocytes. J Biol Chem 273:22014–22020
102. Michalek M, Melican D, Brunke-Reese D, et al (1998) Activation of rat macrophages by Betafectin® PGG-glucan requires cross-linking of membrane receptors distinct from complement receptor three (CR3). J Leuk Biol 64:337–344
103. Brunke-Reese D, Gu Y, Crotty K, Fisette L, Mackin WM (1994) Enhanced microbicidal activities of human peripheral blood monocytes and neutrophils (PMN) after pre-treatment with PGG-glucan (Betafecin™). FASEB J 8:488
104. Cisneros RL, Gibson FC, Tzianabos AO (1996) Passive transfer of poly-[1–6]-β-D-glucopyranosyl-[1–3]-β-D-lucopyranose glucan protection against lethal infection in an animal model of intra-abdominal sepsis. Infect Immun 64:2201–2205
105. Poutsiaka DD, Mengozzi M, Vannier E, Sinha B, Dinarello CA (1993) Crosslinking of the β-glucan receptor on human monocytes results in interleukin-1 receptor antagonist but not interleukin-1 production. Blood 82:3695–3700

106. Adams DS, Pero SC, Petro JB, Nathans R, Mackin WM, Wakshull E (1997) PGG-glucan activates NF-κB-like and NF-IL-6-like transcription factor complexes in a murine monocytic cell line. J Leuk Biol 62:865–873
107. Bone RC (1991) The pathogenesis of sepsis. Ann Intern Med 115:457–469
108. Fenton MJ, Golenbock DT (1998) LPS-binding proteins and receptors. J Leuk Biol 64:25–32
109. Yang RB, Mark MR, Gray A, et al (1998) Toll-like receptor-2 mediates lipopolysaccharide-induced cellular signaling. Nature 395:284–288
110. Glauser MP, Zanetti G, Baumgartner JD, Cohen J (1991) Septic shock: pathogenesis. Lancet 338:732–736
111. Rowley D (1955) Stimulation of natural immunity to *Escherichia coli* infections. Lancet 1: 232–234
112. Landy M (1956) Increase in resistance following administration of bacterial lipopolysaccharides. Ann NY Acad Sci 66:292–303
113. Vuopio-Varkila J, Nurminen M, Pyhala L, Makela PH (1988) Lipopolysaccharide-induced non-specific resistance to systemic *Esherichia coli* infection in mice. J Med Microbiol 25: 197–203
114. Chase JJ, Kubey W, Dulek MH, et al (1986) Effect of monophosphoryl lipid A on host resistance to bacterial infection. Infect Immun 53:711–712
115. Nakano Y, Onozuka K, Terada Y, Shinomiya H, Nakano M (1990) Protective effect of recombinant tumour necrosis factor-α in murine salmonellosis. J Immunol 144:1935–1941
116. Chedid L, Parant M, Damais C, Parant F, Juy D, Galalli A (1976) Failure of endotoxin to increase non-specific resistance to infection of lipopolysaccharide low-responder mice. Infect Immun 13:722–727
117. Zuckerman SH, Evans GF (1991) Endotoxin tolerance: in vivo regulation of tumour necrosis factor and interleukin-1 synthesis at a transcriptional level. Cell Immunol 140:513–519
118. Czuprynski CJ, Brown JF, Young KM, Cooley J, Kurtz RS (1988) Effects of murine recombinant interleukin-1α on the host response to bacterial infection. J Immunol 140:962–968
119. Minami A, Fujimoto K, Ozaki Y, Nakamura S (1988) Augmentation of host resistance to microbial infections by recombinant human interleukin-1α. Infect Immun 56:3116–3120
120. Morikage T, Mizushima Y, Sakamoto K, Yano S (1990) Prevention of fatal infections by recombinant human interleukin-1α in normal and anti-cancer drug-treated mice. Cancer Res 50:2099–2104
121. Van Der Meer JWM, Barza M, Wolff SM, Dinarello CA (1988) A low dose of recombinant interleukin 1 protects granulocytopaenic mice from lethal Gram-negative infection. Proc Natl Acad Sci USA 85:1620–1623
122. McIntyre KW, Unowsky J, DeLorenzo W, Benjamin W (1989) Enhancement of antibacterial resistance of neutropanic, bone marrow suppressed mice by interleukin-1α. Infect Immun 57:48–54
123. Gladue R, Girard A, Newborg M (1988) Enhanced antibacterial resistance in neutropenic mice treated with human recombinant interleukin-1β. Agents Actions 24:130–136
124. Kullberg BJ, van't Wout JW, van Furth R (1990) Role of granulocytes in increased host resistance to *Candida albicans* induced by recombinant interleukin-1. Infect Immun 58:3319–3324
125. Sullivan GW, Gelrud AK, Carper HT, Mandell GL (1996) Interaction of tumour necrosis factor-α and granulocyte colony-stimulating factor on neutrophil apoptosis, receptor expression and bactericidal function. Proc Assoc Am Physicians 108:455–466
126. Vogels MTE, Cantoni L, Carelli M, Sironi M, Ghezzi P, van der Meer JWM (1993) Role of acute-phase proteins in interleukin-1-induced nonspecific resistance to bacterial infections in mice. Antimicrob Agents Chemother 37:2527–2533
127. Vogels MT, Mensink EJ, Ye K, et al (1994) Differential gene expression for IL-1 receptor antagonist, IL-1 and TNF receptors and IL-1 and TNF synthesis may explain IL-1 induced resistance to infection. J Immunol 153:5772–5780
128. Vogels MT, Eling WM, Otten A, van der Meer JW (1995) Interleukin-1 (IL-1)-induced resistance to bacterial infection: role of the type I IL-1 receptor. Antimicrob Agents Chemother 39:1744–1747
129. Larrick J, Graham D, Toy K, Lin LS, Senyk G, Fendly BM (1987) Recombinant tumour necrosis factor causes activation of human granulocytes. Blood 69:640–644

130. Desiderio JV, Kiener PA, Lin PF, Warr GA (1989) Protection of mice against *Listeria monocytogenes* infection by recombinant human tumour necrosis factor alpha. Infect Immun 57: 1615–1617
131. Dalrymple SA, Lucian LA, Slattery R, et al (1995) Interleukin-6 deficient mice are highy susceptible to *Listeria monocytogenes* infection: correlation with inefficient neutrophilia. Infect Immun 63:2262–2268
132. van der Poll T, Keogh C, Guirao X, Buurman WA, Kopf M, Lowry SF (1997) Interleukin-6 gene deficient mice show impaired defense against pneumococcal pneumonia. J Infect Dis 176:439–444
133. van der Meer JWM, Helle M, Aarden L (1989) Comparison of the effects of recombinant interleukin 6 and recombinant interleukin 1 on nonspecific resistance to infection. Eur J Immunol 19:413–416
134. Czuprynski CJ, Haak-Frendscho M, Maroushek N, Brown JF (1992) Effects of recombinant human interleukin-6 alone and in combination with recombinant interleukin-1α and tumor necrosis factor alpha on antibacterial resistance in mice. Antimicrob Agents Chemother 36:68–70
135. van Damme J (1991) Interleukin 8 and related molecules. In: Thompson A (ed) The Cytokine Handbook. Academic Press Inc, San Diego, pp 201–214
136. Vogels MTE, Lindley IJD, Curfs JHAJ, Eling WMC, van der Meer JWM (1993) Effects of interleukin-8 on nonspecific resistance to infection in neutropenic and normal mice. Antimicrob Agent Chemother 37:276–280
137. Morrissey PJ, Charrier K, Vogel SN (1995) Exogenous tumor necrosis factor alpha and interleukin-1 alpha increase resistance to *Salmonella typhimurium*: efficacy is influenced by the Ity and Lps loci. Infect Immun 63:3196–3198
138. Gaar E, Naziri W, Cheadle WG, Pietsch JD, Johnson M, Polk HC (1994) Improved survival in simulated surgical infection with combined cytokine, antibiotic and immunostimulant therapy. Br J Surg 81:1309–1311
139. Zeni F, Freeman B, Natanson C (1997) Anti-inflammatory therapies to treat sepsis and septic shock: a reassessment. Crit Care Med 25:1095–1100
140. Babineau TJ, Marcello P, Swails W, Kenler A, Bistrian B, Armour Forse R (1994) Randomized phase I/II trial of a macrophage specific immunomodulator (PGG-glucan) in high-risk surgical patients. Ann Surg 220:601–609
141. Astiz ME, Rackow EC, Still JG, et al (1995) Pretreatment of normal humans with monophosphoryl lipid A induces tolerance to endotoxin: A prospective, double-blind, randomized, controlled trial. Crit Care Med 23:9–17

Cytokines as Mediators of Lung Innate Immunity

T. J. Standiford, B. Merhad, and W. C. Tsai

Introduction

The emergence of multi-drug resistant microbes in the immunocompromised host has made the treatment of bacterial, fungal, and mycobacterial infections of the lung increasingly difficult [1–3]. This rather ominous trend underscores the need to better understand the immune host response in order to develop immunotherapies directed at these responses. Effective host defense against common bacterial pathogens of the respiratory tract is primarily dependent upon the rapid clearance of the etiologic agent from the lung [4, 5]. Innate, or natural immunity, is the principal pathway for effective elimination of bacterial organisms that have reached the alveolus. The three principal phagocytic cells that constitute innate immunity in the lung include resident alveolar macrophages, recruited neutrophils, and mononuclear phagocytes. In addition, these cells, as well as resident T cells (particularly γδ-T cells) and natural killer (NK) cells, participate in innate immune responses in the lung via the elaboration of important activating and/or chemotactic cytokines. In contrast to bacterial infection, host responses to intracellular bacteria, fungi, mycobacterium and viruses are more complex and require both the phagocytic system, as well as antibody-mediated and cell-mediated immunity [4–7]. While neutrophils play a role in host defense against some of these pathogens, the recruitment and/or activation of macrophages and $CD4^+$ T cells is essential for the effective clearance of many intracellular pathogens from the lung.

Cytokines as Mediators of Pulmonary Innate Immunity

The generation of inflammation in the setting of infectious challenge is a complex and dynamic process which involves the balanced expression of both pro- and anti-inflammatory cytokines [8, 9]. The elaboration of activating and/or chemotactic cytokines is necessary to generate sufficient leukocyte recruitment/activation required for eradication of the particular pathogen. However, the magnitude of inflammatory cytokine expression must be appropriately controlled and compartmentalized to prevent excessive tissue injury and 'spill-over' of cytokine effects into the systemic circulation. Such is the case for tumor necrosis factor-alpha (TNF-α), a cytokine which is absolutely required for effective innate and adaptive immunity, but can also trigger a cascade of events that results in substantial hemodynamic instability and end-organ injury when TNF-α is released systemically [10–12].

Cytokines participate in innate and acquired immune responses by either directly or indirectly mediating leukocyte recruitment, or by serving as important signals in the activation of leukocytes that have accumulated at specific sites of microbial invasion. Cytokines that directly or indirectly influence both leukocyte recruitment and activation include TNF-α, granulocyte-colony stimulating factor (G-CSF), granulocyte-macrophage colony stimulating factor (GM-CSF), and members of the chemokine family, whereas cytokines that predominantly regulate the state of leukocyte activation include interferon-gamma (IFN-γ), interleukin-10 (IL-10), and IL-12. Cytokines can also influence microbial clearance by inducing or regulating the expression of other effector molecules, which can occur

Table 1. Direct experimental evidence supporting the contribution of specific cytokines to innate immune responses directed against bacterial pathogens of the lung

Cytokine	*Biologic Effect in Bacterial Pneumonia*
TNF-α	- neutralization impairs bacterial clearance and survival in murine bacterial pneumonia [10, 17–20] - compartmentalized intrapulmonary overexpression enhances clearance and survival in murine *Klebsiella* pneumonia [55]
CXC Chemokines	- neutralization of specific CXC chemokines or common receptor (CXCR2) impairs neutrophil influx, bacterial clearance and survival in murine gram-negative bacterial and aspergillus pneumonia [23] - lung transgenic expression of specific CXC chemokines (KC) enhances bacterial clearance and survival in murine *Klebsiella* pneumonia [24]
G-CSF	- neutralization impairs microbial clearance and neutrophil influx in rodent bacterial pneumonia [9] - administration or overexpression of G-CSF enhances bacterial clearance and survival in rodent [57] or rabbit [58] Gram-negative pneumonia
IL-6	- impaired clearance of *S. pneumoniae* in IL-6 deficient mice [59]
IL-12	- neutralization impairs bacterial clearance and decreases survival in murine *Klebsiella* pneumonia [33] - transient intrapulmonary overexpression increases neutrophil influx and survival in murine *Klebsiella* pneumonia [33]
IFN-γ	- impaired bacterial clearance and increased lethality in IFN-γ deficient mice after intrapulmonary challenge with *S. pneumoniae* [29] or *K. pneumoniae* - transient overexpression of IFN-γ enhances intrapulmonary clearance of *P. aeruginosa* [30]
IL-10	- neutralization enhances bacterial clearance and survival in murine *Klebsiella* pneumonia [40] and reverses sepsis-induced impairment in clearance of intrapulmonary *P. aeruginosa* [50] - administration of IL-10 impairs bacterial clearance and decreases survival in murine pneumococcal pneumonia [41] but attenuates lung injury and enhances survival in mice administered cytotoxic strains of *P. aeruginosa* intratracheally [51]

in either an autocrine or paracrine fashion. Cytokines that have been shown to play an instrumental role in mediating innate immune responses in the setting of lung bacterial challenge are listed in Table 1, and this chapter focuses on cytokines which have been investigated in our laboratory.

Cytokines that Influence Leukocyte Recruitment and Activation

TNF-α

Of all cytokines studied to date, TNF represents one of the most important components of cytokine-mediated host defense against bacteria, mycobacteria, fungi and parasites. Specifically, TNF-α is a 17 kDa protein produced predominantly by myeloid cells that activates both neutrophils and macrophages, leading to enhancement of protease release, stimulation of the respiratory burst, and enhanced leukocyte phagocytic and microbicidal activity [13–15]. Although not directly chemotactic by itself, TNF-α can mediate the influx of leukocytes (both neutrophils and mononuclear phagocytes) by stimulating the expression of adhesion molecules on the surface of leukocytes and vascular endothelial cells [13–15]. Moreover, TNF-α serves as a potent endogenous signal for the expression of a number of chemotactic cytokines, particularly chemokines [11]. Finally, TNF-α is expressed in increased amounts in the airspace of humans with bacterial pneumonia [16], and in the lungs of animals after intrapulmonary challenge with various respiratory pathogens [10, 11, 17–20]. The inhibition of TNF-α has been shown to impair lung bacterial clearance, and in some but not all studies, to attenuate lung neutrophil influx in response to aerosolized or intratracheally administered *Pseudomonas aeruginosa*, *Klebsiella pneumoniae*, and *Streptococcus pneumoniae*, resulting in markedly decreased survival in animals with bacterial pneumonia [10, 17–19]. We have shown that the administration of a soluble TNF receptor:Fc immunoglobulin construct intraperitoneally in murine *Klebsiella* pneumonia results in a 10–20 fold increase in *K. pneumoniae* organisms recovered from blood and lung, as compared to control animals, and a marked increase in mortality from 10% in control animals administered *K. pneumoniae* 10^2 colony forming units (CFU) to 80% in *Klebsiella*-challenged animals depleted of TNF-α [10].

TNF also appears to be a necessary component of lung innate and cell-mediated immunity against intracellular pathogens. TNF-α is produced and is required for effective clearance of *Legionella pneumophilia* in mice, which appears to be dependent upon the ability of TNF-α to stimulate the production of nitric oxide (NO) [18]. Likewise, TNF-α is expressed in a time-dependent manner within the lungs of immunocompetent and immunocompromised mice intratracheally challenged with *Aspergillis fumigatus* conidia, and neutralization of TNF in these settings results in the development of invasive pulmonary aspergillus infection in normally resistant mice, and marked worsening of infection in immunocompromised (cytoxan-treated) mice [20]. In addition, the early expression of TNF-α is required for the development of acquired immunity in murine lung cryptococcal infection, as treatment of *Cryptococcus neoformans*-infected mice with anti-TNF at the onset of infection results in a significant reduction in pulmonary inflammation, impaired pulmonary clearance, and early dissemination of infection to the central nervous system [11].

Chemokines

Six closely related subfamilies of chemotactic cytokines, referred to as chemokines, have now been characterized. Of these, members of at least two subfamilies contribute to pulmonary antimicrobial host defense [28, 29]. The CXC chemokine family members, which include IL-8, macrophage inflammatory protein (MIP)-2, cytokine-induced neutrophil chemo-attractant (KC), epithelial cell-derived neutrophil activating peptide (ENA)-78, neutrophil activating protein (NAP)-2, granulocyte chemotactic protein (GCP)-2, LPS-induced CXC chemokine (LIX), and lungkine, have predominant neutrophil stimulatory and chemotactic activities, whereas the CC family, which includes monocyte chemotactic protein (MCP)-1, MCP-2, MCP-3, regulated on activation, normal T cells expressed and secreted (RANTES), MIP-1α, and MIP-1β, exerts predominant chemotactic and/or activating effects on macrophages, lymphocytes, and eosinophils [28]. A number of infectious agents, or cellular components of these agents, have been shown to induce the production of CXC or CC chemokines from mononuclear phagocytes and stromal cells. In addition, chemokines, in particular IL-8, have been detected in increased amounts within the lungs of patients with a variety of pulmonary infections.

In order to establish direct causal relationships between chemokines and specific biologic events in pneumonia, we have employed murine pneumonia models to begin to assess the role of the CXC chemokines MIP-2 and KC, functional murine homologs of IL-8, to innate immunity in murine *Klebsiella* pneumonia [23, 24]. Incubation of neutrophils with murine MIP-2 *in vitro* has been shown to enhance both the ingestion and killing of bacterial organisms by these cells. *In vivo*, challenge with intratracheal *K. pneumoniae* resulted in a time-dependent increase in MIP-2 mRNA and protein within the lung. The neutralization of MIP-2 using rabbit anti-murine MIP-2 antibody resulted in an approximately 60% decrease in lung neutrophil influx, as compared to animals receiving control IgG. In addition, treatment with anti-MIP-2 antibodies resulted in a modest but significant impairment in clearance of *K. pneumoniae* from the lungs of these animals, as well as increased early dissemination of *K. pneumoniae* to both blood and liver [23]. As compared to animals receiving control IgG, passive immunization with anti-MIP-2 antibody resulted in a 40–50% increase in early (24–48 hour) mortality, but no change in survival past 72 hours. Like MIP-2, KC is expressed within the lung in response to intrapulmonary challenge with *K. pneumoniae*, although the peak expression of KC occurs at an earlier time point than the maximal expression of MIP-2 [24]. A KC transgenic mouse has been developed in which the KC gene is linked to a Clara cell-specific promoter (CC10), whereby the transgenic expression of KC occurs only in the lung (the unique site of Clara cells). Interestingly, as compared to wildtype control mice, KC transgenic mice display greatly enhanced clearance of bacteria from the lung and substantially increased survival when challenged with *K. pneumoniae* 3×10^3 CFU (10% survival in wildtype versus 80% survival in KC transgenic animals). This enhanced resistance to bacterial challenge occurred in association with a marked increase in the recruitment (and possibly activation) of airway and airspace neutrophils.

Given that significant redundancy in CXC chemokine expression exists in the setting of pneumonia, inhibition of an individual CXC chemokine may have only modest effects on neutrophil dependent clearance of respiratory pathogens. To this end, we have performed studies to evaluate the effect of blocking CXCR2, the common shared receptor of MIP-2, KC, and other glutamic acid-leucine-arginine (ELR)-containing CXC chemokines [25]. Treatment of C57BL/6 mice with a single administration of goat antimouse CXCR2 antiserum markedly increased the susceptibility of mice to invasive pulmonary infection due to *Pseudomonas aeruginosa* (Fig. 1), *Nocardia asteroides*, and *Aspergillis fumigatus*, pathogens which are highly dependent on the influx of neutrophils for adequate pulmonary clearance. In fact, anti-CXCR2-treated animals develop invasive disease with 10–50-fold less *P. aeruginosa* or *N. asteroides* than that required in control animals.

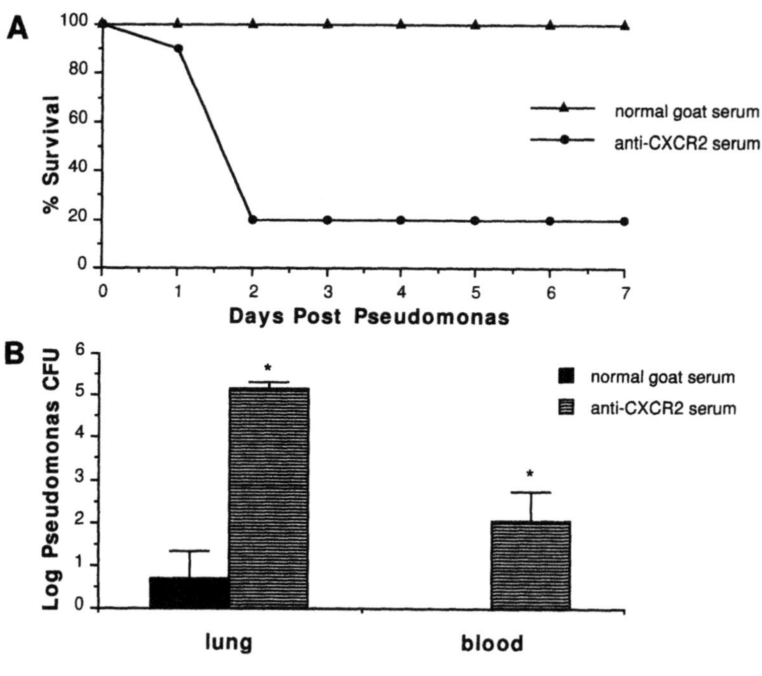

Fig. 1. Effect of CXCR2 neutralization on survival (A) and lung and blood *Pseudomonas* colony forming units (CFU) after intratracheal challenge with *P. aeruginosa* (8×10^5 CFU). Animals were administered goat antimouse CXCR2 antiserum 2 hours prior to *P. aeruginosa* administration. Blood and whole lung CFU determined 24 hours after *Pseudomonas* administration and expressed as $\log_{10}$. * $p < 0.01$

These findings indicate that CXC chemokines collectively play a major role in innate immunity against a variety of respiratory pathogens.

Cytokines that Influence Leukocyte Activation

IFN-γ

IFN-γ is a cytokine produced by T cells and NK cells that is instrumental in cell-mediated immunity against a broad spectrum of pulmonary pathogens. This cytokine activates several macrophage effector cell activities, including stimulation of respiratory burst, the ability to present antigen, priming of macrophage-derived TNF release, and enhanced *in vitro* macrophage antimicrobial activity against bacterial, fungal, and mycobacterial organisms [26]. *In vivo*, IFN-γ depletion using specific neutralizing antibodies has resulted in impaired pulmonary clearance of *Mycoplasma*, *Chlamydia*, and *Histoplasma* [9]. In addition, the aerosolized administration of recombinant murine IFN-γ reduced the intensity of *P. carinii* pneumonia in $CD4^+$ depleted mice [27], whereas intratracheal, but not intraperitoneal administration of recombinant murine IFN-γ has been shown to enhance the clearance of *L. pneumophilia* from the lungs of corticosteroid-treated rats [28]. In these studies, treatment with IFN-γ did not alter, or in fact decreased, the intra-alveolar influx of inflammatory cells, suggesting that the beneficial effects of IFN-γ in these models was likely attributable to direct leukocyte activation rather than augmenting lung leukocyte recruitment. Furthermore, compartmentalized IFN-γ therapy via intratracheal administration appeared to be more efficacious than that observed when IFN-γ was delivered systemically.

IFN-γ also appears to be a critical signal in innate immunity against extracellular bacterial pathogens of the lung. Specifically, IFN-γ knockout mice have recently been shown to be particularly susceptible to aerosolized challenge with *S. pneumoniae*, which is due, in part, to an impaired ability of these animals to produce TNF *in vivo* [29]. Similarly, we have shown that IFN-γ knockout mice (on both a BALB/c and C57BL/6 background) displayed impaired bacterial clearance and increased mortality when challenged intratracheally with *K. pneumoniae*. IFN-γ also appears to contribute to anti-pseudomonal host defense, as the intratracheal administration or systemic overexpression of murine IFN-γ using adenovirally-mediated gene therapy results in improved clearance of aerosolized *P. aeruginosa* [30]. Similar to observations made in IFN-γ deficient animals, the beneficial effects of IFN-γ on innate immunity appear to be partially mediated by the enhanced production of TNF in the lungs of these animals.

IL-12

Like IFN-γ, IL-12 is a cytokine that was initially recognized as a critical component of 'Th1' phenotype cell-mediated immune responses [31]. More recent studies, however, indicate that this cytokine is not only instrumental in the modulation of acquired immunity against a variety of intracellular pathogens, but IL-12 also plays a major role in the innate immune response against common extracellular bacterial pathogens.

IL-12 is a heterodimeric protein consisting of two subunits (p35 and p40) that promotes Th1-type immune responses by stimulating the development of Th1 T cells and NK cells, increasing the cytolytic activity of $CD8^+$ cells and NK cells, and most importantly, serving as the major signal for IFN-γ expression from T cells and NK cells [31]. In addition to its role in host defense against tumors, IL-12 has been increasingly recognized for its central role in antimicrobial immunity [31]. The systemic administration of IL-12 to mice has been shown to increase host resistance to several intracellular pathogens, including *Leishmania major*, *Toxoplasma gondii*, *Listeria monocytogenes*, *Mycobacterium tuberculosis*, and *Plasmodium chabaudi* [31]. In addition, the systemic administration of IL-12 to mice with cryptococcal pneumonia has been shown to result in improved pulmonary clearance, decreased dissemination to the brain, and increased survival [32].

Our laboratory has demonstrated that IL-12 represents an integral component of innate immunity against bacterial pathogens of the lung [33]. Specifically, IL-12 p35 and p40 mRNA, as well as intact IL-12 protein are expressed within the lungs of mice challenged with *K. pneumoniae*, and the passive immunization of *Klebsiella*-challenged mice with anti-IL-12 antibodies results in an approximately 12-fold increase in the numbers of *K. pneumoniae* CFU isolated from lung homogenates at 48 hours post-inoculation, as compared to animals receiving preimmune serum. Furthermore, *in vivo* neutralization of IL-12 significantly decreased long-term survival in animals challenged with *K. pneumoniae.*

IL-10

In distinct contrast to IL-12, IL-10 promotes the development of Th2-type immune responses, while inhibiting cell-mediated (Th1-type) immune responses [34]. Notably, this cytokine has been shown to exert potent anti-inflammatory properties, in part by directly de-activating neutrophils and macrophages, and by down-regulating the expression of TNF, IFN-γ, and members of both the CXC and CC chemokine families [35–37]. Importantly, IL-10 can attenuate the overzealous production of cytokines in states of systemic immune cell activation, as occurs in the sepsis syndrome [38, 39]. However, in the setting of pneumonia the generation of a vigorous inflammatory response is essential for effective clearance of microbes from the lung, and IL-10-mediated suppression of activating and chemotactic cytokines has been shown to be detrimental to the host in the setting of pneumonia. The inoculation of mice with *K. pneumoniae* resulted in the early expression of both IL-10 mRNA and protein, with maximal expression occurring at 48 hours post-inoculation [40]. Passive immunization with anti-IL-10 antibodies significantly enhanced bacterial clearance from the lung, and resulted in a greater than 100-fold reduction in the numbers of *K. pneumoniae* recovered from the bloodstream. This enhanced bacterial clearance was associated with an improvement in both early and long-term survival. While the mechanism by which inhibition of IL-10 protects animals has not been defined, additional studies have demonstrated that treatment with anti-IL-10 antibodies results in a maximal 2- to 4-fold increase in TNF, MIP-2 and IFN-γ protein levels in lung homogenates, as compared to animals receiving control. Consistent with our observations, van der Poll and colleagues have demonstrated that IL-10 administration to mice with pneumococcal pneumonia substantially impairs lung bacterial clearance and increased lethality [41].

IL-10 as a Mediator of Sepsis-Induced Immunosuppression

There is now compelling evidence to indicate that the sepsis syndrome results in a prolonged and profound state of immunosuppression, which is characterized by substantially diminished monocyte/macrophage effector cell function. Specific monocyte/macrophage defects in septic patients include a reduced human leukocyte antigen (HLA)-DR expression, loss of antigen-presenting capacity, and a striking decrease in the ability to produce important activating and regulatory cytokines, including TNF-α, IL-1β, and IL-6 [42–44]. Monocyte/macrophage deactivation appears to be of considerable functional significance, as higher rates of infection and increased mortality have been observed in post-operative or septic patients who display evidence of monocyte deactivation, either in the form of decreased monocyte HLA-DR expression or impaired delayed-type hypersensitivity responses [45, 46]. Septic patients are especially susceptible to nosocomial infections of the lung, particularly pneumonia secondary to *P. aeruginosa* [47].

Recent studies indicate that the expression of IL-10 may contribute to sepsis-induced leukocyte deactivation. For example, the production of TNF from endotoxin-desensitized blood monocytes and monocytes isolated from septic patients can be nearly completely restored when treated in culture with anti-IL-10 antibodies [48]. Furthermore, we have observed that IL-10 levels are increased greater than 50-fold in CD-1 mice undergoing cecal ligation and 26 gauge needle puncture (a commonly used model of abdominal sepsis syndrome), and levels of IL-10 remain elevated significantly longer than do the levels of pro-inflammatory cytokines (e.g., TNF, MIP-2, IL-12 [49]). In order to reproduce the common clinical scenario whereby critically-ill patients develop *Pseudomonas* pneumonia in the post-septic period, we induced sepsis sydrome in mice by performing cecal ligation and 26 gauge needle puncture (CLP), then administered *P. aeruginosa* intratracheally 24 hours after CLP or sham abdominal surgery [50]. In animals undergoing sham surgery, *P. aeruginosa* was rapidly and completely cleared from the lung within 24 hours. In contrast, mice undergoing CLP readily developed pneumonia, *P. aeruginosa* bacteremia, and death as early as 48 hours after *Pseudomonas* challenge. Interestingly, no induction of IL-10 was observed in sham-operated animals challenge with *P. aeruginosa*, whereas a similar challenge in CLP mice resulted in a 3.5-fold increase in lung IL-10 levels at 24 hours post *P. aeruginosa* administration. Importantly, administration of rabbit anti-murine IL-10 serum intraperitoneally at the time of *P. aeruginosa* challenge significantly improved survival in CLP animals as compared to *Pseudomonas*-challenged CLP mice receiving non-immune serum (62% survival vs. 32% survival), which occurred in association with a 19- and 26-fold reduction in *P. aeruginosa* CFU isolated from blood and lung respectively (Fig. 2). The mechanism(s) by which anti-IL-10 therapy increased bacterial clearance in animals undergoing CLP has not been completely defined. However, the *in vivo* neutralization of IL-10 resulted in significantly improved alveolar macrophage phagocytic and bactericidal activity when cultured *ex vivo*. These observations provide rather convincing evidence that IL-10 is a major mediator of sepsis-induced immunosuppression.

Collectively, the observations made in murine models of pneumonia due to *K. pneumoniae*, *S. pneumoniae*, and CLP followed by *P. aeruginosa*, indicate that the expression of IL-10 can attenuate antibacterial host defense by down-regulating the magnitude of the inflammatory response. However, a recent study examining acute pneumonia utilizing two cytotoxic strains of *P. aeruginosa* suggests that a delicate balance between local, organ specific inflammatory responses and systemic inflammatory responses exists. Sawa and colleagues found that two cytotoxic strains rapidly induced acute lung epithelial injury, blood dissemination,

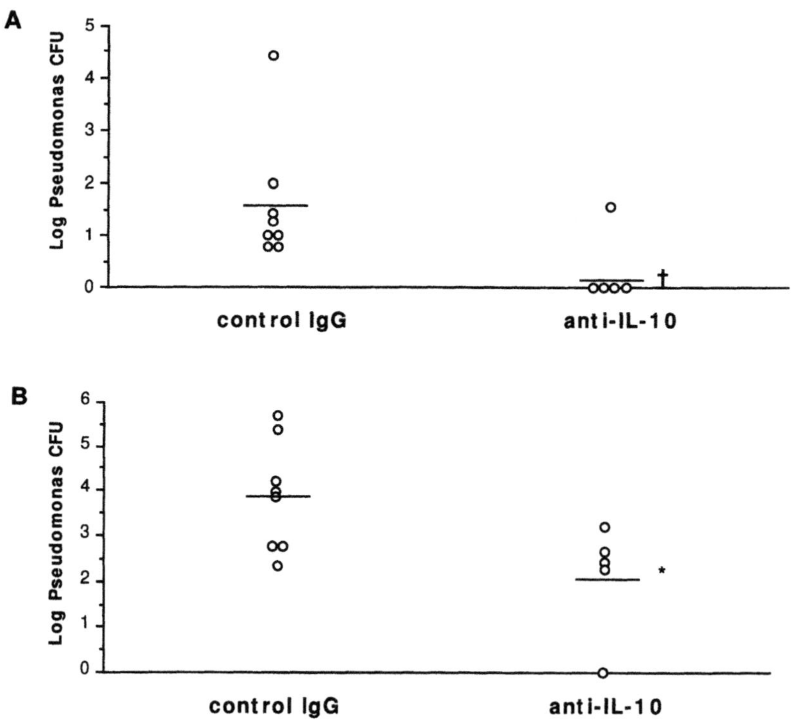

Fig. 2A, B. Effect of IL-10 neutralization on lung and plasma *P. aeruginosa* CFU in cegal ligation and puncture (CLP) mice administered *P. aeruginosa* (4×10^5 CFU) 24 hours post-CLP or sham surgery. Rabbit antimurine IL-10 serum or control rabbit serum (control IgG) was administered 2 hours prior to *P. aeruginosa* inoculation. Experimental n=5–8 per group. Line represents mean CFU value. * $p<0.05$, † $p<0.01$ as compared to animals receiving control IgG and mortality (within 2 days) while non-cytotoxic strains were non-injurious or lethal. Cytotoxic strains induced rapid lung and blood IL-10 levels, whereas the non-cytotoxic strains failed to induce IL-10 [51]. Interestingly, the systemic administration of IL-10 significantly decreased lung injury and mortality induced by these cytotoxic *P. aeruginosa* strains. These results would suggest that the cytotoxic strains of *P. aeruginosa* are inducing an overwhelming, unregulated proinflammatory response resulting in excessive tissue injury and rapid death, and in this setting IL-10 is required to keep this response in check. Therefore, the overall effect of a specific cytokine (whether beneficial or detrimental) can be organism-dependent, and observations made using one particular organism cannot necessarily be extrapolated to models employing different microbes.

Compartmentalized Cytokine Immunotherapy Using Intrapulmonary Adenoviral Gene Therapy

Most previous approaches to immunotherapy have involved the systemic augmentation or neutralization of specific cytokines and/or cytokine receptors. Unfortunately, this form of immunotherapy is often complicated by significant dose-limiting toxicity or specific immune effects that are undesirable when they occur systemically. This is especially true for the systemic administration of cytokines such as TNF, IL-2, and IL-12 [12, 52]. Therefore, in instances where the disease process is focal, local and compartmentalized delivery of specific immunotherapy is the most rational approach to treatment. A limitation of this form of therapy is that cytokines may not be adequately delivered to poorly ventilated alveolar units, and that intermittent therapy results in therapeutic levels of cytokines for inadequate periods of time. Despite these potential drawbacks, aerosolized or intratracheally-administered IFN-γ has been employed effectively in the treatment of several lung pathogens, including *P. carinii* and *L. pneumophilia* [26, 27]. We have recently administered a TNF agonist peptide (consisting of the 11 amino acid binding site of TNF to its receptor) intratracheally, which protected mice challenged with *K. pneumoniae* when given 3 or 7 days before bacterial administration, but not when given concomitant with bacterial challenge or when given by the intraperitoneal route [53].

To overcome problems with variability and, at times, inadequacy of cytokine delivery by the intrapulmonary route, we have employed a novel approach to compartmentalized cytokine delivery using adenoviral gene therapy. The use of intratracheal gene therapy in the treatment of lung infection has several attractive features. In particular, the human type 5 adenovirus used has specific tropism for the respiratory epithelium, resulting in relatively efficient infectivity and gene transfer [54]. Moreover, the E1 region of the viral genome has been deleted, rendering the virus unable to replicate *in vivo*. Therefore, the expression of a specific gene is transient, resulting in acute desirable effects of transgene expression (i.e., rapid microbial clearance) without the untoward complications of persistent cytokine overexpression [33]. Finally, (and most importantly) the expression of a specific gene can be compartmentalized to the lung, avoiding toxic effects of systemic therapy. We have constructed a recombinant adenovirus that contains the murine TNF gene incorporated into the E1 region of the viral genome (referred to as Ad5mTNF), and the administration of this vector results in the dose-dependent expression of bioactive TNF protein within the lung as early as 24 hours post administration, with continued expression to 7–10 days. Interestingly, the administration of Ad5mTNF intratracheally at a dose of 1×10^8 plaque forming units (PFU) to animals co-challenged with *K. pneumoniae* increased survival by approximately 2-fold as compared to those mice receiving control adenovirus (Ad5LacZ) or vehicle alone, and survival in Ad5mTNF-treated mice was associated with significant improvements in lung bacterial clearance and decreased bacterial dissemination to the blood [55]. However, this beneficial effect was dose-dependent, as administration of Ad5mTNF at a dose of 5×10^8 PFU effected lesser survival advantages than that observed with lesser doses of Ad5mTNF, and control vector at that dose actually increased lethality over that observed in animals co-treated with *K. pneumoniae* and vehicle.

We have similarly employed a recombinant human type 5 adenoviral vector containing the murine IL-12 p35 and IL-12 p40 cDNAs inserted into the E1 and E3 region of the viral genome, respectively, in mice with Gram-negative pneumonia [33, 56]. Importantly, the transient lung IL-12 transgene expression resulted in significantly enhanced survival in animals co-infected with *K. pneumoniae* intratracheally, as compared to animals treated with control vector or *K. pneumoniae* alone (Fig. 3). The beneficial effects of IL-12 overexpression was partially mediated by endogenously-produced IFN-γ and TNF, as the *in vivo* depletion of these cytokines partially abrogated the survival benefits of IL-12 overexpression in animals concomitantly challenged with *K. pneumoniae.* Recombinant adenoviruses have also been administered intraperitoneally, resulting in the systemic overexpression of IFN-γ to successfully treat murine *P. aeruginosa* pneumonia [29]. Thus, the use of gene therapy to deliver specific cytokines

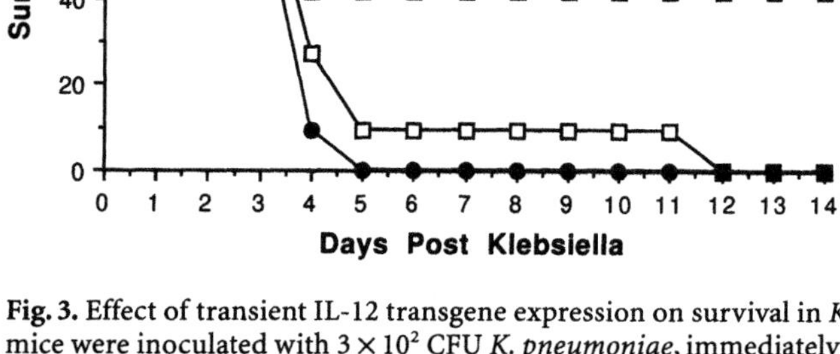

Fig. 3. Effect of transient IL-12 transgene expression on survival in *Klebsiella pneumonia.* CBA/J mice were inoculated with 3×10^2 CFU *K. pneumoniae*, immediately followed by administration of 5×10^8 pfu Ad5LacZ (control vector) or Ad5mIL-12

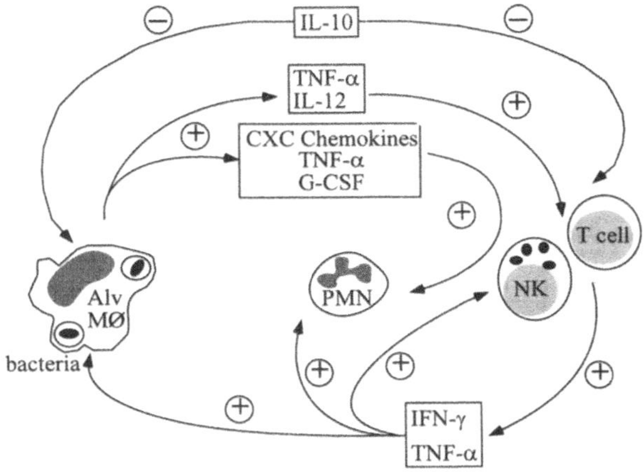

Fig. 4. Schematic diagram depicting the contribution of specific cells and cytokines to lung antibacterial host immunity. – denotes inhibitory effect, whereas + denotes stimulatory effect

and/or cytokine inhibitors in either a systemic fashion, or preferably compartmentalized fashion, appears to be an exciting and realistic approach to immune intervention in the treatment of pneumonia. Implementation of such an approach will likely require the development of improved vector systems to deliver genes of interest to the lung.

Conclusions

In this chapter, we have reviewed the contribution of specific cytokines as mediators of innate immunity against bacterial pathogens of the lung, as depicted in Fig. 4. While the cytokines discussed have clearly been implicated in cytokine-mediated lung host defense, other candidate cytokines include GM-CSF, IL-1β, and IL-6. IL-15 and IL-18 may also be of some importance, given that these cytokines have been shown to be important endogenous co-stimulatory signals in the induction of IFN-γ. It is becoming increasingly clear that we cannot rely solely on the development of new classes of antibiotics, but rather we must continue to search for novel approaches to immunotherapy that may serve as important adjuvants in the treatment of immunocompromised and/or immunocompetent patients with severe bacterial, mycobacterial, fungal, and parasitic infections of the lung.

References

1. Davies J (1994) Inactivation of antibiotics and dissemination of resistance genes. Science 264:375–382
2. Wunderink R (1995) Ventilator-associated pneumonia. Clin Chest Med 16:173–193
3. Center for Disease Control (1997) Update: *Staphylococcus aureus* with reduced susceptibility to Vancomycin – United States. Morb Mortal Wkly Rep 46:813–815

4. Toews GB, Gross GN, Pierce AK (1979) The relationship of inoculum size to lung bacterial clearance and phagocytic cell response in mice. Am Rev Respir Dis 120:559–566
5. Nelson S, Mason CM, Kolls JK (1995) Pathophysiology of pneumonia. Clin Chest Med 16:1–12
6. Murphy J (1989) Cryptococcosis. In: Cox RA (ed) Immunology of the fungal diseases. CRC Press, Boca Raton, pp 93–138
7. DesPrez RM, Heim CR (1990) Mycobacterium tuberculosis. In: Mandell GL, Douglas RG, Bennett JE (eds) Principles and practice of infectious diseases, edn 3. Churchill Livingstone, New York, pp 1877–1905
8. Standiford TJ, Huffnagle GB (1997) Cytokines in host defense against pneumonia. J Invest Med 45:335–345
9. Kolls JK, Nelson S, Summer WR (1993) Recombinant cytokines and pulmonary host defense. Am J Med Sci 306:330–335
10. Laichalk LL, Kunkel SL, Strieter RM, Danforth JM, Bailie M, Standiford TJ (1996) Tumor necrosis factor mediates lung antibacterial host defense in murine Klebsiella pneumonia. Infect Immun 64:5211–5218
11. Huffnagle GB, Toews GB, Burdick MD, et al (1996) Afferent phase production of TNF-α is required for the development of protective T cell immunity to Cryptococcus neoformans. J Immunol 157:4529–4536
12. Tracey KJ, Beutler B, Lowry SF, Cerami A (1986) Shock and tissue injury induced by recombinant human cachectin. Science 234:470–474
13. Le J, Vilcek J (1987) Tumor necrosis factor and interleukin-1: Cytokines with multiple overlapping biological activities. Lab Invest 56:234–248
14. Oswald IP, Wynn TA, Sher A, James SL (1992) Interleukin 10 inhibits macrophage microbicidal activity by blocking endogenous production of tumor necrosis factor α required as a costimulatory factor for interferon-γ-induced activation. Proc Natl Acad Sci USA 89: 8676–8680
15. Tan AM, Ferrante A, Goh DH, Robertson DM, Cripps AW (1995) Activation of the neutrophil bactericidal activity for non typeable *Haemophilus* influenza by tumor necrosis factor and lymphotoxin. Pediatr Res 37:155–159
16. Dehoux MS, Boutten A, Ostinelli J, et al (1994) Compartmentalized cytokine production within the human lung in unilateral pneumonia. Am J Respir Crit Care Med 150:710–716
17. Gosselin D, DeSanctis J, Boule M, Skamene E, Matouk C, Radzioch D (1995) Role of tumor necrosis factor alpha in innate resistance to mouse pulmonary infection with Pseudomonas aeruginosa. Infect Immun 63:3272–3278
18. Brieland J, Remick D, Freeman P, Hurley M, Fantone J, Engleberg N (1995) In vivo regulation of replicative Legionella pneumophila lung infection by endogenous tumor necrosis factor alpha and nitric oxide. Infect Immun 63:3253–3258
19. Takashima K, Tateda K, Matsumoto T, Lizawa Y, Nakao M, Yamaguchi K (1997) Role of tumor necrosis factor alpha in pathogenesis of pneumococcal pneumonia in mice. Infect Immun 65:257–260
20. Kolls JK, Lei D, Nelson S, Summer WR, Greenberg S, Beutler B (1995) Adenovirus-mediated blockade of tumor necrosis factor in mice protects against endotoxic shock yet impairs pulmonary host defense. J Infect Dis 171:570–575
21. Baggiolini M, Dewald B, Moser B (1997) Human chemokines: an update. Annu Rev Immunol 15:675–705
22. Huffnagle GB, Strieter RM, Kunkel SL, Toews GB, Standiford TJ (1996) The role of chemokines in pneumonia. In: Koch A, Strieter R (eds) Chemokines in disease. R. G. Landis Co, Texas, pp 151–168
23. Greenberger MJ, Strieter RM, Kunkel SL, et al (1996) Neutralization of MIP-2 attenuates neutrophil recruitment and bacterial clearance in murine *Klebsiella* pneumonia. J Infect Dis 173:159–165
24. Tsai WC, Strieter RM, Wilkowski JM, et al (1998) Lung-specific transgenic expression of KC enhances resistance to *Klebsiella pneumoniae* in mice. J Immunol 161:2435–2440
25. Murphy PM (1997) Neutrophil receptors for interleukin-8 and CXC chemokines. Semin Hematol 34:311–318

26. Jenson W, Rose R, Wasserman A, Kalb T, Anton K, Remold H (1987) In vitro activation of the antibacterial activity of human pulmonary macrophages by recombinant gamma interferon. J Infect Dis 155:574–577
27. Beck J, Liggitt H, Brunette E, Fuchs H, Shellito J, Debs R (1991) Reduction in intensity of Pneumocystis carinii pneumonia in mice by aerosol administration of gammma interferon. Infect Immun 59:3859–3862
28. Skerrett S, Martin T (1994) Intratracheal interferon-γ augments pulmonary defenses in experimental legionellosis. Am J Respir Crit Care Med 149:50–58
29. Rubins JB, Pomeroy C (1997) Role of gamma interferon in the pathogenesis of bacteremic pneumococcal pneumonia. Infect Immun 65:2975–2977
30. Kolls JK, Lei D, Nelson S, Summer WR, Shellito JE (1997) Pulmonary cytokine gene therapy. Adenoviral-mediated murine interferon gene transfer compartmentally activates alveolar macrophages and enhances bacterial clearance. Chest 111 (suppl 6): 104S
31. Chehimi J, Trinchieri G (1994) Interleukin-12: a bridge between innate resistance and adaptive immunity with a role in infection and acquired immunodeficiency. J Clin Immunol 14:149–159
32. Kawakami K, Tohyama M, Xie Q, Saito A (1996) IL-12 protects mice against pulmonary and disseminated infection caused by Cryptococcus neoformans. Clin Exp Immunol 104: 208–214
33. Greenberger MJ, Kunkel SL, Strieter RM, et al (1996) IL-12 gene therapy protects mice in lethal Klebsiella pneumonia. J Immunol 157:3006–3012
34. Howard M, O'Garra A, Ishida H, Malefyt RD, De Vries J (1992) Biological properties of interleukin 10. J Clin Immunol 12:239–247
35. Laichalk LL, Danforth JM, Standiford TJ (1996) Interleukin-10 inhibits neutrophil phagocytic and bactericidal activity. FEMS Immunol Med Microbiol 15:181–187
36. Rolph P, Nakoinz I, Sampson-Johannes A, et al (1992) IL-10, T lymphocyte inhibitor of human blood cell production of IL-1 and tumor necrosis factor. J Immunol 148:808–814
37. Kasama T, Strieter RM, Lukacs NW, Burdick MD, Kunkel SL (1994) Regulation of neutrophil-derived chemokine expression by IL-10. J Immunol 152:3559–3569
38. Howard M, Muchamuel T, Andrade S, Menon S (1993) Interleukin 10 protects mice from lethal endotoxemia. J Exp Med 177:1205–1208
39. Standiford TJ, Strieter RM, Lukacs NW, Kunkel SL (1995) Neutralization of IL-10 increases lethality in endotoxemia. Cooperative effects of macrophage inflammatory protein-2 and tumor necrosis factor. J Immunol 155:2222–2229
40. Greenberger MJ, Strieter RM, Kunkel SL, Danforth J, Goodman R, Standiford TJ (1995) Neutralization of IL-10 increases survival in a murine model of Klebsiella pneumonia. J Immunol 155:722–729
41. van der Poll T, Marchant A, Keogh C, Goldman M, Lowry S (1996) Interleukin-10 impairs host defense in murine pneumococcal pneumonia. J Infect Dis 174:994–1000
42. Volk HD, Reinke P, Krausch D, et al (1996) Monocyte deactivation – rationale for a new therapeutic strategy in sepsis. Intensive Care Med 22 (suppl 4): S474–S481
43. Docke WD, Randow F, Syrbe U, et al (1997) Monocyte deactivation in septic patients: Restoration by IFN-γ treatment. Nat Med 3:678–681
44. Munoz CJ, Carlet C, Fitting C, Misset B, Bleroit JP, Cavaillon JM (1991) Dysregulation of in vitro cytokine production by monocytes during sepsis. J Clin Invest 88:1747–1754
45. Wakefield CH, Cary PD, Foulds S J, Monson RT, Guillou PJ (1993) Changes in major histocompatibility complex class II expression in monocytes and T cells of patients developing infection after surgery. Br J Surg 80:205–209
46. Christou NV (1985) Host-defense mechanisms in surgical patients: a correlative study of the delayed hypersensitivity skin-test response, granulocyte function and sepsis. Can J Surg 28:39–49
47. Brun-Buisson C, Doyon F, Carlet J, et al (1995) Incidence, risk factors, and outcome of severe sepsis and septic shock in adults. JAMA 274:968–973
48. Randow F, Syrbe U, Meisel C, et al (1995) Mechanism of endotoxin desensitization: involvement of interleukin 10 and transforming growth factor β. J Exp Med 181:1887–1892

49. Walley KR, Lukacs NW, Standiford TJ, Strieter RM, Kunkel SL (1996) Balance of inflammatory cytokines related to severity and mortality of murine sepsis. Infect Immun 64:4733–4738
50. Steinhauser ML, Hogaboam CM, Kunkel SL, Lukacs NW, Strieter RM, Standiford TJ (1999) IL-10 is a major mediator of sepsis-induced impairment in lung antibacterial host defense. J Immunol 161:2435–2440
51. Sawa T, Corry DB, Gropper MA, Ohara M, Kurahashi K, Wiener-Kronish JP (1997) IL-10 improves lung injury and survival in *Pseudomonas aeruginosa* pneumonia. J Immunol 159: 2858–2866
52. Cohen J (1995) IL-12 deaths: Explanation and a puzzle. Science 270:908
53. Laichalk LL, Bucknell KA, Huffnagle GB, et al (1998) Intrapulmonary delivery of tumor necrosis factor agonist peptide augments host defense in murine gram-negative bacterial pneumonia. Infect Immun 66:2822–2826
54. Wilson JM (1995) Molecular medicine. Adenoviruses as gene-delivery vehicles. N Engl J Med 334:1185–1187
55. Standiford TJ, Wilkowski JM, Sisson TH, et al (1999) Intrapulmonary tumor necrosis factor gene therapy increases bacterial clearance and survival in murine gram-negative pneumonia. Hum Gene Ther 10:899–909
56. Bramson J, Hitt M, Gallichan WS, Rosenthal K, Gauldie J, Graham FL (1995) Construction and characterization of an adenovirus expressing IL-12. Hum Gene Ther 7:333–340
57. Preheim LC, Snitily MU, Gentry MJ (1996) Effects of granulocyte colony-stimulating factor in cirrhotic rats with pneumococcal pneumonia. J Infect Dis 174:225–228
58. Smith WS, Sumnicht GE, Sharpe RW, Samuelson D, Millard FE (1995) Granulocyte colony-stimulating factor versus placebo in addition to penicillin G in randomized blinded study of gram-negative pneumonia sepsis: Analysis of survival and multisystem organ failure. Blood 86:1301–1309
59. van der Poll T, Keogh CV, Guirao X, Buurman WA, Kopf M, Lowry SF (1997) Interleukin-6 gene-deficient mice show impaired defense against pneumococcal pneumonia. J Infect Dis 176:439–444

Fetuin Opsonizes Macrophage-Deactivating Cations

H. Wang and K. J. Tracey

Introduction

The macrophage is a central participant in the development of septic shock, acute respiratory distress syndrome (ARDS), inflammatory bowel disease, and rheumatoid arthritis. In these, and other inflammatory diseases, macrophages release excessive quantities of pro-inflammatory mediators including nitric oxide (NO), tumor necrosis factor (TNF), interleukin (IL)-1, and IL-6. Exogenous stimulating factors can cause an overexpression of macrophage-derived mediators, as for instance in Gram-negative sepsis caused by bacterial lipopolysaccharide (LPS). In this case, monocytes/macrophages respond to extremely low concentrations of LPS-LPS binding protein (LBP) complexes by interacting with CD14 on the cell membrane, or by internalizing the LPS-LBP-CD14 complex through endosomal pathways [1]. Although CD14 is a glycosylphosphatidylinositol (GPI)-anchored membrane protein, it is also a soluble serum protein which can be adopted onto the cell surface to confer LPS sensitivity to unresponsive cells [1–3]. Membrane-bound CD14-LPS-LBP interacts with specific receptors, recently identified as members of the toll-like receptor (TLR) family, that activate intracellular signaling pathways [4]. It appears that one function of CD14 is to opsonize the LPS-LBP complex, enabling the macrophage to efficiently recognize an invasive threat signaled by the presence of LPS.

Mammals have evolved a number of counterregulatory mechanisms to prevent the inadvertent or excessive release of pro-inflammatory mediators. For instance, glucocorticoid hormones, which are released as a component of the stress response to injury or infection, suppress macrophage cytokine synthesis by stabilizing the cytoplasmic form of nuclear factor-kappa B (NF-κB) [5]. Another class of macrophage deactivating factors is the anti-inflammatory cytokines, including transforming growth factor-β (TGF-β), IL-4 and IL-10. These anti-inflammatory cytokines effectively inhibit macrophage activation and prevent the release of pro-inflammatory cytokines. Ultimately, the balance between the activities of the pro-inflammatory and anti-inflammatory mediator cascades determines whether the net effects of macrophage activation will participate in the benefit or the detriment of the host.

We recently identified a previously unrecognized macrophage counterregulatory mechanism that is dependent upon spermine, an abundant biogenic polyamine [6]. Spermine, which is released from dying and injured cells and accumulates at sites of inflammation and injury, effectively deactivates macrophages by inhibiting the translation of pro-inflammatory cytokine mRNA [6]. This provides an important, localized feed-back mechanism that restrains innate inflammation. We were subsequently surprised to find that macrophage recognition of spermine is dependent on fetuin, a ubiquitous negative acute phase serum protein that is found on the macrophage cell surface [7]. Cationic macrophage-deactivating molecules bind to sialic acid moieties on fetuin, and the resultant fetuin-cationic complex inhibits macrophage activation and cytokine release. In this chapter we summarize these and other results implicating fetuin as an opsonic participant in a macrophage deactivating pathway that contributes to the counterregulation of inflammation.

Deactivation of Macrophage Activities by CNI-1493

Our original interest in macrophage-deactivation stemmed from studies addressing the molecular mechanism of action of CNI-1493, a tetravalent guanylhydrazone inhibitor of macrophage TNF synthesis [8, 9]. CNI-1493 prevents phosphorylation of p38 mitogen-activated protein kinase (MAPK), a signaling pathway that is required for the efficient translation of TNF mRNA [10]. When macrophages are stimulated in the presence of CNI-1493, TNF mRNA accumulates, but TNF protein synthesis is blocked [11]. The suppression of cytokine release by CNI-1493 is reversible, because when CNI-1493 is removed from the macrophage cultures, TNF release in response to LPS stimulation is restored [9]. CNI-1493-mediated cytokine suppression is specific, because the synthesis of TGF-β is not inhibited by TNF-suppressing concentrations of CNI-1493, and there is no significant suppression of either generalized protein or RNA synthesis [9]. Moreover, CNI-1493 does not prevent either the release of TGF-β, or the increased expression of major histocompatibility complex (MHC) class II mediated by interferon (IFN)-γ [9]. In pharmacological doses that prevent phosphorylation of macrophage p38 MAPK, CNI-1493 does not interfere with LPS-stimulated translocation of the transcription factor NF-κB [10, 11]. The 3′-untranslated region (3′-UTR) of TNF mRNA, which has been implicated in the regulation of TNF protein translation, participates in CNI-1493-mediated suppression of TNF protein translation [10]. CNI-1493 exhibits macrophage specificity for pro-inflammatory cytokine inhibition, because pharmacological concentrations of CNI-1493 do not inhibit the release of cytokines from activated T cells [12].

The anti-inflammatory activities of CNI-1493 *in vivo* have been characterized in animal models including carrageenan-induced inflammation in mice, LPS lethality, cecal ligation and puncture, cerebral ischemia, pancreatitis, and IL-2 toxicity [13]. A Phase I clinical trial of intravenous CNI-1493, in which CNI-1493 was administered to patients receiving IL-2 for the treatment of renal cell cancer and melanoma, is nearing completion. At the completion of this trial it may be possible to determine whether CNI-1493 can suppress the release of TNF, which has been implicated as a mediator of IL-2 toxicity. Despite the wealth of information concerning the molecular mechanism of action and the pharmacological effects of CNI-1493, until recently it was unclear whether a specific binding protein was required for CNI-1493-mediated TNF suppression.

Identification of Fetuin as a Macrophage Protein that is Required for the Deactivating Effects of CNI-1493

With this background, we initiated a research effort to study the molecular interaction of CNI-1493 with macrophages. We accidentally discovered that murine macrophage-like RAW264.7 cells became unresponsive to CNI-1493-mediated TNF suppression when pre-cultured under conditions of partial serum-starvation [14]. That is, despite the addition of cytokine-suppressing concentrations of CNI-1493, LPS-stimulated TNF synthesis was not inhibited in serum-deprived macrophage cultures. Reasoning that these unresponsive macrophage cultures may have become depleted of a factor that is required for macrophage deactivation by CNI-1493, we used these cells in a bioassay, and screened proteins derived from normal 'CNI-1493-responsive' macrophages for an activity that could restore the suppressive activity of CNI-1493. Fractionation and purification of the active principle revealed that a 65–67 kDa protein, which is normally present in macrophages, specifically restored the TNF-suppressing activity of CNI-1493 when added to serum-deprived macrophage cultures. N-terminal amino acid sequencing analysis identified this 65–67 kDa protein as fetuin [14].

The macrophage requirement for fetuin in order to be deactivated by CNI-1493 was confirmed by addition of highly purified, LPS-free fetuin in combination with CNI-1493 to LPS-stimulated macrophage cultures [14]. Exogenous fetuin fully restored the sensitivity of serum-starved macrophages to CNI-1493, as evidenced by CNI-1493-mediated inhibition of both p38 MAPK phosphorylation and of TNF synthesis in serum-deprived macrophage cultures. Evidence of specificity was obtained by addition of other serum glycoproteins (glycophorin, α1-acid glycoprotein, human glycoprotein, and albumin). None of these glycoproteins restored the TNF-suppressing activities of CNI-1493 in macrophage cultures. Partial serum starvation significantly depletes the levels of cell-associated fetuin as compared to normally cultured macrophages, as determined by measuring fetuin levels in cell lysates with a specific immunoassay [14].

Fetuin is required for the deactivation of primary human monocytes by CNI-1493, because when neutralizing anti-fetuin antibodies were added to cultures of LPS-stimulated peripheral blood mononuclear cells, we observed no significant suppression of TNF release as compared to peripheral blood mononuclear cells not exposed to CNI-1493. Co-administration of fetuin with CNI-1493 to BALB/c mice significantly decreased the peak levels of serum TNF, indicating that this pathway participates in regulating the state of LPS-stimulated macrophage activation *in vivo* [14]. Thus, fetuin is required in the CNI-1493-mediated inhibition of TNF release by the murine macrophage-like RAW 264.7 cell line, peripheral blood mononuclear cells, and *in vivo*.

Fetuin as a Carrier of Biologically Active Molecules

Fetuin, a 65 kDa serum glycoprotein, was first described by Pedersen in 1944 as a fetal plasma protein [15]. In 1987, Dziegielewska and colleagues showed that human fetuin is homologous to a serum protein known as 'α2-HS-glycoprotein'. Subsequent cloning of the complete cDNA confirmed the identity of human fetuin as a member of the cystatin superfamily (including the stefins, cystatins, kininogens, and histidine-rich glycoprotein [16, 17]). Southern blot analysis indicates that there is a single human fetuin gene located on chromosome 3, but the gene product undergoes extensive post-translational modifications [18].

Human fetuin contains N-linked and O-linked oligosaccharide chains, whose terminal sugar residues are rich in sialic acid moieties [19]. Fetuin has been implicated as a carrier of biologically active molecules such as fatty acids, thyroid hormone, and calcium ions [20]. A hydrophobic core (the D3a domain) consisting of 28–32 amino acids is evolutionarily conserved, suggesting that it may be the lipid-binding region. A separate domain shares homology with the consensus sequence, Ca^{++} binding domain, of the cystatin protein family, which may be a Ca^{++} binding site on fetuin [20]. We recently demonstrated that the sialic acid moieties of fetuin are responsible for binding cationic molecules, since when the sialic acid residues were removed by treatment of fetuin with neuraminidase, asialofetuin failed to bind CNI-1493 under *in vitro* conditions [14]. Moreover, asialofetuin failed to restore the responsiveness of serum-deprived macrophage cultures to CNI-1493, indicating that the sialic acid moieties are required for mediation of macrophage deactivation [14].

Fetuin is normally found on the external surface of many cells including macrophages, and its relative abundance in crude membrane factions of serum-deprived macrophage cultures is decreased by 30–50% as compared to normally cultured macrophages [14, 21, 22]. To address whether fetuin acts as a receptor-like protein or a carrier-like protein on macrophages, we measured macrophage binding of radioiabeled CNI-1493 at 4°C and 37°C. 'CNI-1493-unresponsive' macrophages failed to incorporate radiolabeled CNI-1493, but cell incorporation of CNI-1493 was significantly increased by addition of fetuin to the cultures [14]. Fetuin did not significantly increase the binding of CNI-1493 to the macrophages at 4°C, indicating that fetuin restores the response of macrophages to CNI-1493 by facilitating the cellular uptake of CNI-1493, not by increasing cell surface binding [14]. Although the mechanism by which fetuin interacts with the cell surface is not known, our results indicate that macrophage-associated fetuin binds cationic deactivating molecules via sialic acid moieties, which facilitates the suppression of cytokine synthesis.

Fetuin-CNI-1493 Activity Recapitulated by Fetuin-Spermine

The potent macrophage deactivating effects of CNI-1493 led us to consider whether the anti-inflammatory activities of this cationic molecule might be attributable to molecular mimicry with some endogenous, cationic macrophage deactivating compound. The molecular structure of CNI-1493 is characterized by four positive charges linked by a flexible aliphatic chain. Spermine, a ubiquitous tetravalent biogenic amine that is present in all eukaryotic cells, is characterized structurally by four positive charges separated by an aliphatic chain. Addition of spermine to LPS-stimulated primary human monocytes dose-dependently suppresses the synthesis of pro-inflammatory cytokines including TNF, IL-1, IL-6, macrophage inflammatory protein (MIP)-1α, and MIP-1β [6]. Treatment of LPS-simulated macrophage cultures with spermine does not significantly affect the levels of TNF mRNA, providing evidence that the mechanism by which spermine suppresses TNF release is post-transcriptional [6]. Local application of spermine into the footpad of rats *in vivo* significantly suppressed the development of carrageenan-induced edema, indicating that the release of spermine from dying and injured cells can down-regulate the host response to infection or invasion by counterregulating pro-inflammatory cytokine synthesis [6].

Fetuin-depleted, partially starved macrophage cultures (human peripheral blood monocytes or RAW cells) continue to produce TNF despite addition of exogenous spermine, indicating that fetuin is also required for macrophage responses to spermine. The TNF suppressing effects of spermine are completely restored by addition of highly purified, exogenous fetuin, but not by other serum glycoproteins [7, 14]. One molecule of fetuin binds 4–6 molecules of spermine, but asialofetuin, which fails to restore spermine responses in macrophages, does not bind spermine. Treatment of peripheral blood mononuclear cells with neutralizing anti-fetuin antibodies prevents the cytokine-suppressing activity of spermine, indicating that macrophage-associated fetuin normally participates in spermine-mediated deactivation [7]. While fetuin is required for both spermine and CNI-1493 to suppress TNF synthesis, recent evidence suggests that the intracellular molecular targets may be distinct. For instance, CNI-1493 suppresses TNF synthesis by more than 95%, but spermine blocks only 50% of TNF release. One possibility is that these cations act through separate molecular targets which are as yet unidentified.

Interactions of Cells with Fetuin

A specific cell surface receptor for fetuin has not been described, but macrophage receptors for asialoglycoproteins have been extensively studied [23–26]. These asialoglycoprotein receptors are present on the surface of various cells, including Kupffer cells and macrophages, where they serve to bind, internalize, and dispose of desialylated serum glycoproteins [23]. It is plausible, though unproven, that cationic molecules such as spermine or CNI-1493 bind and neutralize the terminal sialic acid residues of fetuin, and that the fetuin/cation complex then interacts with the asialoglycoprotein receptor. The cell-associated complex may then be either internalized to interact with an intracellular target(s), or may interact with an unidentified protein on the macrophage surface. For instance, Demetriou and colleagues found that fetuin shares homology with the cytokine-binding domain (TRH1) of the Type II TGF-β receptor, suggesting that fetuin may be a TGF-β-binding protein, which could theoretically function as a natural antagonist or reservoir of TGF-β [27].

We considered whether fetuin itself is required for inhibiting signal transduction via the MAPK in activated macrophages, but our results argue against this interpretation [14]. First, LPS-induced TNF synthesis in fetuin-depleted macrophages can be inhibited by addition of the pyridinyl imidazole SB203580 inhibitor of p38 MAPK, indicating that fetuin is not required directly for inactivating TNF synthesis via this p38 pathway. Second, fetuin alone does not inhibit the release of TNF from LPS-stimulated macrophages, suggesting that it does not function as a direct inhibitor of LPS-induced signal transduction cascades. Finally, in the presence of fetuin, maximal TNF-suppressing concentrations of spermine only reduce TNF release by 50%, as compared to a 95% reduction of TNF synthesis by CNI-1493. Accordingly, it is likely that macrophages share a requirement for fetuin in order to be deactivated by either CNI-1493 or spermine, but that fetuin functions to facilitate interaction of the macrophage by opsonizing these cations, and not as an integral component of the intracellular signal transduction pathway. It is also intriguing to consider however, that fetuin has been implicated as an inhibitor of insulin receptor tyrosine kinase, because it shares homology with a 63 kDa glycoprotein (pp63) originally identified as a natural inhibitor of this kinase [28–30]. It is unclear whether this previously described kinase-inhibiting activity of fetuin may actually be dependent upon an associated cation.

Fetuin in Pregnancy and Inflammation

Fetuin is a negative acute phase reactant protein in rats and humans, and serum levels fall during acute inflammatory responses [31]. Serum fetuin is produced primarily by hepatocytes, and analysis of the fetuin promoter region reveals the presence of an IL-6-response element (5′-CTGGGAA-3′) [32]. Hepatocyte syn-

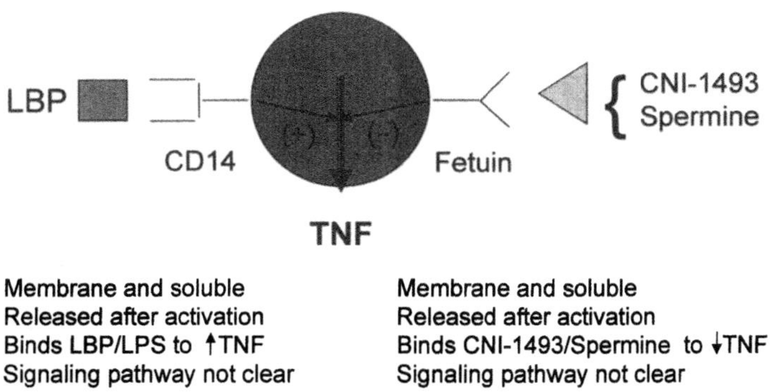

Fig. 1. Regulation of tumor necrosis factor (TNF) production by fetuin and CD14. Low concentrations of lipopolysaccharide (LPS) bind strongly to LPS binding protein (LBP), and surface CD14 facilitates interaction with toll-like receptors, increasing expression of TNF. In contrast, spermine or CNI-1493 are opsonized by fetuin on the macrophage surface, and this interaction is required for inhibition of TNF synthesis

thesis of fetuin is down-regulated by IL-6, TNF, and IL-1, suggesting that the release of pro-inflammatory cytokines underlies the decline in serum fetuin levels [33]. An opsonic role for fetuin in bacterial phagocytosis has been observed in neutrophils, and fetuin can also increase endocytosis by mouse macrophages [34]. Fetuin can also inhibit mitogen-induced lymphoblast transformation, and suppress T- and B-lymphocyte response to lectins [19]. Interpretation of these results has been hampered by the affinity of fetuin for binding other molecules. For instance, we have found that highly purified fetuin is frequently contaminated by LPS, which must be removed by exhaustive extraction over a polymyxin B affinity column.

Based on these results, we predicted that the macrophage-deactivating role of fetuin is important in pregnancy, because high levels of fetuin and spermine in the periamnion can interact to suppress TNF release by maternal macrophages [7]. TNF is a powerful abortifacient, so fetal viability may be, in part, dependent upon fetuin and spermine preventing the release of maternal TNF to maintain a viable pregnancy. In agreement with this, Dzieglielewska and Andersen administered fetuin to pregnant rats, and found that it conferred significant protection against LPS-induced lethality and abortion [35].

It is quite likely that macrophages utilize fetuin in assessing the abundance of extracellular spermine in other inflammatory conditions as well. This feedback mechanism can operate to down-regulate the synthesis of pro-inflammatory cytokines and to prevent excessive tissue damage. It is notable that decreased levels of human fetuin have been observed in patients with acute lymphocytic leukemia, rheumatoid arthritis, acute alcoholic hepatitis, chronic active hepatitis, acute and chronic pancreatitis, inflammatory bowel disease, and trauma [19, 31]. Low fetuin levels may theoretically render macrophages insensitive to deactivation by endogenous spermine, thereby contributing to an overproduction of pro-inflammatory cytokines. On the contrary, when fetuin levels are extremely high, as in the fetus and in some tumors, this system is poised to counterregulate TNF production.

Conclusion

It is instructive to compare and contrast the roles of fetuin and CD14 in regulating the state of macrophage activation (Fig. 1). Both serum proteins are synthesized by hepatocytes and macrophages, and under the control of the acute phase response to inflammation. Each is associated with the macrophage cell surface, and both can function as a carrier for other biologically active molecules. Whereas CD14 serves to opsonize LPS-LBP, activate the macrophage, and stimulate TNF release, it now appears that fetuin functions as part of an intrinsic system of macrophage deactivation that can restrain the innate immune response and protect the host from excessive tissue injury. It is plausible that a relative deficiency of fetuin during critical illness would contribute to the excessive release of pro-inflammatory cytokines from macrophages. It is also worth considering that fetuin supplementation may suppress an overactivated phase of immune dysfunction in critical illness.

References

1. Ulevitch RJ, Tobias PS (1995) Receptor-dependent mechanisms of cell stimulation by bacterial endotoxin. Annu Rev Immunol 13:437–457
2. Ulevitch RJ, Tobias PS (1994) Recognition of endotoxin by cells leading to transmembrane signaling. Curr Opin Immunol 6:125–130
3. Ziegler-Heitbrock HW, Ulevitch RJ (1993) CD14: cell surface receptorand differentiation marker. Immunol Today 14:121–125
4. Ulevitch RJ (1999) Endotoxin opens the Toligates to innate immunity. Nat Med 5:144–145
5. Auphan N, DiDonato JA, Rosette C, Helmberg A, Karin M (1995) Immunosuppression by glucocorticoids: inhibition of NF-kappa B activity through induction of I kappa B synthesis. Science 270:286–290
6. Zhang M, Caragine T, Wang H, et al (1997) Spermine inhibits proinflammatory cytokine synthesis in human mononuclear cells: A counterregulatory mechanism that restrains the immune response. J Exp Med 185:1–10
7. Wang H, Zhang M, Soda K, Sama A, Tracey KJ (1997) Fetuin protects the fetus from TNF. Lancet 350:861–862
8. Bianchi M, Ulrich P, Bloom O, et al (1995) An inhibitor of macrophage arginine transport and nitric oxide production (CNI-1493) prevents acute inflammatory and endotoxin lethality. Mol Med 1:254–266
9. Bianchi M, Bloom O, Raabe T, et al (1996) Suppression of proinflammatory cytokines in monocytes by a tetravalent guanylhydrazone. J Exp Med 83:927–936
10. Cohen PS, Schmidtmayerova H, Dennis J, et al (1997) The critical role of p38 MAP kinase in T cell HIV-1 replication. Mol Med 3:339–346
11. Cohen PS, Nakshaatri H, Dennis J, et al (1996) CNI-1493 inhibits monocyte/macrophage tumor necrosis factor by suppression of translation efficiency. Proc Natl Acad Sci USA 93: 3967–3971
12. Bjork L, Tracey KJ, Ulrich P, et al (1997) Targeted suppression of cytokine production in monocytes but not in T lymphocytes by a tetravalent guanylhydrazone (CNI-1493). J Infect Dis 176:1303–1312
13. Tracey KJ (1998) Suppression of TNF and other proinflammatory cytokines by the tetravalent guanylhydrazone CNI-1493. Prog Clin Biol Res 397:335–343
14. Wang H, Zhang M, Bianchi M, Sherry B, Sama A, Tracey KJ (1998) Fetuin (alpha2-HS-glycoprotein) opsonizes cationic macrophage-deactivating molecules. Proc Natl Acad Sci USA 95:14429–14434
15. Pedersen KO (1944) Fetuin, a new globulin isolated from serum. Nature 154:575–576
16. Christie DL, Dziegielewska KM, Hill RM, Saunders NR (1987) Fetuin: the bovine homologue of human alpha 2HS glycoprotein. FEBS Lett 214:45–49
17. Dziegielewska KM, Brown WM, Casey SJ, et al (1990) The complete cDNA and amino acid sequence of bovine fetuin. Its homology with alpha 2HS glycoprotein and relation to other members of the cystatin superfamily. J Biol Chem 265:4354–4357
18. Lee CC, Bowman BH, Yang FM (1987) Human alpha 2-HS-glycoprotein: the A and B chains with a connecting sequence are encoded by a single mRNA transcript. Proc Natl Acad Sci USA 84:4403–4407
19. Dziegielewska KM, Brown WM (1995) Fetuin. RG Landes Co, Austin
20. Brown WM, Saunders NR, Mollgard K, Dziegielewska KM (1992) Fetuin – an old friend revisited. Bioessays 14:749–755
21. Chertov OY, Ermolaeva MV, Satpaev DK, et al (1994) Inhibitory effect of calf fetuin on the cytotoxic activity of LAK cell-derived factors and tumor necrosis factor Immunol Lett 42: 97–100
22. Rohrlich ST, Rifkin DB (1981) Isolation of the major serine protease inhibitor from the 5-day serum-free conditioned medium of human embryonic lung cells and demonstration that it is fetuin. J Cell Physiol 109:1–15
23. Stockert RJ (1995) The asialoglycoprotein receptor: relationships between structure, function, and expression. Physiol Rev 75:591–609

24. Geffen I, Fuhrer C, Leitinger B, et al (1993) Related signals for endocytosis and basolateral sorting of the asialoglycoprotein receptor. J Biol Chem 268:20772–20777
25. Geffen I, Spiess M (1992) Asialoglycoprotein receptor. Int Rev Cytol 137B:181–219
26. Geffen I, Fuhrer C, Spiess M (1991) Endocytosis by the asialoglycoprotein receptor is independent of cytoplasmic serine residues. Proc Natl Acad Sci USA 88:8425–8429
27. Demetriou M, Binkert C, Sukhu B, Tenenbaum HC, Dennis JW (1996) Fetuin/alpha2-HS glycoprotein is a transforming growth factor-beta type II receptor mimic and cytokine antagonist. J Biol Chem 271:12755–12761
28. Haasemann M, Nawratil P, Muller-Esterl W (1991) Rat tyrosine kinase inhibitor shows sequence similarity to human alpha 2-HS glycoprotein and bovine fetuin. Biochem J 274: 899–902
29. Rauth G, Poschke O, Fink E, et al (1992) The nucleotide and partial amino acid sequences of rat fetuin. Identity with the natural tyrosine kinase inhibitor of the rat insulin receptor. Eur J Biochem 204:523–529
30. Srinivas PR, Wagner AS, Reddy LV, et al (1993) Serum alpha 2-HS-glycoprotein is an inhibitor of the human insulin receptor at the tyrosine kinase level. Mol Endocrinol 7:1445–1455
31. Lebreton JP, Joisel F, Raoult JP, Lannuzel B, Rogez JP, Humbert G (1979) Serum concentration of human alpha 2 HS glycoprotein during the inflammatory process: evidence that alpha 2 HS glycoprotein is a negative acute-phase reactant. J Clin Invest 64:1118–1129
32. Banine F, Gangneux C, Lebreton JP, Frebourg T, Salier JP (1998) Structural and functional analysis of the 5′-transcription control region for the human alpha2-HS glycoprotein gene. Biochim Biophys Acta 1398:1–8
33. Daveau M, Christian-Davrinche, Julen N, Hiron M, Arnaud P, Lebreton JP (1988) The synthesis of human alpha-2-HS glycoprotein is down-regulated by cytokines in hepatoma HepG2 cells. FEBS Lett 241:191–194
34. van Oss CJ, Gillman CF, Bronson PM, Border JR (1974) Opsonic properties of human serum alpha-2 HS glycoprotein. Immunol Commun 3:329–335
35. Dziegielewska KM, Andersen NA (1998) The fetal glycoprotein, fetuin, counteracts ill-effects of the bacterial endotoxin, lipopolysaccharide, in pregnancy. Biol Neonate 74:372–375

LPS Receptors

E. Lien, H. Heine, and D. T. Golenbock

Introduction

Invasive Gram-negative bacterial infections often result in the development of septic shock. This syndrome is always serious, and often fatal. While the best estimates of the incidence of Gram-negative sepsis in the United States are almost a decade old, Gram-negative sepsis may account for as many as 50 000 deaths annually [1, 2]. Once patients exhibit the septic shock syndrome, almost 40% will die. A major challenge is identifying drug targets that can be manipulated therapeutically in order to reduce the high mortality associated with sepsis.

Endotoxin or lipopolysaccharide (LPS) is an amphipathic glycolipid which constitutes the major portion of the outermost membrane of Gram-negative bacteria [3]. The lipid A portion of LPS contains all of the pro-inflammatory activity observed with the entire molecule. Interaction of lipid A with macrophage LPS receptors results in the release of systemically active pro-inflammatory molecules, which in turn mediate systemic toxicity. LPS is an extremely potent toxin: Macrophages can be activated at concentrations of LPS as low as 1 pg/ml. A greater understanding of the nature of host receptors for LPS is essential before we can hope to design effective anti-LPS therapies.

LPS Receptors

The lipid A portion of LPS is conserved among Gram-negative bacteria and causes the biological toxicity of LPS [3, 4]. Although few molecules have been studied with the intensity of LPS, an important advance in the understanding of LPS biology was the remarkably recent elucidation of the correct structure of the lipid A portion of the molecule [5]. The discovery of certain lipid A precursors in *E. coli* allowed for structural and functional studies to be carried out, which were complemented by major advances in the synthetic chemistry of lipid A [6]. A variety of natural and synthetic LPS agonists and antagonists are now available for the study of LPS-animal cell interactions, thus making possible an entirely new approach to the therapy of endotoxin mediated disease.

Three cloned molecules expressed on the surface of monocytes and macrophages are known to bind the lipid A moiety of LPS. These include CD14, the macrophage scavenger receptor (SR), and the β2 leukocyte integrins (CD11a/

CD18, CD11b/CD18, and CD11c/CD18; this family of receptors herein will be referred to as CD11/18). Both CD14 and CD11/18 are capable of initiating signals to cells, resulting in phagocyte activation, bacterial internalization (phagocytosis, endocytosis), and the activation of bactericidal defenses. The scavenger receptor does not appear to function as a signaling receptor for LPS, although studies of scavenger receptor knockout mice have demonstrated a role for the scavenger receptor in host defense [7] Lastly, CD14 and the β2 leukocyte integrins interact with LPS in conjunction with soluble blood products that appear to function as sensitizers to the presence of extracellular LPS. These include both soluble CD14 (sCD14) and LPS-binding protein (LBP), but additional LPS binding proteins with biological activity (e.g., soluble toll-like receptor 2 [TLR2]) also may exist.

The earliest cell-mediated events following endotoxin release appear to involve the transfer of LPS to CD14, the LPS 'binding receptor' (for the purposes of this review, any surface molecule that interacts with CD14 and/or LPS resulting in a signal transduction event is referred to as an LPS receptor or receptor component). Evidence supporting a central role for CD14 in LPS-mediated responses includes the findings that:

1) LPS binds CD14 [8]
2) monoclonal antibodies (mAb) to CD14 inhibit the response to LPS stimulation [9–13]
3) sCD14 is present in blood [14] and facilitates the activation of cells which do not express membrane CD14 such as endothelia [15–18]
4) transfection of CD14 enhances the responsiveness of a variety of cell types to LPS by more than 1000-fold [19] and in some cases changes the phenotype from non-responder cell to responder cell [20, 21]
5) a CD14-deficient 'knockout' mouse was reported to be 10 000-fold less sensitive to LPS than its control littermates [22, 23], confirming the central importance of CD14 in biological responses to LPS.

LPS is an amphiphilic membrane phospholipid that forms aggregates in aqueous environments such as tissue culture medium or blood. Spontaneous diffusion of LPS monomers from these aggregates to CD14 occurs at a very slow rate [8]. Tobias and colleagues [24] described a plasma protein known as LBP, which bound LPS with apparent high affinity. While it was initially thought that LBP was somehow involved in LPS detoxification and metabolism, it ultimately became clear that LBP had many roles in host responses to LPS. We now know that LBP dramatically accelerates the binding of LPS CD14 [8], thereby enhancing the sensitivity of cells to LPS [8, 9, 25, 26]. LBP acts as a lipid transfer protein (this function might have been predicted based upon the homology of LBP with phospholipid transfer protein and cholesterol ester transfer protein); more recent studies have demonstrated that LBP co-purifies with high density lipoprotein (HDL) particles [27, 28], and can transfer LPS to lipoproteins [28], resulting in functional neutralization [29–32]. Thus, LBP has two opposing roles with respect to LPS; it moves LPS onto the LPS receptor CD14, and it helps neutralize LPS.

The clue to why LBP might have these dual and opposing roles may relate to the observation that LBP does not maintain a constant level in blood. LBP concentrations have been reported in the range of 2–20 μg/ml [33–35]; however, during sepsis [33–35], and other inflammatory states characterized by the acute phase response), LBP functions as an acute phase reactant [24], and plasma levels rise dramatically. While LBP appears to have a primary source in the liver, local production of LBP might account for many of its biological effects. For example, levels of LBP are markedly increased (64-fold) in the bronchoalveolar space of patients with acute respiratory distress syndrome (ARDS) compared with controls [36]. We have found that gonococci isolated directly from the cervical secretions of female patients with pelvic inflammatory disease are heavily opsonized by LBP. We are currently testing an LBP-knockout mouse in both infectious models of lung disease and pelvic inflammatory disease to determine if LBP has an important functional role in these localized infections of animals.

While it is established that LBP moves LPS onto CD14 [8, 9, 25, 26], the role of LBP as an opsonin may be less appreciated. The CD11/18 integrins also appear to participate in responses to LPS [37, 38]. LBP has been observed to act as an opsonin for Gram-negative bacteria [39]. We recently reported that LBP enhanced the binding of Gram-negative bacteria to a Chinese hamster ovary (CHO) cell line transfected with CD11b/CD18 and enhanced LPS-induced activation of these cells by approximately 30-fold [40]. The physiological relevance of this observation needs to be explored, but may be important under circumstances where both cytokine production and the engulfment of LPS particles (such as bacterial membranes) is necessary for survival.

LPS Antagonists: Tools for Characterizing LPS Receptors and Potential Therapeutic Agents for Septic Shock

The identification of compounds that have the biological properties of LPS antagonists made the pharmacological characterization of the LPS receptor system possible (reviewed in [41]). These compounds are derived from lipid A precursors and products (e.g., lipid IVa and deacylated LPS), inactive lipid A species from non-pathogenic bacteria (e.g., *R. sphaeroides* lipid A [RSLA]). Recently, synthetic lipid A analogs have been made available for study; advances in process chemistry have made the large scale production and clinical applications of LPS antagonists a real possibility for the near future. Phase 1 studies have demonstrated that E5531, an analog of *R. capsulatum* lipid A, is an effective inhibitor of injected LPS in human volunteers [42]. The LPS antagonists behave as competitive antagonists, and studies have demonstrated that inhibition is reversible by adding excess ligand. The target of the LPS antagonists appears to be located on the cell membrane, presumably a trans-membrane protein [41]. We have worked most extensively with the LPS antagonists lipid IVa and RSLA, which both competitively inhibit the effects of LPS on human cells, thereby preventing the induced release of cytokines and all other effects of LPS that have been tested. Our previous results demonstrated that the species from which CD14 is obtained does not determine the agonist/antagonist action of either lipid IVa or RSLA [43]. Instead, we found a common pattern of agonism and antagonism which was dependent on the genetic background of the host cell. Thus, we concluded that these LPS-analogs act by interacting with a molecule which is unique from CD14 and which exhibits species-specific recognition of lipid IVa and RSLA and proposed the existence of a second LPS recognition molecule which is the target of the LPS antagonists.

Cellular Activation by LPS and Toll Proteins as LPS Signal Transducers

While the role of CD14 as the most proximal portion of the LPS receptor is no longer controversial, there is still considerable controversy about how CD14 generates a transmembrane signal. CD14 is a glycosyl phosphatidylinositol (GPI)-linked protein, and thus it is not likely that the protein directly activates cells after binding LPS. The species-specific experiments with CD14-transfected CHO cells cited above suggested the existence of a signal transducer. Furthermore, careful experiments by Kitchens and Munford [12, 44] gave even greater support to the idea that LPS did not directly activate cells as a result of CD14 binding. These investigators found that LPS inhibitors suppressed LPS signaling at concentrations of inhibitor that were too low to inhibit LPS-binding to CD14. Furthermore, LPS is not the only ligand that binds and activates cells via CD14, but these other ligands have different pharmacological characteristics, suggesting that they have unique signal transduction complexes. For example, mycobacterial lipoarabinomannan (LAM) has been shown to activate macrophages and CD14-transfected 70Z/3 B cells. Unlike LPS, LAM fails to activate CD14-transfected fibroblasts [45, 46]. This finding suggested that fibroblasts lack a CD14-associated signal transducer that can be engaged by LAM, or alternatively, that LAM signaling requires an additional factor that confers LAM-responsiveness on the LPS receptor complex (i.e., CD14 and a signal transducer). We believe that fibroblasts lack sufficient levels of one or more TLRs necessary for LAM signal transduction.

Recent studies from several laboratories support the hypothesis that CD14 is the first portion of a larger signaling complex involving a transmembrane signal transducer. Toll is a Drosophila receptor whose cytoplasmic domain resembles the human interleukin-1 receptor [47]. Toll activation in flies results in the production of anti-microbial peptides, and is a key feature of the primitive innate immune system. At least five mammalian TLRs have recently been described [48]. Given the greater complexity of the human genome, many more TLRs are likely to be discovered soon.

Yang et al. [49] and Kirschning et al. [50] observed that transfection of human TLR2 into HEK 293 cells renders these otherwise LPS non-responsive cells, responsive to LPS. However, TLR2 is not the only potential LPS signal transducer. The C3H/HeJ mouse is a spontaneous LPS resistant mutant. Poltorak et al. have mapped the *Lps* gene, which has previously been shown to be necessary for LPS responses in LPS non-responder C3H/HeJ mice, to TLR4 [51]. This observation has been confirmed by other investigators [52]. TLR4 from the C3H/HeJ mouse has a single point mutation at amino acid 712 (pro to his) that changes the function of the receptor dramatically. In addition, in collaboration with others, our own lab has found an LPS signaling role for TLR4 [53]. Furthermore, we suggest that this molecule functions with CD14 to transduce signals when bound by LPS. The studies of Chow et al. [53] on TLR4 transfected HEK293 cells demonstrated that this protein could function as a signal transducer. The LPS antagonist E5531 inhibited LPS in TLR4 transfected HEK293 cells. Thus, TLR4 is at least one target of LPS antagonists. Thus, it appears that the LPS signaling complex consists of CD14, and several TLRs, perhaps in a manner analogous to the signaling pathways utilized by the IL-1 receptor.

TLR2 versus TLR4

The finding that more than one TLR is involved in LPS signal transduction leaves open the question: Is TLR2 or TLR4 the dominant LPS receptor, or are they both important? Clearly, the C3H/HeJ mouse is highly LPS resistant, so any response to this question cannot be correct if a central role for TLR4 is not part of the answer, at least in the mouse. TLRs are homologous to the IL-1 receptor, which signals via ligand-dependent formation of a heterodimer [54].

We sought to identify the role of TLR2 in LPS signal transduction by first deriving mutants in LPS signal transduction, and then learning what the role of TLR2 was in this LPS non-responder state. We constructed CHO/CD14 cells that express CD14, and that 'report' to LPS by expressing CD25 on their surface. Mutant cells were enriched by stimulating cells with LPS, and then cell sorting for the rare cell that failed to 'report' [55] in response to LPS. Cells were cloned and clonal LPS non-responder cells were analyzed genetically. To date, we have identified two complementation groups of LPS non-responsive CHO/CD14 cells. Both complementation groups respond to tumor necrosis factor(TNF)-α and interleukin(IL)-1β, suggesting that the mutations are in very proximal portions of the LPS signal transduction apparatus.

We transfected TLR2 into these mutant cell lines and derived clonal cell lines. When the cells were stimulated with LPS, they were not complemented until the concentrations of LPS exceeded 1 microgram/ml. In comparison, wild-type cells were activated at 1 ng/ml. Preliminary experiments suggest that TLR4 functions similarly. These results suggest that both TLR2 and TLR4 can function as LPS signal transducers, but additional components to the signal transduction apparatus are yet to be discovered.

In an effort to determine the genetic basis of the responses to LPS in CHO cells, we cloned TLR2 and TLR4 from the wild-type cell lines (we are currently cloning and sequencing these genes from the mutants). We also cloned mouse TLR2 from the RAW 264.7 monocyte/macrophage cell line. Sequence analysis of CHO-TLR2, compared to mouse and human TLR2, revealed a single base pair deletion, resulting in a frame-shift mutation in the extracellular portion of the molecule. Consequently, an alternative stop codon occurs, encoding a protein devoid of transmembrane and intracellular domains. This sequence analysis was extended to several TLR2 clones, from three different cell lines. In all cases, only a truncated protein sequence was observed.

We cloned CHO-TLRs into a mammalian expression vector. CHO-TLR2 cDNA failed to enable LPS-signaling upon transient transfection into human epithelial kidney (HEK) 293 cells. Site-directed mutagenesis of CHO-TLR2 was performed to insert an 'A' at bp 1758 of its cDNA, enabling expression of a presumed full-length hamster TLR2. Over-expression of the 'repaired' hamster cDNA conferred LPS-responsiveness in HEK293 cells, similar to mouse and human TLR2.

Finally, we analyzed TLR2 in native Chinese hamsters. TLR2 transcripts isolated from primary hamster macrophages also contained the frame-shift mutation found in CHO fibroblasts. We performed sequence analysis on genomic DNA, in order to determine if an alternative cDNA might potentially exist. No alternative sequence was found for TLR2, suggesting that CHO cells are not unique in the type of TLR2 mRNA that they transcribe. Nevertheless, hamster peritoneal macrophages were found to respond normally to LPS, as evidenced by the induction of IL-1β, IL-6, and TNF-α. These results imply that expression of TLR2 is sufficient but not essential for mammalian responses to endotoxin. We predict that

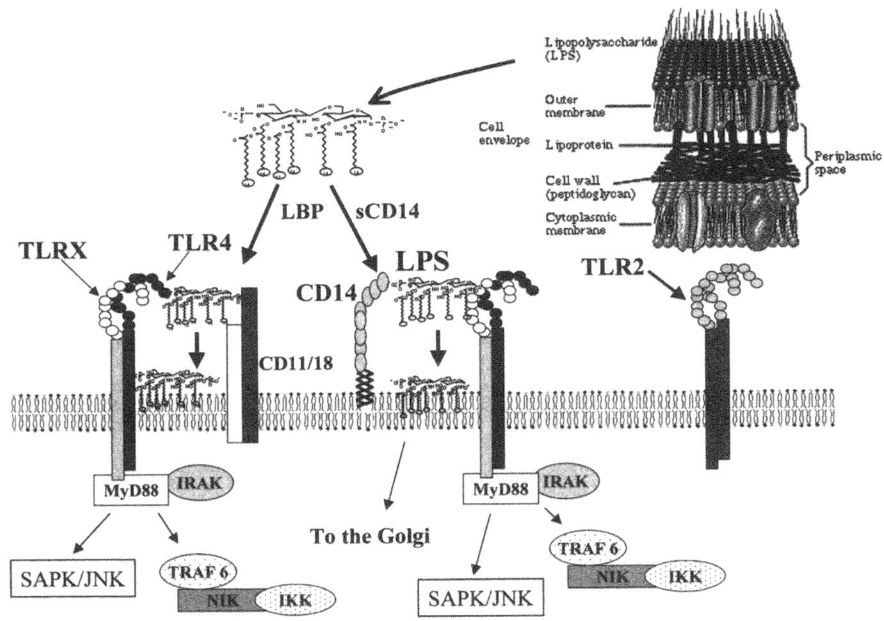

Fig. 1. Proposed model for LPS activation and uptake. The figure shows putative interactions in the LPS signaling pathway. Toll-like receptor (TLR) 4 may be able to homodimerize, or heterodimerize with other members of the TLR family (including TLR2). The relative role of TLR2 and TLR4 in LPS signaling for different species and cell types is not clear. Intracellular signaling pathways for TLRs can lead to activation of nuclear factor-kappa B (NF-κB) and stress-activated protein kinase/c-Jun N-terminal protein kinase (SAPK/JNK)

the more important role of TLR2 will be shown to relate to the recognition of alternative LPS-like ligands.

Conclusions

The LPS receptor system is extraordinarily complex. It appears to have important components in serum that present LPS to a cell-bound receptor, CD14, especially LPS binding protein and soluble CD14. CD14, in turn, appears to present LPS to a signal transducer, probably TLR4. Our current understanding of how LPS activates cells is summarized in Fig. 1.

Acknowledgments. This work was supported in part by NIH grants GM54060, AI38515, and DK50305 (to D. T. G. and H. H.), by The Research Council of Norway and The Norwegian Cancer Society (E. L.).

References

1. Bone RC (1991) The pathogenesis of sepsis. Ann Intern Med 115:457–469
2. Martin MA (1991) Epidemiology and clinical aspects of Gram-negative sepsis. Infect Dis Clin North Am 5:739–752
3. Raetz CRH (1990) Biochemistry of endotoxins. Annu Rev Biochem 59:129–170
4. Rietschel ET, Brade H (1992) Bacterial endotoxins. Sci Am 267:26–31
5. Strain SM, Fesik SW, Armitage IM (1983) Characterization of lipopolysaccharide from a heptoseless mutant of *Escherichia coli* by carbon-43 nuclear magnetic resonance. J Biol Chem 258:2906–2910
6. Imoto M, Kusumoto S, Shiba T, et al (1983) Chemical structure of *E. coli* Lipid A: Linkage site of acyl groups in the disaccharide backbone. Tetrahedron Lett 24:4017–4020
7. Haworth R, Platt N, Keshav S, et al (1997) The macrophage scavenger receptor type A is expressed by activated macrophages and protects the host against lethal endotoxic shock. J Exp Med 186:1431–1439
8. Hailman E, Lichenstein HS, Wurfel MM, et al (1994) Lipopolysaccharide (LPS)-binding protein accelerates the binding of LPS to CD14. J Exp Med 179:269–277
9. Wright SD, Ramos RA, Tobias PS, Ulevitch RJ, Mathison JC (1990) CD14, a receptor for complexes of lipopolysaccharide (LPS) and LPS-binding protein. Science 249:1431–1433
10. Wright SD, Ramos RA, Hermanowski-Vosatka AH, Rockwell P, Detmers PA (1991) Activation of the adhesive capacity of CR3 on neutrophils by endotoxin: Dependence on lipopolysaccharide binding protein and CD14. J Exp Med 173:1281–1286
11. Lynn WA, Raetz CR, Qureshi N, Golenbock DT (1991) Lipopolysaccharide-induced stimulation of CD11b/CD18 expression on neutrophils. Evidence of specific receptor-based response and inhibition by lipid A-based antagonists. J Immunol 147:3072–3079
12. Kitchens RL, Ulevitch RJ, Munford RS (1992) Lipopolysaccharide (LPS) partial structures inhibit responses to LPS in a human macrophage cell line without inhibiting LPS uptake by a CD14-mediated pathway. J Exp Med 176:485–494
13. Kirkland TN, Finley F, Leturcq D, et al (1993) Analysis of lipopolysaccharide binding by CD14. J Biol Chem 268:24818–24823
14. Bazil V, Baudys M, Hilgert I, et al (1989) Structural relationship between the soluble and membrane-bound forms of human monocyte surface glycoprotein CD14. Mol Immunol 26:657–662
15. Frey EA, Miller DS, Jahr TG, et al (1992) Soluble CD14 participates in the response of cells to lipopolysaccharide. J Exp Med 176:1665–1671

16. Arditi M, Zhou J, Dorio R, Rong GW, Goyert SM, Kim KS (1993) Endotoxin-mediated endothelial cell injury and activation: role of soluble CD14. Infect Immun 61:3149–3156
17. Haziot A, Rong GW, Silver J, Goyert SM (1993) Recombinant soluble CD14 mediates the activation of endothelial cells by lipopolysaccharide. J Immunol 151:1500–1507
18. Pugin J, Schurer MC, Leturcq D, Moriarty A, Ulevitch RJ, Tobias PS (1993) Lipopolysaccharide activation of human endothelial and epithelial cells is mediated by lipopolysaccharide-binding protein and soluble CD14. Proc Natl Acad Sci USA 90:2744–2748
19. Lee J-D, Kato K, Tobias PS, Kirkland TN, Ulevitch RJ (1992) Transfection of CD14 into 70Z/3 cells dramatically enhances the sensitivity to complexes of lipopolysaccharide (LPS) and LPS binding protein. J Exp Med 175:1697–1705
20. Golenbock D, Liu Y, Millham F, Freeman M, Zoeller R (1993) Surface expression of human CD14 in Chinese hamster ovary fibroblasts imparts macrophage-like responsiveness to bacterial endotoxin. J Biol Chem 268:22055–22059
21. Viriyakosol S, Kirkland TN (1995) A region of human CD14 required for lipopolysaccharide binding. J Biol Chem 270:361–368
22. Haziot A, Ferrero E, Kontgen F, et al (1996) Resistance to endotoxin shock and reduced dissemination of gram-negative bacteria in CD14-deficient mice. Immunity 4:407–414
23. Haziot A, Ferrero E, Lin XY, Stewart CL, Goyert SM (1995) CD14-deficient mice are exquisitely insensitive to the effects of LPS. Prog Clin Biol Res 392:349–351
24. Tobias PS, Soldau K, Ulevitch RJ (1986) Isolation of a lipopolysaccharide-binding acute phase reactant from rabbit serum. J Exp Med 164:777–793
25. Mathison JC, Tobias PS, Wolfson E, Ulevitch RJ (1992) Plasma lipopolysaccharide (LPS)-binding protein. A key component in macrophage recognition of gram-negative LPS. J Immunol 149:200–206
26. Hailman E, Vasselon T, Kelley M, et al (1996) Stimulation of macrophages and neutrophils by complexes of lipopolysaccharide and soluble CD14. J Immunol 156:4384–4390
27. Park CT, Wright SD (1996) Plasma lipopolysaccharide-binding protein is found associated with a particle containing apolipoprotein A-I, phospholipid, and factor H-related proteins. J Biol Chem 271:18054–18060
28. Wurfel MM, Kunitake ST, Lichenstein H, Kane JP, Wright SD (1994) Lipopolysaccharide (LPS)-binding protein is carried on lipoproteins and acts as a cofactor in the neutralization of LPS. J Exp Med 180:1025–1035
29. Skarnes RC (1966) The inactivation of endotoxin after interaction with certain proteins of normal serum. Ann NY Acad Sci 133:644–662
30. Skarnes RC (1968) In vivo interaction of endotoxin with a plasma lipoprotein having esterase activity. J Bacteriol 95:2031–2034
31. Munford RS, Hall CL, Lipton JM, Dietschy JM (1982) Biological activity, lipoprotein-binding behavior, and in vivo disposition of extracted and native forms of *Salmonella typhimurium* lipopolysaccharides. J Clin Invest 70:877–888
32. Ulevitch RJ, Johnston AR, Weinstein DB (1979) New function for high density lipoproteins. Their participation in intravascular reactions of bacterial lipopolysaccharides. J Clin Invest 64:1516–1524
33. Gallay P, Barras C, Tobias PS, Calandra T, Glauser MP, Heumann D (1994) Lipopolysaccharide (LPS)-binding protein in human serum determines the tumor necrosis factor response of monocytes to LPS. J Infect Dis 170:1319–1322
34. Calvano SE, Thompson WA, Marra MN, et al (1994) Changes in polymorphonuclear leukocyte surface and plasma bactericidal/permeability-increasing protein and plasma lipopolysaccharide binding protein during endotoxemia or sepsis. Arch Surg 129:220–226
35. Myc A, Buck J, Gonin J, Reynolds B, Hammerling U, Emanuel D (1997) The level of lipopolysaccharide-binding protein is significantly increased in plasma in patients with the systemic inflammatory response syndrome. Clin Diagn Lab Immunol 4:113–116
36. Martin TR, Rubenfeld GD, Ruzinski JT, et al (1997) Relationship between soluble CD14, lipopolysaccharide binding protein, and the alveolar inflammatory response in patients with acute respiratory distress syndrome. Am J Respir Crit Care Med 155:937–944
37. Ingalls RR, Golenbock DT (1995) CD11c/CD18, a transmembrane signaling receptor for lipopolysaccharide. J Exp Med 181:1473–1479

38. Ingalls RR, Arnaout MA, Golenbock DT (1997) Outside-in signaling by lipopolysaccharide through a tailless integrin. J Immunol 159:433–438
39. Wright SD, Tobias PS, Ulevitch RJ, Ramos RA (1989) Lipopolysaccharide (LPS) binding protein opsonizes LPS-bearing particles for recognition by a novel receptor on macrophages. J Exp Med 170:1231–1241
40. Ingalls RR, Monks BG, Savedra R Jr, et al (1998) CD11/CD18 and CD14 share a common lipid A signaling pathway. J Immunol 161:5413–5420
41. Lynn WA, Golenbock DT (1992) Lipopolysaccharide antagonists. Immunol Today 13: 271–276
42. Christ W, Asano O, Robidoux AL, et al (1995) E5531, a pure endotoxin antagonist of high potency. Science 268:80–83
43. Delude R, Savedra R, Zhao H, et al (1995) CD14 enhances cellular responses to endotoxin without imparting ligand-specific recognition. Proc Natl Acad Sci USA 92:9288–9292
44. Kitchens RL, Munford RS (1995) Enzymatically deacylated lipopolysaccharide (LPS) can antagonize LPS at multiple sites in the LPS recognition pathway. J Biol Chem 270:9904–9910
45. Pugin J, Heumann ID, Tomasz A, et al (1994) CD14 is a pattern recognition receptor. Immunity 1:509–516
46. Savedra R Jr, Delude RL, Ingalls RR, Fenton MJ, Golenbock DT (1996) Mycobacterial lipoarabinomannan recognition requires a receptor hat shares components of the endotoxin signaling system. J Immunol 157:2549–2554
47. Belvin MP, Anderson KV (1996) A conserved signaling pathway: the Drosophila toll-dorsal pathway. Ann Rev Cell Dev Biol 12:393–416
48. Rock FL, Hardiman G, Timans JC, Kastelein RA, Bazan JF (1998) A family of human receptors structurally related to Drosophila Toll. Proc Natl Acad Sci USA 95:588–593
49. Yang RB, Mark MR, Gray A, et al (1998) Toll-like receptor-2 mediates lipopolysaccharide-induced cellular signalling. Nature 395:284–288
50. Kirschning CJ, Wesche H, Ayres TM, Rothe M (1998) Human toll-like receptor 2 confers responsiveness to bacterial lipopolysaccharide. J Exp Med 188:2091–2097
51. Poltorak A, He X, Smirnova I, et al (1998) Defective LPS signaling in C3H/HeJ and C57BL/10ScCr mice: Mutations in Tlr4 gene. Science 282:2085–2088
52. Qureshi ST, Lariviere L, Leveque G, et al (1999) Endotoxin-tolerant mice have mutations in toll-like receptor 4 (Tlr4). J Exp Med 189:615–625
53. Chow JC, Young DW, Golenbock DT, Christ WJ, Gusovsky F (1999) Toll-like receptor-4 mediates lipopolysaccharide-induced signal transduction. J Biol Chem 274:10689–10692
54. O'Neill LA, Greene C (1998) Signal transduction pathways activated by the IL-1 receptor family: ancient signaling machinery in mammals, insects, and plants. J Leukoc Biol 63: 650–657
55. Delude RL, Yoshimura A, Ingalls RR, Golenbock DT (1998) Construction of a lipopolysaccharide reporter cell line and its use in identifying mutants defective in endotoxin, but not TNF-alpha, signal transduction. J Immunol 161:3001–3009

Regulation of Cellular Responses to Bacterial Endotoxin

R. J. Ulevitch

Introduction

Of late, the innate and adaptive immune systems have been compared and contrasted in a considerable literature; the evolutionary conservation of innate immunity has also been pointed out [1–3]. In particular, there are remarkable parallels when the innate immune responses to microbial pathogens by lower organisms and mammals are compared [4–8]. The innate immune system functions to provide signals to the host that microbial pathogens are present. This response is designed to up-regulate host defense mechanisms that either directly kill the pathogen or keep the infection in check until the adaptive immune response is fully active. In man, and in experimental model systems, infection with Gram-negative bacteria has been extensively studied in order to define the mechanisms that control recognition of this class of bacteria. It is now generally agreed that studies with endotoxin (lipopolysaccharide, LPS) purified from the outer membrane of Gram-negative bacteria offer an alternative and simpler system than that of intact bacteria to define the recognition mechanisms operative within the innate immune system.

As recently as ten years ago the mechanisms controlling cellular responses to the endotoxin or LPS of Gram-negative bacteria were poorly understood. Now a considerable body of evidence has been published to support a model where endotoxin or endotoxin-containing particles (including intact bacteria) form complexes with a serum protein, LPS binding protein (LBP); the LPS present in the LPS-LBP complex is subsequently transferred to another endotoxin binding protein, CD14. This protein is located on the outer leaflet of the plasma membrane of most myeloid lineage cell types as well as in the serum where it is a soluble protein. LPS binding to these two forms of CD14 results in activation of myeloid or non-myeloid lineage cell types respectively.

While differences between challenge with intact organism versus purified LPS most certainly exist, this chapter will focus exclusively on studies where LPS is used to activate cells. Further, this discussion will be limited to studies of LPS interactions with myeloid lineage cells and will include data obtain in studies of primary explants of cells as well as with continuous cell lines. The purpose of this chapter is to discuss the current level of understanding of the LBP/CD14 pathway in so far as it is the physiological recognition pathway for LPS and how this pathway impacts cellular signaling pathways that transfer information from the cell surface to the interior.

LPS Recognition via the LBP/CD14 Pathway

A full understanding of the physiological pathway for LPS recognition eluded scientists for many decades in part due to the ability of LPS to interact with proteins through what are now known to be non-specific interactions. It was, however, reasonable to hypothesize that LPS is recognized by a non-redundant set of proteins to produce its diverse biologic effects. Lewis Thomas described the drama of the interactions of Gram-negative bacteria and LPS with what we know to be the host innate immune system. Thomas wrote that; "It is the information carried by the bacteria that we cannot abide. The gram-negative bacteria are the best examples of this. They display lipopolysaccharide endotoxin in their walls, and these macromolecules are read by our tissues as the very worst of bad news. When we sense lipopolysaccharide, we are likely to turn on every defense at our disposal ...." [9].

A complete understanding of the chemical structure of LPS has been available for more than ten years [10,11]. Nonetheless, the recognition of LPS by serum proteins and/or cells has only been understood at the molecular level for a short period of time. This warning that Thomas so aptly described was not understood in molecular terms until the beginning of this decade. The seminal discovery of LBP by Tobias, Ulevitch and co-workers, and the subsequent elucidation of its structure and function [12, 13], provided a basis for deciphering the steps involved in LPS recognition. The identification of CD14 as an LPS receptor [14] provided the means to systematically investigate the mechanisms of LPS-induced cell activation in a variety of *in vivo* or *in vitro* model systems [15,16]. Sub-picomolar LPS concentrations trigger direct responses from cells; as summarized below such responses require both LBP and CD14. Most recently members of the family of human toll-like receptors (TLRs) have also been linked to LBP/CD14-dependent responses to LPS [17–21].

The biologically active structure of all LPS isolates is the lipid A moiety that is comprised of a diglucosamine backbone containing ester and amide-linked long chain fatty acids. The glucosamine residues may be substituted with a variety of side groups including phosphate and amino-arabinose [10, 11]. Nonetheless, it is the basic diglucosamine backbone with its fatty acid substituents that makes up the chemical structure recognized by cells. Both LBP and CD14 bind to LPS via the lipid A portion of the molecule. The biochemical properties of LBP and CD14 have recently been described in reviews [15, 16, 22, 23] and will also be considered in other sections of this volume. Nonetheless some recent data regarding these proteins will be considered here as additional background to the main issue of LPS signaling pathways.

The development of a working model for structure-function relationships in LBP received a substantive boost from the X-ray crystallographic structural analysis of bactericidal/permeability increasing protein (BPI) [24]. BPI and LBP have long been recognized as closely related LPS binding proteins; thus information from BPI structure is likely to be informative for understanding LBP [25]. BPI has a boomerang shape with two similar arms. Both arms are crystallized together with phospholipids, suggesting locations for LPS binding sites. Basic residues in the sequences of BPI and LBP between positions 90–100 are thought to be important for LPS binding [26]. However, the pockets where the bound phospholipids reside are not large enough to accommodate lipid A. Moreover it must be emphasized that BPI and LBP have very different effects on LPS; BPI inhibits LPS delivery to monocyte CD14 and appears to condense LPS aggregates while LBP promotes LPS delivery to monocyte CD14 and disaggregates LPS [27].

Some new insights into the function of LBP derive from understanding its ability to act as a phospholipid transfer protein and its role in LPS internalization. Consistent with the homology between cholesterol ester transfer protein and phospholipid transfer protein and LBP, LBP catalyzes the movement of LPS from LPS aggregates to phospholipid micelles [28]. This observation led to the suggestion that LBP and CD14 functioned in cellular activation by delivering LPS to the plasma membrane. An alternative function for the ability of LBP to transfer phospholipids to CD14 is raised by the observation that phosphatidylinositides in serum bind to plasma membrane CD14 on monocytes, this binding inhibits LPS action and is enabled by LBP [29]. The significance of this finding is not entirely clear, but suggests that competition of activating and inhibitory ligands for CD14 is important.

Role of LPS Binding Protein and CD14 *in Vivo*

Although LPS binds to multiple plasma proteins, only one, LBP, is known to bind to LPS via lipid A and to modulate subsequent interactions of LPS with CD14. LBP has a non-redundant function in so far as initiation of host defense responses to minute amounts of LPS and thus for elimination and/or killing of Gram-negative organisms. Data to support this claim are derived from two independent reports describing experiments with mice containing a targeted deletion of the LBP gene [30, 31]. Targeted gene deletion of murine CD14 has revealed a very similar phenotype in that the absence of CD14 results in a mouse that is resistant to the lethal effects of LPS [30].

The totality of data from targeted gene deletion studies of both LBP and CD14 support the contention that these proteins are essential parts of a physiological recognition pathway used by the innate immune system to mount responses to the presence of Gram-negative bacteria. The LBP/CD14 pathway seems to be non-redundant; thus it seems reasonable that modulation of this pathway might provide a new means of controlling responses to infection. This would be especially useful in the setting of Gram-negative sepsis where septic shock and its complications cause serious clinical problems [32–34]. In this regard CD14 has been a target, and recent studies performed in rabbits confirm the potential utility of CD14 blockade [35]. LPS-induced organ damage and lethality is caused by multiple injections of LPS given over 24 hours; lethality and organ injury occur during 24–48 hours. The administration of a monoclonal antibody to rabbit

CD14 after one or two LPS exposures resulted in protection suggesting the possibility of a therapeutic window in Gram-negative sepsis in man. In contrast anti-rabbit tumor necrosis factor (TNF) monoclonal antibody had no such therapeutic benefit when tested in comparative studies [35]. Testing in humans will be needed to determine if findings from animal model studies predict outcomes in the clinical situation.

LPS Signaling from A Membrane Receptor

The discovery of the LBP-CD14 dependent pathways of LPS-induced cell activation allowed the design of experiments to study LPS signaling with *in vitro* cellular model systems under conditions that reflected physiological conditions. Previously, studies were performed with concentrations of LPS that were up to three logs higher than the amounts needed to trigger cellular responses via an LBP-CD14 pathway. Thus some data in the older literature may reflect cellular changes resulting from non-specific effects of LPS, rather than those resulting from the initiation of a transmembrane signal via the biologically relevant LPS receptor.

LPS directly activates cells of the myeloid and non-myeloid lineage. In either case CD14 is involved; membrane bound CD14 (mCD14) for myeloid and soluble CD14 (sCD14) for other cell types. Most investigators accept a model for an LPS receptor that involves CD14 as a ligand binding protein that serves to transfer LPS to a transmembrane protein that, while capable of binding LPS, only does so efficiently when the LPS is presented via CD14 [36, 37]. This model differs from others that invoke membrane perturbations resulting from insertion of LPS into the lipid bilayer of the membrane [38]. Thus CD14 does not directly participate in signaling, consistent with its role as a glycosylphosphatidyl-inositol (GPI) anchored membrane protein of myeloid cells or as a soluble serum protein. The localization of CD14 in lipid-rich domains of the plasma membrane suggested that complexes of signaling molecules on the inner face of the plasma membrane might participate in CD14-dependent cell activation [39]. This view is not widely held now due to recent discoveries of the role of TLRs in LPS signaling.

Following the discovery of the function of CD14 in LPS-induced cell activation substantial efforts were made to identify additional components of the LPS receptor. Such efforts yielded little information until recently. The cloning of the first member of the human TLR family was noted, followed by additional reports describing new members of this family and some properties of individual members of the TLR family [17–21]. Recently two groups reported that expression of human TLR2 in HEK293 cells resulted in a LPS-responsive cell line that is activated by an LBP/CD14-dependent pathway [20, 21]. These studies also provided information about intracellular signaling pathways used by LPS. Important data from Poltorak and co-workers suggests that in addition to TLR2 there is a role for TLR4 in LPS signaling, at least in the mouse [19]. This contention is supported by the finding that the *Lps* gene is that encoding murine TLR4 and is distinct from murine TLR2. Thus the defect in LPS-hyporesponsive mouse strain, C3H/HeJ, is in the gene encoding TLR4; a null mutation in TLR4 was also reported for another LPS non-responsive strain, C57Bl/10ScCr. Precisely how the members of the TLR family are involved in LPS signaling in myeloid and non-myeloid lineage cell types will require additional study. Furthermore it will be very important to determine if there are species-dependent utilization of individual members of the TLR family.

Intracellular Signaling Pathways Used by LPS

Although numerous claims for atypical signaling mechanisms have been advanced in the past, it is not surprising that LPS signaling from the membrane to the nucleus uses intracellular signaling pathways that overlap with those of cytokines and extra-cellular stimuli. Following is a summary of information about the activation of intracellular kinase cascades following binding of LPS to its membrane receptor. Here the focus is on two divergent pathways; nuclear factor-kappa B (NF-κB) and the mitogen activated protein kinase (MAPK) pathways.

Weinstein, DeFranco and co-workers first linked LPS stimulation to increased protein tyrosine phosphorylation and activation of MAPK pathways [40, 41]. They showed that LPS treatment of macrophages induced protein tyrosine phosphorylation including the MAPK family members known as ERK1/ERK2 (extra-cellular signal-regulated kinases). In subsequent studies this group documented that protein tyrosine phosphorylation occurred via CD14-dependent mechanisms and that in addition to ERK1/ERK2, the c-Jun-N-terminal kinase (JNK) is also activated by LPS [42, 43].

An important advance in the ability to analyze LPS-induced cell activation came from establishment of cell lines where mCD14 is expressed following transfection [36, 37, 44]. Such lines include 70Z/3 and CHO-K1 cells. In particular the 70Z/3 cells expressing human mCD14, 70Z/3-hCD14 cells, have been of great value in analyzing various aspects of LPS signaling. With this line Ulevitch, Lee and colleagues provided evidence that the GPI-anchoring mechanism for CD14 is not essential for CD14 to bind LPS and to support cell activation [36, 37]. Based on the work of Weinstein and DeFranco, we analyzed lysates from LPS-treated 70Z/3-hCD14 cells for protein tyrosine phosphorylation profiles. In this particular cell line a protein with an apparent molecular weight of 38-kDa was phosphorylated on tyrosine after LPS treatment but not after exposure of the same cells to phorbol 12-myristate 13-acetate (PMA) [45]. Purification of this protein and microsequencing led to the cDNA cloning and discovery of a new member of the MAPK pathway termed p38 [46]. In most, if not all LPS-responsive cell lines, p38 is activated and has been shown to play a role regulating a variety of cellular functions. In some cell types LPS treatment leads to activation of three MAPK family members; ERK1/ERK2, p38 and JNK. However in other cell types only selective activation is noted. Moreover there are no data to suggest that the fourth MAPK family member, BMK1/ERK5, is ever activated by LPS treatment [47, 48].

All MAPK are activated by phosphorylation on adjacent threonine and tyrosine residues [49, 50] and this is regulated by a conserved set of upstream protein kinases. Each MAPK pathway is controlled by distinct upstream enzymes that in turn are thought to be regulated by small guanosine triphosphate (GTP)-binding proteins. There are some data to indicate how LPS activates each of the MAPK family members, particularly at the MAPK kinase (MKK, MEK) level. For example biochemical analyses suggest that of the two known activators of p38, MKK3 and MKK6, MKK6 is the favored enzyme in LPS treated THP-1 cells [51]. For ERK1/ERK2 activation pharmacologic inhibitors suggest that MEK1 is involved in at least some LPS-dependent signaling [52, 53]. Of the two known JNK activators, MKK4 and MKK7, there are no data to suggest that LPS favors one over the other. Events upstream of the MKKs are even less well understood and will require further study to define the pathways utilized during LPS signaling. Such studies will have to include an analysis of the MAPK kinase kinase family members and the various low molecular weight GTP-binding proteins. In addition to the MAPKs several other kinases have been shown to be activated following LPS treatment and these include members of the protein kinase C family and kinases involved in phosphatidyl inositol phosphorylations [54, 55].

Activation of intracellular kinase cascades leads to new gene expression primarily though effects on the activity of transcription factors. The MAPKs participate in such events as do members of a family of transcription factors known as NF-κB [56]. In the past two years a remarkable amount of information has emerged about the steps leading to activation of this latter group of transcription factors [57, 58]. The establishment of model systems to evaluate the role of human TLRs in LPS signaling has also led to the beginnings of an understanding of LPS signaling mechanisms that result in NF-κB activation. Two groups have provided data suggesting that LPS uses pathways that overlap with those used by interleukin (IL)-1 and involve MyD88, IL-1 receptor-associated kinase (IRAK) and TNF receptor-associated factor 6 (TRAF6) [20, 21]. The similarities between LPS and IL-1 signaling are not surprising given the homology in the cytoplasmic tail of the IL-1 receptor and the human TLRs [17, 18]. Undoubtedly in the coming year significant new information will accrue about LPS-induced signaling pathways.

The importance of members of the NF-κB family in regulating LPS-induced gene expression is widely appreciated. The role of MAPKs in such events has received much less study. Mainly through the use of pharmacologic inhibitors of the pyridinyl imidazole family has an appreciation for the role of p38 in both transcriptional and post-transcriptional regulatory mechanisms been appreciated. In the case of p38 a number of downstream targets have been identified that provide mechanistic explanations for how this MAPK regulates LPS-induced events; such downstream targets include transcription factors and other protein kinases. A full understanding of these pathways may result in the identification of new targets for the development of therapeutics to intervene in septic shock.

Conclusion

During the past decade, research has provided the molecular basis of the 'sensing' mechanism used to detect the presence of Gram-negative bacteria through their product known as endotoxin. This progress has provided numerous new opportunities to consider methods to intervene when activation of the innate immune system causes serious human disease. Moreover a new chapter has been opened with the discovery of the roll of the human TLR family in recognition of LPS. This promises to provide the means to fully understanding the signaling pathways used by LPS and perhaps to determine a genetic basis for susceptibility to septic shock. At a minimum there will be an increasing awareness of new ways to modulate the response of the innate immune system to infection.

Acknowledgments. This is publication number 12176-IMM from the Department of Immunology of The Scripps Research Institute. This work was supported in part by National Institutes of Health grants GM37696, AI15136 and GM28485.

References

1. Fearon DT (1997) Seeking wisdom in innate immunity. Nature 388:323–324
2. Medzhitov R, Janeway CA Jr (1997) Innate immunity: The virtues of a nonclonal system of recognition. Cell 91:295–298
3. Medzhitov R, Janeway CA Jr (1998) Self-defense: The fruit fly style. Proc Natl Acad Sci USA 95:429–430
4. Ip YT, Reach M, Engstrom Y et al (1993) Dif, a dorsal-related gene that mediates an immune response in Drosophila. Cell 75:753–763
5. Lemaitre B, Nicolas E, Michaut L, Reichhart JM, Hoffmann JA (1996) The dorsoventral regulatory gene cassette spatzle/Toll/cactus controls the potent antifungal response in Drosophila adults. Cell 86:973–983
6. Hultmark D (1994) Ancient relationships. Nature 367:116–117
7. Dushay MS, Asling B, Hultmark D (1996) Origins of immunity: Relish, a compound Rel-like gene in the antibacterial defense of Drosophila. Proc Natl Acad Sci USA 93:10343–10347
8. Hultmark D (1993) Immune reactions in Drosophila and other insects: a model for innate immunity. Trends Genet 9:178–183
9. Thomas L (1974) The Lives of a Cell. Notes of a Biology Watcher. The Viking Press, New York
10. Raetz CRH (1990) Biochemistry of endotoxins. Annu Rev Biochem 59:129–170
11. Jann K, Jann B (1984) Structure and biosynthesis of O-antigens. In: Rietschel ET (ed) Handbook of endotoxin, Vol. I. Chemistry of endotoxin. Elsevier, Amsterdam, pp 138–186
12. Tobias P, Soldau K, Ulevitch R (1986) Isolation of a lipopolysaccharide-binding acute phase reactant from rabbit serum. J Exp Med 164:777–793
13. Schumann RR, Leong SR, Flaggs GW, et al (1990) Structure and function of lipopolysaccharide binding protein. Science 249:1429–1431
14. Wright SD, Ramos RA, Tobias PS, Ulevitch RJ, Mathison JC (1990) CD14 serves as the cellular receptor for complexes of lipopolysaccharide with lipopolysaccharide binding protein. Science 249:1431–1433
15. Ulevitch RJ (1993) Recognition of bacterial endotoxins by receptor-dependent mechanisms. Adv Immunol 53:267–289
16. Ulevitch RJ, Tobias PS (1994) Recognition of endotoxin by cells leading to transmembrane signalling. Curr Opin Immunol 6:125–130
17. Medzhitov R, Preston-Hurlburt P, Janeway CA Jr (1997) A human homologue of the Drosophila Toll protein signals activation of adaptive immunity. Nature 388:394–397
18. Rock FL, Hardiman G, Timans JC, Kastelein RA, Bazan JF (1998) A family of human receptors structurally related to Drosophila toll. Proc Natl Acad Sci USA 95:588–593
19. Poltorak A, He X, Smirnova I, et al (1998) Defective LPS signalling in C3H/HeJ and C57BL/10ScCr mice: Mutations in Tlr4 gene. Science 282:2085–2088

20. Kirschning CJ, Wesche H, Ayres TM, Rothe M (1998) Human Toll-like receptor 2 confers responsiveness to bacterial lipopolysaccharide. J Exp Med 188:2091–2097
21. Yang RB, Mark MR, Gray A et al (1998) Toll-like receptor-2 mediates lipopolysaccharide-induced cellular signalling. Nature 17:284–288
22. Fenton MJ, Golenbock DT (1998) LPS-binding proteins and receptors. J Leukoc Biol 64: 25–32
23. Kirkland TN, Viriyakosol S (1998) Structure-function analysis of soluble and membrane--bound CD14. Prog Clin Biol Res 397:79–87
24. Beamer LJ, Carroll SF, Eisenberg D (1997) Crystal structure of human BPI and two bound phospholipids at 2.4 angstrom resolution. Science 276:1861–1864
25. Tobias PS, Mathison JC, Ulevitch RJ (1988) A family of lipopolysaccharide binding proteins involved in responses to gram-negative sepsis. J Biol Chem 263:13479–13481
26. Lamping N, Hoess A, Yu B, et al (1996) Effects of site-directed mutagenesis of basic residues (Arg 94, Lys 95, Lys 99) of lipopolysaccharide (LPS)-binding protein on binding and transfer of LPS and subsequent immune cell activation. J Immunol 157:4648–4656
27. Tobias PS, Soldau K, Iovine NM, Elsbach P, Weiss J (1997) Lipopolysaccharide (LPS)-binding proteins BPI and LBP form different types of complexes with LPS. J Biol Chem 272: 18682–18685
28. Wurfel MM, Wright SD (1997) Lipopolysaccharide-binding protein and soluble CD14 transfer lipopolysaccharide to phospholipid bilayers: preferential interaction with particular classes of lipid. J Immunol 158:3925–3934
29. Wang PY, Kitchens RL, Munford RS (1998) Phosphatidylinositides bind to plasma membrane CD14 and can prevent monocyte activation by bacterial lipopolysaccharide. J Biol Chem 273:24309–24313
30. Jack RS, Fan X, Bernheiden M, et al (1997) Lipopolysaccharide-binding protein is required to combat a murine Gram-negative bacterial infection. Nature 389:742–745
31. Wurfel MM, Monks BG, Ingalls RR, et al (1997) Targeted deletion of the lipopolysaccharide (LPS)-binding protein gene leads to profound suppression of LPS responses ex vivo, whereas in vivo responses remain intact. J Exp Med 186:2051–2056
32. Glauser MP, Zanetti G, Baumgartner JD, Cohen J (1991) Septic shock: pathogenesis. Lancet 338:732–736
33. Cohen J, Glauser MP (1991) Septic shock: treatment. Lancet 338:736–739
34. Gutierrez-Ramos JC, Bluethmann H (1997) Molecules and mechanisms operating in septic shock: lessons from knockout mice. Immunol Today 8:329–334
35. Schimke J, Mathison J, Morgiewicz J, Ulevitch RJ (1998) Anti-CD14 mAb treatment provides therapeutic benefit after in vivo exposure to endotoxin. Proc Natl Acad Sci USA 95: 13875–13880
36. Lee JD, Kato K, Tobias PS, Kirkland TN, Ulevitch RJ (1992) Transfection of CD14 into 70Z/3 cells dramatically enhances the sensitivity to complexes of lipopolysaccharide (LPS) and LPS binding protein. J Exp Med 175:1697–1705
37. Lee JD, Kravchenko V, Kirkland TN, et al (1993) GPI-anchored or integral membrane forms of CD14 mediate identical cellular responses to endotoxin. Proc Natl Acad Sci USA 90: 9930–9934
38. Thieblemont N, Thieringer R, Wright SD (1998) Innate immune recognition of bacterial lipopolysaccharide: Dependence on interactions with membrane lipids and endocytic movement. Immunity 8:771–777
39. Stefanova I, Horejsi V, Ansotegui IJ, Knapp W, Stockinger H (1991) GPI-anchored cell-surface molecules complexed to protein tyrosine kinases. Science 254:1016–1019
40. Weinstein SL, Sanghera JS, Lemke K, DeFranco AL, Pelech SL (1992) Bacterial lipopolysaccharide induces tyrosine phosphorylation and activation of mitogen-activated protein kinass in macrophages. J Biol Chem 267:14955–14962
41. Weinstein SL, Gold MR, DeFranco AL (1991) Bacterial lipopolysaccharide stimulates protein tyrosine phosphorylation in macrophages. Proc Natl Acad Sci USA 88:4148–4152
42. Hambleton J, Weinstein SL, Lem L, DeFranco AL (1996) Activation of c-Jun N-terminal kinase in bacterial lipopolysacchride-stimulated macrophages. Proc Natl Acad Sci USA 93: 2774–2778

43. Weinstein SL, June CH, DeFranco AL (1993) Lipopolysaccharide-induced protein tyrosine phosphorylation in human macrophages is mediated by CD14. J Immunol 151:3829–3838
44. Zoeller RA, Liu Y, Millham FH, Freeman MW, Golenbock DT (1993) Surface expression of human CD14 in Chinese hamster ovary fibroblasts imparts macrophage-like responsiveness to bacterial endotoxin. J Biol Chem 268:22055–22059
45. Han J, Lee JD, Tobias PS, Ulevitch RJ (1993) Endotoxin induces rapid protein tyrosine phosphorylation in 70Z/3 cells expressing CD14. J Biol Chem 268:25009–25014
46. Han J, Lee JD, Bibbs L, Ulevitch RJ (1994) A MAP kinase targeted by endotoxin and hyperosmolarity in mammalian cells. Science 265:808–811
47. Lee JD, Ulevitch RJ, Han J (1995) Primary structure of BMK1: A new mammalian MAP kinase. Biochem Biophys Res Comm 213:715–724
48. Zhou G, Bao ZQ, Dixon JE (1995) Components of a new human protein kinase signal transduction pathway. J Biol Chem 270:12665–12669
49. Dhanasekaran N, Premkumar Reddy E (1999) Signaling by dual specificity kinases. Oncogene 17:1447–1455
50. Keyse SM (1998) Protein phosphatases and the regulation of MAP kinase activity. Semin Cell Dev Biol 9:143–152
51. Cuenda A, Alonso G, Morrice N, et al (1996) Purification and cDNA cloning of SAPKK3, the major activator of RK/p38 in stress- and cytokine-stimulated monocytes and epithelial cells. EMBO J 15:4156–4164
52. Scherle PA, Jones EA, Favata MF, et al (1998) Inhibition of MAP kinase kinase prevents cytokine and prostaglandin E2 production in lipopolysaccharide-stimulated monocytes. J Immunol 161:5681–5686
53. Rawadi G, Ramez V, Lemercier B, Roman-Roman S (1998) Activation of mitogen-activated protein kinase pathays by Mycoplasma fermentans membrane lipoproteins in murine macrophages: Involvement in cytokine synthesis. J Immunol 160:1330–1339
54. Herrera-Velit P, Knutson KL, Reiner NE (1997) Phosphatidylinosil 3-kinase-dependent activation of protein kinase C-zeta in bacterial lipopolysaccharide-treated human monocytes. J Biol Chem 272:16445–16452
55. Liu MK, Herrera-Velit P, Brownsey RW, Reiner NE (1994) CD14-dependent activation of protein kinase C and mitogen-activated protein kinases (p42 and p44) in human monocytes treated with bacterial lipopolysaccharide. J Immunol 153:2642–2652
56. Baeuerle PA, Baltimore D (1996) NF-κB: Ten years after. Cell 87:13–20
57. Verma IM, Stevenson J (1997) IκB kinase: Beginning, not the end. Proc Natl Acad Sci USA 94:11758–11760
58. Stancovski I, Baltimore D (1999) NF-κB activation: the IκB kinase revealed? Cell 91:299–302

The Role of Nitric Oxide in the Initiation of Inflammation in Shock

R. T. Villavicencio and T. R. Billiar

Introduction

Inadequate tissue perfusion occurs in a number of settings in critically ill patients. Septic patients experience bouts of hypotension and inadequate perfusion and may experience regional ischemia due to dysregulation of the microcirculation. Organ ischemia may result from vascular occlusive events such as myocardial infarction or stroke, or from transient vascular occlusion during surgical procedures. Multisystem trauma involving both tissue destruction and hemorrhage can result in localized tissue ischemia at the site of injury as well as systemic hypoperfusion due to blood loss. Hemorrhagic shock in the absence of infection or tissue damage due to injury or surgical procedures is the purest form of global ischemia. Common to all events involving sustained, reduced organ perfusion is organ damage and inflammation that becomes evident upon reperfusion. Efforts to understand how ischemia and reperfusion initiate inflammation and lead to organ damage have focused on models of isolated organ ischemia and reperfusion in hemorrhagic shock.

Direct tissue damage resulting from toxic radical production during reperfusion has been demonstrated. However, the mechanisms for activation of inflammatory cascades are not so apparent. Compared to sepsis where the activation of inflammatory gene expression clearly occurs as a result of a specific interaction between a septic agent (e.g., bacterial toxins) and a host, no such inflammatory agent has been shown to exist for hemorrhagic shock. Bacterial products from the gut [1], activation of neurohumoral pathways [2], and activation of hypoxia or redox sensitive transcription factors have all been proposed as inflammatory inciting events in hemorrhagic shock. Here we will summarize the activation of inflammation in hemorrhagic shock with a focus on the role of nitric oxide (NO) in the activation of nuclear factor-kappa B (NF-κB).

Cytokine Up-regulation in Hemorrhagic Shock

Hemorrhagic shock and resuscitation produces acute inflammation. Hemorrhagic shock and resuscitation, in mouse models, has been reported to increase, within one hour of blood loss, mRNA levels of multiple cytokines, including interleukin (IL)-1α, IL-1β, IL-5, tumor necrosis factor (TNF)-α, and transforming growth factor (TGF)-β1 [3], and protein levels of IL-1β [2]. IL-6 and interferon (IFN)-γ mRNA levels were also elevated in lung lymphocyte populations within 4 h of hemorrhage [3]. Additional rodent studies report increases in the following cytokines: TNF serum levels [4], myocardial TNF-α protein levels [5], and IL-6 and granulocyte colony-stimulating factor (G-CSF) mRNA [6,7]. Immunoregulatory proteins such as intercellular adhesion molecule (ICAM)-1 and P-selectin also rapidly increase after resuscitated hemorrhagic shock [8]. Many upregulated cytokines and mediators, including TNF-α, IL-1β, IL-6, ICAM-1, and inducible NO synthase (iNOS), have transactivating binding sites for the upstream transcription NF-κB in the regulatory segments of their genes. Consequently, elucidating the functional role(s) of NF-κB in this setting of redox stress is one approach to possibly regulate excessive cytokine expression after hemorrhagic shock.

NF-κB regulation is part of a swift cellular response system to many different noxious and pro-inflammatory stimuli. The genes regulated by the NF-κB family of transcription factors include more than 60 pro-inflammatory genes involved in controlling, for example, cell adhesion, immune stimulation, apoptosis, chemoattraction, differentiation, extracellular matrix degradation, redox metabolism, and production of mediators [9]. NF-κB is sequestered in the cytoplasm by its tight association with a class of specific inhibitory proteins, called IκBs, that prevent nuclear translocation and DNA binding of the transcription factor [9]. In response to pro-inflammatory stimuli, IκB is phosphorylated, ubiquitinylated, and degraded, allowing NF-κB to be transported into the nucleus, where it will initiate gene transcription upon binding its cognate DNA motifs in regulatory segments of genes [9]. NF-κB is required for maximal transcription of many cytokines including TNF-α, IL-1, IL-6, and IL-8, which are thought to be important in the generation of acute inflammatory responses [10]. The diversity of NF-κB inducers highlights an intriguing aspect of its regulation, namely the ability of many different signal transduction pathways emanating from a wide variety of induction mechanisms to converge on a single target: The cytosolic NF-κB-IκB complex [11].

NF-κB Activation in Hemorrhagic Shock

NF-κB activation has been mostly reported in models of hemorrhagic shock and resuscitation and not in models employing only hemorrhagic shock [5, 7, 12–15]. In many studies, rats and mice were cannulated, briefly hemorrhaged to 30–40 mm Hg, resuscitated, and then sacrificed to harvest organs [5, 7, 12, 14, 15]. Alternatively, in other models, mice were quickly hemorrhaged by cardiac puncture, resuscitated, and then sacrificed [2, 13, 16, 17]. After various periods of resuscitation, ranging from 15 min [17] to 4 hours [13], NF-κB activation has been reported. The observation of NF-κB activation in widespread tissues (heart, lung, liver, spleen) is consistent with the activation of a systemic inflammatory response [2, 5, 7, 15]. Inhibition of NF-κB activation post-hemorrhagic shock and resuscitation has been reported to reduce immediate post-hemorrhage events such as cytokine up-regulation [2, 7] in addition to later post-hemorrhage events such as organ injury (i.e., reduced neutrophil accumulation, pulmonary edema formation, and plasma liver enzyme levels) [7, 14].

Mechanisms of NF-κB Activation in Hemorrhagic Shock

Mechanisms of NF-κB activation in hemorrhagic shock and resuscitation include reactive oxygen intermediates, α-adrenergic stimulation, iNOS, and changes in IκB inhibitory protein levels. At least six IκB proteins are involved in controlling the activity of NF-κB dimers [9]. The stimulus-dependent regulators include IκBα. In mouse lung cells, xanthine oxidase-dependent mechanisms may produce alterations in IκBα levels which regulate the state of NF-κB activation [13]. Another mechanism of NF-κB activation may involve reactive oxygen intermediates which are rapidly generated in resuscitated hemorrhagic shock [18–20]. Xanthine oxidase-derived O_2 radicals may have an important role since xanthine oxidase is not required for NF-κB activation in lung mononuclear cells taken from mice 15 min after hemorrhage but is required for NF-κB activation in lung cells taken from mice one hour after hemorrhage [16, 17]. Hemorrhage may thus be followed by two phases of NF-κB activation: One which is xanthine oxidase-independent and occurs immediately after blood loss, and a second phase which is xanthine oxidase-dependent and takes place at later post resuscitation time points [17]. A third mechanism for NF-κB activation may involve α-adrenergic stimulation [2, 12]. Treatment of mice with the α-adrenergic receptor antagonist phentolamine, prevented not only the elevation in mRNA levels of IL-1β, TNF-α, and TGF-β1, but also the increase in NF-κB which occurred in lung cells of untreated animals during the first hour after hemorrhage [2]. In hemorrhaged mice pretreated with phentolamine, the level of NF-κB activation was markedly lower than that observed in untreated, hemorrhaged mice, and was even lower than that present in unmanipulated mice [2].

We have identified a key role for iNOS in the activation of NF-κB in the lungs, liver, and gut following resuscitated shock [7, 21]. Using the iNOS inhibitor N-6-(iminoethyl)-L-lysine (L-NIL), or iNOS knockout mice, we found that the activation of NF-κB and signal transducer and activator of transcription (STAT) 3 and increases in IL-6 and G-CSF mRNA levels in the lungs and livers, measured four hours after hemorrhagic shock and resuscitation, were iNOS dependent [7]. Each parameter was between 40–60% lower when iNOS was absent (knockout mice) or when iNOS was inhibited. Furthermore, iNOS inhibition resulted in a marked reduction of lung (reduced polymorphonuclear cell [PMN] accumulation and edema formation) and liver injury (reduced plasma levels of liver enzymes) produced by hemorrhagic shock. Subsequent studies have shown that iNOS inhibition results in similar findings in the gastrointestinal tract. Interestingly gut smooth muscle function was preserved when iNOS was absent or inhibited [21]. How NO up-regulates NF-κB and whether the resulting inflammation leads to organ damage is unknown; however the lack of PMN influx does suggest that the activation of NF-κB and PMN influx are limited. It should be noted that this activation of iNOS was not expressed in the stomach in rats subjected to hemorrhagic shock and that PMN influx and damage were not NO dependent (Tsukada et al., unpublished data). Thus, induced NO is essential for the up-regulation of the inflammatory response under conditions of redox stress, such as hemorrhagic shock, and participates in end organ damage under these conditions.

The Expression of iNOS in Hemorrhagic Shock

NO is one of many effector molecules produced by the vascular endothelium and helps mediate its functions such as regulating blood vessel tone, permeability, adhesion and diapedesis of leukocytes, coagulation, and growth of surrounding tissues [22]. NO is synthesized from L-arginine and oxygen in small amounts by constitutive NO synthases (NOS-1 or nNOS and NOS-3 or eNOS) and in large amounts by NOS-2 or iNOS. In most cell types, iNOS is expressed only when cells are exposed to pro-inflammatory cytokines, microbial products (i.e., endotoxin, peptidoglycan, lipoteichoic acid), or hypoxia [23]. iNOS differs considerably from the constitutive isoforms in its pattern of expression and regulation. While nNOS and eNOS are expressed in a limited number of cell types, iNOS can be expressed in a wide variety of cell types, and its expression is regulated predominantly at the level of transcription. The basal release of eNOS-generated NO regulates vasomotor tone by maintaining vasodilatation in small resistance arteries by activating soluble guanylate cyclase in smooth muscle cells leading to relaxation of the vessel wall. This basal release also reduces the adhesion of platelets and PMNs to the endothelium. In contrast, the sustained production of iNOS-generated NO contributes to antimicrobial activities, tissue protection, or conversely, tissue injury depending on the setting. Once synthesized, NO can rapidly move from cell to cell independent of membrane channels or receptors and react with a wide array of molecular targets [24]. Because of the reactivity of NO, it has a short half-life, and therefore, diffuses only short distances [24]. NO is rapidly inactivated by hemoglobin which keeps the action of NO localized [24]. Nitrite and nitrate are the stable end products of NO oxidation.

Pathophysiologic alterations resulting from hemorrhagic shock include redistribution of blood flow, vascular decompensation due to a fall in peripheral vascular resistance, adhesion of PMNs to the capillary endothelium, vascular hyporeactivity to vasoconstrictor agents, myocardial dysfunction, and cell dysfunction [25]. NOS activity is most likely suppressed although not completely inhibited during hemorrhagic shock although this has not been proven [26]. Data showing that arginine administration has salutory effects in hemorrhagic shock raise the possibility that eNOS activity would be limited by substrate [27]. Amazingly, iNOS expression can be detected in just one hour following initiation of shock (below). iNOS expression and NO production in hemorrhagic shock have been reported in both humans and animals [26, 28–30]. These studies show that iNOS activity is increased in various tissues (lung, liver, spleen) after prolonged hemorrhagic shock in rats, and this would suggest that hemodynamic decompensation and hyporeactivity to vasoconstrictor agents may be mediated by iNOS [31]. Further studies in rat models demonstrate that hemorrhagic shock may induce iNOS expression in circulating and bronchoalveolar macrophages resulting in significantly increased NO production [32]. NO may also contribute to the maintenance of hepatic blood flow after resuscitation from hemorrhagic shock in rats [33]. In humans, low level iNOS expression has been detected by reverse transcriptase polymerase chain reaction (RT-PCR) in liver biopsies from 18 hypotensive trauma patients who underwent laparotomy for control of acute hemorrhage and abdominal injuries, but not in controls undergoing laparotomy without hypotension [29]. Biopsies were performed within two hours of presentation to the emergency room. In summary, animal and human studies demonstrate that hemorrhagic shock can induce iNOS expression. Proposed mechanisms by which hemorrhagic shock induces iNOS expression include:

1) cytokine (TNF-α, IL-1β) stimulation of iNOS expression [28]
2) hypoxia-inducible factor-1 activation of iNOS expression [34]
3) endotoxin stimulation of iNOS expression via bacterial translocation [35].

Although iNOS is up-regulated during hemorrhagic shock, it is unknown when and where this gene is up-regulated following the initiation of shock. In rodent studies, we tested the hypothesis that hemorrhagic shock and/or resuscitation up-regulates iNOS expression. Rats were subjected to hemorrhagic shock for 1, 2.5, and 5 hours. In separate experiments, after 2.5 hours of hemorrhagic shock, rats were resuscitated for 1 and 4 hours. Liver samples were studied for evidence of iNOS mRNA expression using RT-PCR. Comparisons were made with similarly instrumented time-matched sham rats. iNOS expression was detectable as early as one hour after hemorrhagic shock (the earliest timepoint studied) and all further timepoints. iNOS localization studies in the liver identified abundant iNOS protein in hepatocytes adjacent to the central vein (Zone 3). The iNOS inhibitor L-NIL did not inhibit iNOS mRNA expression during hemorrhagic shock indicating that iNOS did not regulate its own expression.

NO and Redox Signaling

In current conceptual frameworks, NO freely diffuses from endothelium to vascular smooth muscle and platelet and across neuronal synapses to evoke biological responses [36]. NO reacts in biological systems with oxygen (O_2), superoxide (O_2^-), and transition metals [37]. Each of the products of these reactions – NOx, peroxynitrite ($OONO^-$), and metal-NO adducts, respectively – support additional nitrosative or oxidative reactions [38, 39]. Accordingly, metal- and thiol-containing proteins serve as major target sites for NO; the essential components of the NO-responsive signaling circuitry – signaling proteins, ion channels, receptors, enzymes, and transcription factors – contain either allosteric or active sites [37]. NO has been reported to activate G proteins [40] and ion channels [41], to affect redox-sensitive kinases [42], and to induce activation of NF-κB [40].

Hemorrhagic shock is a condition of redox stress due to hypoxia and reactive oxygen species production. In previously reported lab studies in rats subjected to hemorrhagic shock, significant differences in cytokine mRNA levels [43] between the shock and sham groups were seen only after resuscitation, indicating that reperfusion was required [7]. This suggests that redox-sensitive mechanisms were responsible for the NO-mediated signaling [7]. NO has been reported to activate $p21^{ras}$ in the human T cell line, Jurkat, through S-nitrosylation leading to NF-κB activation and that this occurs more efficiently under conditions of oxidative stress [44, 45]. Thus, in hemorrhagic shock where iNOS-generated NO is produced, S-nitrosylation of $p21^{ras}$ may be a redox signaling mechanism leading to NF-κB activation. Another intriguing possibility for the up-regulation of inflammation by NO is via the activation of poly(ADP-ribose) synthetase (PARS). Szabo and colleagues have presented evidence that NO dependent activation of PARS takes place in hemorrhagic shock [46] and evidence, in zymosan- and carrageenan-triggered rat models of local inflammation and wild-type and PARS knockout mice, that PARS activation can regulate PMN recruitment [47]. Therefore, PARS activation resulting from peroxynitrite formation could contribute to pro-inflammatory signaling in addition to direct tissue toxicity.

Conclusion

In summary, NF-κB activation has been observed in rodent models of resuscitated hemorrhagic shock and not in clinical studies. In addition, mechanisms underlying its activation, its role in cytokine up-regulation, and the functional effects of its inhibition in this setting of redox stress have been investigated. Due to a lack of studies, it is unknown if NF-κB modulation, or transcriptional control, is a promising therapeutic approach to reduce shock-induced inflammation. Our studies have identified a role for iNOS in the up-regulation of NF-κB in resuscitated hemorrhagic shock. Combined, the available data support a paradigm where iNOS is up-regulated early during shock in a number of organs including the lung, liver, and bowel. Resuscitation in the face of low level iNOS expression results in redox mediated activation of NF-κB that then promotes downstream pro-inflammatory signaling events. We postulate that NO mediates damage via the up-regulation of inflammation as well as by direct toxicity [48]. Approaches to suppress iNOS or remove NO via scavengers at the time of resuscitation from hemorrhagic shock or during reperfusion of ischemic vascular beds may prove beneficial.

References

1. Jiang J, Bahrami S, Leichtfried G, Redl H, Ohlinger W, Schlag G (1995) Kinetics of endotoxin and tumor necrosis factor appearance in portal and systemic circulation after hemorrhagic shock in rats. Ann Surg 221: 100–106
2. Tulzo YL, Shenkar R, Kaneko D, et al (1997) Hemorrhage increases cytokine expression in lung mononuclear cells in mice: involvement of catecholamines in NF-κB regulation and cytokine expression. J Clin Invest 99: 1516–1524
3. Shenkar R, Abraham E (1993) Effects of hemorrhage on cytokine gene transcription. Lymphokine Cytokine Res 12: 237–247

4. Bauer C, Roth W, Bahrami S, Marzi I (1996) Attenuation of shock-induced inflammation in the rat liver depends on the time of TNF-α inhibition. J Mol Med 74:51–58
5. Meldrum DR, Shenkar R, Sheridan BC, Cain BS, Abraham E, Harken AH (1997) Hemorrhage activates myocardial NF-κB and increases TNF-α in the heart. J Mol Cell Cardiol 29: 2849–2854
6. Hierholzer C, Kelly E, Tsukada K, et al (1997) Hemorrhagic shock induces G-CSF expression in bronchial epithelium. Am J Physiol 273:L1058–L1064
7. Hierholzer C, Harbrecht B, Menezes JM, et al (1998) Essential role of induced nitric oxide in the initiation of the inflammatory response after hemorrhagic shock. J Exp Med 187:917–928
8. Shenkar R, Cohen AJ, Vestweber D, Miller YE, Tuder R, Abraham E (1995) Hemorrhage and resuscitation alter the expression of ICAM-1 and P-selectin in mice. J Inflamm 45:248–259
9. Baeuerle PA (1998) IκB-NF-κB structures: at the interface of inflammation control. Cell 95: 729–731
10. Blackwell TS, Christman JW (1997) The role of NF-κB in cytokine gene regulation. Am J Respir Cell Mol Biol 17:3–9
11. May MJ, Ghosh S (1998) Signal transduction through NF-κB. Immunol Today 19:80–88
12. Meldrum DR, Cleveland JC, Sheridan BC, et al (1997) α-adrenergic activation of myocardial NFκB during hemorrhage. J Surg Res 69:268–276
13. Moine P, Shenkar R, Kaneko D, Tulzo YL, Abraham E (1997) Systemic blood loss affects NF-κB regulatory mechanisms in the lungs. Am J Physiol 273:L185–L192
14. Fan J, Marshall JC, Jimenez M, Shek PN, Zagorski J, Rotstein OD (1998) Hemorrhagic shock primes for increased expression of cytokine-induced neutrophil chemoattractant in the lung: role in pulmonary inflammation following lipopolysaccharide. J Immunol 161: 440–447
15. Samy Anantha TS, Ayala A, Catania RA, Chaudry IH (1998) Trauma-hemorrhage activates signal transduction pathways in mouse splenic T cells. Shock 9:443–450
16. Shenkar R, Schwartz MD, Terada LS, Repine JE, McCord J, Abraham E (1996) Hemorrhage activates NF-κB in murine lung mononuclear cells in vivo. Am J Physiol 270:L729–L735
17. Shenkar R, Abraham E (1997) Hemorrhage induces rapid in vivo activation of CREB and NF-κB in murine intraparenchymal lung mononuclear cells. Am J Respir Cell Mol Biol 16: 145–152
18. Anderson BO, Moore EE, Moore FA, et al (1991) Hypovolemic shock promotes neutrophil sequestration in the lungs by a xanthine oxidase-related mechanism. J Appl Physiol 71: 1862–1865
19. Tan S, Yokoyama Y, Dickens E, Cash TG, Freeman BA, Parks DA (1993) Xanthine oxidase activity in the circulation of rats following hemorrhagic shock. Free Rad Biol Med 15:407–414
20. Schwartz MD, Repine JE, Abraham E (1995) Xanthine oxidase-derived oxygen radicals increase lung cytokine expression in mice subjected to hemorrhagic shock. Am J Respir Cell Mol Biol 12:434–440
21. Hierholzer C, Menezes JM, Kalff JC, et al (1998) Essential role of inducible nitric oxide in intestinal inflammation and stasis following hemorrhagic shock. Surg Forum 49:78–80
22. Cain BS, Meldrum DR, Selzman CH, et al (1997) Surgical implications of vascular endothelial physiology. Surgery 122:516–526
23. Geller DA, Billiar TR (1998) Molecular biology of nitric oxide synthases. Cancer Metastasis Rev 17:7–23
24. Tzeng E, Billiar TR (1997) Nitric oxide and the surgical patient. Arch Surg 132:977–982
25. Wang P, Ba ZF, Chaudry IH (1993) Endothelial cell dysfunction occurs very early following trauma-hemorrhage and persists despite fluid resuscitation. Am J Physiol 265:H973–H979
26. Kelly E, Shah NS, Morgan NN, Watkins SC, Peitzman AB, Billiar TR (1997) Physiologic and molecular characterization of the role of NO in hemorrhagic shock: evidence that type II nitric oxide synthase does not regulate vascular decompensation. Shock 7:157–163
27. Angele MK, Smail N, Wang P, Cioffi WG, Bland KI, Chaudry IH (1998) L-arginine restores the depressed cardiac output and regional perfusion after trauma-hemorrhage surgery. Surgery 124:394–401
28. Szabo C, Thiemermann C (1994) Invited opinion: role of nitric oxide in hemorrhagic, traumatic, and anaphylactic shock and thermal injury. Shock 2:145–155

29. Kelly E, Hierholzer C, Harbrecht BG, Billiar TR, Peitzman AB (1996) Traumatic shock induces type 2 nitric oxide synthase mRNA expression in the human liver. Surg Forum 47:32–33
30. Sato S, Miyabe M, Saito S, Yamaguchi H (1997) Nitric oxide in the brain increased during a short period of hemorrhagic shock in the rabbit. Shock 8:136–140
31. Thiemermann C, Szabo C, Mitchell JA, Vane JR (1993) Vascular hyporeactivity to vasoconstrictor agents and hemorrhagic decompensation in hemorrhagic shock is mediated by nitric oxide. Proc Natl Acad Sci USA 90:267–271
32. Naziri W, Pietsch JD, Appel SH, Cheadle WG, Bergamini TM, Polk HC (1995) Hemorrhagic shock-induced alterations in circulating and bronchoalveolar macrophage nitric oxide production. J Surg Res 59:146–152
33. Pannen BHJ, Bauer M, Nolde-Schomburg GFE, et al (1997) Regulation of hepatic blood flow during resuscitation from hemorrhagic shock: role of NO and endothelins. Am J Physiol 272:H2736–H2745
34. Guillemin K, Krasnow MA (1997) The hypoxic response: huffing and HIFing. Cell 89:9–12
35. LaRocco MT, Rodriguez LF, Chen Y, et al (1993) Reevaluation of the linkage between acute hemorrhagic shock and bacterial translocation in the rat. Circ Shock 40:212–220
36. Lancaster JR (1994) Simulation of the diffusion and reaction of endogenously produced nitric oxide. Proc Natl Acad Sci USA 91:8137–8141
37. Stamler JS (1994) Redox signaling: nitrosylation and related target interactions of nitric oxide. Cell 78:931–936
38. Stamler JS, Singel DJ, Loscalzo J (1992) Biochemistry of nitric oxide and its redox-activated forms. Science 258:1898–1902
39. Mohr S, Stamler JS, Brune B (1994) Mechanism of covalent modification of glyceraldehyde-3-phosphate dehydrogenase at its active site thiol by nitric oxide, peroxynitrite and related nitrosating agents. FEBS Lett 348:223–227
40. Lander HM, Sehajpal PK, Novogrodsyk A (1993) Nitric oxide signaling: a possible role for G proteins. Immunology 151:7182–7187
41. Bolotina VM, Najibi S, Palacino JJ, Pagano PJ, Cohne RA (1994) Nitric oxide directly activates calcium-dependent potassium channels in vascular smooth muscle. Nature 368:850–853
42. Gopalakrishna R, Chen ZH, Gundimeda U (1993) Nitric oxide and nitric oxide-generating agents induce a reversible inactivation of protein kinase C activity and phorbol ester binding. J Biol Chem 268:27 180–27 185
43. Hierholzer C, Kelly E, Billiar TR, Tweardy DJ (1997) Granulocyte colony-stimulating factor (G-CSF) production in hemorrhagic shock requires both the ischemic and resuscitation phase. Arch Orthop Trauma Surg 116:173–176
44. Lander HM, Milbank AJ, Tauras JM, et al (1996) Redox regulation of cell signaling. Nature 381:380–381
45. Lander HM, Ogiste JS, Teng KK, Novogrodsky A (1995) $p21^{ras}$ as a common signaling target of reactive free radicals and cellular redox stress. J Biol Chem 270:21 195–21 198
46. Szabo C (1998) Potential role of the peroxynitrite-poly(ADP-ribose) synthetase pathway in a rat model of severe hemorrhagic shock. Shock 9:341–344
47. Szabo C, Lim LH, Cuzzocrea S, et al (1997) Inhibition of poly (ADP-ribose) synthetase attenuates neutrophil recruitment and exerts anti-inflammatory effects. J Exp Med 186:1041–1049
48. Szabo C (1996) The pathophysiological role of peroxynitrite in shock, inflammation, and ischemia-reperfusion injury. Shock 6:79–88

Regulation of Neutrophil Activation in Acute Lung Injury and SIRS

J. Kruger, Q. Dong, and G. Downey

Introduction

The primary function of neutrophils is host defense but, paradoxically, unregulated activation of these phagocytes may result in tissue damage in conditions such as acute lung injury and the systemic inflammatory response syndrome (SIRS). Despite extensive research into the physiological and cellular basis of inflammatory injury and increasingly sophisticated intensive care, the morbidity and mortality of these syndromes remains distressingly high. The purpose of this chapter is to summarize recent developments in our understanding of the signaling pathways regulating leukocyte activation relevant to neutrophil-mediated tissue injury. Two main concepts will be explored: 1) that defective regulation of protein tyrosine phosphatases (PTPs) that function primarily in signal termination may predispose to uncontrolled neutrophil activation, and 2) that signals from adhesion receptors contribute to enhanced release of cytotoxic compounds by neutrophils during adhesion to endothelium, epithelium, or extracellular matrix proteins in the interstitium. This 'adhesion-dependent activation' of leukocytes can greatly potentiate the effects of soluble mediators on activation. Recent studies from our laboratory that illuminate these signaling pathways will be reviewed. It is hoped that the results of these studies will provide insights into the pathogenesis of lung injury and eventually lead to novel therapeutic strategies to prevent or ameliorate tissue injury.

Acute Lung Injury and SIRS

Under most circumstances inflammation is self-limiting and beneficial. However, under certain conditions, the inflammatory response can spiral out of control resulting in severe organ dysfunction, as is seen in acute lung injury [1]. This syndrome is the end result of a variety of local or systemic insults culminating in diffuse damage to the pulmonary parenchyma (Fig. 1). Despite intensive research into the physiological and cellular basis of lung injury and increasingly sophisticated intensive care, improvements in prognosis have lagged behind and patients frequently die from progressive multi-organ failure (MOF) [2, 3]. This latter sequence of events, termed SIRS, is attributable to generalized activation of the inflammatory response, most commonly due to infection, leading to diffuse endothelial injury and microcirculatory dysfunction [3]. Many of the manifestations of this syndrome result from a complex interplay between pro-inflammatory (e.g., lipopolysaccharide [LPS], cytokines, and eicosanoids) and anti-inflammatory (e.g., interleukin [IL]-10, IL-1 receptor antagonist [IL-1ra], prostaglandin I_2 [PGI_2]) mediators and their effects on leukocytes, endothelial, and epithelial cells [4]. A more complete understanding of the complexities of the inflammatory response and the mechanisms of tissue damage is essential if we are to improve the prognosis of acute lung injury and SIRS.

Induction of the Acute Inflammatory Response

Histological examination of lungs and other organs (kidney, gut) from patients with acute lung injury and SIRS reveals extensive infiltration with neutrophils associated with evidence of diffuse endothelial and epithelial injury defining this as an acute inflammatory response. It is currently believed that some inciting event (trauma, sepsis, transfusion, etc.) initiates the inflammatory cascade that spirals out of control leading to tissue injury. This is to be contrasted with the situation in most localized infections, such as, for example, uncomplicated pneumonia, where inflammation proceeds in a more regulated fashion and resolves once the inciting cause (i.e., the bacteria) has been removed, leaving the tissue intact [5]. It is evident that under most circumstances, counter-regulatory mechanisms limit inflammatory damage and allow reparative processes to prevail. However, in acute lung injury and SIRS (Fig. 1), where the inflammatory response progresses to become generalized (i.e., systemic) and self-propagating despite removal of the inciting cause, these regulatory mechanisms fail [6, 7]. This highlights one of the main paradoxes in the field of inflammation research; why neutrophils, cells which usually serve an important host defense function, can induce tissue injury under some circumstances? The primary purpose of this chapter is to provide insights into the mechanisms responsible for this apparent loss of regulation of leukocyte activation.

Sequestration of Neutrophils in the Pulmonary Microvasculature

The capillaries (and primarily those of the lung) are the major site of the marginated pool of neutrophils which serve as a rapidly mobilizable reserve of phagocytes [8, 9]. Work from many laboratories including our own, has demonstrated that activation of neutrophils by inflammatory mediators leads to their microvascular sequestration as a consequence of several factors including: i) the unique geometric and hydrodynamic conditions in the microvasculature [9, 10]; ii) decreased deformability [10–12]; and iii) increased adhesion between neutrophils and endothelial cells [13, 14]. Neutrophils subsequently emigrate into the tissue parenchyma where they are in contact with extracellular matrix proteins or epithelium. In this location they can be induced to release cytotoxic compounds in

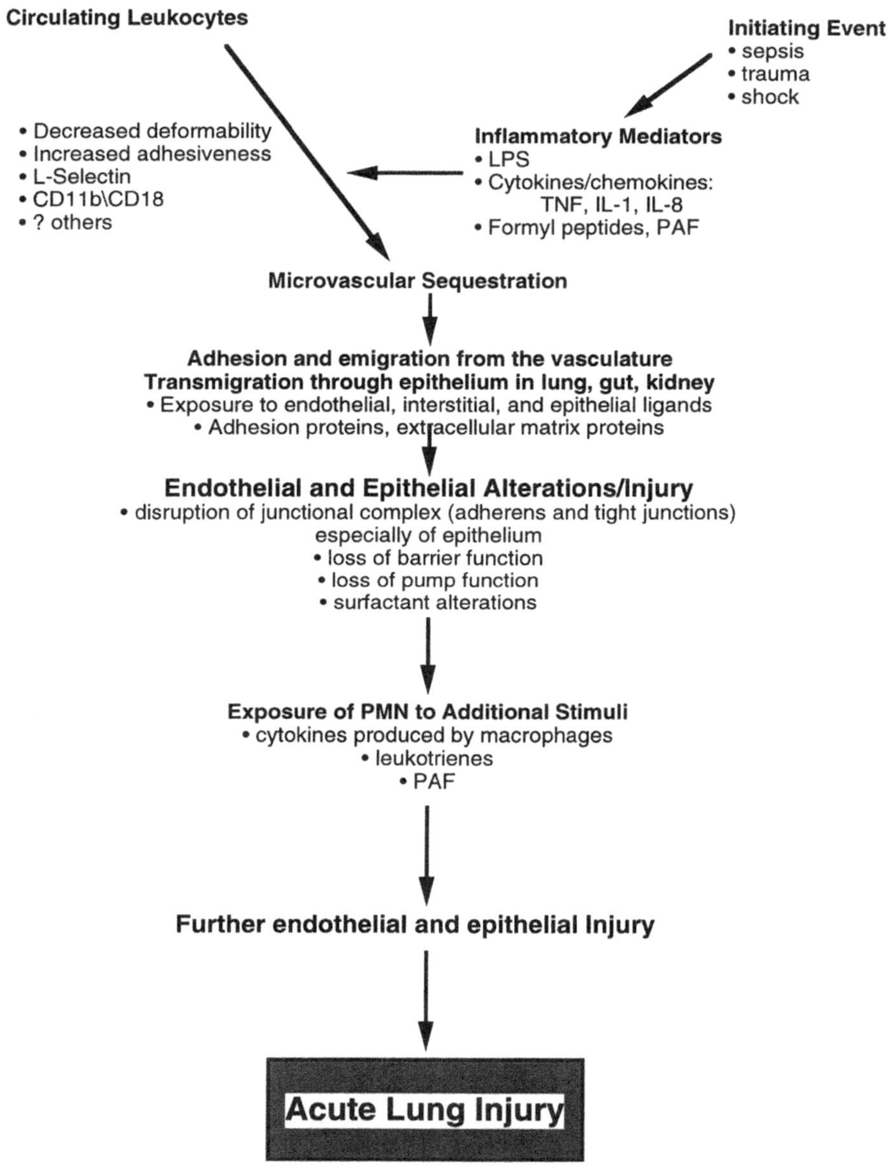

Fig. 1. Mechanisms of leukocyte-mediated lung injury in sepsis. A variety of initiating events leads to activation of the inflammatory response on a systemic level leading to tissue injury

response to mediators (e.g., cytokines) produced by resident cells, such as macrophages, promoting further tissue injury [15].

Regulation of Leukocyte Activation: Intracellular Signaling Pathways

The functional role of myeloid leukocytes in host defense is achieved through a series of rapid and coordinated responses that include chemotaxis, phagocytosis, secretion of a variety of granules/vesicles, and production of reactive oxygen intermediates [16, 17]. These responses are initiated by the interaction of cell surface receptors with specific ligands found on microbial targets or in the inflammatory milieu and the consequent induction of intracellular signaling pathways that couple such activating stimuli to physiologic responses [16–18]. To maintain homeostasis and minimize tissue damage, leukocyte microbicidal responses must be tightly regulated by processes including selective triggering and rapid termination of activation cascades once the initial stimulus has been removed.

The most basic signaling paradigm involves interaction of a ligand with its cognate surface membrane receptor leading to the generation of intracellular signals. One of the earliest events is the cleavage of membrane phospholipids by phospholipases with generation of inositol phosphates (IP_3), leading to changes in intracellular Ca^{2+} and diacylglycerols and consequent activation of protein kinase C [19]. Over the last decade this field has witnessed an explosion of developments and it has become apparent that complexity exists at many levels of the signaling cascades. For example, there are multiple membrane receptors that include members of the seven transmembrane spanning domain family ('serpentine') (e.g., formyl peptide receptors, complement receptors, and chemokine receptors), receptors linked to tyrosine kinases (e.g., phagocytic receptors such as Fc receptors), as well as receptors that are themselves primarily tyrosine kinases (e.g., growth factor receptors).

Downstream of the receptors are complex and interconnected signaling pathways. Figure 2 illustrates some of the signaling pathways that have been characterized recently. Although at first glance these pathways appear complex, it is helpful to think of them as being grouped in several levels or tiers of signaling molecules (enzymes and adapters). Serpentine family receptors (e.g., receptors for N-formyl-methionyl-leucyl-phenylalanine [fMLP], C5a, platelet activating factor [PAF], leukotriene B_4 [LTB_4]) are linked to heterotrimeric guanosine triphosphate (GTP) binding proteins that confer some specificity and amplification to a signal resulting from receptor occupation. Cytosolic tyrosine kinases including Hck, Fgr, and Src are activated very early after neutrophil activation by phagocytic receptors and appear to be involved in activation of subsequent microbicidal responses [20, 21]. A variety of intermediary 'adapter' molecules such as Shc and Grb-2 serve to transmit signals by protein-protein interactions. Somewhat downstream of these juxtamembrane events lie small GTPases, such as Ras, and a series of enzymes, such as Raf, leading to the canonical mitogen-activated protein kinase kinase-mitogen activated protein kinase (MEK-MAPK) signaling

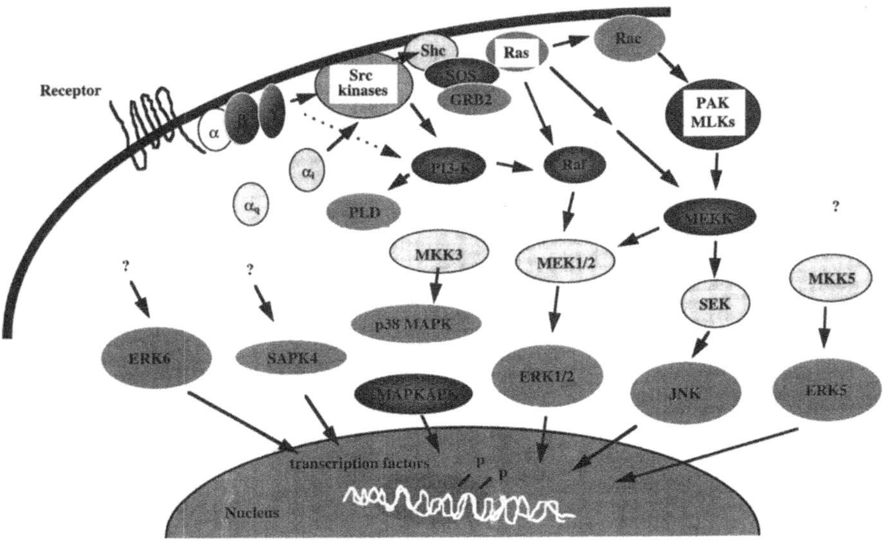

Fig. 2. Divergent protein kinase cascades link plasma membrane receptors to the nucleus. Parallel kinase cascades control the activity of members of the mitogen-activated protein kinase (MAPK) superfamily family of serine-threonine kinases that include Erk, C-Jun kinases (JNKs), and p38 MAP. The pathway connecting G protein-coupled receptors to low molecular weight GTP-binding proteins and to additional members of the MAPK superfamily are outlined and shown in tiers of signaling molecules

pathway [22]. In addition, recent evidence suggests that Ras is also located upstream of Rac, a small GTPase of the Rho subfamily, which also regulates protein kinases including the p21-activated kinases (PAKs) and two other members of the MAPK family, Jun N-terminal kinase (JNK) and p38 MAPK [23]. Although the relevant targets of these MAPK family members are not completely understood, it is well described that certain transcription factors (e.g., Elk-1, c-Fos, c-Jun) can be phosphorylated by MAPKs leading to gene transcription.

In human neutrophils, activation of the extracellular signal regulated kinase (ERK) family of MAPKs is prominent after stimulation by a variety of soluble agonists including fMLP, PAF and phorbol myristate acetate (PMA). A new and expanding family of soluble pharmacological inhibitors targeting specific enzymes in this signaling pathway is being developed. One of these compounds, PD98059, is a potent and selective inhibitor of MEK, the enzyme directly upstream of, and responsible for, the activation of ERKs. Pre-treatment of neutrophils with this compound essentially abrogates agonist-induced stimulation of ERKs. Utilizing this compound, we and others have demonstrated that ERK is involved in regulation of the oxidative burst, chemotaxis, phagocytosis, apoptosis, with a more minor role in adhesion, activation of phospholipase A_2, and apoptosis [24, 25]. Analagous studies investigating the physiological importance of P38 MAPK using other pharmacological inhibitors (e.g., SK&F 86002 and SB203580), have demonstrated the importance of this kinase in activation of the NADPH oxidase, chemotaxis, adhesion, and regulation of stress-induced apoptosis [24, 26, 27].

Regulation of Intracellular Signaling by Protein Tyrosine Phosphorylation

Myeloid cell receptor engagement leads to the rapid phosphorylation of cellular proteins on tyrosine residues [28, 29]. Increases in tyrosine phosphorylation can be elicited by a variety of soluble and particulate stimuli and correlate temporally with the appearance of cellular responses [30–32]. The importance of tyrosine phosphorylation to leukocyte function is underscored by the observation that inhibitors of tyrosine kinases block many microbicidal responses, including adhesion [33], chemotaxis [34], phagocytosis [35] and production of reactive oxygen intermediates [32, 36, 37].

Protein Tyrosine Phosphatases and Regulation of Neutrophil Activation

Phosphorylation of tyrosine residues is regulated by the competing activities of protein tyrosine kinases and PTPs. In neutrophils, activation of tyrosine kinases occurs in response to chemotactic peptides [38], cytokines [39, 40] and multiple other ligands [41], and is pivotal to the increased tyrosine phosphorylation observed following stimulation with these agents. Alternatively, decreases in the activity of PTPs may contribute to an increase in cellular tyrosine phosphorylation following stimulation. Thus for example, stimulation with the chemoattractant fMLP or with phorbol esters, is associated with decreases in global neutrophil phosphotyrosine phosphatase activity, although the identity of the particular phosphatases responsible for this effect has not been determined [42, 43]. Similarly, inhibition of tyrosine phosphatases with vanadate or its peroxides has been shown to potentiate fMLP-induced superoxide production in intact cells [44] and to activate a respiratory burst in electroporated cells [45, 46], providing additional evidence that a reduction of phosphatase activity may lead to microbicidal responses in neutrophils.

While the importance of tyrosine phosphatases in regulating neutrophil function is accepted, comparatively little is known about the identity and role of specific tyrosine phosphatases in modulating the outcome of myeloid leukocyte signal transduction pathways. Indeed, to date only CD45 and src homology 2 (SH-2) domain-containing phosphatase-1 (SHP-1) have been identified in neutrophils but, based on information available in other cell types, it is likely that additional types are expressed. We sought to identify additional (and perhaps novel) tyrosine phosphatases expressed by neutrophils. To accomplish this, we took advantage of the highly conserved catalytic domain of all known tyrosine phosphatases ('signature' domain) to design degenerate primers for use in reverse transcription polymerase chain reaction (RT-PCR). This technique has been used successfully by others to identify messenger ribonucleic acid (mRNA) which contain such highly conserved sequences of interest including phosphatases [47]. Degenerate primers targeted at highly conserved regions within the catalytic domain of tyrosine phosphatases were utilized in the reaction to amplify RNA from human peripheral blood neutrophils. This strategy yielded sequences corresponding to four known PTPs: CD45, SHP-1, PTP1B, and MEG2. The expression of CD45 and SHP-1 in neutrophils has previously been reported by our laboratory and others [48–50]. PTP1B is expressed in a wide array of cells making it less likely to have a myeloid-specific functions. Accordingly, we focused our attention on MEG2, a cytosolic phosphatase about which little is known.

Functional MEG2 protein is expressed by neutrophils

A polyclonal anti-MEG2 peptide antibody was generated and Western analysis of protein extracts of neutrophils resulted in a 68 kDa band corresponding to the predicted molecular weight of MEG2. To determine if MEG2 endogenously expressed in neutrophils possessed enzymatic activity, affinity-purified anti-MEG2 peptide serum was used for immunopreciptiation from cell lysates. The immunoprecipitates demonstrated significant phosphatase activity using a phosphopeptide as the substrate and malachite green as the detection system. At present we are investigating the role of MEG2 in leukocyte activation.

Importance of SHP-1 in Leukocyte Activation

We and others have previously demonstrated that SHP-1, an SH2-domain containing phosphatase, is expressed in leukocytes of myelo-monocytic lineages including HL-60 cells [51], THP-1 cells [52], and human peripheral blood neutrophils [50]. SHP-1 has now been implicated in the negative regulation of a broad spectrum of growth-promoting receptors including receptor tyrosine kinases such as the c-kit [53, 54], colony stimulating factor-1 (CSF-1) receptor [55], TrkA [56], and the epidermal growth factor (EGF) receptor [57], cytokine receptors such as the IL-3 [53], the interferon α/β [58], and the erythropoietin [59, 60] receptors, and receptors of the immune system containing the immune receptor tyrosine-based inhibitory motif (ITIM) such as CD22 [61] and the FcγRIIB [61, 62]. SHP-1 inhibitory effects on receptor tyrosine kinases are mediated by direct dephosphorylation of the activated receptors [53, 55, 57, 63], while its effects on suppression of cytokine receptor signaling are mediated by binding of the phosphatase to noncatalytic subunits of the receptors and dephosphorylation of the associated Janus (JAK) family tyrosine kinase [58, 59]. In some instances, the negative modulatory effects of SHP-1 on receptor signaling have been linked to its capacity to interact with multiple receptor and cytosolic signaling effectors. For example SHP-1 down-regulates antigen receptor signaling in T-cells by interactions and/or dephosphorylation of T-cell antigen receptor (TCR) components, the Lck [64, 65] and zeta-associated protein (ZAP)-70 [66] protein tyrosine kinases, and the guanine exchange factor, Vav [67]. Similarly in B cells, SHP-1 binds

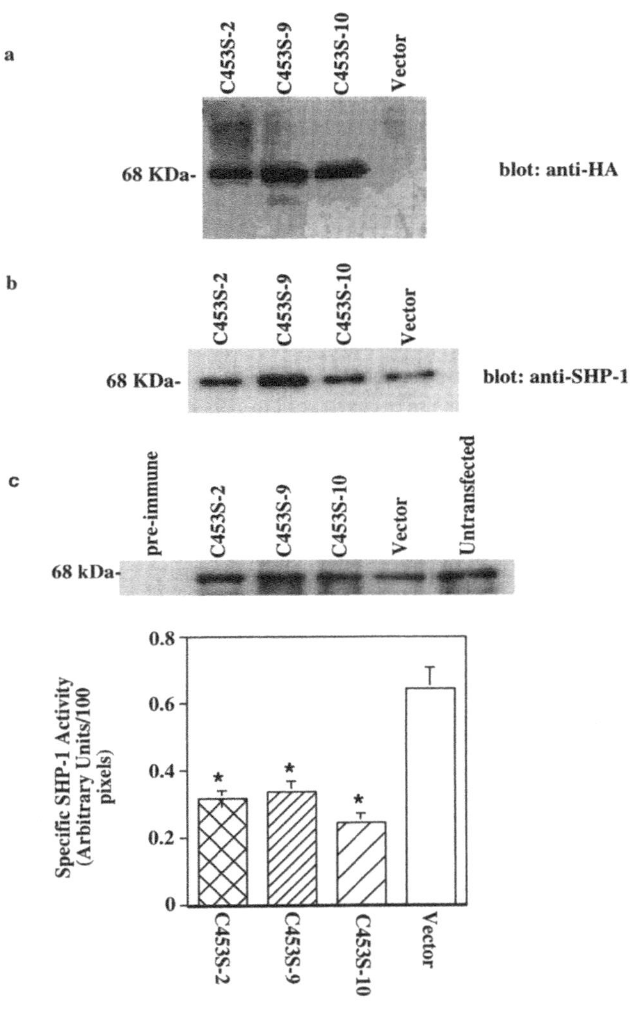

Fig. 3a–c. Identification of HA-SHP-1^{C453S} protein in U937 cells and inhibition of SHP-1 activity. **a, b** Equal amounts of protein from whole cell lysates of U937 cells transfected with HA-SHP-1^{C453S} (clones C453S-2, C453S-9, C453S-10) or empty vector (vector) were separated by SDS-PAGE gels and subjected to immunoblotting with anti-HA antibodies (**a**) or affinity purified anti-SHP-1 antibodies (**b**). **c** *In vitro* phosphatase assay using anti-SHP-1 immunoprecipitates from each of the clones as indicated using a phosphopeptide (RRLIEDAEpYAARG) as the substrate and the malachite green phosphatase assay kit (UBI, Lake Placid, NY) normalized for the amount of SHP-1 protein present in each of the immunoprecipitates (i.e., specific activity). SHP-1 phosphatase activity (OD) was divided by the intensity of the corresponding SHP-1 band in immunoblots quantitated using IPLab Gel-D10, * $p < 0.05$

and likely dephosphorylates the BCR [67], FcγRIIB [68] Vav [69], and CD22 [61, 70]. While SHP-1 roles in myeloid cell biology are not yet well defined, the pivotal role for SHP-1 in regulatory development and function of this lineage is highlighted by the enormous myelo-monocytic expansion found in motheaten (*me*/*me*) and motheaten viable (*me*^{v}/ *me*^{v}) mice in which expression of PTP activity is essentially abrogated [71–73].

Accordingly, as a step toward delineating the role of tyrosine phosphatases in initiation and/or modulation of myeloid leukocyte responses, we explored the roles of SHP-1 in myeloid cell signaling by assessing the impact of overexpressing an enzymatically inactive mutant of SHP-1 (SHP-1^{C453S}) on specific functions of the myelo-monocytic cell line U937. We derived stable clones of a myelo-monocytic cell line U937 expressing recombinant SHP-1, enzymatically inactivated by substitution of the highly conserved cysteine residue in the catalytic domain for serine (SHP-1^{C453S}). To distinguish recombinant from endogenous SHP-1, the protein was tagged with an HA-epitope at the NH2 terminus. The construct was ligated into the pcDNA3 vector, transfected into U937 cells, and multiple G418-resistant clones were isolated and expanded. Clones expressing HA-SHP-1^{C453S} were identified by RT-PCR and by Western blotting with anti-HA antibodies. The three clones showing highest levels of HA-SHP-1^{C453S} protein, designated C453S-2, C453S-9, C453S-10 respectively, were selected for further study. In these clones, estimation of the specific activity of SHP-1 (done by correcting the enzymatic activity for the amount of immunoreactive SHP-1 protein) revealed overexpression of HA-SHP-1^{C453S} to be associated with an almost 50% decrease in SHP-1 specific activity compared to that detected in clones transfected with vector alone (Fig. 3).

Expression of HA-SHP-1^{C453S} Increases Cell Proliferation and Decreases Apoptosis

Expansions of cell populations following various growth stimuli are known to reflect the net effects of both proliferation and death rate. The possible relevance of SHP-1 to regulation of cell proliferation and death was studied by comparing rates of ^{3}H-thymidine incorporation and apoptosis in clones overexpressing HA-SHP-1^{C453S} and control clones. Apoptosis was examined after 24 hours of serum starvation by flow cytometry using propidium iodide staining. As shown in Figure 4 there was an enhanced ^{3}H-thymidine incorporation and diminished rates of apoptosis in clones overexpressing HA-SHP-1^{C453S} compared to control cells. These observations suggest that PTPs such as SHP-1 regulate myeloid proliferation in the bone marrow and rates of death in the peripheral tissues; both of these effects are of potential importance during the acute inflammatory response.

Expression of HA-SHP-1^{C453S} Potentiates the Oxidative Burst

The microbicidal function of myeloid cells is dependent on their ability to produce reactive oxygen intermediates such as superoxide (O_2^-) and hydrogen per-a

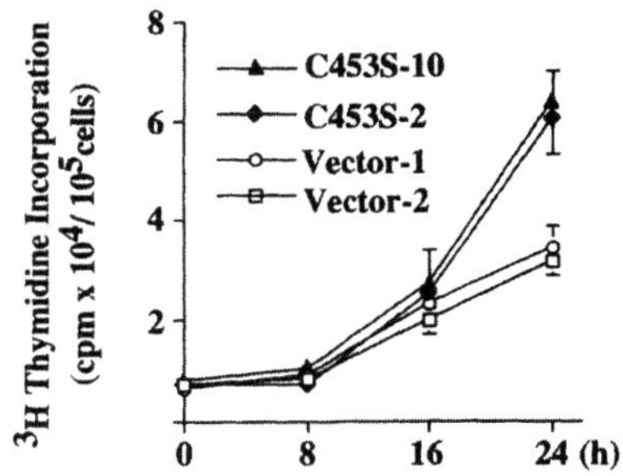

b

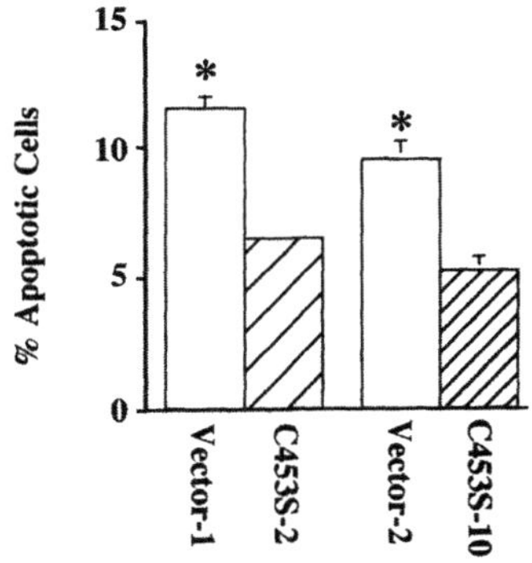

Fig. 4a, b. Expression of HA-SHP-1^{C453S} in U937 cells enhances cell proliferation and diminishes apoptosis. **a** One $\times 10^5$ cells from each clone were serum starved for 24 hours followed by the addition of 20% FBS. The amount of (^{3}H) thymidine incorporation was measured during 8 hours epochs over a period of 24 hours (i.e., from 0–8 hours, 8–16 hours, and 16–24 hours) by addition of 1 μCi/ml (^{3}H) thymidine to the appropriate wells at the beginning of the epoch. **b** One $\times 10^5$ cells from each clone were serum starved for 24 hours followed by the addition of 20% FBS. After an additional 24 hours, cells were fixed and stained using propidium iodide and the apoptotic cells (hypodiploid) were quantified by flow cytometry, * $p < 0.05$

oxide (H_2O_2) and to secrete lytic enzymes. Reactive oxygen intermediate production is in turn mediated by a multi-component enzyme complex, termed NADPH oxidase, that is known to be functional in U937 cells [74]. To determine the importance of SHP-1 in regulation of this important effector function, the production of H_2O_2 was compared in clones overexpressing HA-SHP-1^{C453S} and controls. As illustrated in Figure 5, clones overexpressing HA-SHP-1^{C453S} displayed

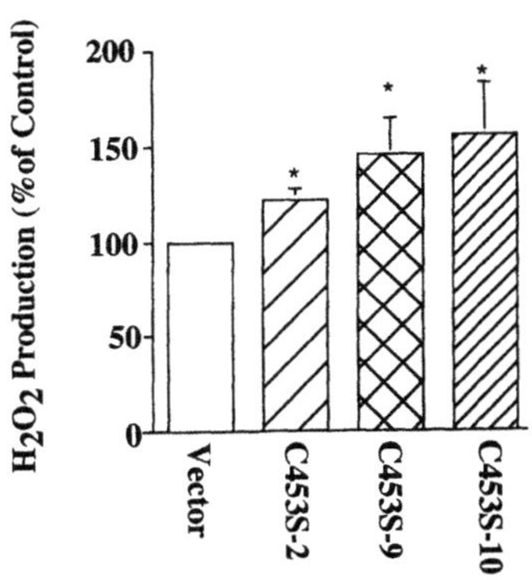

Fig. 5. Expression of HA-SHP-1^{C453S} in U937 cells increases oxidant production. Equal numbers of U937 cells transfected with HA-SHP-1^{C453S} (clones C453S-2, C453S-9, C453S-10) or empty vector (vector) were stimulated with 10^{-7} M PMA for 2 hours at 37°C in buffer containing 10.4 mM scopoletin, 9.6 U/ml horseradish peroxidase, 4 mM sodium azide for 2 hours. Reduction in fluorescence of scopoletin was measured by a fluorescence spectrophotometer (Hitachi F-2000) with excitation wavelength = 365 nm and emission wavelength = 473 nm. Standard curves were generated using known amounts of H_2O_2, * $p < 0.05$

increased oxidant production when compared to controls after treatment with phorbol ester 12-phorbol-13 myristate acetate (PMA), a direct activator of protein kinase C and potent agonist of the NADPH oxidase. The effects on oxidant production of other agonists including the formyl peptide fMLP, the phagocytic stimulus opsonized zymosan, and cross linking of FcγRI receptors, were also studied in these cells, but none of these agents induced a significant increase in oxidant production in either the control or HA-SHP-1^{C453S} overexpressing clones (not illustrated).

Expression of HA-SHP-1^{C453S} Enhances Cell Adhesion

Adhesive interactions between leukocytes and endothelial cells are paramount in the emigration of circulating polymorphonuclear cells (PMN) from the blood into inflamed tissues [75, 76]. To determine the importance of SHP-1 in regulation of this important leukocyte function, HA-SHP-1^{C453S} overexpressing and control cells were compared with respect to their adhesion to serum-coated plastic following treatment with PMA, fMLP, or C5a, known stimuli for leukocyte adhesion [77–79]. Figure 6 illustrates that clones overexpressing HA-SHP-1^{C453S} displayed increased adhesion to serum-coated plastic when compared to controls. As adhesion of myeloid leukocytes to extracellular matrix proteins is mediated predominantly by β2 integrins [13, 80], the HA-SHP-1^{C453S} overexpressing cells and control clones were also evaluated for surface expression of CD18 by flow cytometry utilizing IB4, a monoclonal antibody that recognizes the common β chain (CD18) [81]. This analysis revealed CD18 expression to be relatively increased in the clones overexpressing HA-SHP-1^{C453S}. To ensure that the enhanced adhesion of the HA-SHP-1^{C453S} overexpressing clones was in fact β2 integrin-mediated, adhesion was assayed in the presence of the blocking anti-CD18 antibody, IB4. As shown in Figure 6, this analysis revealed adhesiveness of HA-SHP-1^{C453S} overexpressing cells to be diminished in the presence of IB4 to a level indistinguishable from that detected in clones transfected with vector alone. In addition, the basal adhesion of the clones transfected with vector alone was diminished by this antibody suggesting that a portion of the basal adhesion of these U937 cells was mediated by β2 integrins.

The effects of HA-SHP-1^{C453S} overexpression on other cell functions including phagocytosis of serum-opsonized zymosan and motility as assayed by chemotaxis through methylcellulose/nitrocellulose filters in response to fMLP, recombinant C5a and zymosan-activated serum, were also studied. However, no significant differences were observed between clones overexpressing HA-SHP-1^{C453S} and controls with respect to these functional properties (data not shown).

Activation of Leukocytes by Signals from Adhesion Receptors

A pivotal concept in the understanding of leukocyte-mediated tissue injury is that neutrophils do not cause damage while suspended in the blood stream; rath-

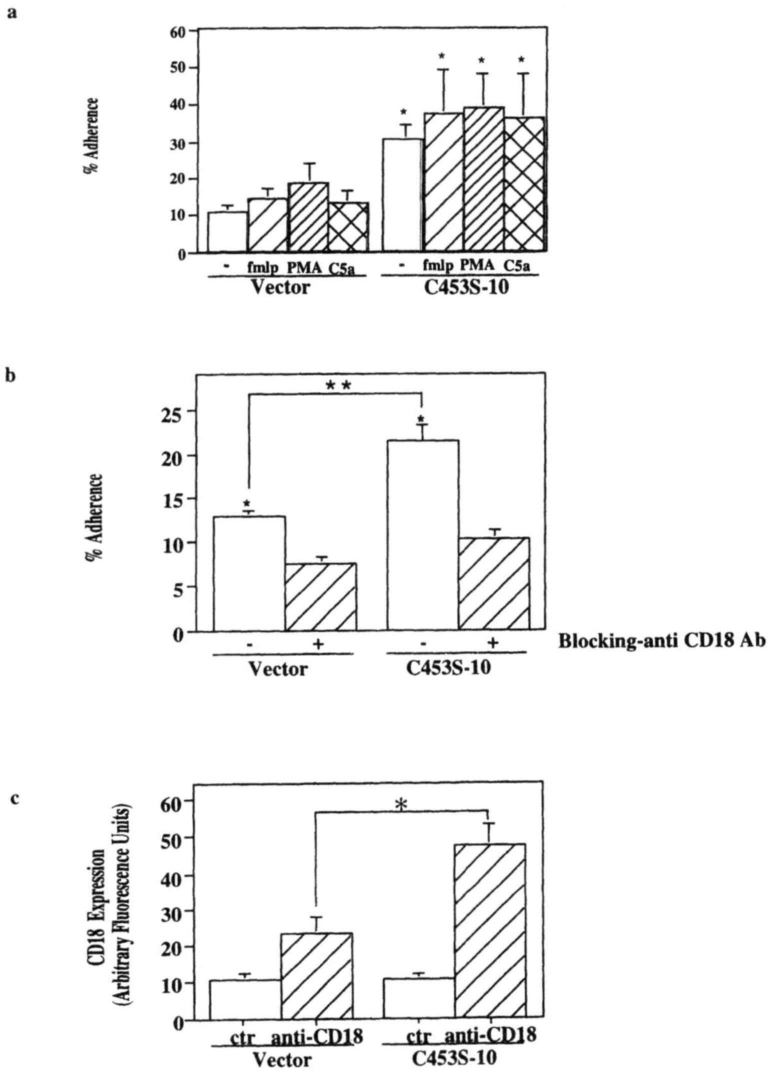

Fig. 6a–c. Expression of HA-SHP-1^{C453S} in U937 cells increases adhesion and surface expression of CD18. **a, b** The adhesion of U937 cells transfected with HA-SHP-1^{C453S} (clone C453S-10) or empty vector (vector) to serum-coated plastic was assayed as described in the text in the absence (**a**) or presence of blocking concentrations (44 μg/ml) of the anti-CD18 antibody IB4. In (**a**), the adhesion in the absence or presence of 10^{-6} M fMLP, 10^{-7} M PMA, and 10^{-6} M C5a is illustrated. **c** Surface expression of CD18 as determined by flow cytometry using an anti-CD18 Ab and indirect immunofluorescence. The geometric mean of fluorescence was calculated for each group and compared statistically. * $p < 0.05$, ** $p < 0.01$ for vector vs cells from the C453S-9 clone

er release of cytotoxic compounds occurs primarily while they are adherent to endothelium or epithelium or in contact with extracellular matrix proteins in the interstitium. Thus, it is the behavior of adherent cells that is most germane to inflammatory tissue injury. In this regard, it has become apparent that in addition to functioning in attachment of leukocytes to surfaces, adhesion receptors also participate in cell activation. In fact, adhesion can greatly potentiate the effects of soluble mediators on activation of the respiratory burst and release of granule contents by neutrophils [82–84]. As is illustrated in Figure 7, the amount of oxidant production by neutrophils adherent to a substrate can be increased from 50 up to 1000 (!!) fold when compared with cells stimulated in suspension. Signals from integrins are primarily responsible for this enhanced activation during adhesion because the effect can be blocked by antibodies to CD11b/CD18 (85) and is absent in neutrophils from patients deficient in β2 integrins [86]. In addition, signals from other adhesion molecules such as L-selectin can also enhance the oxidative burst of neutrophils [87–89] indicating that signaling and activation occurs even during the earliest adhesive interactions.

Elucidation of the molecular signals from adhesion receptors is important in understanding this hyperactivatable state of adherent neutrophils. One of the ways of dissecting the importance of various adhesion receptors and signaling pathways involved in these processes is by the use of monoclonal antibodies directed at specific adhesion receptors. When these antibodies are allowed to bind to the cell surface followed by the addition of a secondary ('cross-linking') antibody that leads to clustering of receptors, intracellular signals are generated. This is thought to model some of the events that occur when leukocytes bind to adhesive ligands bound to substrates. Using this model system, we and others have demonstrated that signals from β2 integrins and L-selectin can activate a variety of intracellular signaling pathways, including cleavage of membrane polyphosphoinositides with release of Ca^{2+} from intracellular stores, activation of cytosolic tyrosine kinases, tyrosine phosphorylation and activation of the ERK and JNK members of the MAPK family [39, 87, 90–90]. Importantly, cross linking either β2 integrins or L-selectin leads to activation of physiologically important responses including alterations in the actin cytoskeleton, decreases in cell deformability, enhanced adhesivity, potentiation of the oxidative burst, and cytokine (e.g., tumor necrosis factor [TNF]-α) gene expression [87, 88, 90, 94].

Since neither integrins nor selectins posses enzymatic activity, studies on adhesion receptor signaling have focused on proteins that interact with the cytoplasmic domains of the receptors. The intracellular domain of L-selectin is very short (18 amino acids) and while it has not been shown to bind directly to any '-signaling' molecules, it is known to bind to α-actinin [95], a cytoskeletal protein, which may provide a link to intracellular signaling pathways [96]. The cytoplasmic domain of the β chain of integrins also interacts directly with cytoskeletal elements such as α-actinin [97] and talin [98]. However, in contrast to L-selectin, the β chain of integrins is known to bind signaling molecules including integrin associated protein (IAP, CD47) [99], focal adhesion kinase (FAK) [100, 101], cytohesin-1 [102], and the integrin-linked kinase (ILK) [103]. These molecules are presumably involved in regulation of the affinity state of the receptor ('inside-out

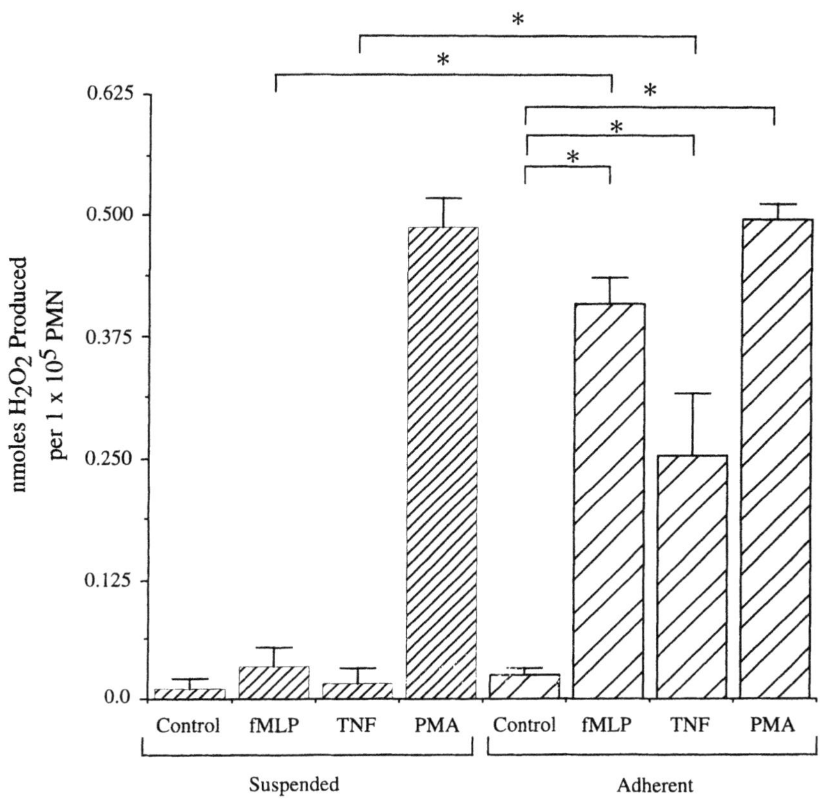

Fig. 7. Effect of adhesion on the neutrophil oxidative burst. **a** 7.5×10^6 human neutrophils were stimulated in suspension with 10^{-6} M fMLP, 10^{-7} M PMA, or DMSO and incubated for 120 min. The production of H_2O_2 was monitored by measurement of the reduction of scopoletin. **b** 7.5×10^6 human neutrophils were first allowed to adhere to tissue culture plastic coated with fetal bovine serum then stimulated with 10^{-6} M fMLP, 10^{-7} M PMA, or DMSO and incubated for an additional 120 min. Data are means ± SE of 4 experiments. Note the pronounced amplification of the oxidative burst in response to fMLP stimulation in the cells adherent to the serum-coated surface, * $p < 0.05$

signaling') or of signals emanating from the receptors ('outside-in signaling'). Calreticulin binds to the integrin α chain and participates in regulation of Ca^{2+}-dependent events during adhesion [104, 105]. In addition, association of integrins with other membrane proteins such as Fc receptors and transmembrane-4 superfamily proteins [106, 107] may participate in transmission of intracellular signals. Lastly, cytosolic factors such as integrin modulating factor-1 (IMF-1) can increase the avidity of the β2 integrin CD11b/CD18 [108].

Our recent studies have focused on ILK, a serine/threonine kinase that was identified in a yeast 2-hybrid screen using the cytoplasmic domain of β1 integrin as 'bait' [103]. ILK has been shown to bind directly to the cytoplasmic domain of β1 integrins *in vitro* indicating that the kinase may function at a very proximal (if not the first) step in transmission of signals from integrins. The substrate(s) of ILK are, at present, incompletely characterized although protein kinase B (PKB/AKT) and glycogen synthase kinase 3 (GSK-3) can be phosphorylated and activated by ILK [109]. In epithelial cell lines, overexpression of ILK resulted in profound alterations in cell morphology, diminished adhesion to the substratum, enhanced deposition of extracellular matrix, and anchorage-independent proliferation [103]. Taken together, these results imply that ILK regulates both inside-out and outside-in integrin signals.

We undertook studies to determine if ILK (or a related kinase) participated in adhesion-dependent signaling in leukocytes. Western blotting demonstrated that neutrophils and leukocyte cell lines express a prominent immunoreactive band at 56 kDa, the predicted Mr of ILK, and immunofluorescence studies demonstrated that ILK was localized diffusely in the cytosol of quiescent neutrophils in suspension. Importantly, when neutrophils were adhered to a surface coated with fibrinogen (a β2 integrin ligand), a fraction of ILK migrated to the basal (adherent) surface and co-localized with CD18, the common β2 chain. This adhesion-dependent co-localization suggests an important link between ILK and β2 integrins. Moreover, the activity of ILK was increased by 60% in cells adherent to surfaces coated with integrin ligands. Given the profound influence that adhesion has on neutrophil function, and the range of important functions influenced by ILK in epithelial cells, by analogy we believe that ILK will play a pivotal role in adhesion-dependent signaling pathways in neutrophils.

Conclusion

Acute lung injury and SIRS are the end result of a wide variety of initiating events. The clinical picture is rather stereotypical implying that the pathways leading to injury converge on a final common pathway leading to tissue injury. This concept holds out the possibility that selective interventions may be possible to ameliorate the untoward effects of leukocyte activation. It is our belief that, in the vast majority of cases, acute lung injury and SIRS are the end result of an acute inflammatory response that has become unregulated because of the overwhelming nature of the insult and an inappropriate host response to the inciting event. We have described how inflammation may spiral our of control and have focused on the potential mechanisms by which neutrophil activation may become unregulated including diminution of negative signals from tyrosine phosphatases and enhanced positive signals from adhesion receptors. The challenge for the next decade will be to unravel at the cellular and molecular level the complexities of the inflammatory response and regulation of neutrophil function in order to target our therapeutic interventions so that they will lessen the injurious consequences of inflammation while leaving the beneficial effects intact.

Acknowledgment. This work was supported by operating grants from the Ontario Thoracic Society, the Medical Research Council of Canada, the Neil Winter Fund from the Toronto General Hospital, and the National Institutes of Health.

References

1. Schuster DP, Kollef MH (1996) Acute respiratory distress syndrome. Dis Mon 42:270–326
2. Montgomery BA, Stager MA, Carrico CJ, Hudson LD (1985) Causes of mortality in patients with the adult repiratory distress syndrome. Am Rev Respir Dis 132:485–489
3. Bone RC (1994) Sepsis and its complications: the clinical problem. Crit Care Med 22:S8–S11
4. Donnelly SC, Haslett C (1992) Cellular mechanisms of acute lung injury: Implications for future treatment in the adult respiratory distress syndrome. Thorax 47:260–263
5. Reynolds HY (1987) Lung inflammation: normal host defense or a complication of some diseases. Annu Rev Med 38:295–323
6. Balk RA, Bone RC (1989) The septic syndrome. Definition and clinical implications. Crit Care Clin 5:1–8
7. St. John RC, Dorinsky PM (1993) Immunologic therapy for ARDS, septic shock, and multiple organ failure. Chest 103:932–943
8. Doerschuk CM, Allard MF, Martin BA, MacKenzie A, Autor AP, Hogg JC (1987) Marginated pool of neutrophils in rabbit lungs. J Appl Physiol 63:1806–1815
9. Hogg JC, Doerschuk CM (1995) Leukocyte traffic in the lung. Annu Rev Physiol 57:97–114
10. Downey GP, Worthen GS (1988) Neutrophil retention in model capillaries: deformability, geometry, and hydrodynamic forces. J Appl Physiol 65:1861–1871
11. Worthen GS, Schwab BD, Elson EL, Downey GP (1989) Mechanics of stimulated neutrophils: cell stiffening induces retention in capillaries. Science 245:183–186
12. Inano H, English D, Doerschuk CM (1992) Effect of zymosan-activated plasma on the deformability of rabbit polymorphonuclear leukocytes. J Appl Physiol 73:1370–1376
13. Bevilacqua MP, Nelson RM, Mannori G, Cecconi O (1994) Endothelial-leukocyte adhesion molecules in human disease. Annu Rev Med 45:361–378
14. Doerschuk CM, Winn RK, Coxson HO, Harlan JM (1990) CD18-dependent and -independent mechanisms of neutrophil emigration in the pulmonary and systemic microcirculation of rabbits. J Immunol 144:2327–2333
15. Rinaldo JE, Christman JW (1990) Mechanisms and mediators of the adult respiratory distress syndrome. Clin Chest Med 11:621–632
16. Sha'afi R, Molski T (1988) Activation of the neutrophils. In: Becker EL (ed) Progress in Allergy, vol. 42. Karger, Basel, pp 1–64
17. Downey GP, Fukushima T, Fialkow L, Waddell TK (1995) Intracellular signaling in neutrophil priming and activation. Semin Cell Biol 6:345–356
18. Gerard C, Gerard NP (1994) The pro-inflammatory seven-transmembrane segment receptors of the leukocyte. Curr Opin Immunol 6:140–145
19. Huang KP (1990) The mechanism of protein kinase C activation. Trends Neuro Sci 12:425–431
20. Hamada F, Aoki M, Akiyama T, Toyoshima K (1993) Association of immunoglobulin G Fc receptor II with Src-like protein-tyrosine kinase Fgr in neutrophils. Proc Natl Acad Sci USA 90:6305–6309
21. Greenberg S (1995) Signal transduction of phagocytosis. Trends Cell Biol 5:93–99
22. Gutkind JS (1998) The pathways connecting G protein-coupled receptors to the nucleus through divergent mitogen-activated protein kinase cascades. J Biol Chem 273:1839–1842
23. Kieran MW, Zon LI (1996) Stress- and mitogen-activated signal transduction in hematopoietic cells. Curr Opin Hematol 3:27–34
24. Nick JA, Avdi NJ, Young SK, et al (1997) Common and distinct intracellular signaling pathways in human neutrophils utilized by platelet activating factor and fMLP. J Clin Invest 99: 975–986
25. Downey GP, Butler JR, Tapper H, et al (1998) Importance of the MEK/MAP kinase pathway in neutrophil microbicidal responsiveness. J Immunol 160:434–443
26. Krump E, Sanghera JS, Pelech SL, Furuya W, Grinstein S (1997) Chemotactic peptide N-formyl-met-leu-phe activation of p38 mitogen-activated protein kinase (MAPK) and MAPK-activated protein kinase-2 in human neutrophils. J Biol Chem 272:937–944
27. Frasch SC, Nick JA, Fadok VA, Bratton DL, Worthen GS, Henson PM (1998) p38 mitogen-activated protein kinase-dependent and -independent intracellular signal transduction pathways leading to apoptosis in human neutrophils. J Biol Chem 273:8389–8397

28. Dusi S, Donini M, Della Bianca V, Rossi F (1994) Tyrosine phosphorylation of phospholipase C-gamma2 is involved in the activation of phosphoinositide hydrolysis by Fc receptors in human neutrophils. Biochem Biophys Res Commun 201:1100–1108
29. Greenberg S, Chang P, Silverstein SC (1993) Tyrosine phosphorylation is required for Fc receptor-mediated phagocytosis in mouse macrophages. J Exp Med 177:529–534
30. Huang C, Laramee G, Casnellie J (1988) Chemotactic factor induced tyrosine phosphorylation of membrane associated proteins in rabbit peritoneal neutrophils. Biochem Biophys Res Commun 151:794–801
31. Gomez-Cambronero J, Huang C, Bonak V, Wang E, Casnellie J (1989) Tyrosine phosphorylation in human neutrophil. Biochem Biophys Res Commun 162:1478–1485
32. Berkow RL, Dodson RW, Kraft AS (1989) Human neutrophils contain distinct cytosolic and particulate tyrosine kinase activities: possible role in neutrophil activation. Biochim Biophys Acta 997:292–301
33. McGregor PE, Agrawal DK, Edwards JD (1994) Attenuation of human leukocyte adherence to endothelial cell monolayers by tyrosine kinase inhibitors. Biochem Biophys Res Commun 198:359–365
34. Gaudry M, Caon AC, Gilbert C, Lille S, Naccache PH (1992) Evidence for the involvement of tyrosine kinases in the locomotory responses of human neutrophils. J Leukocyte Biol 51: 103–108
35. Kobayashi K, Takahashi K, Nagasawa S (1995) The role of tyrosine phosphorylation and Ca^{2+} accumulation in Fcgamma-receptor-mediated phagocytosis of human neutrophils. J Biochem (Tokyo) 117:1156–1161
36. Grinstein S, W Furuya (1991) Tyrosine phosphorylation and oxygen consumption induced by G proteins in neutrophils. Am J Physiol 260:C1019–C1027
37. Kusunoki T, Higashi H, Hosoi S, et al (1992) Tyrosine phosphorylation and its possible role in superoxide production by human neutrophils stimulated with FMLP and IgG. Biochem Biophys Res Commun 183:789–796
38. Ptasznik A, Prossnitz ER, Yoshikawa D, Smrcka A, Traynor-Kaplan AE, Bokoch GM (1996) A tyrosine kinase signaling pathway accounts for the majority of phosphatidylinositol 3,4,5-trisphosphate formation in chemoattractant-stimulated human neutrophils. J Biol Chem 271:25204–25207
39. Berton G, Fumagalli L, Laudanna C, Sorio C (1994) β2 integrin-dependent protein tyrosine phosphorylation and activation of the FGR protein tyrosine kinase in human neutrophils. J Cell Biol 126:1111–1121
40. Corey S, Eguinoa A, Puyana-Theall K, et al (1993) Granulocyte macrophage-colony stimulating factor stimulates both association and activation of phosphoinositide 3OH-kinase and src-related tyrosine kinase(s) in human myeloid derived cells. EMBO J 12:2681–2690
41. Asahi M, Taniguchi T, Hashimoto E, Inazu T, Maeda H, Yamamura H (1993) Activation of protein-tyrosine kinase $p72^{syk}$ with concanavalin A in polymorphonuclear neutrophils. J Biol Chem 268:23334–23338
42. Kraft AS, Berkow RL (1987) Tyrosine kinase and phosphotyrosine phosphatase activity in human promyelocytic leukemia cells and human polymorphonuclear leukocytes. Blood 70:356–362
43. Kansha M, Takeshige K, Minakami S (1993) Decrease in the phosphotyrosine phosphatase activity in the plasma membrane of human neutrophils on stimulation by phorbol 12-myristate 13-acetate. Biochim Biophys Acta Mol Cell Res 1179:189–196
44. Lloyds D, Hallett MB (1994) Neutrophil "priming" induced by orthovanadate: Evidence of a role for tyrosine phosphorylation. Biochem Pharmacol 48:15–21
45. Grinstein S, Furuya W, Lu DJ, Mills GB (1990) Vanadate stimulates oxygen consumption and tyrosine phosphorylation in electropermeabilized human neutrophils. J Biol Chem 265: 318–327
46. Mitsuyama T, Takeshige K, Minakami S (1993) Tyrosine phosphorylation is involved in the respiratory burst of electropermeabilized human neutrophils at a step before diacylglycerol formation by phospholipase C. FEBS Lett 322:280–284
47. Rotin D, Goldstein BJ, Fladd CA (1994) Expression of the tyrosine phosphatase LAR-PTP2 is developmentally regulated in lung epithelia. Am J Physiol 267:L263–L270

48. Pulido R, Alvarez V, Mollinedo F, Sánchez-Madrid F (1992) Biochemical and functional characterization of the leucocyte tyrosine phosphatase CD45 (CD45RO, 180 kD) from human neutrophils. In vivo upregulation of CD45RO plasma membrane expression on patients undergoing haemodialysis. Clin Exp Immunol 87:329–335
49. Fialkow L, Chan CK, Downey G (1997) Regulation of protein tyrosine phosphatase activity in neutrophils: Modulation by oxidants. J Immunol 158:5409–5417
50. Brumell J, Chan CK, Butler J, et al (1997) Regulation of SHP-1 during activation of human neutrophils: Role of protein kinase C. J Biol Chem 272:875–882
51. Uchida T, Matozaki T, Matsuda K, et al (1993) Phorbol ester stimulates the activity of a protein tyrosine phosphatase containing SH_2 domains (PTP1C) in HL-60 leukemia cells by increasing gene expression. J Biol Chem 268:11845–11850
52. Knutson KL, Hmama Z, Herrera-Velit P, Rochford R, Reiner NE (1998) Lipoarabinomannan of *Mycobacterium tuberculosis* promotes protein tyrosine dephosphorylation and inhibition of mitogen-activated protein kinase in human mononuclear phagocytes; Role of the src homology 2 containing tyrosine phosphatase 1. J Biol Chem 273:645–652
53. Yi T, Ihle J (1993) Association of hematopoietic cell phosphatase with c-Kit after stimulation with c-Kit ligand. Mol Cell Biol 13:3350–3358
54. Paulson RF, Vesely S, Siminovitch KA, Bernstein A (1996) Signalling by the W/Kit receptor tyrosine kinase is negatively regulated in vivo by the protein tyrosine phosphatase Shp1. Nature Genet 13:309–315
55. Chen HE, Chang S, Trub T, Neel BG (1996) Regulation of colony-stimulating factor 1 receptor signaling by the SH2 domain-containing tyrosine phosphatase SHPTP1. Mol Cell Biol 16:3685–3697
56. Vambutas V, Kaplan DR, Sells MA, Chernoff J (1995) Nerve growth factor stimulates tyrosine phosphorylation and activation of Src homology-containing protein-tyrosine phosphatase 1 in PC12 cells. J Biol Chem 270:25629–25633
57. Tomic S, Greise RU, Lammers R, et al (1995) Association of SH2 domain protein tyrosine phosphatases with the epidermal growth factor receptor in human tumor cells. Phosphatidic acid activates receptor dephosphorylation by PTP1C. J Biol Chem 270:21277–21284
58. David M, Chen HE, Goelz S, Larner AC, Neel BG (1995) Differential regulation of the alpha/beta interferon-stimulated Jak/Stat pathway by the SH2 domain-containing tyrosine phosphatase SHPTP1. Mol Cell Biol 15:7050–7058
59. Klingmüller U, Lorenz U, Cantley LC, Neel BG, Lodish HF (1995) Specific recruitment of SH-PTP1 to the erythropoietin receptor causes inactivation of JAK2 and termination of proliferative signals. Cell 80:729–738
60. Klingmüller U (1997) The role of tyrosine phosphorylation in proliferation and maturation of erythroid progenitor cells – signals emanating from the erythropoietin receptor. Eur J Biochem 249:637–647
61. Law CL, Sidorenko SP, Chandran KA, et al (1996) CD22 associates with protein tyrosine phosphatase 1C, Syk, and phospholipase C-gamma(1) upon B cell activation. J Exp Med 183:547–560
62. Nadler MJS, Chen B, Anderson JS, Wortis HH, Neel BG (1997) Protein-tyrosine phosphatase SHP-1 is dispensable for FcgammaRIIB-mediated inhibition of B cell antigen receptor activation. J Biol Chem 272:20038–20043
63. Vogel W, Lammers R, Huang J, Ullrich A (1993) Activation of a phosphotyrosine phosphatase by tyrosine phosphorylation. Science 259:1611–1614
64. Binstadt BA, Brumbaugh KM, Dick CJ, et al (1996) Sequential involvement of Lck and SHP-1 with MHC-recognizing receptors on NK cells inhibits FcR-initiated tyrosine kinase activation. Immunity 5:629–638
65. Lorenz U, Bergemann AD, Steinberg HN, et al (1996) Genetic analysis reveals cell type-specific regulation of receptor tyrosine kinase c-Kit by the protein tyrosine phosphatase SHP1. J Exp Med 184:1111–1126
66. Plas DR, Johnson R, Pingel JT, et al (1996) Direct regulation of ZAP-70 by SHP-1 in T cell antigen receptor signaling. Science 272:1173–1176
67. Pani G, Kozlowski M, Cambier JC, Mills GB, Siminovitch KA (1995) Identification of the tyrosine phosphatase PTP1C as a B cell antigen receptor-associated protein involved in the regulation of B cell signaling. J Exp Med 181:2077–2084

68. D'Ambrosio D, Hippen KL, Minskoff SA, et al (1995) Recruitment and activation of PTP1C in negative regulation of antigen receptor signaling by FcgammaRIIB1. Science 268: 293–297
69. Kon-Kozlowski M, Pani G, Pawson T, Siminovitch KA (1996) The tyrosine phosphatase PTP1C associates with Vav, Grb2, and mSos1 in hematopoietic cells. J Biol Chem 271: 3856–3862
70. Doody GM, Justement LB, Delibrias CC, et al (1995) A role in B cell activation for CD22 and the protein tyrosine phosphatase SHP. Science 269:242–244
71. Tsui HW, Siminovitch KA, de Souza L, Tsui FW (1993) Motheaten and viable motheaten mice have mutations in the haematopoietic cell phosphatase gene. Nature Genet 4:124–129
72. Kozlowski M, Mlinaric-Rascan I, Feng GS, Shen R, Pawson T, Siminovitch KA (1993) Expression and catalytic activity of the tyrosine phosphatase PTP1C is severely impaired in motheaten and viable motheaten mice. J Exp Med 178:2157–2163
73. Bignon JS, Siminovitch KA (1994) Identification of PTP1C mutation as the genetic defect in motheaten and viable motheaten mice: a step toward defining the roles of protein tyrosine phosphatases in the regulation of hemopoietic cell differentiation and function. Clin Immunol Immunopathol 73:168–179
74. Obermeier H, Sellmayer A, Danesch U, Aepfelbacher M (1995) Cooperative effects of interferon-gamma on the induction of NADPH oxidase by retinoic acid or 1,25(OH)2-vitamin D3 in monocytic U937 cells. Biochim Biophys Acta 1269:25–31
75. Granger DN, Kubes P (1994) The microcirculation and inflammation: Modulation of leukocyte-endothelial cell adhesion. J Leukoc Biol 55:662–675
76. Springer TA (1994) Traffic signals for lymphocyte recirculation and leukocyte emigration: The multistep paradigm. Cell 76:301–314
77. Lundgren-Akerlund E, Berger E, Arfors KE (1992) Effect of divalent cations on adhesion of polymorphonuclear leukocytes to matrix molecules in vitro. J Leukoc Biol 51:603–608
78. Albelda SM, Smith CW, Ward PA (1994) Adhesion molecules and inflammatory injury. FASEB J 8:504–512
79. Firestein GS, Bullough DA, Erion MD, et al (1995) Inhibition of neutrophil adhesion by adenosine and an adenosine kinase inhibitor: The role of selectins. J Immunol 154:326–334
80. Brown EJ, Lindberg FP (1996) Leucocyte adhesion molecules in host defence against infection. Ann Med 28:201–208
81. Wright SD, Rao PE, Van Voorhis WC, et al (1983) Identification of the C3bi receptor of human monocytes and macrophages by using monoclonal antibodies. Proc Natl Acad Sci USA 80:5699–5703
82. Nathan CF (1987) Neutrophil activation on biological surfaces. Massive secretion of hydrogen peroxide in response to products of macrophages and lymphocytes. J Clin Invest 80: 1550–1560
83. Berton G, Yan SR, Fumagalli L, Lowell CA (1996) Neutrophil activation by adhesion: mechanisms and pathophysiological implications. Int J Clin Lab Res 26:160–177
84. Suchard SJ, Boxer LA (1994) Exocytosis of a subpopulation of specific granules coincides with H_2O_2 production in adherent human neutrophils. J Immunol 152:290–301
85. Nathan C, Srimal S, Farber C, et al (1989) Cytokine-induced respiratory burst of human neutrophils: dependence on extracellular matrix proteins and CD11/CD18 integrins. J Cell Biol 109:1341–1349
86. Nauseef WM, De Alarcon P, Bale JF, Clark RA (1986) Aberrant activation and regulation of the oxidative burst in neutrophils with Mol glycoprotein deficiency. J Immunol 137: 636–642
87. Waddell TK, Fialkow L, Chan CK, Kishimoto TK, Downey GP (1994) Potentiation of the oxidative burst of human neutrophils. A signaling role for L-selectin. J Biol Chem 269: 18485–18491
88. Laudanna C, Constantin G, Baron P, et al (1994) Sulfatides trigger increase of cytosolic free calcium and enhanced expression of tumor necrosis factor-α and interleukin-8 mRNA in human neutrophils. Evidence for a role of L-selectin as a signaling molecule. J Biol Chem 269:4021–4026
89. Crockett-Torabi E, Sulenbarger B, Smith CW, Fantone JC (1995) Activation of human neutrophils through L-selectin and Mac-1 molecules. J Immunol 154:2291–2302

..ddell TK, Fialkow L, Chan CK, Kishimoto TK, Downey GP (1995) Signaling functions of L-selectin. Enhancement of tyrosine phosphorylation and activation of MAP kinase. J Biol Chem 270:15403–15411
91. Brenner B, Grassme HU, Muller C, Lang F, Speer CP, Gulbins E (1998) L-selectin stimulates the neutral sphingomyelinase and induces release of ceramide. Exp Cell Res 243:123–128
92. Brenner B, Weinmann S, Grassme H, Lang F, Linderkamp O, Gulbins E (1997) L-selectin activates JNK via src-like tyrosine kinases and the small G- protein Rac. Immunology 92: 214–219
93. Brenner B, Gulbins E, Busch GL, Koppenhoefer U, Lang F, Linderkamp O (1997) L-selectin regulates actin polymerisation via activation of the small G- protein Rac2. Biochem Biophys Res Commun 231:802–807
94. Tsang YT, Neelamegham S, Hu Y, et al (1997) Synergy between L-selectin signaling and chemotactic activation during neutrophil adhesion and transmigration. J Immunol 159: 4566–4577
95. Pavalko FM, Walker DM, Graham L, Goheen M, Doerschuk CM, Kansas GS (1995) The cytoplasmic domain of L-selectin interacts with cytoskeletal proteins via α-actinin: Receptor positioning in microvilli does not require interaction with α-actinin. J Cell Biol 129: 1155–1164
96. Hynes RO (1992) Integrins: variety, versatility, and interactions in cell adhesion. Cell 69: 11–25
97. Burridge K, Fath K, Kelly G, Nuckols G, Turner C (1988) Transmembrane junctions between the extracellular matrix and the cytoskeleton. Annu Rev Cell Biol 4:487–525
98. Horwitz A, Duggan K, Buck C, Beckerle MC, Burridge K (1986) Interaction of plasma membrane fibronectin receptor with talin-a transmembrane linkage. Nature 320:531–533
99. Lindberg FP, Gresham HD, Schwarz E, Brown EJ (1993) Molecular cloning of integrin-associated protein: An immunoglobulin family member with multiple membrane-spanning domains implicated in $\alpha_v\beta_3$-dependent ligand binding. J Cell Biol 123:485–496
100. Lipfert L, Haimovich B, Schaller MD, Cobb BS, Parsons JT, Brugge JS (1992) Integrin-dependent phosphorylation and activation of the protein tyrosine kinase $pp125^{FAK}$ in platelets. J Cell Biol 119:905–912
101. Dedhar S, Hannigan GE (1996) Integrin cytoplasmic interactions and bidirectional transmembrane signalling. Curr Opin Cell Biol 8:657–669
102. Kolanus W, Nagel W, Schiller B, et al (1996) αLβ2 integrin/LFA-1 binding to ICAM-1 induced by cytohesin-1, a cytoplasmic regulatory molecule. Cell 86:233–242
103. Hannigan GE, Leung-Hagesteijn C, Fitz-Gibbon L, et al (1996) Regulation of cell adhesion and anchorage-dependent growth by a new beta 1-integrin-linked protein kinase. Nature 379:91–96
104. Coppolino M, Leung-Hagesteijn C, Dedhar S, Wilkins J (1995) Inducible interaction of integrin alpha 2 beta 1 with calreticulin. Dependence on the activation state of the integrin. J Biol Chem 270:23132–23138
105. Coppolino MG, Woodside MJ, Demaurex N, Grinstein S, St-Arnaud R, Dedhar S (1997) Calreticulin is essential for integrin-mediated calcium signalling and cell adhesion. Nature 386:843–847
106. Zhou M, Todd RF, Van de Winkel JGJ, Petty HJ (1993) Cocapping of the leukoadhesion molecules complement receptor type 3 and lymphocyte function-associated antigen-1 with Fcgamma receptor III on human neutrophils: possible role of lectin-like interactions. J Immunol 150:3030–3041
107. Berditchevski F, Tolias KF, Wong K, Carpenter C, Hemler M (1997) A novel link between integrins, transmembrane-4 superfamily proteins (CD63 and CD81), and phosphatidylinositol 4-kinase. J Biol Chem 272:2595–2598
108. Hermanowski-Vosatka A, Van Strijp JA, Swiggard WJ, Wright SD (1992) Integrin modulating factor-1: a lipid that alters the function of leukocyte integrins. Cell 68:341–352
109. Delcommenne M, Tan C, Gray V, Rue L, Woodgett J, Dedhar S (1998) Phosphoinositide-3-OH kinase-dependent regulation of glycogen synthase kinase 3 and protein kinase B/AKT by the integrin-linked kinase. Proc Natl Acad Sci USA 95:11211–11216

Neutrophils and Acute Lung Injury

C. Haslett, S. Donnelly, and N. Hirani

Introduction

The first detailed clinical-pathological description of 'acute respiratory distress in adults' [1] was provided by Asbaugh and colleagues, who, in 1967, identified a group of patients that could be differentiated from the majority of patients requiring intensive care management for severe respiratory failure on the following features:

- Tachypnea and cyanosis refractory to oxygen treatment
- Markedly reduced lung compliance upon mechanical ventilation
- Diffuse alveolar shadowing on the chest radiograph
- Pulmonary edema, congestion and hyaline membranes on histological examination of necropsy specimens

In a later study this condition was termed 'adult respiratory distress syndrome' (ARDS) to distinguish it from a similar pathological condition in premature neonates [2].

It has become clear over the ensuing years that the term ARDS embraces a spectrum of acute lung injury (ALI) of varying disease severity – a continuum rather than a quantifiably definable entity – and it is perhaps not surprising that stringent diagnostic criteria have been difficult to set. Murray's expanded criteria [3] have provided a useful definition for many epidemiological and basic research studies, but almost certainly have excluded some individuals with mild disease. The North American/European Consensus Criteria [4] for ARDS have effectively amplified these criteria to include all patients with $PaO_2/FiO_2 < 200$ and recommend that the criteria are linked to the precipitating event. In this chapter, it will be made clear whether Murray's [3], or the Consensus [4], criteria were used to define ARDS in the various studies that are discussed.

ARDS is now recognized as a syndrome of inflammatory lung injury which is a central part of a systemic microvascular injury response that often causes failure of other organs including the kidneys and liver (multiple organ failure [MOF]). In a currently unpredictable fashion, ARDS usually becomes clinically overt after a 'latent period' of several hours or days following a wide range of predisposing events, many of which (e.g., multiple trauma, sepsis, pancreatitis) affect the lung indirectly. Despite the varied underlying causes, a small percentage of patients develop overt lung injury with the apparently common histopathological picture characterized as 'diffuse alveolar damage'. Most patients with ARDS require mechanical ventilation and, in the absence of specific therapy, treatment is supportive only. In some centers there is a trend towards improvement in mortality figures, perhaps as a result of refinement in intensive care, but at least 50% of patients still die in an unpredictable fashion, usually as a result of MOF, nosocomial infection in the injured lung and episodes of septicemia. Remarkably, in about 80% of those who survive, pulmonary function either returns to normal or is greatly improved within a year. These patients represent a remarkable example of the potential, under some circumstances, for extensive, severe lung inflammation and injury to resolve and repair.

Recent advances in our understanding of the inflammatory mechanisms of ALI and the likely pivotal role of the neutrophil in its early stages are likely to generate novel and incisive mechanism-based therapies which could perhaps be applied in the early stages of disease.

Evidence for Neutrophil Involvement in ARDS

The association between neutrophils in histological sections of lungs from patients in the early stages of ARDS and the lung injury process has long been recognized [5], and bronchoalveolar lavage (BAL) cytology reveals large numbers of neutrophils, the products of which (e.g., the granule enzyme myeloperoxidase [MPO]) correlate with the development and severity of ARDS [6].

Other potentially injurious neutrophil products, including neutrophil elastase [6] and collagenase [7], are also prominent. External imaging of radiolabeled neutrophils has demonstrated neutrophil accumulation in the lungs of patients with ARDS [8] and a variety of studies of ALI in experimental animal models have highlighted the pathogenetic role of neutrophil granulocytes. In a sheep model [9], neutrophil depletion abrogated endotoxin-induced lung injury, and in a rabbit model of lung injury induced by a combination of endotoxic lipopolysaccharide (LPS) and the complement fragment C5a, lung injury was abolished by neutrophil depletion and re-constituted by replenishment of neutrophils [10]. This is not to suggest that other inflammatory cells are unimportant in the pathogenesis of human ARDS. ARDS has been described in neutropenic patients [11], but the histological examination of lungs in neutropenic patients reveals the presence of significant numbers of neutrophils, and it is not certain how many neutrophils are needed for the injurious signal. Certainly in the neutrophil replenishment experiment cited above [10] only a small proportion of the total neutrophil complement needed to be re-constituted in neutropenic animals in order to re-constitute the injury signal. Nevertheless, the occurrence of a syndrome indistinguishable from ARDS in neutropenic patients does raise the possibility that other cells, perhaps monocytes in particular which possess most, if not all, of the injurious potential of neutrophils, play an important ancillary role or may even substitute for neutrophils under poorly understood circumstances.

However, notwithstanding these provisos, there is now a large body of evidence which has led a number of observers to implicate the neutrophil granulocyte as a centrally important player in the pathogenesis of ARDS [12–15], a premise which is supported by our own recent studies of the early risk period (latent period) in subgroups of patients with conditions that place them at very high risk of developing this devastating form of ALI.

Studies of the Early ARDS Risk Period

In order to try to identify which of the plethora of mediators and inflammatory cell products (see below) are involved in the development of ARDS, we have, in Edinburgh, embarked upon a series of studies on well-defined subgroups of patients at risk of ARDS (e.g., severe multiple trauma in which the timing of the initiating event can usually be well-defined) at the earliest possible stage of the latent period – less than 2 hours (with a median of 70 minutes). In these patients, we investigated a wide range of inflammatory mediators which have been implicated in inflammatory cell recruitment, adhesion, activation and secretion and correlated these with whether or not the patients subsequently developed full-blown ARDS (by Murray's criteria [3]). Despite the large number of mediators and events so far studied, we have found that only the following have strongly correlated with ARDS development:

i) neutrophil elastase levels of peripheral blood [15];
ii) levels of the powerful neutrophil chemokine interleukin (IL)-8 [16];
iii) an inverse correlation with levels of the soluble form of the adhesion molecule L-selectin in peripheral blood [17].

It will readily be appreciated that two of these elements are directly related to neutrophil behavior and function and provide further persuasive evidence implicating the neutrophil in the early pathogenesis of ARDS. The relationship with IL-8 levels is particularly strong and continues to hold up in our extended studies (unpublished data, Table 1). This relationship is not seen with any other neutrophil chemotaxin or chemokine.

We are developing the hypothesis (see below) that the IL-8 signal, perhaps induced by hypoxia/re-oxygenation in the very early risk period and later amplified by other factors such as LPS known to induce macrophage IL-8 production, is pivotal in determining which patients develop full-blown ARDS.

Table 1. Lavage IL-8 levels and patients at-risk of ARDS

• patients at risk of ARDS	90
• those progressing to ARDS	21
• those not developing ARDS	69
• High IL-8 levels in lavage predicts ARDS ($P = 0.00001$)	
• No relationship with other chemokines (e.g., ENA 78; $P = 0.16$)	

ENA: epithelial cell-derived neutrophil activator.

Mechanisms of Neutrophil-Mediated Pulmonary Microvascular Injury

In summary, it is widely accepted that in most cases of ARDS the neutrophil, which is able to generate a range of reactive oxygen intermediates (ROI) and potentially histotoxic granule contents, e.g., elastase and collagenase, plays a key role in the pathogenesis of ARDS. It is now generally believed that one of the earliest initiation mechanisms is damage to the capillary endothelial cells and the airway epithelial cells that form the delicate alveolar gas exchange membrane, caused by toxic products of inflammatory cells that have become sequestered and activated as a result of inflammatory mediators generated as a consequence of the initiating insult (Fig. 1). It is uncertain why lung injury is so prominent and often the first clinically obvious event in the multi-system microvascular injury of MOF. However, it may in part be due to the fact that the major part of the 'marginating pool' of neutrophils resides in lung capillaries and, even in the healthy state, neutrophils (average diameter 7.5 µm) are required to 'squeeze' through lung capillaries (mean diameter 5.5 µm), thus presenting a massive surface area of contact between this potentially injurious cell and the at-risk gas exchange membrane. With regard to this interaction, it is now clear that neutrophils cannot injure cells or degrade matrix proteins without extremely close apposition, and definition of the mechanisms that relate to this critical interaction is essential for us to gain a full appreciation of the pathogenesis of ALI. Finally, it is now clear that neutrophil secretion is not necessarily an all-or-nothing phenomenon; it is likely to be tightly controlled and, for maximum release of ROI or granule enzymes, the neutrophil needs to be exposed to agents that 'prime' the cell (see below) together with those that activate the cell. Therefore, in order to simplify the complex mechanisms that are likely to be involved in neutrophil-mediated tissue injury the discussion below will be divided as follows:

i) The involvement of mediators - particularly those involved in neutrophil sequestration and activation in the lung.
ii) Neutrophil-endothelial interaction - the creation of an injury-favoring microenvironment.

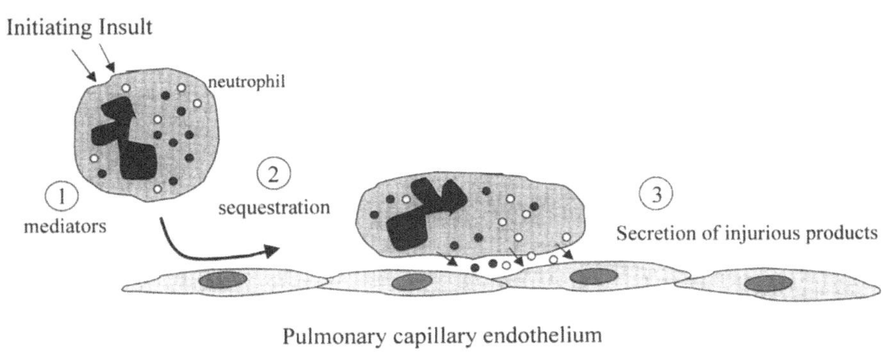

Fig. 15.1. Mechanisms of acute-neutrophil-mediated injury

iii) Potentially injurious neutrophil products released from primed and triggered neutrophils.

Mediators

A very large number of mediators, from several mediator cascades, are known to activate neutrophils and have been implicated in the pathogenesis of ARDS.

Endotoxin. Endotoxic LPS is the main 'active' ingredient of the cell walls of *E. coli* and other Gram-negative organisms that cause sepsis syndrome, septic shock and ARDS. When injected into animals, LPS causes many of the pathophysiological features of septic shock, and in some animals, e.g., sheep, ALI [9]. Low concentrations of LPS may enter the circulation of patients with circulatory shock by the process of 'translocation' of the compromised gut lining [18–20]. LPS exerts a number of direct influences on neutrophils and very low concentrations (pg/ml) are required in the presence of serum when LPS interacts with a protein called LBP (LPS-binding protein) to ligate CD14 on the neutrophil surface [20–23]. LPS alone is not a good neutrophil secretagogue, but it is a very powerful priming agent (see below) and it directly causes enhanced expression of neutrophil surface adhesion molecules which bind the activated endothelium, and a reduction in neutrophil deformability [24], both of these events being critical for neutrophil sequestration in pulmonary microvessels (see below). LPS also causes macrophages to release chemokines and cytokines including IL-8, IL-1 and tumor necrosis factor (TNF)-α which further modulate neutrophil function. Endotoxin may play an early role in the pathogenesis of ARDS [25]; it can certainly be detected in patients at risk of ARDS [26,27] and in cases of established ARDS [28], but so far anti-endotoxin therapeutic strategies have proven disappointing.

Peptide Mediators. Endotoxin is a potent activator of the complement cascade, and for some years the peptide C5a was assumed to be centrally involved in neutrophil attraction to the lung in ARDS since it is an effective neutrophil chemotaxin and secretagogue *in vitro* and is found in the blood of patients at risk of ARDS in addition to those with established disease [25]. However, lung macrophages do not produce C5a and levels in at-risk patients do not correlate with ARDS development [29]. Most researchers in this field now believe that chemokines, especially IL-8 (see below) play the key role in neutrophil chemoattraction to the lung in ARDS. However C5a, like many other mediators, may well influence ARDS pathogenesis especially in combination with other agents such as LPS [10].

There has been much less recent study of the role of the contact system which activates bradykinin, and the clotting and fibrinolytic cascades, but these are likely to be important in the pathogenesis of ARDS. Activated kinins are vasoactive and cause increased vascular permeability. They can also act as secretagogues for neutrophils and other inflammatory cells.

Cytokines. Cytokines are a diverse group of soluble, hormone-like, polypeptides produced by leukocytes and also by some constitutive tissue cells, especially macrophages, endothelial cells, epithelial cells and fibroblasts. TNF-α and IL-1 are generated by alveolar macrophages on exposure to LPS and other stimuli of relevance to ARDS pathogenesis and are likely to play important roles in the initiation of inflammation [30–33]. These cytokines cause other resident cells, particularly epithelial and microvascular endothelial cells, to release IL-8 and other potent neutrophil chemokines. They also act on capillary endothelial cells to induced expression and activation of adhesion molecules necessary for neutrophil sequestration and for the creation of an 'injury-promoting' microenvironment (see below). Elevated levels of these agents are found in association with ARDS [34]. Although TNF-α is not a good neutrophil secretagogue, like LPS it is a potent priming agent for subsequent neutrophil secretory responses (see below).

Chemokines. This new family of small molecular weight peptides has received much recent attention. Depending on the position of cysteine in the molecule they have been subdivided into CXC and CC chemokines (Table 2). The CXC subgroup contains a variety of peptides that are powerful neutrophil chemoattractants and activators, whereas the CC group exert their chemotactic influences on monocytes and/or eosinophils. It is now generally agreed that IL-8, a CXC chemokine, and its family members are more likely to be responsible for neutrophil attraction to the lung in ARDS than C5a. IL-8 is an 8.0 kDa polypeptide that is a potent neutrophil chemoattractant [35, 36] and a powerful stimulus for endothelial cell chemotaxis and angiogenesis [37]. In our studies of patients at risk of ARDS at the earliest stage of the risk period, IL-8, of a plethora of candidates studied, was the only mediator to correlate with ARDS development [16].

The IL-8 signal, which we believe may be pivotal in determining whether or not patients at risk of developing ARDS progress to full-blown disease, occurs very early in the latent period. In our studies all patients were assessed in less than two hours (median 70 minutes) and one patient who went on to develop ARDS had markedly elevated BAL IL-8 levels as early as 45 minutes after multi-

Table 2. The Chemokine Family of Small Peptides

Some Members of the Chemokine Family	
CXC Subgroup	**CC Subgroup**
IL-8 (NAP-1)	MIP-1α
NAP-2	MIP-1β
ENA-78	RANTES
gro-α	MCP-1
PF-4	MCP-2
	MCP-3

IL: interleukin; NAP: neutrophil activating peptide; ENA: epithelial cell-derived neutrophil activator; PF: platelet factor; MIP: macrophage inflammatory protein; RANTES: regulated upon activation, normal T lymphocyte expressed and secreted; MCP: monocyte chemoattractant protein.

ple trauma. The mechanism of this early release of IL-8 into lung secretions, presumably from lung macrophages or other constitutive cells, is uncertain. Although LPS is a powerful stimulator of IL-8 secretion *in vitro*, we detected no *in vivo* correlation with lavage or blood LPS levels at this early time point, but there was a strong correlation between IL-8 levels and the PO_2/FiO_2 ratios (unpublished data) suggesting that early shock/hypoxemia might be an important early trigger. This has led to a new series of observations (unpublished) that hypoxemia and re-oxygenation are powerful activators of the IL-8 gene, and a novel hypothesis (Fig. 2) for a stepwise amplification of IL-8 generation which begins with hypoxemia and is subsequently augmented by re-oxygenation and perhaps later by LPS as a result of endotoxin translocation from the gut.

Membrane Phospholipid Derivatives. Membrane-derived phospholipid products including platelet activating factor (PAF), leukotrienes, prostaglandins and prostacyclin, stimulate inflammatory cells (PAF is an important neutrophil priming agent and leukotriene [LT] B_4 is a neutrophil chemotaxin, for example), but they also exert major influences on local blood vessels, and promote the generation of edema fluid.

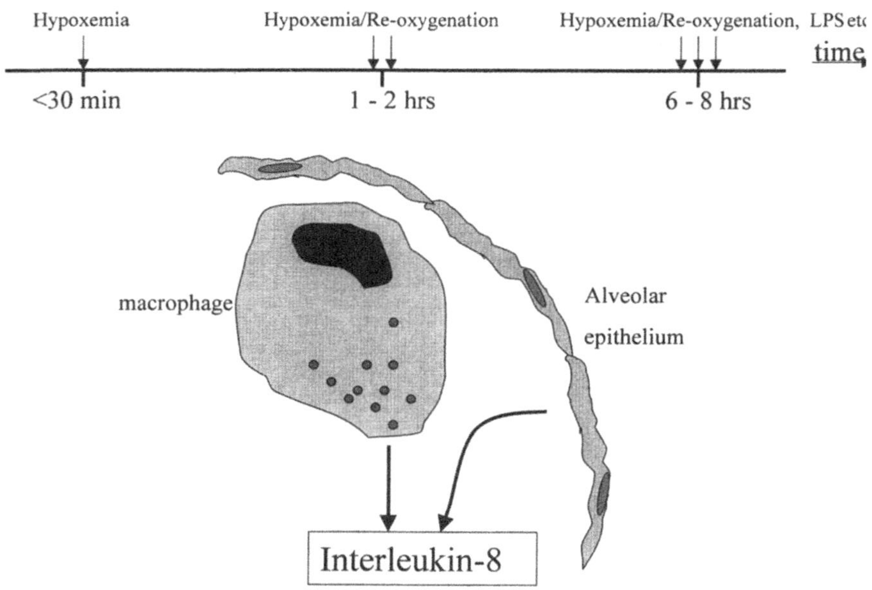

Fig. 15.2. Time-related amplification of lung IL-8 signal

An Injury-Promoting Microenvironment Between Abnormally Sequestered Neutrophils and Pulmonary Capillary Endothelial Cells

Stimulated neutrophils do not injure endothelial cells *in vitro* unless they are in close contact, and it is likely that, *in vivo*, neutrophils interact with endothelium in a fashion which leads to the formation of a specialized intercellular microenvironment (Fig. 3) within which concentrations of histotoxic agents, such as enzymes and ROI are generated in very high local concentrations whereas their inhibitors are relatively excluded. Furthermore, many potent neutrophil enzymes such as elastase are preferentially located on the 'leading' surface of the cell and would need close apposition in order to cause effects. Finally, some of the most reactive ROI are so labile that they are likely to have a very short tissue distance of activity. This concept of a restricted intercellular microenvironment, necessary for neutrophil-mediated injury, is supported by experiments showing that matrix degradation, occurring in areas where stimulated neutrophils are tightly adherent, continues in the presence of the large molecule weight antiproteinase α-1 proteinase inhibitor [38]. The creation of such a microenvironment between neutrophils and endothelial cells in lung capillaries is likely to occur by a combination of adhesion mechanisms and alterations of neutrophil rheological properties, particularly a reduction in deformability.

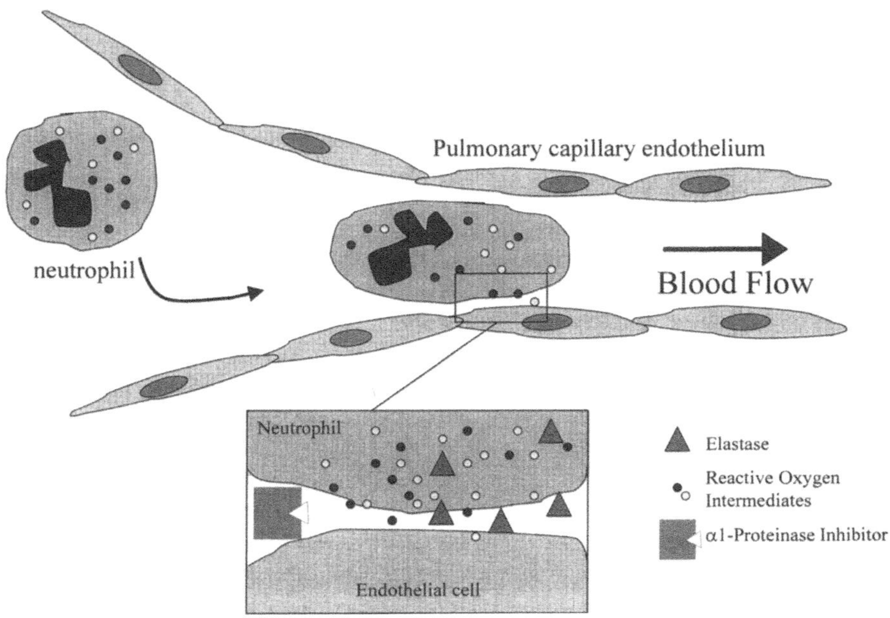

Fig. 15.3. Creation of an injury-promoting microenvironment

Neutrophil-Endothelial Surface Adhesion Molecules. Adhesion between neutrophils and endothelial cells *in vitro* is greatly enhanced within minutes of the addition of inflammatory mediators such as C5a or PAF [39]. Much of this enhanced adhesion can be abolished by monoclonal antibodies directed against the CD11/18 group of adhesive molecules on the neutrophil surface. A number of inflammatory cytokines have the capacity to increase the expression of neutrophil adhesion molecules that are of relevance for their interaction with endothelial cells. Similarly, endothelial cells that have been activated by LPS or by cytokines express adhesion molecules on their surface and others that are already expressed become activated. *In vivo*, it is likely that neutrophil adhesion to endothelial cells in microvessels occurs by a complex process which involves at least two phases. In the first, transient phase of adhesion (which is nevertheless necessary for the second phase), interactions between molecules of the selectin family on neutrophils and endothelial cells are particularly important. In the second phase of 'tight' adhesion which is necessary for the creation of an injurious microenvironment and also for capillary transmigration of neutrophils, integrin molecules play the central role (Table 3). In considering this 'pro-injury' microenvironment it is also important to consider its kinetic aspects. For example an actively secreting neutrophil in contact with a pulmonary capillary endothelial cell for a few microseconds is a very different proposition than the same cell in contact with the endothelium for several seconds. Experiments in which the combination of low concentrations of endotoxin and chemotactic peptides induce ALI in the rabbit [10] show that these agents, when combined, greatly enhance the time of contact of neutrophils with the lung microvessels [40].

Reduced Neutrophil Deformability. As discussed above, neutrophils are normally required to 'squeeze' through the narrow lung capillaries, and any factors that reduce neutrophil deformability would significantly increase their time of sequestration and thereby increase the time of contact between activated or secreting neutrophils and the at-risk gas exchange membrane. Although it has been widely considered that abnormal sequestration occurs mainly by up-regulation of neutrophil and endothelial surface adhesive molecules, alteration in neutrophil deformability is also likely to play an especially important role in the pulmonary microcirculation. It has been shown that neutrophils treated with relevant inflammatory mediators are retained abnormally in filters with a pore diameter of 5 μm by a mechanism which does not involve CD11/18 but which is abolished by cytochalasin D suggesting a role for the cytoskeleton [24, 41]. Direct measurements show that these cells displayed markedly reduced deformability *in vitro* and when injected intravenously have prolonged residence time in the pulmonary microcirculation [42]. The mechanisms involved in neutrophil deformability are much less well understood than the molecular mechanisms related to the expression of adhesion molecules. However, a full understanding of ARDS pathogenesis and its potential therapeutic manipulation requires that these mechanisms receive more attention in research.

Table 3. Adhesion molecules in granulocyte/endothelial interaction

Family	Receptor	Distribution	Ligand/Counter Receptor	Promotes Adhesion to
Integrin Family	LFA-1 (CD11a/CD18)	All leukocytes	ICAM-1, ICAM-2, ICAM-3	Endothelial cells
	MAC-1/CR3 (CD11b/CD18)	granulocytes monocytes lymphocytes	ICAM-1, C3bi, Factor X	Endothelial cells Opsonized particles
	P150.95 (CD11c/CD18)	granulocytes monocytes	Endothelial ligand?	Endothelial cells
Selectin Family	L-selectin (CD)	neutrophils monocytes lymphocytes	?E selectin ?P selectin CD15 C5(ex)	Endothelial cells
	P-selectin (CD 62)	endothelium	Sialyl Lewis X (CD15)	Neutrophils
	ICAM-1 (CD54)	endothelium epithelium	LFA-1 (CD11a/CD18) Mac-1 (CD11b/CD18)	All leukocytes
Immunoglobulin Superfamily	ICAM-2	monocytes lymphocytes endothelium	LFA-1 (CD11a/CD18)	All leukocytes
	VCAM-1	activated endothelium	VLA-4	Monocytes Eosinophils

LFA: leukocyte function-associated antigen ; ICAM: intercellular adhesion molecule; VCAM: vascular cell adhesion molecule; VLA: very late antigen.

Neutrophil Priming, Triggering and Secretion of Injurious Products

Even when neutrophils are tightly apposed to matrix proteins or 'target' endothelial cells *in vitro*, the induction of neutrophil-mediated injury is not a single-step, or 'all-or-nothing' phenomenon. When neutrophils are prepared by stringent methods which avoid their exposure to ubiquitous LPS or other agents that might influence their function, subsequent deliberate stimulation with secretagogues such as C5a or n-formyl-methionyl-leucyl-phenylalanine (fMLP) cause little or no release of ROI or enzymes [43, 44]. However, if these cells have been previously exposed to low concentrations of LPS, which itself does not cause secretion, subsequent exposure to fMLP causes major release of ROI and granule enzymes [43,44]. These priming and triggering phenomena have a number of implications for tissue injury. Firstly, the presence *per se* of neutrophils in tissue does not equate with injury; it is likely that they require to be primed and triggered to achieve a maximal secretory state. Secondly, when examined in this context, many of the mediators implicated in ARDS pathogenesis (see above) exert different effects e.g., LPS, TNF-α [45] and PAF [46] are poor secretagogues but highly effective priming agents, whereas C5a, IL-8 and LTB4 together with other neutrophil chemotaxins are potent secretagogues for primed cells. Furthermore, in studies of neutrophil-mediated injury *in vitro* using stringently prepared neutrophils, it was found that both LPS and C5a (or fMLP) were required for injury to occur [47] and *in vivo* this combination of agents was required to induce neutrophil-mediated endothelial injury [10].

Therefore, rather than seeking a 'single common neutrophil mediator', it is perhaps more important to define how certain key mediators act together to influence critical mechanistic events, e.g., neutrophil secretion. In this regard, the intracellular pathways responsible for neutrophil activation and secretion are partially understood but little is known of how agents that prime neutrophils influence these events. While priming agents including LPS do not in themselves cause significant secretion, they do exert other influences on neutrophil behavior, including reduction in deformability [29] and increased adhesivity [44] which may be extremely important in determining the degree and longevity of neutrophil sequestration in pulmonary capillaries. Indeed, in one of the *in vivo* studies mentioned above, the addition of LPS which was necessary for C5a-induced lung injury greatly increased the time of contact between neutrophils (presumably primed and triggered) and pulmonary capillary endothelium [45].

When the vast array of potentially injurious neutrophil products is considered it is clear that we have another problem with a remarkable redundancy of the inflammatory response. Most of these products have probably evolved to assist the neutrophil in its rapid passage to the inflamed/infected site, and in its effective killing of bacteria, but in neutrophil-mediated tissue injury and disease processes the difficulty of identifying centrally important toxic agents cannot be exaggerated. Over the years, much circumstantial evidence has accrued to support a role for neutrophil-generated ROI in ARDS [20]. However, our studies early in the ARDS risk period suggest that neutrophil elastase is also an important agent [15] and in an *in vitro* study of neutrophil-mediated endothelial injury using neutrophil stimuli of relevance to the pathogenesis of ARDS [47], we found that inhibitors of ROI alone were not effective in blocking injury, whereas a specific neutrophil elastase inhibitor exerted major inhibitory effects. At present it seems that an effective therapeutic strategy directed against neutrophil toxic products would need to include both antiproteinase and antioxidant elements.

Prospects For New Mechanism-Based Therapy in ARDS

Most of the steady improvement in ARDS mortality over recent years is probably the result of gradual improvement in intensive care management. Attempts at anti-inflammatory therapy have not been helpful so far. The use of corticosteroids in early established disease and in the risk period has proved disappointing and even been associated with detrimental effects, and treatment remains supportive. However, recent advances in our understanding of the role of the neutrophil in the early mechanisms of disease may provide opportunities to develop new therapeutic approaches, which could be applied in high risk subgroups of patients particularly in the risk period before the full-blown, complex disease is established. A number of approaches could be taken:

i) Certain key mediators could be targeted. However, it will be important to establish the stage of disease pathogenesis when that particular link in the chain of critical events is most vulnerable, for example anti-LPS strategies have probably been applied too late in the pathogenesis of septic shock. Based on recent evidence it appears that IL-8 may be centrally important in ARDS pathogenesis, but again it would probably need to be inhibited early in the risk period.

ii) The processes whereby neutrophils sequester in pulmonary capillaries including those by which they adhere to endothelial cells could be manipulated. The mechanisms responsible for reduced deformability are poorly understood at present, but the molecular characterization of adhesion molecules that are required for neutrophil/endothelial adherence are receiving much attention (Table 3). The use of monoclonal antibodies that block adhesion molecules is an expensive approach and perhaps the antibody molecules may be too large for effective accessibility to the intercellular micro-environments. However, the molecular engineering of peptides that block key sites of adhesion molecule ligation may provide new drugs in the near future. There have been suggestions that different components of the adhesion molecule repertoire may be employed during different physiological processes in different organs. This suggests the exciting possibility that in the longer term it may be possible to block neutrophil adhesion molecules needed for migration to sites where they are involved in disease pathogenesis, but perhaps retain their ability to migrate to other sites for the purpose of host defense.

iii) It may be possible to block key neutrophil injurious products, but again, in this prime example of redundancy, which ones should be targeted? There is much circumstantial evidence that ROI generated by neutrophils and other inflammatory cells are centrally important in pathogenesis and there is increasing recent evidence that neutrophil elastase may be an important target.

By now it will be appreciated that there is a 'down side' to any approach (including all three mentioned above) that would effectively ablate the neutrophil effector pathway, namely the loss of these highly effective mechanisms in host defense, particularly against bacteria. While this consideration may be more important in chronic inflammatory diseases and may represent less of a problem in acute tissue injury syndromes such as ARDS in which patients could be supported during the application of such therapies for a few days, it must be remembered that injured, burned and septic patients are likely to be particularly at risk from potentially life threatening infections and it is of interest that much of the increased morbidity and mortality observed in the multicenter studies of corticosteroid therapy in ARDS were associated with infectious complications. As we learn more about the inflammatory response it seems clear that the very same mechanisms that evolved to protect the host against bacterial invasion are turned against us in the pathogenesis of inflammatory diseases and it is unlikely that we will be able to 'dissect away' mainly detrimental mechanisms from those that are crucially involved in host defense. This paradox of inflammation being a 'double-edged sword', together with its very many redundant mechanisms, is perhaps the biggest problem in the design of anti-inflammatory strategies.

Nevertheless, other approaches could be taken which might not have the same implications for host defense:

i) Constitutive lung cells including endothelial cells and epithelial cells have the capacity to resist a certain amount of oxidative and/or protease-mediated damage *in vitro* and *in vivo*. We are beginning to learn more about these cyto-protective mechanisms, e.g., the role of glutathione and small molecular weight antiproteinases such as secretory leukoproteinase inhibitor (SLPI) and elafin. In the future it may be possible, in the latent period for example, to augment such protective mechanisms by 'at-risk' endothelial and epithelial cells themselves, by pharmacological or gene-therapeutic approaches. In this regard we have recently shown (Simpson, Haslett and Sallenave, unpublished data) that transfection of lung epithelial cells with the gene for elafin, using an adenoviral vector, protects not only against elastase injury but also against injury caused by primed and activated neutrophils.

ii) It may be possible to harness the poorly understood mechanisms whereby acute inflammation normally resolves spontaneously. By contrast with initiation mechanisms, this side of the inflammatory equation has been subjected to far less research. However, it now seems clear that apoptosis is a key mechanism controlling the functional longevity of neutrophils and other granulocytes at the inflamed sites. As discussed elsewhere, (see chapter by Taneja et al., pp 264–279), granulocyte apoptosis leads to shutdown of granulocyte secretion and their silent removal by local macrophages. When more is known of the selective use of different death receptors or the induction of apoptosis in different cell types it may be possible to induce the selective removal of neutrophil granulocytes at an appropriate stage in ARDS.

Conclusion

There is persuasive evidence that the neutrophil granulocyte is centrally involved in the pathogenesis of ARDS, particularly its early stages. Recent advances in our understanding of the mediators that attract neutrophils to the lungs and mechanisms whereby they adhere to, and injure, microvascular endothelial cells have opened up new therapeutic avenues. However, in designing and applying new therapies it must be remembered that inflammation is a 'double-edged sword' that evolved to protect us against bacterial infection, and powerful anti-neutrophil strategies may also enhance the risk of serious infective morbidity and mortality.

References

1. Asbaugh DG, Bigelow DB, Petty TL, Levine BE (1967) Acute respiratory distress in adults. Lancet ii: 319–323
2. Petty TL, Asbaugh DG (1971) The adult respiratory distress syndrome : clinical features, factors influencing prognosis and principles of management. Chest 60:233–239
3. Murray JF, Matthay MA, Luce JM, Flick MR (1988) An expanded definition of the adult respiratory distress syndrome. Am Rev Respir Dis 138:720–723
4. Bernard GR, Artigas A, Brigham KL, et al (1994) The American-European consensus conference on ARDS. Definitions, mechanisms, relevant outcomes, and clinical trials co-ordination. Am J Respir Crit Care Med 149:818–824
5. Rinaldo JE, Rogers RM (1982) Adult respiratory distress syndrome: changing concepts of lung injury and repair. N Eng J Med 306:900–910
6. Lee CT, Fein AM, Lippmas M, Hotzmann IF, Kimbel P, Weinbum E (1981) Elastolytic activity in pulmonary lavage fluid from patients with adult respiratory distress syndrome. N Eng J Med 304:192–196
7. Christner P, Fein AM, Goldberg S, et al (1985) Collagenase in the lower respiratory tract of patients with adult respiratory distress syndrome. Am Rev Respir Dis 131:690–695
8. Warshawski F, Sibbald W, Driedger A, Cheung H (1986) Abnormal neutrophil-pulmonary interaction in the adult respiratory distress syndrome: qualitative and quantitative assessment of pulmonary-neutrophil kinetics in humans with in vivo indium-111 neutrophil scintigraphy. Am Rev Respir Dis 133:792–804
9. Brigham KL, Bowers R, Haynes J (1979) Increased sheep lung vascular permeability caused by E.Coli endotoxin. Circ Res 45:292–297
10. Worthen G, Haslett C, Rees A, et al (1987) Neutrophil-mediated pulmonary vascular injury. Synergistic effect of trace amounts of lipopolysaccharide and neutrophil stimuli on vascular permeability and neutrophil sequestration within the lung. Am Rev Respir Dis 136:19–28
11. Braude S, Apperley J, Goldman JM (1985) Adult respiratory distress syndrome after allogeneic bone marrow transplantation: evidence for a neutrophil-independent mechanism. Lancet i:1239–1243
12. Donnelly SC, Haslett C (1992) Cellular mechanisms of acute lung injury: implications for treatment in the adult respiratory distress syndrome. Thorax 47:250–263
13. Owen CA, Campbell EJ (1996) Proteinases. In: Evans TW, Haslett C (eds) ARDS – Acute Respiratory Distress in Adults, Chapman and Hall Medical, pp 140–165
14. Repine JE (1992) Scientific perspectives on adult respiratory distress syndrome. Lancet 339: 469–472
15. Donnelly SC, MacGregor I, Zamani A, et al (1995) Plasma elastase levels and the development of the adult respiratory distress syndrome (ARDS). Am J Resp Crit Care Med 125: 191–196

16. Donnelly SC, Strieter RM, Kunkel SL, et al (1993) Interleukin-8 and development of adult respiratory distress syndrome in at-risk patient groups. Lancet 341:643–647
17. Donnelly SC, Haslett C, Dransfield I, et al (1994) Role of selectins in development of adult respiratory distress syndrome. Lancet 344:215–219
18. Ziegler T, Smith R, O'Dwyer S, et al (1988) Increased intestinal permeability associated with infection in burn patients. Arch Surg 123:1313–1319
19. Baker J, Deitch E, Berg R, et al (1988) Hemorrhagic shock induces bacterial translocation from the gut. J Trauma 28:896–906
20. Deitch E, Winterton J, Berg R (1987) The gut as a portal of entry for bacteremia. Ann Surg 205:681–692
21. Wright S, Ramos R, Hermanowski-Vasatka A, et al (1991) Activation of the adhesive capacity of CR3 on neutrophils by endotoxin: dependence on lipopolysaccharide-binding protein and CD14. J Exp Med 173:1281–1286
22. Wright SD, Ramos RA, Tobias PS, et al (1990) CD14 a receptor for complexes of lipopolysaccharide (LPS) and LBP-binding protein. Science 249:1431–1433
23. Weingarten R, Sklar L, Mathison J, et al (1993) Interaction of lipopolysaccharide with neutrophils in blood via CD14. J Leuk Biol 53:518–524
24. Erzurum S, Downey G, Schwab B, et al (1992) Cell mechanics of neutrophils: induction of stiffness and actin by lipopolysaccharide. J Immunol 149:154–162
25. Parsons P (1996) Complement, endotoxin and acute lung injury. In: Evans TW, Haslett C (eds) ARDS – Acute Respiratory Distress in Adults. Chapman and Hall Medical, pp 70–84
26. Brandtzaeg P, Kierulf P, Gaustad P, et al (1989) Plasma endotoxin as a predictor of multiple organ failure and death in meningococcal disease. J Infect Dis 159:195–204
27. Donner RL, Elin RJ, Hossein SM, et al (1991) Endotoxin in human septic shock. Chest 99: 169–175
28. Parrillo JE (1993) Pathogenetic mechanisms of septic shock. N Engl J Med 328:1471–1477
29. Parsons PE, Giclas PC (1990) The terminal complement complex (sC5b-9) is not specifically associated with the development of the adult respiratory distress syndrome. Am Rev Respir Dis 141:98–103
30. Larrick JW, Kunkel SL (1988) The role of tumor necrosis factor and interleukin-1 in the immunoinflammatory response. Pharmacol Res 5:129–139
31. Le J, Vilcek J (1987) TNF and IL-1: cytokines with multiple overlapping biological activities. Lab Invest 56:234–282
32. Sherry B, Cerami A (1988) Cachectin/tumor necrosis factor exerts endocrine, paracrine, and autocrine control of the inflammatory responses. J Cell Biol 107:1269–1277
33. Girardin E, Grau GE, Dayer JM, et al (1988) Tumor necrosis factor and interleukin-1 in the serum of children with severe infectious purpura. New Engl J Med 319:397–400
34. Marks JD, Marks CB, Luce JM, et al (1990) Plasma tumor necrosis in patients with septic shock: mortality rate, incidence of adult respiratory distress syndrome. Am Rev Respir Dis 141:94–97
35. Matsushima K, Oppenheim JJ (1989) Interleukin-8 and MCAF: novel inflammatory cytokines inducible by IL-1 and TNF. Cytokine 1:2–13
36. Baggiolini M, Walz A, Kunkel SL (1989) Neutrophil-activating peptide-1/interleukin-8, a novel cytokine that activates neutrophils. J Clin Invest 84:1045–1049
37. Koch AE, Polverini PJ, Kunkel SL et al (1992) Interleukin-8 as a macrophage-derived mediator of angiogenesis. Science 258:1798–1801
38. Campbell EJ, Campbell MA (1988) Pericellular proteolysis by neutrophils in the presence of proteinase inhibitors: effects of substrate opsonization. J Cell Biol 106:667–676
39. Tonnesen MG, Anderson DC, Springer TA, et al (1989) Adherence of neutrophils to cultures human microvascular endothelial cells. Stimulation by chemotactic peptides and lipid mediators and dependence upon the Mac-1, LFA-1, p150, 95 glycoprotein family. J Clin Invest 83:637–646
40. Haslett C, Worthen G, Giclas P, et al (1987) The pulmonary vascular sequestration of neutrophils in endotoxemia is initiated by an effect of endotoxin on the neutrophil in rabbits. Am Rev Respir Dis 136:9–18

41. Worthen GS, Schwab B, Elson EL, Downey GP (1989) Mechanics of stimulated neutrophils: cell stiffening induces retention in capillaries. Science 245:183–185
42. Selby C, Drost E, Lannan S, Wraith PK, MacNee W (1991) Neutrophil retention in the lungs of patients with chronic obstructive pulmonary disease. Am Rev Respir Dis 143:1359–1364
43. Guthrie LA, McPhail LC, Henson PM, Johnston RB Jr (1984) The priming of neutrophils for enhanced release of oxygen metabolites by bacterial lipopolysaccharide: evidence for increased activity of the superoxide-producing enzyme. J Exp Med 160:1656–1671
44. Haslett C, Guthrie LA, Kopaniak MM, Johnston RJ, Henson PM (1985) Modulation of multiple neutrophil functions by preparative methods of by trace concentrations of bacterial lipopolysaccharide. Am J Pathol 119:101–110
45. Berkow RL, Wang D, Larrick JW, et al (1987) Enhancement of neutrophil superoxide production by preincubation with recombinant human tumor necrosis factor. J Immunol 139: 3783–3791
46. Worthen GS, Seccombe JF, Guthrie LA, et al (1988) Priming of neutrophils by lipopolysaccharide for enhanced production of platelet-activating factor: potential role in mediation of enhanced superoxide secretion. J Immunol 140:3553–3559
47. Smedly LA, Tonnesen MG, Sandhaus RA, et al (1986) Neutrophil-mediated injury to endothelial cells. Enhancement by endotoxin and essential role of neutrophil elastase. J Clin Invest 77:1233–1243

Lymphocyte Activation, Anergy, and Apoptosis in Polymicrobial Sepsis

A. Ayala, C. S. Chung, and G. Y. Song

Introduction

Sepsis and multiple organ failure (MOF) are reported to be responsible for upwards of 60% of the deaths which occur in the surgical intensive care unit [1], despite the use of specific antibiotics, aggressive operative intervention and nutritional support, and also the use of new therapeutic agents in clinical trails, such as antibodies to endotoxin and the pro-inflammatory cytokines [1,2]. A number of studies have suggested that the link between cell and organ dysfunction associated with MOF lies in the initial presentation of sepsis (Gram-negative, Gram-positive, and/or fungal in nature) [3]. In this respect, it has been reported that patients exposed to various forms of trauma and soft tissue injury as well as those with sepsis exhibit a broad spectrum of alterations in both innate and acquired immunity which are eventually deleterious to host survival.

The process of lymphocyte (T- and B-cell) activation is fundamental to the competent development of the reactions to opportunistic foreign pathogens associated with the development of sepsis (Fig. 1). Microbial antigens derived from such pathogens typically must undergo some form of processing mediated by the antigen presenting cell (APC, e.g., macrophages/monocytes, dendritic cells, B-cells). The antigen presenting cell then expresses the processed antigen associated with either the major histocompatibility (MHC) class II (for presentation to helper T-lymphocytes [Th-cell], $CD3^+CD4^+$) or MHC class I (for presentation by target cells to cytotoxic T-lymphocytes [Th-cell, $CD3^+CD8^+$). On recognition of foreign antigen associated with the MHC class II molecule via interaction with the T-cell receptor (TCR) complex, and upon receipt of the appropriate co-stimulatory signals (via B7-1/2:CD28 and/or intercellular adhesion molecule-1/leukocyte function associated antigen-1 [ICAM-1/LFA-1] interaction, and/or soluble co-stimuli such as interleukin [IL]-1, IL-6, etc.), the Th-cell is typically induced to secrete a variety of lymphokines, such as IL-2, interferon (IFN)-γ, IL-4, IL-10, etc. These cytokines in turn not only drive the differentiation of the T-cell and its proliferative expansion but eventually serve to up-regulate the effector arms of cellular immunity by activating mononuclear cell microbiocidal activity. These same lymphokines released by the activated Th-cell also augment the humoral response to antigen binding through the B-cell surface Ig receptor (BCR) complex, thus potentiating antibody secretion (Fig. 1). The intricacies of T- and B-cell activation have been reviewed extensively [4–7].

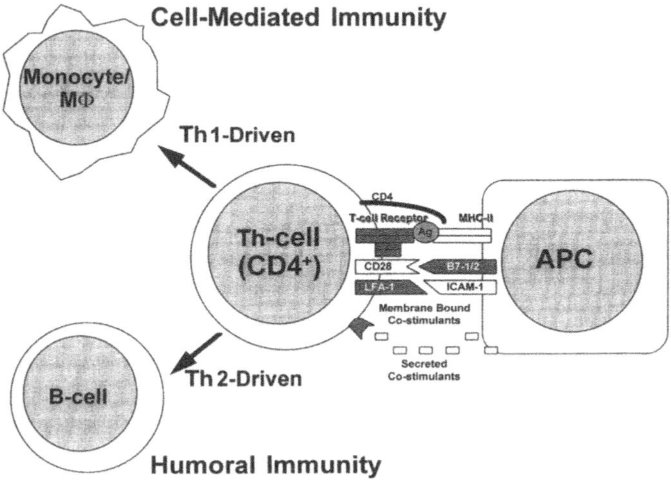

Fig. 1. Central role of T-cell activation in the development of acquired immunity (either cell-mediated and/or humoral) in response to foreign antigen (Ag) presented by an antigen presenting cell (APC). MΦ: macrophage; LFA: leukocyte function associated antigen; ICAM: intercellular adhesion molecule; MHC: major histocompatibility complex

The present chapter provides a brief overview of the more prominent features of the signal transduction systems which may impact on the capacity of the normal mature-resting T-cell to respond to antigen presentation. The possible pathways or second messengers which may facilitate this response in the septic animal lymphocytes will be described (Fig. 2) [4].

T Cell Activation

T cell receptor ligation via presented antigen or mitogen cross-linking appears to induce the activation of a family of tyrosine kinases (i.e., *src*-family members, Lck or Fyn; *syk*-family member, ZAP-70) which act primarily to phosphorylate a variety of adapter proteins (e.g., son of sevenless protein [SOS], growth factor receptor-bound protein 2 [GRB2], Snc, signal transducer and activator of transcription protein 5 [STAT5], etc.) which interact with the cytoplasmic domain of the CD3 molecule. This in turn leads to the recruitment of various effector molecules such as various guanosine triphosphate (GTP)-binding proteins (e.g., Ras, Rac, and various G-proteins [G-α, β, γ]) and phospholipase C-γ (PLC-γ). PLC-γ, through the release of diacylglycerol (DAG) and inositol triphosphate (IP3), mobilizes calcium (Ca^{2+}) from intracellular stores, which acts typically through calcineurin to up-regulate the transcriptional factor NF-AT (nuclear factor of activated T cells) or to further stimulate protein kinase C (PKC). PKC activation stimulates activation of nuclear factor-κB (NF-κB), the inhibitor factor(s), IκB, dissociates and the NF-κB complex translocates to the nucleus where it can bind the appropriate desoxyribonucleic acid (DNA) promoter sequences (Fig. 2). Concomitantly, the other GTP-binding proteins such as Ras and Rac regulate the activation of serine/threonine kinase pathways, also known as the mitogen activated protein kinase (MAPK) cascades, of which there are three primary systems (extracellular signal-regulated kinase [ERK]-1/2, c-Jun N-terminal kinase/stress-activated protein kinase [JNK/SAPK], and p38). These MAPK pathways in turn activate transcriptional regulatory factors such as Fos, Jun and/or activating transcription factor (ATF)-1 which serve to stimulate the binding of the activated protein (AP)-1 sites on various cytokine promoters. Together, these pathways serve to up-regulate the transcription of genes for the inflammatory cytokines IL-2, IFN-γ, IL-4, IL-10, etc.

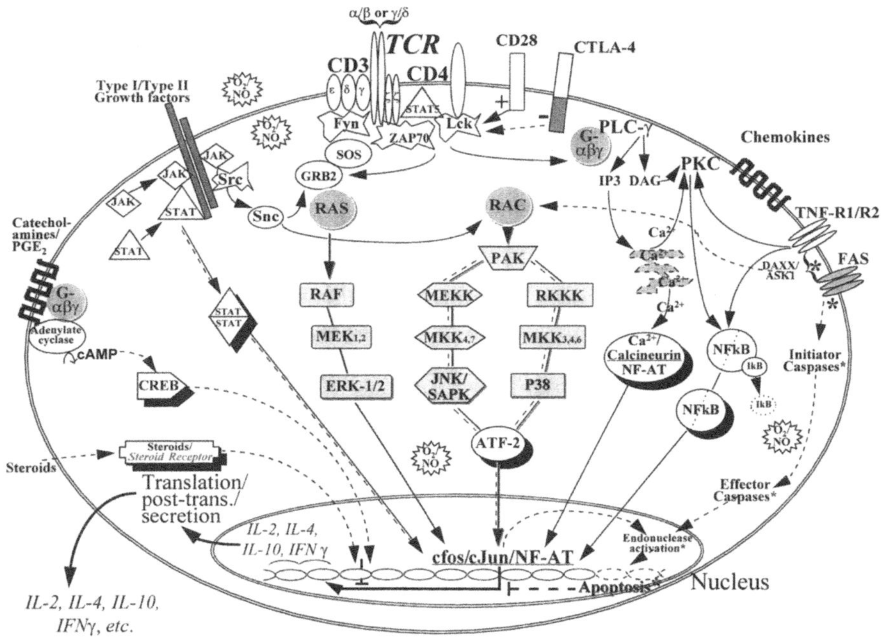

Fig. 2. Diagrammatic representation of the various activation signal pathways (——►) induced by presentation of antigen (or mitogenic stimulant) through the T-cell receptor complex (TCR/CD3/CD4), in the presence or absence of co-stimulatory receptor signaling via CD28, various type I/II growth factors, chemokines, as well as antagonistic signals (- - - -►) which inhibit activation, via CTLA-4 (phosphatase activity), catecholamines, prostaglandins, steroids, apoptotic stimuli (e.g., Fas and TNF-R1) or anti-inflammatory cytokines, such as IL-4 and IL-10, which act through alternate growth factor receptor signaling pathways. Pathways which appear to be involved in transmitting signals which both stimulate or inhibit cell activation are indicated by ═══►. Tyrosine kinase family members are indicated by ☆, reactive oxygen species and/or nitric oxide ✪, phosphorylated adapter proteins by ○, regulatory GTP-binding proteins are illustrated by ●, janus kinase (JAK) family members by ◊, signal transduction and transcription (STAT) family members by Δ, mitogen activated kinase pathway family members (i.e., ERK-1/2, JNK/SAPK or P38) by ■, and various transcription factors are depicted by ❍. The apoptotic pathways stimulated by Fas and/or TNF are indicated by a * and given in greater detail in Fig. 4

There are, however, a number of mechanisms by which these pathways can be affected by signals transduced through pro-inflammatory cytokine receptors such as tumor necrosis factor (TNF) [4], type I/II growth factors such as IL-1, IL-2, IL-6, IL-4, IL-10, IFN-γ [8], prostaglandins/catecholamines [7], membrane associated co-stimulants such as cytotoxic T lymphocyte associated antigen (CTLA)-4 vs CD28 [9], steroids [7], as well as signaling through cell death receptors such as Fas antigen, TNFR1, TNF-related apoptosis-inducing ligand (TRAIL) receptors [10]. Such mechanisms must also be considered if we are to understand the altered responsiveness seen in lymphocytes from septic animals (Fig. 2). With this in mind, it is clear that knowledge of the changes in any single signal transduction system, let alone the effects of any one mediator, will be insufficient to understand the complex alterations induced in the cells obtained from the septic/traumatized animal patient. Therefore, integrational approaches are needed if we are to understand the complex pathobiology of this activation process in lymphocytes let alone any other cell type, tissue or organ.

It is also evident that defects or dysfunction in any component involved in T-cell activation can inhibit the process of T-cell activation resulting in a condition commonly referred to as immune suppression or 'anergy'. In the clinical setting, or *in vivo*, this is reflected as a diminished delayed-type hypersensitivity response to common recall antigens, while in the laboratory setting or *in vitro*, this is typically evidenced by either a mixed-lymphocyte response or diminished T-cell help. The inability of the lymphocyte to respond to appropriate stimuli during exposure to antigen is, therefore, a critical component of the host's ability to mount either a cell-mediated or humoral response to foreign pathogens. However, the impact of dysfunction of APCs in the process of lymphocyte activation has been described elsewhere [11].

Studies suggest that the lymphoid response to presented antigen is regulated at a number of levels [5]. In this respect, aspects of the direct interaction between components of MHC-class II-antigen complex and TCR complex, such as antigen concentration, avidity of antigen-TCR complex binding, and the antigen's ability to cross-link (soluble versus complexed or membrane associated) can affect the signal induced by the TCR complex [4, 12]. Similarly, the timing or duration of antigen exposure also plays a role in regulating the response of the cell to such stimuli. Alterations in such antigen-TCR complex/BCR complex have been documented to produce states of partial activation, reflected in incomplete T-cell signaling [4]. This same concept also applies to the timing and to the duration of exposure of the lymphocyte to co-stimulants such as B7-1/2 or ICAM-1 surface antigen family, IL-1 and IL-6, which potentiate the response to antigen, and immune suppressants such as IL-4, IL-10, transforming growth factor (TGF)-β, prostaglandin E_2 (PGE_2), nitric oxide (NO), CTLA-4, etc., irrespective of the competency of antigen recognition (Fig. 1). An antigen can induce markedly different states of activation of cell-mediated immunity or anergy depending not only on the maturational status of the cell but also on the nature of the prior signal(s) perceived by the lymphocyte. The anergic lymphocyte does not lose all its functional properties simultaneously. A number of examples of decreased T-cell help (IL-2/IFN-γ, etc.) can be documented while the same general cell population does not appear to lose the capacity to produce immune suppressants such as IL-4 and/or IL-10 (Fig. 3), and also seems to up-regulate components of the cell suicide machinery, such as Fas-Fas ligand (FasL) (Fig. 2). This apparent dichotomy, however, may be a reflection of the activation of distinct T-cell sub-populations, such as Th0-, Th1-, Th2-, Th3?-, or Tc1-, Tc2-cells, which are defined primarily by their lymphokine release patterns (Fig. 3) [12–14]. Considerable effort has gone into trying to understand the ontogeny of such T-cell types, in both animal models [12–14] and humans, relative to their abilities to either augment or suppress the cell-mediated immune response.

T-cells differ with respect to maturational status (maturing T-cells in the thymus as compared to mature peripheral lymphoid T-cells; $CD4^+$ vs $CD8^+$ T-cells; $\alpha\beta TCR^+$- vs $\gamma\delta TCR^+$-T-cells) [15, 16] and the differentiation status (resting T-cell, Th0 vs Th1, Th2, Th3?, etc.) [12–14] (Fig. 3). Furthermore, some defects in the capacity to activate lymphocytes may also be the result of less specific (receptor independent) mediators, such as reactive oxygen/reactive nitrogen [17, 18], changes in cellular adenosine triphosphate (ATP) levels [19], altered cellular pH [20] as well as calcium dyshomeostasis [21].

The induction of lymphocyte activation sets in motion a process which initiates the eventual suicide of the activated cell itself. This process has been re-

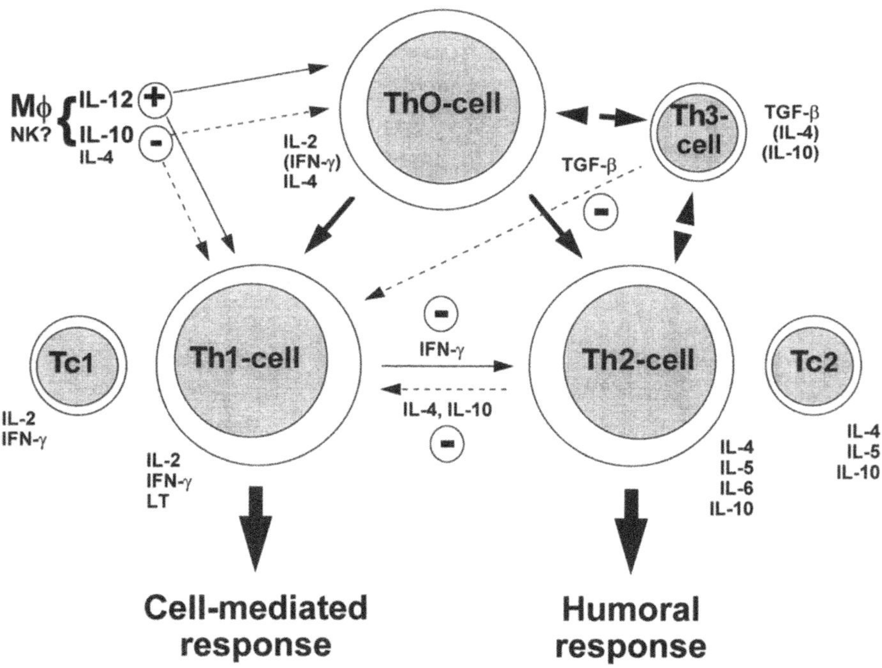

Fig. 3. Postulated inter-relationship of Th0-, Th1-, Th2-, Th3?-, or Tc1-, Tc2-cells and the cytokines they express to the regulation/development of a competent cell-mediated immune response. MΦ: macrophage

ferred to as apoptosis or programmed cell death (Fig. 4). Programmed cell death is a process by which selected cell populations can be actively deleted from specific tissues [22]. This concept has been extended by immunologists to include any cell in which a programmed series of biochemical events occurs, in some cases requiring *de novo* gene expression [22]. A number of these proteins, such as Fas-FasL are up-regulated not only in cells competently stimulated to produce T-cell help and thus amplify the cell-mediated immune response, but are also up-regulated in cells which exhibit anergic/immune suppressed responses [23, 24].

The induction of programmed cell death via apoptosis has been proposed as a mechanism whereby the immune system can remove (deselect) auto-reactive lymphocytes [22] or regulate the extent of immune cell activation [23] (Fig. 5). Apoptosis of activated lymphocytes, therefore, protects the host from an uncontrolled, overzealous response to activating stimuli or response to inappropriate antigens (self), thus allowing processes such as wound tissue remodeling to progress. This same process can contribute to the pathophysiology of disease states such as human immunodeficiency virus (HIV) immune depression, cancer, autoimmune disorders, neurodegenerative diseases and ischemic injury [25–27]. However, until recently the contribution of the process of apoptosis in sepsis-induced immune dysfunction had not been examined.

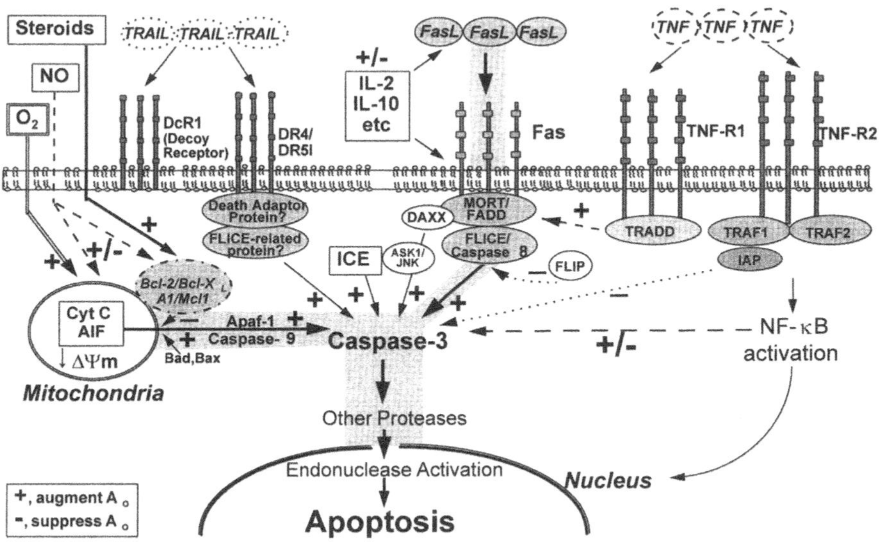

Fig. 4. Some of the mediators and the pathways which have been implicated in the induction and suppression of lymphocyte apoptosis. Pathways (caspase 3 & 9 activation; ICE [interleukin-1β converting enzyme/caspase 1] activation; steroids/reactive oxygen [O_2] /nitric oxide [NO] induced suppression of Bcl-family vs. increased Bax/Bad-family genes) or receptor-ligand (FasL-Fas antigen; TNF-TNF-R1; TRAIL-DR4/DR5I) interactions which are reported to increase or lead to lymphocyte apoptosis (mediated by caspases 8, 9 & 3 and/or activation of DAXX-SAPK pathways) are indicated with a '+', whereas, those which suppress (augmented Bcl-gene family expression; TNF-TNF-R2 activation of IAP [inhibitor of apoptosis protein]; TRAIL-DcR1 [non-signal transducing decoy receptor]) the induction of apoptosis are indicated by a '–'

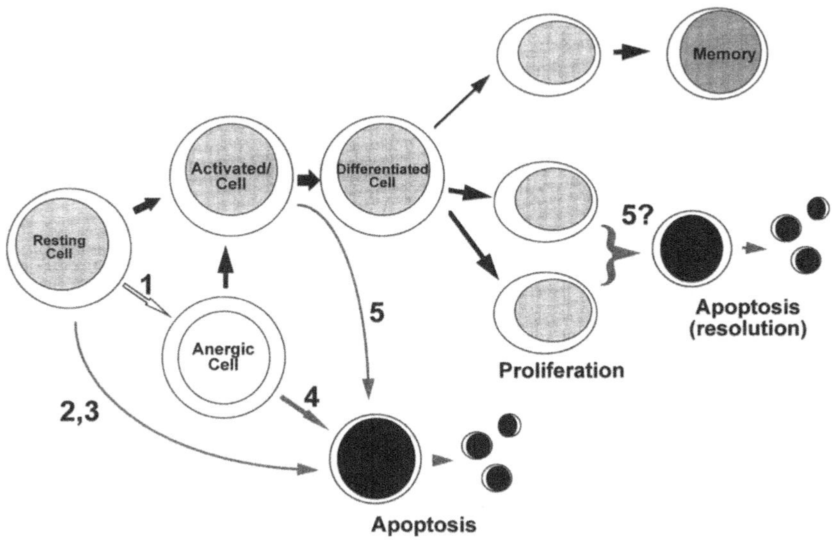

Fig. 5. Postulated steps at which the process of lymphocyte activation/differentiation might be inhibited by various agents associated with polymicrobial sepsis which could result in apparent lymphocyte anergy and/or apoptosis. 1) Direct inhibition of the activation/differentiation of immune cells produced by the action of immune suppressive agent(s) which produce an anergic state but do not lead to the induction of cell death via apoptosis. 2) Indirect inhibition of the activation/differentiation of immune cells (due to their loss), produced by the overt induction of cell death via apoptosis by mediator(s). 3) Direct/indirect inhibition of the activation/differentiation of immune cells (due to their loss), produced by the inadvertent induction of cell death via apoptosis due to loss or removal of required growth factor(s). 4) Incomplete antigenic stimulation due to lack of co-stimulatory signal, etc., and/or 5) superantigen (e.g., exotoxin) overstimulation leading to activation-induced apoptosis

Much has been learned about the initial signal transduction events following the engagement of Fas antigen (receptor for FasL) (Fig. 4). This area has been covered in great detail by other reviews [23, 28]; therefore, we will only summarize the salient events initiated by Fas receptor engagement. Typically FasL is synthesized and secreted and expressed on the cell surface of the activated T-lymphocyte [23, 24]. The activation of resting T- or B-cells also induces increased expression of cell surface receptors (Fas antigen) for FasL [23]. However, for some immature lymphocytes higher densities of Fas antigen are consistently expressed (e.g., thymocytes). The regulation of FasL or Fas antigen expression is poorly understood, although pathways leading to NF-kB, NFAT-RE3 appear to stimulate FasL gene expression [29], while stimulation of PKC [30] seems to lead to the activation of a novel regulatory factor, TDAG51 [30], which augments Fas antigen expression. The expression of Fas-FasL is also affected by cytokines such as IL-2 and IL-10 [31, 32]. Thus, there is a commonality between the signaling pathways and mediators which affects the apoptotic process and those events which are involved in mediating T-cell activation and regulation of cell-mediated immunity. In view of this, it is not difficult to perceive how dysfunction in T-cell responses as reflected by anergy may be the result of inappropriate activation of apoptotic processes or, alternatively, the induction of the anergic state could eventually result in the induction of apoptosis.

Evidence of Lymphocyte Anergy in Polymicrobial Sepsis

Sepsis commonly manifests clinically as a two phase process in which the patient initially goes through a hyperdynamic-hypermetabolic phase (fever, increased cardiac output, enhanced metabolic rate) and subsequently through a hypodynamic-hypometabolic state [33]. The latter stage of this process is typically referred to as 'septic shock', in which the circulatory system is compromised, organ function becomes more depressed, and the animal or patient eventually dies. However, a major deficiency in models which have thus far been utilized to study sepsis is that they rarely exhibit both the hyper- and hypo-dynamic states of sepsis [34, 35]. The murine model of cecal ligation and puncture (CLP) produces both the early hyper- and late hypo-dynamic metabolic phases of peritonitis [34, 35]. The CLP model also produces a more chronic disease, as mortality develops over days (not hours). This delayed onset of pathology makes this more comparable to the clinical conditions associated with sepsis syndrome [35] and allows for delayed therapeutic interventions.

Studies from a number of laboratories indicate that the immune system exhibits a biphasic response, comparable to the metabolic and circulatory responses seen in sepsis [3, 33]. Initially there is evidence of an exaggerated systemic inflammatory response, thought to be due to immune cell stimulation by microbes and their products [36, 37]. Mediators released in response to trauma, shock or sepsis, may be the nidus for the hyperdynamic-hypermetabolic response [38]. Over time, however, this stage gives way to a state of generalized immune cell hyporesponsiveness [19, 21, 39–42].

The early stage of sepsis is characterized by the presence of circulating, monocyte-derived pro-inflammatory cytokines, such as TNF, IL-1, IL-6, and chemokines [36, 37]. Elevated circulating levels of TNF and IL-6 appear in both the mouse and rat model of CLP [39, 43, 44]. Hadjiminas et al. [45], using CLP, further documented that enhanced TNF-α release following the onset of sepsis was a reflection of both increased secretion and elevated transcriptional activity of the gene following CLP. We have also found that both endotoxin-tolerant C3H/HeJ mice and endotoxin-sensitive C3H/HeN mice exhibit a similar systemic pro-inflammatory cytokine response (increased TNF and IL-6), and comparable rates of mortality in response to CLP [40]. These findings not only demonstrate the capacity of this murine polymicrobial sepsis model to mimic/produce this early systemic inflammatory response, but suggest that sensitivity and/or responsiveness to endotoxin does not markedly alter this response.

With the progression of sepsis, i.e., more than 12 hours after CLP, there is a marked decline in the capacity of lymphocytes from the spleen to respond to stimulation that is not evident prior to this period. This loss of splenic responsiveness does not appear to be a result of prior antigenic stimulation *in vivo*, as there is little overt evidence of such *ex vivo* activation in the absence of added *in vitro* stimulant. The cells harvested late following CLP, therefore, appear to become dysfunctional (anergic) or immunocompromised. Recent findings from our laboratory [19] as well as others [21] indicate that reduced splenic lymphocyte responsiveness appears to be related to a concomitant decrease in cellular ATP stores [19] and an increase in cellular calcium levels [21]. Studies by Choudhry et al. [21] indicated that depression of splenocyte IL-2 release and mitogen responsiveness following a Gram-negative septic insult in the rat was associated with increased basal intracellular calcium and changes in calcium mediated signal transduction mediated through the Fyn kinase family (Fig. 2). We have also reported that by 24 hours post-CLP, there is a marked reduction in IL-2 and IFN-γ release capacity by mouse lymphocytes [42], and that this may be a response to altered signal transduction involving the differential activation of the MAPK family (Fig. 2). We have recently observed alterations in P38 MAPK, rather than ERK-1/2 or JNK/SAPK in septic mouse splenocytes, responding to mitogens in association with reduced IL-2 and IFN-γ release [46]. Whether these changes translate into alterations in transcriptional regulation still remains to be established in the lymphocytes from the septic mouse.

Recent studies examining *ex vivo* (unstimulated) lymphocyte populations in the small intestine following the onset of polymicrobial sepsis indicate that these tissues exhibit a marked increase in mRNA for IL-2, IL-10 and IL-15. This is an important finding, since the phenotypic make-up of the intra-epithelial lymphocyte compartment differs significantly from that of the peripheral blood or secondary lymphoid tissues. These mucosal tissues have a high incidence of $CD3^+CD8^+$ lymphocytes in contrast to the $CD3^+CD4^+$ cells typically encountered in the blood or spleen [15]. This may be a reflection of the presence of a higher frequency of ontologically distinct $\gamma\delta TCR^+$-T-cells seen in the intestinal mucosa as compared to $\alpha\beta TCR^+$-T-cells seen in the spleen, thymus, blood and most non-mucosal lymph nodes [16] (Fig. 2). Whether these lymphocytes if subsequently challenged/stimulated will exhibit an anergic response comparable to that seen in splenic lymphocytes is not known. This, however, may be more difficult to discern, since intra-epithelial and lamina propria T-cells survive poorly following isolation [15], perhaps reflecting that these cells are already activated by enteric antigens [15].

Together, these findings indicate that differences are evident in intracellular functions, such as signal transduction level and basal metabolic capacity, and in their ability to perceive stimuli. However, it is unclear whether these differences serve as an underlying cause of the anergic response seen or are a response to extracellular anergic stimuli.

Exogenous/Endogenous Mediators of Lymphoid Function in Sepsis

The Role of Endotoxin

Studies have shown that if animals are exposed to μg doses of endotoxin *in vivo*, their *ex vivo* macrophage response to endotoxin is reduced [47]. This has been referred to as 'endotoxin tolerance'. However, the extent to which endotoxin is responsible for producing the hypo-responsiveness to mitogenic stimuli seen in the septic animals' splenic lymphocytes is not clear. Therefore, we attempted to determine whether or not the administration of low dose endotoxin in mice, at levels comparable to those encountered during polymicrobial sepsis (CLP), produced a similar dysfunction in the ability of splenic lymphocytes to release lymphokines [48]. The results indicated that sepsis induced by CLP caused a marked suppression of IL-2 and IFN-γ release, lymphokines characteristic of Th1-cells, while potentiating the release of the immunosuppressive, Th2-cell products, IL-4 and IL-10 in splenocytes harvested 24 hours following the septic insult [42] (Fig. 3). However, chronic exposure (24 hours) to endotoxin, at a level comparable to that seen in CLP, caused no depression in release of these Th1 lymphokines. Our most recent assessments of splenic and peritoneal macrophage cytokine release capacity indicate that a comparable inversion of this pro- vs anti-inflammatory cytokine response may also be evident in macrophages, as we have demonstrated a decrease in IL-12 secretion in the presence of increased and/or unchanged IL-10 production [49].

The lethality rate following CLP in endotoxin-tolerant C3H/HeJ mice and endotoxin-sensitive C3H/HeN mice is comparable [50], suggesting that a bacterial component other than endotoxin mediates the differential alterations observed in lymphocyte responsiveness and cytokine release during polymicrobial sepsis.

Contribution of the Response to Tissue Injury

While the majority of studies have focused on the contribution of microbes to the changes seen during sepsis, little attention has been paid to the role of devitalized or necrotic tissue and its impact on the changes seen in the septic animal immune cell response. It may well be that tissue wounding itself is sufficient to induce marked suppression in lymphocyte responsiveness [51], and that necrotic/devascularized cecal tissue may also be a stimulant which is capable of mediating the induction of macrophage/lymphocyte immunosuppression. Wichterman et al. [34] reported that cecal ligation alone, in the absence of puncture, did not cause mortality. Furthermore, these rodents showed no overt physiological signs of sepsis, were blood culture negative, and upon sacrifice for necropsy had walled off the necrotic cecal tissue. Interestingly, our initial findings using C3H/HeN mice indicate that cegal ligation alone is sufficient to induce the augmented production of the anti-inflammatory (Th2) cytokine, IL-10 [49] (Fig. 3). This is associated with a marked decrease in splenic lymphocyte IL-2/IFN-γ and macrophage IL-6/IL-12 production. This change does not appear to be due to leakage/contribution of endotoxin from the ligated cecum, since peritoneal implantation of a sterile source of devitalized/necrotic/injured tissue, for example, syngenec donor muscle, is capable of producing a macrophage phenotype with suppressive characteristics comparable to that seen in cecal ligation [49]. Taken together, these findings of suppressed cell-mediated immune responsiveness are in keeping with the general observation that soft-tissue trauma alone [51], as well as shock [52] or burn [53], also produce states of immune suppression following which survival to septic infectious microbial challenge is diminished.

The Role of Pro-inflammatory Cytokine Mediators

A number of investigators have suggested that, irrespective of the nidus of stimulation, it is the systemic pro-inflammatory mediator response that is the motor for the developing host cell dysfunction. The results of studies from several laboratories indicate that pro-inflammatory cytokines, particularly TNF, IL-1 and IL-6, might be the agents which initiate the development of cell and organ dysfunction associated with sepsis and MOF [2]. Support for this suggestion came from early reports [36] that indicated that the morbidity and mortality from sepsis or traumatic injury was associated with the marked elevation of TNF, IL-1 and/or IL-6, and that intravenous administration of these cytokines produced a shock-like state [54, 55] with organ dysfunction [1] comparable to septic shock. However, the majority of these studies used high doses or extended infusion of these cytokines, a stimulus that is not typical of the levels detected in CLP [39, 43, 45, 56] or septic patients [57]. While it has been shown that that there is a marked early (~1 hour peak) elevation in circulating bioactive TNF, followed by IL-6 (~4–24 hours) and later by TGF-β (24 hours) [39, 43], the levels of TNF are markedly lower than that required to produce shock [57]. The question, therefore, arises as to what is the significance of the early low-level TNF response encountered in CLP. Studies by Eskandari et al. [56] indicate that when mice are pretreated with antibodies to TNF prior to CLP, a significant decrease in their survival rate is observed. Further, Hadjimias et al. [45] also reported that passive immunization with antibodies against either TNF-α or IL-1β did not inhibit sequestration of neutrophils in the lung following CLP. These data would imply that the early low-level systemic TNF may be insufficient to produce the septic shock response, further suggesting that the early pro-inflammatory mediator response is not necessarily out of control (beyond normal limits) but reflects the animal's initial attempts to contain the infection. However, in the animal/patient when a chronic septic insult persists, we suggest that there is a sustained anti-inflammatory response at a local and/or systemic level which eventually pushes the immune system towards suppression (Fig. 3).

The Contribution of the Anti-inflammatory Cytokine IL-10

Studies from our laboratory [42] have shown that in late sepsis the decrease in splenic lymphocyte IL-2 and IFN-γ release capacity is associated with an elevated ability to produce the anti-inflammatory cytokines IL-4 and IL-10. Furthermore, our data [49] indicate that a similar state of decreased IL-12, as opposed to enhanced IL-10, release is also evident in macrophages from mice undergoing CLP or cecal ligation as well as implanted necrotic muscle tissue alone (Fig. 3).

However, in these studies neither the contribution of IL-4 nor IL-10 was directly linked to the observed suppression of Th1-lymphocyte lymphokine release.

The role of IL-10 in the mortality of CLP, therefore, is controversial. Work by Hogaboam et al. [58] indicates that mice pre-treated with polyclonal antibody to IL-10 exhibit a decreased survival to subsequent CLP. Studies by Ertel et al. [59] indicated that IL-10 administered following the induction of sepsis in mice, had the capacity to suppress the early pro-inflammatory cytokine response but suppressed their Th1 lymphokine response and decreased the animals' overall survival.

We have recently assessed the *in vitro* and *in vivo* effects of either anti-IL-10 antibody treatment or IL-10 gene deficiency on lymphocyte Th1 cytokine release and survival following a lethal septic challenge [60]. The results indicated that IL-10 gene deficiency prevented the sepsis induced depression of Th1 lymphokine production. The role of IL-10 in sepsis-induced splenic immune suppression *in vitro* was further confirmed by the capacity of anti-IL-10 monoclonal antibody treatment to restore Th1 cytokine productive capacity. Interestingly, we found that *in vivo* treatment of animals with antibody to IL-10 had a salutary effect on animal survival only when administered following the pro-inflammatory/hyper-dynamic/hyper-metabolic phase, but not when given during pro-inflammation. Thus, our results document not only IL-10's role in septic immune dysfunction, but illustrate that anti-IL-10 administration beyond the initial pro-inflammatory state of polymicrobial sepsis improves survival.

We have also recently shown that administration of antibodies to IL-10 during mitogen stimulation of septic mouse splenic lymphocytes markedly attenuated the rise in P38 MAPK expression in these cells while restoring their ability to produce IL-2 and IFN-γ [46]. These results, therefore, indicate that IL-10 appears at least in part to mediate its anergic effects by altering the cell's MAPK signal transduction cascade.

The Role of IL-12 in Sepsis

Recent findings by Zisman et al. [61] indicate that pre-treatment of mice with polyclonal antibodies against IL-12, a Th1 stimulating cytokine, while mitigating the lethal effects of endotoxic shock also reduces the capacity of the animal to clear live bacteria. This suggests that the role of IL-12, similar to that previously documented for TNF in CLP [45, 56], may be paramount in mounting an antimicrobial response necessary to survive the lethal effects of CLP.

Studies of the regulatory affects of IL-2, IFN-γ, IL-4, IL-10 and IL-12, suggest that while a number of signal transduction or nuclear factor components mediate these effects, the major regulatory pathway utilized by these particular lymphokines appears to be the activation of the JAK/STAT components. For example, JAK1/3-STAT4 appears to predominate with respect to IL-12 effects, while the JAK2-STAT6 pathway is activated by IL-4 and JAK1/3-STAT5 are activated by IL-2 [8]. IFN-γ acts mainly through JAK1-STAT1 while IL-10 stimulates JAK1-STAT3

[8]. However, the direct contribution of these transcriptional elements to the splenic lymphoid immune suppression seen in sepsis and the nature of the cross-talk between these pathways and those inducing MAPKs or other transcriptional factors has yet to be clarified.

The Contribution of the Anti-inflammatory Cytokine TGF-β

Studies from our laboratory [40] have also demonstrated that immunosuppression during sepsis is associated with the systemic release of the anti-inflammatory cytokine TGF-β [14]. The role of TGF-β and IL-6 (a direct/indirect inducer of TGF-β release) as potential anti-inflammatory agents in sepsis, as well as in trauma, has been documented by the work of Miller-Graziano et al. [62] and Zhou et al. [63]. In the light of this evidence, one can envision a network of systemic effects mediated by agents that induces the release of IL-6, leading to increased TGF-β levels that would in turn directly or indirectly induce the suppression of host responses seen during sepsis. Support for this hypothesis comes from our recent finding that the Kupffer cell appears to be a significant source of systemic IL-6 seen during sepsis. The depletion of Kupffer cells by gadolinium chloride pre-treatment not only markedly attenuated the rise in blood IL-6 levels but also preserved splenic lymphokine release capacity [64].

PGE2 Induced Septic Lymphocyte Anergy

In addition to the anti-inflammatory cytokines, prostaglandins, particularly PGE_2 are important mediators that act on lymphocytes. Their production can be induced not only by microbial components such as endotoxin, but also by complement, or by platelet and leukocyte aggregation. There is also evidence that cytokines such as TNF, IL-1, and TGF-β, may also stimulate the release of PGE_2 [55, 61]. Studies by Ertel et al. [44] in rats subjected to CLP indicated both elevated IL-6 and TNF levels in circulation, and a marked increase in plasma PGE_2 levels. Choudhry et al. [21] have recently reported evidence that prostaglandins appear to mediate lymphocyte dysfunction in rat sepsis model.

Nitric Oxide as a Lymphocyte Immune Suppressant

Another potentially important immunosuppressive agent which may contribute to the suppression of lymphocytic mediated immune response following sepsis is NO (Fig. 2). Hogaboam et al. [58] has shown that NO may play a role in improving survival of female mice subjected to sepsis, although when a non-specific NO antagonist (N^G-nitro-L-arginine methyl ester, L-NAME) was used they found that such post-treatment also increased the peritoneal exudate fluid IL-10 levels, though not the capacity of the peritoneal macrophage to make IL-10. However, it is not known if these effects would be comparable if male mice had been used. Thus, NO's contribution to septic immune depression remains to be established.

The Effect of Gender

With respect to these findings, as well as a number of those mentioned earlier, it is important to keep in mind that a potential limitation of these studies is the contribution of differences in gender driven immune responses. The impact of such differences with respect to sepsis has recently been documented by studies done by Zellweger et al. [65] who documented that proestrus female mice survived septic challenge better then age-matched males. Since the proestrus state in rodents is associated with high prolactin and estrogen levels it is conceivable that these agents (or their lack) would alter lymphocyte responsiveness. Alternatively, androgens present in males might also contribute to this divergence. This, however, has not been extensively addressed in sepsis.

Evidence of Sepsis-Induced Lymphoid Apoptosis

Thymic Apoptosis in Sepsis

Zhang et al. [66] reported that thymic apoptosis could be increased by exposure of mice to high dose endotoxin ($\geq$50 µg/mouse). An increased frequency of apoptosis in the thymus of septic mice can be detected as early as 4 hours post-CLP, increasing up through 24 hours [67]. Furthermore, this increase in apoptosis in the thymuses of the CLP mice appears to be primarily a response to glucocorticoids and not to TNF [68, 69]. Interestingly, studies from our laboratory have also indicated that mice with a combined deficiency in FasL and endotoxin sensitivity exhibit a comparable increase in thymic apoptosis following the induction of sepsis [70] (Fig. 4). These findings differ from those of Zhang et al. [66], who reported that acute endotoxin-induced apoptosis was mediated through both glucocorticoids and TNF. Studies by Wang et al. [71] using monospecific bacterial infection reported that the capacity of antibodies directed against TNF-α to inhibit apoptosis in the thymus of bacteremic mice was markedly reduced in animals receiving a Gram-positive agent versus Gram-negative microbes. We speculate that the mixed nature of a polymicrobial septic insult, i.e., CLP, might account for the ineffectiveness of the TNF inhibitor we utilized [67]. Interestingly, studies by Hiramatsu et al. [72] have shown that antibodies against TNF were sufficient to inhibit endotoxin induced thymic apoptosis but not to block apoptosis induced by CLP. These studies further support the notion that sepsis, as produced by CLP, encompasses more than endotoxin *per se*.

Apoptosis of Mucosal Lymphoid Tissue in Sepsis

A number of other lymphoid tissues also appear to be actively undergoing increased apoptosis following the onset of sepsis. However, this does not appear until later ($>$12 hours) during hypodynamic sepsis, unlike that occurring in the thymus in which it is evident as early as 4 hours post-CLP. Our studies indicate that mixed bone marrow cells showed an increase in apoptosis at 24, but not at 4 hours, following CLP [73]. Changes in apoptosis were not evident in splenocytes at 24 hours. Phenotypic as well as morphological assessment indicated that most of the increase in apoptosis in the thymus was in the immature T-cell population, $CD4^+CD8^+$ and $CD8^-CD4^-$ cells. In contrast, the increase in bone marrow cell apoptosis was associated with only the $B220^+$ cells (B-lymphocytes), with no significant contribution from myeloid cells. However, unlike with thymocytes, treatment of CLP mice *in vivo* with antagonists of glucocorticoids or TNF failed to suppress the increased apoptosis in the bone marrow.

Intestinal lymphoid tissue, such as the Peyer's patches, also exhibit increased apoptosis in polymicrobial sepsis at 24 but not 12 hours [74]. Phenotypically, these changes were also restricted to the B-cell population, and also exhibited a marked increase of Fas antigen expression. Increased apoptosis is associated with endogenous stimulation of IgA production by B-lymphocytes and increased nuclear c-Rel expression (a component of the NF-κB complex). It could, therefore, be postulated that the increased IgA production is a response to altered exposure to enteric antigens present due to increased gut permeability seen during sepsis [3]. This would, thus, appear to be an example of activation induced lymphocyte apoptosis in Peyer's patch B-cells [23].

Augmented B-cell apoptosis might be a peculiarity of Peyer's patches. We have recently observed that the $B220^+$ lymphocyte subset of the lamina propria also exhibit a marked increase in apoptosis during sepsis. Whether this is a reflection of the teleological linkage which is thought to exist in the development of a mucosal B-cell IgA mediated response [75] or is a reflection of a global non-specific cellular intestinal response, remains to be determined.

Further assessment of lamina propria mononuclear cell preparations from septic mice *ex vivo* indicate not only that there are marked increases in B-cell apoptosis but also increases in apoptosis of the $CD4^+$ (Th-cell), $CD8^+$ (cytotoxic T-cell), and F4/80^+ macrophage cell populations at both 4 (except for $CD4^+$) and 24 hours [76]. This is associated with a significant increase in lamina propria mononuclear cell IL-2, -10, and -15 gene expression observed at 24 hours but not 4 hours after CLP. Thus, the early phenotypic-apoptotic changes may be a reflection of localized immune cell activation in early sepsis which stimulates the increased cytokine gene expression seen in late sepsis. This localized activation may contribute to localized inflammation and/or immune dysfunction in sepsis. These findings correlate well with the *in situ* observations by Hiramatsu et al. [72] who reported evidence of increased apoptosis at 24 hours after CLP in both mouse Peyer's patches and in lymphoid cells lining the small and large intestine.

Most intriguingly, we [77] have also recently shown that the phenotypically distinct (high incidence of $\gamma\delta TCR^+$-lymphocytes, versus the more common $\alpha\beta TCR^+$-T-cell, as well as a higher $CD8^+:CD4^+$ T-cell ratio [15, 16]) intestinal intraepithelial lymphocyte (IEL) population also exhibits changes associated with increased apoptosis which may be a reflection of localized immune cell activation in response to sepsis, as increased cytokine gene expression is also seen in late sepsis. Interestingly this appears to be a FasL-Fas antigen mediated process which is independent of endotoxin sensitivity (Fig. 4); late mortality is reduced in C3H/HeJ-$FasL^{gld}$ (FasL deficient mice/endotoxin tolerant) versus

C3H/HeJ (endotoxin tolerant) mice subject to CLP [77]. Preliminary findings by Hotchkiss et al. [78] indicate that transgenic mice expressing the anti-apoptosis gene, Bcl-2, show a reduction in thymic apoptosis and a survival advantage following CLP.

Increased Activation-Induced Lymphocyte Apoptosis in Sepsis

The findings provided above indicate that apoptosis is evident in a variety of lymphoid tissues in the septic mouse, and this appears, at least in mucosal tissue sites, to be associated with markers of lymphocyte activation. Nonetheless, the link between lymphokine release to direct or indirect induction of *in situ* apoptosis has not been clearly established.

Increased apoptosis may be associated with immune hyporesponsiveness, reflected in decreased proliferative response and diminished IL-2/IFN-γ release capacity [42], since mitogenic stimulation of splenocytes isolated from mice 24 hours post-CLP causes a significant increase in the rate of lymphoid apoptosis [79]. This increase in apoptosis also appears to be restricted to T-cells of the helper ($CD4^+$) lineage [79]. Furthermore, our preliminary data [79] suggests that FasL may be involved in this process (Fig. 4), since animals which are deficient in FasL show a partial restoration of inducible IFN-γ production but not IL-2 following CLP. Interestingly, Castro et al. [80] using a high dose endotoxin model have shown that endotoxin mediates not only an increase in apoptosis but also a change in cytokine productive capacity. These findings are also in keeping with the observations of Oka et al. [81] who reported that inhibition of FasL binding decreased activation induced lymphoid apoptosis in peripheral blood mononuclear cells obtained from surgical trauma patients.

It may be that reduced levels of lymphokines such as IL-2 or granulocyte/macrophage colony-stimulating factor (GM-CSF) are involved in the increase in lymphocyte apoptosis seen in polymicrobial sepsis. Although no clear evidence is as yet available, such a possibility has been documented by the studies of Teodorczyk-Injeyan et al. [82], which indicated that the activation-induced increase in apoptosis seen in peripheral blood lymphocytes from burn patients could be partially restored by supplementation of exogenous IL-2.

Conclusion

The findings described above provide a potential link between the developing dysfunction seen in immune cells obtained from septic animals and suggest ways in which these changes may be mediated by the expression of various pro- (IL-6) and/or anti-inflammatory (i.e., IL-4, IL-10, TGF-β, PGE_2, NO, steroids, etc.) mediators released during sepsis. Furthermore, the nature of this defect in the anergic T-cell is manifested by alterations in a variety of second messengers and in changes in the cell's signal transduction pathways in a suppression of expression of genes associated with T-cell help (Fig. 2). However, the extent of this anergic or apoptotic T-cell response appears to differ depending on whether the cells are derived from mucosal or secondary lymphoid tissues, on their maturational status, and on the T-cell subset (Th1 vs. Th2, Th3?, etc.) (Fig. 3). Many of the mediators which are capable of inducing T-cell activation or anergy are also capable of initiating apoptotic cell death. However, it is also evident that these changes in lymphocyte functional capacity are not simply the results of endotoxemia or rampant pro-inflammation in the polymicrobial septic animal, but are affected by the presence of injured/traumatized tissue and/or varied microbial stimuli.

We propose that the lymphoid immune response might be affected at several points during the process of activation, resulting in the apparent T-cell anergy seen in the septic animal, and that the induction of cell death via apoptotic processes may be both a result and, in some cases, a cause of this immune suppressed state (Fig. 5). Nonetheless, while we have observed that the development of anergy (immune suppression) in this model of sepsis is typically a global response, the same is not consistently seen in apoptosis. Thus, much still needs to be understood about how lymphocyte activation and apoptotic pathways are regulated, and how mediators produced in the response to sepsis interact to produce anergy. Such knowledge, it is hoped, will eventually permit the development of more effective therapeutic modalities for the critically ill septic patient.

Acknowledgments. This investigation was supported by the National Institutes of Health grants R01 GM-46354 and R01 GM-53209.

References

1. Baue AE (1996) MOF/MODS, SIRS: an update. Shock 6: S1–S5
2. Barriere SL, Lowry SF (1995) An overview of mortality risk prediction in sepsis. Crit Care Med 23: 376–393
3. Marshall JC (1993) Immunologic dyshomeostasis in multiple organ failure. In: Faist E, Meakins J, Schildberg FW (eds) Host defense dysfunction in trauma, shock and sepsis. Springer-Verlag, Berlin, pp 243–252
4. Alberola-Ila J, Takaki S, Kerner JD, Perlmutter RM (1997) Differential signaling by lymphocyte antigen receptors. Annu Rev Immunol 15: 125–154
5. Healy JI, Goodnow CC (1998) Positive versus negative signaling by lymphocyte antigen receptors. Annu Rev Immunol 16: 645–670
6. Reth M, Wienands J (1997) Initiation and processing of signals from the B cell antigen receptor. Annu Rev Immunol 15: 453–479
7. Folleta VC, Segal DH, Cohen DR (1998) Transcriptional regulation in the immune system: all roads lead to AP-1. J Leukocyte Biol 63: 139–152
8. Leonard WL, O'Shea JJ (1998) Jaks and Stats: biological implications. Annu Rev Immunol 16: 293–322
9. Lee K, Chuang E, Griffin M, at al (1998) Molecular basis of T cell inactivation by CTLA-4. Science 282: 2263–2266
10. Gulbins E, Brenner B, Koppenhoefer U, Linderkamp O, Lang F (1998) Fas or ceramide induce apoptosis by Ras-regulated phosphoinositide-3-kinase activation. J Leukoc Biol 63: 253–263
11. Ayala A, Ertel W, Chaudry IH (1996) Trauma-induced suppression of antigen presentation and expression of major histocompatibility class II antigen complex. Shock 5: 79–90
12. Constant SL, Bottomly K (1997) Induction of Th1 and Th2 CD4+ T cell responses: the alternative approaches. Annu Rev Immunol 15: 297–322

13. Mosmann TR, Sad S (1996) The expanding universe of T-cell subsets: Th1, Th2 and more. Immunol Today 17:138–149
14. Letterio JJ, Roberts AB (1998) Regulation of immune responses by TGF-beta. Annu Rev Immunol 16:137–161
15. Klein JR, Mosley RL (1993) Phenotypic and cytotoxic characteristics of intraepithelial lymphocytes. In: Kiyono H, McGhee JR (eds) Mucosal immunology: Intraepithelial lymphocytes. Raven Press Ltd., New York, pp 33–47
16. Chien Y, Jores R, Crowley MP (1996) Recognition by gamma/delta T cells. Annu Rev Immunol 14:511–532
17. Nakamura H, Nakamura K, Yodoi J (1997) Redox regulation of cellular activation. Annu Rev Immunol 15:351–369
18. Albina JE, Reichner JS (1995) Nitric oxide in inflammation and immunity. New Horiz 3: 46–64
19. Meldrum DR, Ayala A, Chaudry IH (1994) Energetics of lymphocyte "burnout" in late sepsis: Adjuvant treatment with ATP-$MgCl_2$ improves energetics and decreases lethality. J Surg Res 56:537–542
20. Madshus IH (1988) Regulation of intracellular pH in eukaryotic cells. Biochem J 250:1–8
21. Choudhry MA, Ahmad S, Sayeed MM (1995) Role of Ca2+ in prostaglandin E2-induced T-lymphocyte proliferative suppression in sepsis. Infect Immun 63:3101–3105
22. Schwartz LM, Osborne BA (1993) Programmed cell death, apoptosis and killer genes. Immunol Today 14:582–590
23. Lynch DH, Ramsdell F, Alderson MR (1995) Fas and FasL in the homeostatic regulation of immune responses. Immunol Today 16:569–574
24. Nagata S, Suda T (1995) Fas and Fas ligand: lpr and gld mutations. Immunol Today 16:39–43
25. Sarin A, Clerici M, Blatt SP, Hendrix CW, Shearer GM, Henkart PA (1994) Inhibition of activation-induced programmed cell death and restoration of defective immune responses of HIV^+ donors by cysteine protease inhibitors. J Immunol 153:862–872
26. Liles WC (1997) Apoptosis-role in infection and inflammation. Curr Opin Infect Dis 10: 165–170
27. Reed JC (1996) Mechanism of Bcl-2 family protein and dysfunction in health and disease. Behring Inst Mitt 97:72–100
28. Ashkenazi A, Dixit VM (1998) Death receptors: signaling and modulation. Science 281: 1305–1308
29. Matsui K, Fine A, Zhu B, Marrshak-Rothstein A, Ju S (1998) Identification of two NF-kappaB sites in mouse CD95 ligand (Fas ligand) promoter: functional analysis of T cell hybridoma. J Immunol 161:3469–3473
30. Wang R, Zhang L, Yin D, Mufson RA, Shi Y (1998) Protein kinase C regulating Fas (CD95/APO-1) expression. J Immunol 161:2201–2207
31. Esser MT, Dinglasan RD, Krishnamurthy B, Gullo CA, Graham MB, Braciale VL (1997) IL-2 induces Fas ligand/Fas (CD95L/CD95) cytotoxicity in CD8+ and CD4+ T lymphocytes clones. J Immunol 158:5612–5618
32. Fuss IJ, Strober W, Dale JK, et al (1997) Characteristic T helper 2 T cell cytokine abnormalities in autoimmune lymphoproliferative syndrome, a syndrome marked by defective apoptosis and hunoral autoimmunity. J Immunol 158:1912–1918
33. Cerra FB (1989) Hypermetabolism-organ failure syndrome: A metabolic response to injury. Crit Care Clin 5:289–302
34. Wichterman KA, Baue AE, Chaudry IH (1980) Sepsis and septic shock - A review of laboratory models and a proposal. J Surg Res 29:189–201
35. Chaudry IH, Ayala A, Singh G, Wang P, Hauptman JG (1993) Rodent models of endotoxemia and sepsis. In: Schlag G, Redl H (eds) Pathophysiology of shock, sepsis and organ failure. Springer-Verlag, Berlin, pp 1048–1059
36. Waage A, Brandtzaeg P, Halstensen A, Kierulf P, Espevik T (1989) The complex pattern of cytokines in serum from patients with meningococcal septic shock. Association between interleukin 6, interleukin 1, and fatal outcome. J Exp Med 169:333–338
37. Damas P, Reuter A, Gysen P, Demonty J, Lamy M, Franchimont P (1989) Tumor necrosis factor and interleukin-1 serum levels during severe sepsis in humans. Crit Care Med 17: 975–978

38. Maier RV (1993) The "angry" macrophage and its impact on host response mechanisms. In: Faist E, Meakins J, Schildberg FW (eds) Host defense dysfunction in trauma, shock and sepsis. Springer-Verlag, Berlin, pp 191–197
39. Ayala A, Perrin MM, Kisala JM, Ertel W, Chaudry IH (1992) Polymicrobial sepsis selectively activates peritoneal but not alveolar macrophage to release inflammatory mediators (IL-1, IL-6 and TNF). Circ Shock 36:191–199
40. Ayala A, Knotts JB, Ertel W, Perrin MM, Morrison MH, Chaudry IH (1993) Role of interleukin 6 and transforming growth factor-beta in the induction of depressed splenocyte responses following sepsis. Arch Surg 128:89–95
41. Munoz C, Carlet J, Fitting C, Misset B, Bleriot J, Cavaillon J (1991) Dysregulation of in vitro cytokine production by monocytes during sepsis. J Clin Invest 88:1747–1754
42. Ayala A, Deol ZK, Lehman DL, Herdon CD, Chaudry IH (1994) Polymicrobial sepsis but not low dose endotoxin infusion causes decreased splenocyte IL-2/IFN-gamma release while increasing IL-4/IL-10 production. J Surg Res 56:579–585
43. Ayala A, Kisala JM, Felt JA, Perrin MM, Chaudry IH (1992) Does endotoxin tolerance prevent the release of inflammatory monokines (IL-1, IL-6, or TNF) during sepsis? Arch Surg 127: 191–197
44. Ertel W, Morrison MH, Wang P, Ba ZF, Ayala A, Chaudry IH (1991) The complex pattern of cytokines in sepsis - Association between prostaglandins, cachectin and interleukins. Ann Surg 214:141–148
45. Hadjiminas DJ, McMasters KM, Peyton JC, Cook MD, Cheadle WG (1994) Passive immunization against tumor necrosis factor and interleukin-1 fails to reduce lung neutrophil sequestration in chronic sepsis. Shock 2:376–380
46. Song GY, Chung CS, Schwacha MG, Jarrar D, Chaudry IH, Ayala A (1999) Splenic immune suppression in sepsis: a role for IL-10 induced changes in P38 MAPK signaling. J Surg Res 83:36–43
47. Mathison JC, Virca GD, Wolfson E, Tobias PS, Glaser K, Ulevitch RJ (1990) Adaptation to bacterial lipopolysaccharide controls lipopolysaccharide-induced tumor necrosis factor production in rabbit macrophages. J Clin Invest 85:1108–1118
48. Ayala A, Deol ZK, Lehman DL, Herdon CD, Chaudry IH (1995) Does endotoxin play a major role in inducing the depression of macrophage function during polymicrobial sepsis? Arch Surg 130:1178–1185
49. Song GY, Chung CS, Chaudry IH, Ayala A (1998) Does necrotic tissue depress cell-mediated immune function in polymicrobial sepsis? Surg Forum 49:22–23
50. McMasters KM, Peyton JC, Hadjiminas DJ, Cheadle WG (1994) Endotoxin and tumour necrosis factor do not cause mortality from caecal ligation and puncture. Cytokine 6:530–536
51. Zellweger R, Ayala A, Zhu X, Morrison MH, Chaudry IH (1995) Effect of surgical trauma on splenocyte and peritoneal macrophage immune function. J Trauma 39:645–650
52. Ayala A, Lehman DL, Herdon CD, Chaudry IH (1994) Mechanism of enhanced susceptibility to sepsis following hemorrhage. Arch Surg 129:1172–1178
53. O'Sullivan ST, Lederer JA, Horgan AF, Chin DHL, Mannick JA, Rodrick ML (1995) Major injury leads to predominance of the T helper-2 lymphocyte phenotype and diminished interleukin-12 production associated with decreased resistance to infection. Ann Surg 222: 482–492
54. Okusawa S, Gelfand JA, Ikejima T, Connolly RJ, Dinarello CA (1988) Interleukin-1 induces a shock like state in rabbits. Synergism with tumor necrosis factor and the effects of cyclooxygenase inhibition. J Clin Invest 81:1162–1172
55. Sherry B, Cerami A (1988) Mini-Review. Cachectin/TNF exerts endocrine, paracrine, and autocrine control of inflammatory responses. J Cell Biol 107:1269–1277
56. Eskandari MK, Bolgos G, Miller C, Nguyen DT, DeForge LE, Remick DG (1992) Anti-tumor necrosis factor antibody therapy fails to prevent lethality after cecal ligation and puncture or endotoxemia. J Immunol 148:2724–2730
57. Schlag G, Redl H (1993) Pathophysiology of shock, sepsis and organ failure. Springer-Verlag, Berlin
58. Hogaboam CM, Steinhauser ML, Schock H, et al (1998) Therapeutic effect of nitric oxide inhibtion during experimental fecal peritonitis: role of interleukin-10 and monocyte chemotactic protein 1. Infect Immun 66:650–655

59. Ertel W, Keel M, Steckholzer U, Ungethüm U, Trentz O (1996) Interleukin-10 attenuates the release of proinflammatory cytokines but depresses splenocyte functions in murine endotoxemia. Arch Surg 131:51–56
60. Song GY, Chung CS, Chaudry IH, Ayala A (1999) What is IL-10's role in polymicrobial sepsis: anti-inflammatory agent or immune suppressant? Surgery (in press)
61. Zisman DA, Kunkel SL, Strieter RM, et al (1997) Anti-interleukin-12 therapy protects mice in lethal endotoxemia but impairs bacterial clearance in murine Escherichia coli peritoneal sepsis. Shock 8:349–356
62. Miller-Graziano CL, Szabo G, Griffey K, Metha B, Kodys K, Catalano D (1991) Role of elevated monocyte transforming growth factor beta (TGF-beta) production in posttrauma immunosuppression. J Clin Immunol 11:95–102
63. Zhou D, Munster A, Winchurch RA (1991) Pathologic concentrations of interleukin 6 inhibit T cell responses via induction of activation of TGF-beta. FASEB J 5:2582–2585
64. Ayala A, O'Neill PJ, Uebele SA, Herdon CD, Chaudry IH (1997) Mechanism of splenic immunosuppression during sepsis: key role of kupffer cell mediators. J Trauma 42:882–888
65. Zellweger R, Wichmann MW, Ayala A, Stein S, DeMaso CM, Chaudry IH (1997) Females in proestrus state maintain splenic immune functions and tolerate sepsis better than males. Crit Care Med 25:106–110
66. Zhang Y, Takahashi K, Jiang G, Kawai M, Fukada M, Yokochi T (1993) *In vivo* induction of apoptosis (programmed cell death) in mouse thymus by administration of lipopolysaccharide. Infect Immun 61:5044–5048
67. Ayala A, Herdon CD, Lehman DL, DeMaso CM, Ayala CA, Chaudry IH (1995) The induction of accelerated thymic programmed cell death during polymicrobial sepsis: Control by corticosteroids but not tumor necrosis factor. Shock 3:259–267
68. Ertel W, Morrison MH, Meldrum DR, Ayala A, Chaudry IH (1992) Ibuprofen restores cellular immunity and decreases susceptibility to sepsis following hemorrhage. J Surg Res 53:55–61
69. Wirth JJ, Kierszenbaum F (1984) Variations in expression of markers by populations of adherent cells from *Trypanosoma cruzi*-infected mice. J Protozol 31:147–151
70. Ayala A, Xu YX, Chung CS, Chaudry IH (1999) Does Fas ligand or endotoxin contribute to thymic apoptosis during polymicrobial sepsis? Shock 11:211–217
71. Wang S-D, Huang K-J, Lin Y-S, Lei H-Y (1994) Sepsis-induced apoptosis of the thymocytes in mice. J Immunol 152:5014–5021
72. Hiramatsu M, Hotchkiss RS, Karl IE, Buchman TG (1997) Cecal ligation and puncture (CLP) induces apoptosis in thymus, spleen, lung, and gut by an endotoxin and TNF-independent pathway. Shock 7:247–253
73. Ayala A, Herdon CD, Lehman DL, Ayala CA, Chaudry IH (1996) Differential induction of apoptosis in lymphoid tissues during sepsis: variation in onset, frequency, and the nature of the mediators. Blood 87:4261–4275
74. Ayala A, Xu YX, Ayala CA, et al (1998) Increased mucosal B-lymphocyte apoptosis during polymicrobial sepsis is a Fas ligand but not an endotoxin mediated process. Blood 91: 1362–1372
75. Kagnoff MF (1993) Immunology of the intestinal tract. Gastroenterology 105:1275–1280
76. Chung CS, Xu YX, Chaudry IH, Ayala A (1998) Sepsis induces increased apoptosis in lamina propria mononuclear cells which is associated with altered cytokine gene expression. J Surg Res 77:63–70
77. Chung CS, Xu YX, Wang W, Chaudry IH, Ayala A (1998) Is Fas ligand or endotoxin responsible for mucosal lymphocyte apoptosis in sepsis? Arch Surg 133:1213–1220
78. Hotchkiss R, Swanson P, Osborne D, Cobb JP, Zollner K, Karl IE (1998) Bcl-2 prevents lymphocyte apoptosis and improves survival in sepsis. Shock 9:A65 (abst)
79. Ayala A, Xu YX, Chung CS, Evans TA, Redmond KM, Chaudry IH (1998) Increased inducible apoptosis in CD4+ T-lymphocytes seen during sepsis: mediation by Fas ligand (FasL) not endotoxin. FASEB J 12:A573 (abst)
80. Castro A, Bemer V, Nobrega A, Coutinho A, Truffa-Bachi P (1998) Administration to mouse of endotoxin from gram-negative bacteria leads to activation and apoptosis of T lymphocytes. Eur J Immunol 28:488–495

81. Oka M, Hirazawa K, Yamamoto K, et al (1996) Induction of fas-mediated apoptosis on circulating lymphocytes by surgical stress. Ann Surg 223:434–440
82. Teodorczyk-Injeyan JA, Cembrzynska-Nowak M, Lalani S, Peters WJ, Mills GB (1995) Immune deficiency following thermal trauma is associated with apoptotic cell death. J Clin Immunol 15:318–328

Trauma Mediators Favor Differentiation of Monocytes to Macrophage Rather Than to Dendritic Cells

C. L. Miller-Graziano, A. K. De, and K. Kodys

Introduction

A monocyte antigen presenting cell (APC) dysfunction after trauma has been repeatedly suggested as being involved in post-injury immunosuppression [1, 2]. Conversely, over-activated 'angry' monocytes/macrophages have been implicated in the systemic inflammatory response syndrome as pivotal producers of exaggerated inflammatory cytokines [3–5]. The post-injury development of increased monocyte production of inflammatory cytokines, like interleukin (IL)-1, IL-8, macrophage inflammatory protein (MIP)-1α, IL-6, and tumor necrosis factor (TNF)-α, parallels depressed monocyte antigen presenting functions and decreased immunostimulatory cytokines, like IL-12 and IL-15. This seems to be a paradox. How can severe trauma simultaneously increase and decrease normal monocyte function? Severe tissue trauma generates substance P leakage from disrupted nerve endings, complement activation products, coagulation system products, platelet activating factor (PAF) production after hypoxia, gut derived endotoxin release, and a variety of other mediators [3–12]. One unifying characteristic of these trauma generated products is their ability to activate monocyte/macrophage inflammatory monokines and monocyte to macrophage differentiation [10–16]. However, recent evidence demonstrates that, unlike lipopolysaccharide (LPS) which activates both pro- and anti-inflammatory monokine gene induction, some of the other trauma-induced mediators have a restricted monocyte activation capacity, preferentially inducing a more restricted set of monocyte pro-inflammatory genes [17–19]. These data are consistent with the hypothesis that trauma-generated mediators, like substance P, complement split products, and immunoglobulin complexes, may disproportionately activate monocyte differentiation toward inflammatory activity, rather APC function.

Dendritic Cells Are the Primary Human APCs

Understanding of monocyte APC function has recently been radically altered with the demonstration that circulating peripheral blood monocytes retain enormous differentiation capacity, allowing development of inflammatory macrophage or dendritic cell APCs, depending on the stimulators present in the microenvironment [20–27]. This plasticity allows monocytes to phagocytose and process systemic antigen, then migrate to marginal areas of the nodes, differentiating to mature dendritic cells [20–27]. These monocyte-derived dendritic cells are both the primary APCs for naive T cell activation and the facilitators of long-term survival of memory T cells [22–29]. It is these monocyte derived dendritic cells, not monocytes, which are currently thought of as the primary human APCs [23–30]. At multiple points, a monocyte differentiating toward a dendritic cell can receive other stimuli and redirect its differentiation toward an inflammatory macrophage [20–23]. Conversely, inflammatory macrophages can convert back to dendritic cells under prolonged and appropriate stimuli [20–26]. Macrophage and unactivated monocytes are poor APCs and only those monocytes which can develop into dendritic cells are optimally effective in complete T cell activation [20–22, 28]. Maturation of peripheral blood monocytes to dendritic cells can be initiated by granulocyte/macrophage-colony stimulating factor (GM-CSF) plus IL-4, followed by antigen stimulation, then TNF-α/IL-1 or other cytokines, in a defined sequence and at particular concentrations [20–22]. Alternatively, peripheral blood monocytes can be induced to mature macrophages in the presence of CSF-1 and LPS with consequent increased production of inflammatory monokines and simultaneous high production of mediators, such as complement components, procoagulant activity, substance P, PAF, etc., which stimulate further macrophage-like differentiation [20–25]. Monocyte produced pro-inflammatory mediators can stimulate additional inflammatory monokine production by autocrine and endocrine methods, further driving monocyte differentiation toward inflammatory macrophages, perpetuating an inflammatory response [25]. Consequently, diverse post-injury mediators can contribute to post-trauma monocyte/macrophage deregulation, loss of APC function, and multiple organ dysfunction syndrome (MODS).

Trauma Generated Mediators Can Influence Differentiation of Monocyte to Macrophage versus Monocyte to Dendritic Cell by Altering the Cytokine Environment and Monocyte Receptor Expression

As monocytes respond to trauma-generated mediators, their receptor expression also changes. Triggering of altered receptors by trauma-generated stimulators can dramatically effect the dendritic cell versus inflammatory macrophage maturation equilibrium [20, 25]. Consequently, trauma-generated mediator-induced alterations of monocyte receptor/ligand expression can also affect the balance between monocyte to dendritic cell versus monocyte to macrophage differentiation. In addition, signaling through some receptors selectively activates pro- or anti-inflammatory monokine production, further altering endogenous monokine regulation [17, 18].

Altered Monocyte Receptor Profile in Trauma

Post-trauma altered monocyte/macrophage receptor expression has often been described in the literature [31–34]. For example, the amelioration of post-trauma monocyte TNF-α production by shedding of the 80 kD TNF-α receptor is massively decreased in trauma patients with dysfunctional monokine production [32].

Patient monocytes expressing increased FcγRI are the primary producers of aberrant membrane associated TNF-α, excessive IL-6, increased transforming growth factor (TGF)-β and prostaglandin (PG) E2. Our laboratory originally interpreted these data as indicating post-trauma development of a unique inflammatory monocyte subset [33]. Other investigators also suggested that expansion of a unique $Fc\gamma R^+$ subset was pivotal in post-trauma monocyte dysfunction [34]. Loss of IL-10 production and increased pro-inflammatory monokine production was also a hallmark of this monocyte subset [34]. However, these data are also consistent with a shift in the patient's post-trauma monocyte population toward a macrophage predominant population rather than development of a unique post-trauma monocyte subset.

Receptor Profile of Inflammatory Macrophage versus Dendritic Cell

Different proportions of monocyte subsets, identified by their unique surface receptor profiles, are frequently associated with inflammatory pathology. For example, expression of the calcium binding complex MRP14/8 distinguishes a monocyte subset appearing only in acute inflammation which produces high levels of TNF-α [35, 36]. MRP14/8 is recognized by the monoclonal antibody 27E10 and thought to represent a monocyte differentiating into a mature inflammatory macrophage, just as expression of CD83 indicates a mature dendritic cell [35, 36]. Similarly, increased expression of CD64 (FcγRI) or CD11b/CD11c (C3bR) is a characteristic of monocytes moving toward a macrophage phenotype and away from a dendritic cell phenotype [22]. Decreased CD64 and CD14 expression concomitant to increased CD1a, HLA DR/DQ, and B7 expression, identifies a monocyte moving toward a dendritic cell phenotype [22]. These receptor expression differences, which represent discrete steps in monocyte maturity toward dendritic cell or macrophage, also generate major monocyte functional capacity differences and are the likely basis for many previously defined monocyte subsets. The poor APC capacity and high inflammatory cytokine production of a predominately $Fc\gamma RI^+$ monocyte population may result from the predominance of differentiated macrophages in the monocyte population and, consequently, a reduced potential to develop dendritic cells [33, 37].

Monocyte Receptor Profile Defines Function

The post-trauma increase in monocytes with inflammatory macrophage-like functions but decreased APC capacity may represent a similar skewing of the circulating monocyte population toward predominantly macrophage function.

Both increased monocyte expression of FcγRI and increased expression of the substance P receptor are occurring post-trauma and could be stimulating aberrant cytokine gene activation and exaggerated macrophage development. We have previously described FcγRI up-regulation on post-trauma monocytes and the potential for FcγR crosslinking *in vivo* after trauma [33]. LPS release induces monocyte IL-6 production. IL-6 plus LPS trigger memory B cells to produce antibodies, flooding the system with circulating Ig, which can aggregate and trigger further monocyte induction of IL-6 and FcγRI up-regulation. An increased FcγR expressing subset in post-surgical patients has also been described [34]. Ig complex infusion is a major model of lung injury, is mediated by excessive alveolar macrophage TNF-α production, and is likely to result from monocyte FcγR crosslinking [38]. A number of investigators have suggested monocyte FcγR crosslinking as pivotal in pathologic inflammation, particularly of the lung [39]. Alveolar macrophages produce high levels of membrane-associated, rather than secreted TNF-α during lung inflammation, suggesting aberrant macrophage activation [40]. FcγR crosslinking is a potential inducer of monocyte TNF-α and also, in contrast to LPS, induces significant amounts of membrane associated TNF-α [32, 41]. Substance P (a neuropeptide released during tissue damage) can activate monocyte TNF-α. These TNF-α stimulated monocytes can produce substance P [11, 42]. Thus, substance P, like FcγRI crosslinking, acts in an autocrine loop to both stimulate inflammatory monokines and to perpetuate its own production for continued macrophage-like differentiation [43]. Substance P stimulates monocytes through both a non-neurokinin receptor and a neurokinin receptor (NK-1R) [11, 15]. NK-1R knockout mice are protected against immune complex induced, TNF-α dependent, lung injury, suggesting that monocyte FcγRI crosslinking and substance P stimulation might cooperatively mediate monocyte TNF-α deregulation [43, 44]. Substance P alone does not induce IL-10 but can only augment LPS induced IL-10, suggesting that substance P is an insufficient activator of inflammatory monokine regulation by monocyte production of IL-10 [42]. FcγR crosslinking of monocytes produces membrane associated TNF-α, is involved in post-trauma monocyte aberrant mediator production, and has been already identified as a selective activator of monocyte function [42–45]. Substance P is involved in pulmonary inflarnmation and is involved in autocrine stimulation of monocytes. It is quite conceivable, therefore, that post-injury increases in these and other selective monocyte activators could disrupt the equilibrium between monocyte to dendritic cell and monocyte to macrophage differentiation.

Trauma generated mediators can induce altered mediator production and deregulation by selectively activating or inhibiting monocytes. They can also alter monocyte surface receptor expression, further perturbing the balance of pro-inflammatory vs anti-inflammatory monocyte functions. The monocyte expression of the substance P receptor is upregulated by LPS and IL-1, making post-trauma monocytes more sensitive to substance P activation [43]. Similarly, expression of the MRP 14/8 calcium binding complex is increased in pulmonary inflammation and signaling through this complex alters macrophage activation prolonging TNF-α production [35, 36]. Expression of CD14 is decreased post-injury by shedding of CD14, and monocyte activation through soluble CD14 appears to differ from monocyte activation through CD14 on monocyte surfaces [46]. Complement split product receptors, like CD11b/CD18 complex (CR3) are up-regulated on post-trauma monocytes and after LPS induction [16]. These CR3 receptors appear to augment CD14-induced monocyte TNF-α production but may do so by more restricted activation pathways [47]. Finally, alteration in the expression and shedding of the TNF-α 80 kD and 60 kD receptors can alter the autocrine stimulation/induction of monocytes that accompanies TNF-α production. A p80 TNF receptor deficiency results in dramatically increased polymorphonuclear leukocyte (PMN) accumulation in the lung, exacerbating p60 TNF receptor-dependent pulmonary inflammation, and significantly increasing TNF-α levels after *in vivo* bacterial challenge (*Micropolyspora faeni*) or LPS stimulation [48–50].

Altered Receptor Expression Parallels Altered Dendritic Cell versus Macrophage Maturation Affecting APC Capacity

The level and type of TNF receptor expressed by monocytes also profoundly influences their immunostimulatory capacity. The ability of peripheral blood monocytes to finally differentiate to fully mature dendritic cells is dependent on their late stimulation by secreted TNF-α through the p60 TNF-α receptor [49]. Migration of dendritic cells to the marginal areas of the nodes and spleen to present peripherally captured and processed antigen to T cells is dependent on their expression of the p80 TNF-α receptor [48]. Reduced monocyte APC capacity in post-injury patients and animal models may be exacerbated by both reduced post-injury levels of secreted TNF-α and reduced TNF-α receptor expression. We are now re-interpreting our patient depressed monocyte APC results as

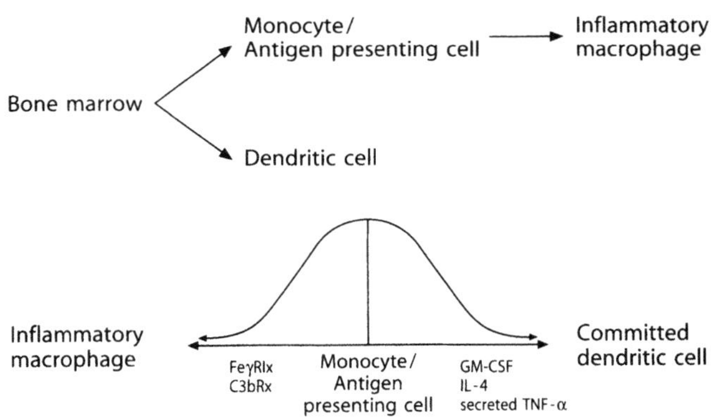

Fig. 1. Dendritic cells can differentiate directly from bone marrow processes or from circulating monocytes. Monocytes stimulated by crosslinking their FcγRI (CD64) receptor or by dimerized complement component 3 are differentiated toward mature macrophage. In contrast, stimulation of monocytes by granulocyte/macrophage-colony stimulating factor (GM-CSF) plus IL-4 favors development of dendritic cells with elevated IL-12 production. Monocyte interaction with Th2 type T cells, therefore, triggers monocyte to dendritic cell differentiation and increased antigen presenting cell activity

indicating that trauma patient monocyte populations have a shifted differentiation capacity favoring activated macrophages. Consequently, this post-trauma peripheral blood monocyte/macrophage population is less able to mature to activated dendritic cells which are the primary APCs in humans [20–25] (Fig. 1). If this hypothesis is valid, then the isolated patient monocyte population should be less able to differentiate to dendritic cells than either normal monocytes or monocytes from trauma patients with normal APCs and inflammatory cytokine levels. These patients' decreased dendritic cell differentiation should also parallel their monocyte receptor changes and functional aberrations.

Trauma Patient Monocytes with Aberrant Cytokine Function and Decreased APC Fail to Develop Into Dendritic Cells

In evaluating the patient monocyte potential to develop dendritic cell antigen presenting activity, it is important to focus primarily on the myeloid derived dendritic cell population. It is now clear that three populations of dendritic cell exist, of which only two are of myeloid origin [21, 51, 52]. These three dendritic cell populations are the myeloid derived Langerhans' cell, the lymphoid derived $CD8\alpha^+$ interdigitating dendritic cell of spleen and thymus, and the monocyte-derived dendritic cell [21, 22, 24, 51, 53, 54]. These three populations have different maturation requirements and different functional activities in the induction of T cell responses [24, 27, 51–54]. All three types of dendritic cell can be generated from bone marrow stem cells [24, 51–54]. The monocyte-derived dendritic cells migrate to nodes and spleen after contact with antigen and are primarily involved in initiating responses to exogenously encountered antigens [22–24, 54]. The lymphoid-derived dendritic cells are primarily involved in responses to endogenously encountered antigens, like viruses and self antigens, and have important immunoregulatory functions [21–24, 54]. A subset of bone marrow-derived dendritic cells migrate to epithelial areas, develop to typical Langerhans' dendritic cells, and are active in contact sensitivity and dermal responses [22, 54]. Different functional activities of these three dendritic cell populations may be responsible for the differences in post-trauma immune functions which are reported for murine splenocyte systems versus human peripheral blood monocyte systems. The murine splenocyte dendritic cell population is 50% lymphoid type [24, 55]. Consequently, the immunoregulatory aspects of lymphoid dendritic cells are emphasized in experiments examining murine splenocyte APC function post-injury.

The maturation requirements for development of the three types of dendritic cell are also different. $CD34^+$ bone marrow precursors can be induced by GM-CSF and TGF-β to differentiate to Langerhans' cell type of dendritic cell [22, 24]. $CD34^+$ differentiation to the lymphoid-derived dendritic cell does not require GM-CSF and these dendritic cells down-regulate T cell responses by Fas mediated killing [24, 55–57]. Peripheral blood monocytes must be induced with GM-CSF plus IL-4/IL-13 to differentiate to immature dendritic cells [20–26]. However, both the Langerhans' cell, and monocyte-derived, dendritic cells must be further stimulated by TNF-α and/or interaction with CD40L$^+$ T cells to become mature APC. Partially mature monocyte-derived dendritic cells immigrate to the lymphoid organs and interact with T cells to maximize their IL-12 production and expression of the T cell co-stimulatory molecule B7.1 and B7.2 [58–60]. Failure to complete these dendritic cell maturation processes can result in dendritic cell differentiation toward inflammatory macrophage or dendritic cell apoptosis [20, 51, 60]. The peripheral blood monocytes provide a pool which can mature toward macrophage or toward dendritic cell [20, 53, 54]. A post-trauma depression of monocyte APC capacity and a depression of IL-12 levels could represent a failure of dendritic cell development. Only dendritic cells can produce IL-12 spontaneously without interferon (IFN)-γ priming [21, 58]. Fully mature dendritic cells lose their ability to produce pro-inflammatory cytokines but retain the ability to produce IL-10 and IL-12 [21, 58]. Inflammatory macrophages are sensitive to IL-10 down-regulation of cytokine production which also down-regulates the inflammatory cytokines which favor monocyte to macrophage differentiation [21–23, 38]. IL-10 can also inhibit initial dendritic cell maturation by inhibiting TNF-α, but has no effect on mature dendritic cell antigen presentation [61]. If maturation of monocyte-derived dendritic cells to mature dendritic cells is prevented so that IL-12 production and co-stimulatory molecules (B7.1/B7.2) are not up-regulated, the immature dendritic cell can anergize rather than activate T cells [23]. Consequently, a trauma patient's monocyte population, which is characterized by reduced secreted TNF-α levels, increased inflammatory receptor levels, and depressed TNF-α receptor expression, would be impaired in its differentiation to mature dendritic cells and enhanced in its maturation toward an inflammatory macrophage.

The receptor expression of monocytes alters as monocytes shift toward dendritic cells or toward macrophages. Up-regulation of CD1a, CD80/86, and HLA-DR is reciprocal to down-regulation of FcγRI, CD14, CD11b (CR3), and CD115 (the CSF-1 receptor). Stimulation of monocytes or DCpl0 through its CD46 receptor, the receptor for complement co-factor 1, by dimerized C3b (complement component 3 split products) results in dramatic depression of both IL-10 and IL-12 production [62, 63]. Since monocyte IL-12 is necessary for IL-10 production by T cells, C3b generated after trauma can simultaneously prevent most IL-12 and IL-10 production, setting the stage for both loss of monocyte APC capacity and loss of endogenous and exogenous inflammatory cytokine control. In addition, monocyte stimulation through FcγRI by circulating Ig aggregates also inhibits dendritic cell and monocyte IL-12 production [39]. Consequently, post-trauma monocytes which express high levels of FcγR, C3R and CD46, can be maximally stimulated by trauma-generated mediators, pushing them toward a terminal differentiation as an inflammatory macrophage, while limiting the normal exogenous and endogenous regulatory mechanisms controlling excessive inflammatory monokine production. Increased expression of some known receptors of inflammatory macrophages, as well as failure to express receptors such as TNF receptor, CD40, and B7.1/B7.2 (CD80/86) which are crucial to dendritic cell APC capacity, should identify a patient monocyte population unable to produce dendritic cells. Simultaneous identification of increased CD46, FcγRI and CD11b/18 should identify patients' monocytes unbalanced toward inflammatory cytokine production.

We have previously published that peripheral blood monocyte TNF receptor expression is depressed in trauma patients with aberrant production of membrane-associated TNF-α [32]. As patient monocytes increase their production of membrane-associated TNF-α, they decrease their production of secreted TNF-α (Table 1) and their production of IL-12 (Table 2). These same patient monocytes

Table 1. TNF-α levels from trauma patients' monocytes

	Median TNF-α levels (ng/10^6 monocytes/ml)[a]	
Groups and Stimuli	Secreted TNF-α	Membrane-Associated TNF-α
Normal controls		
unstim[b]	0.0 (0.0–6.6)	0.0 (0.0–6.5)
+MDP[c]	0.0 (0.0–0.5)	0.0 (0.0–7.2)
+MDP+IFN-γ[d]	4.8 (0.0–167.5)	1.2 (0.0–11.0)
Immunocompetent patients		
unstim	0.0 (0.0–10.3)	1.9 (0.0–234.8)***
+MDP	0.4 (0.0–31.3)*	3.6 (0.0–169.3)***
+MDP+IFN-γ	8.8 (0.0–259.1)*	4.6 (0.0–371.1)***
Immunosuppressed patients		
unstim	0.0 (0.0–0.2)†	16.9 (0.0–578.2)***†††
+MDP	0.0 (0.0–1.9)**††	18.3 (0.0–503.4)***†††
+MDP+IFN-γ	0.4 (0.0–73.0)**††	9.7 (0.0–450.6)***†

Monocyte TNF-α (both secreted and membrane-associated) was determined in a TNF specific LM bioassay.
[a] Values = median (range) of n = 14; TNF measured in: [b] monocytes cultured in medium alone, [c] cultures containing 20 μg/ml muramyl dipeptide (MDP), [d] cultures containing 20 μg/ml MDP + interferon (IFN)-γ.
* $p \leq 0.05$, ** $p \leq 0.005$, *** $p \leq 0.0001$, compared to normals; † $p \leq 0.05$, †† $p \leq 0.005$, ††† $p \leq 0.0001$, compared to immunocompetent patients.

Table 2. Monocyte IL-12 production is depressed concomitant to elevated membrane-associated TNF-α levels

	IL-12 (pg/10^5 monocytes)[a]		sTNF-α/mTNF-α (pg/10^7 monocytes)[b]	
	Normal	Patient	Normal	Patient
Median (n = 11)	435.4	14.3	0.2/0.6	0/28.6
Range	114.2–1968.3	0.0–74.2	0/0–3.8/0	0/16.6–0/241.4

[a] IL-12 level (p70) in the culture supernates of monocytes stimulated with muramyl dipeptide (MDP, 20 μg/ml) + interferon (IFN)-γ (100 U/ml) + staphylococcal enterotoxin B (SEB, 0.5 μg/ml) for 16 hours, were measured by ELISA. [b] secreted TNF-α/membrane-associated TNF-α (sTNF-α/mTNF-α) in the same culture supernate/cell lysate were measured by LM bioassay.

fail *in vitro* to be induced to form dendritic cells under the influence of GM-CSF plus IL-4. Normal monocyte APC activity can be compared to patient APC activity by assessing the isolated monocytes' ability to induce proliferation of allogeneic peripheral blood mononuclear cells in a mixed lymphocyte reaction (MLR). As can be seen in Figure 2b, 4×10^4 normal irradiated monocytes induce a moderate level of proliferation by 2×10^5 third party peripheral blood mononuclear cells. The ability of patients' monocytes producing increased membrane-associated TNF-α but decreased secreted TNF-α to stimulate the same third party MLR is significantly reduced. Almost 100% of normal human monocytes can be converted to dendritic cells after a 6–9 day *in vitro* culture with GM-CSF plus IL-4 or IL-13. However, by approximately three days in culture, the major portion of the monocyte population is committed to the dendritic cell differentiation pathway unless other cytokine signals are received [20, 22, 27].

When we cultured isolated normal monocytes 4–5 days with IL-4 (50 ng/ml) and GM-CSF (50 ng/ml), we differentiated approximately 40–50% of the monocytes to dendritic cells, as determined by their expression of the dendritic cell marker CD1a (Fig. 2a). In addition, these dendritic cells differentiated from monocytes had antigen presenting cell functions in the MLR which were 4–8 fold increased over unstimulated monocytes (Fig. 2b). However, although patient monocytes with aberrant monokine functions (increased membrane-associated TNF-α, decreased secreted TNF-α, and IL-12) also exhibited some increased antigen presenting cell activity in the MLR after *in vitro* culture with IL-4 plus GM-CSF (Fig. 2b), the increase was still dramatically lower than that seen in normal or

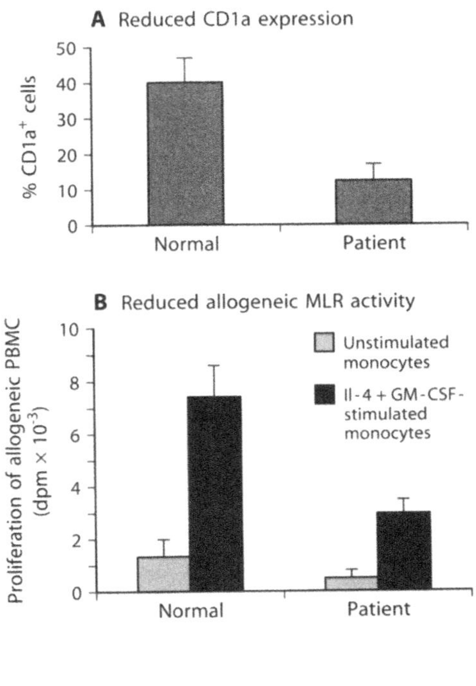

Fig. 2. Normal and patient monocytes were cultured for 4 days in the presence of granulocyte/ macrophage-colony stimulating factor (GM-CSF) (50 ng/ml) + IL-4 (50 ng/ml) and then assessed for (**A**) CD1a expression by flow cytometry and (**B**) mixed lymphocyte reaction (MLR) capacity by culturing these cells (irradiated – 3000 rads) with allogeneic peripheral blood mononuclear cells (PBMC) for 5 days, followed by [^{3}H] TdR incorporation assay

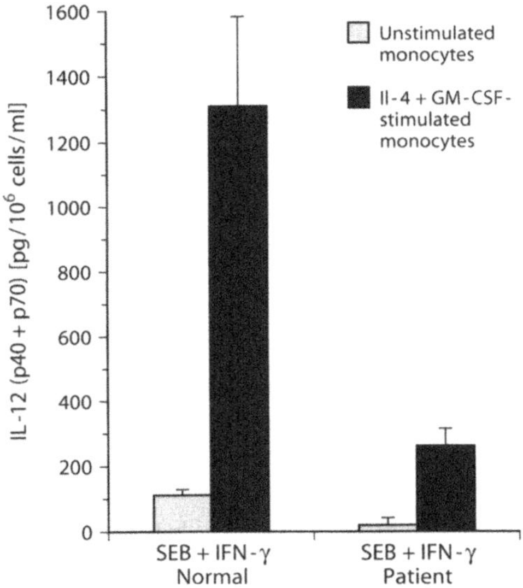

Fig. 3. GM-CSF + IL-4 treated monocytes were then stimulated for 20 hours with staphylococcal enterotoxin B (SEB) (0.5 μg/ml) + IFN-γ (100 U/ml) and assessed for IL-12 (p40 + p70) production by ELISA

patient monocytes with increased secreted TNF-α production (Fig. 2b). The CD1a expression of these patients' monocytes was only 10% compared to >40% in normals (Fig. 2a). Similarly, differentiation of normal monocytes to dendritic cell by GM-CSF plus IL-4 increased their level of IL-12 production by 15 fold (Fig. 3). Although patient monocytes cultured with GM-CSF and IL-4 somewhat increased their IL-12 levels, IL-12 production was still dramatically reduced from that of normal dendritic cells (Fig. 3).

Possible Mechanisms of Diminished Post-Trauma Monocyte to Dendritic Cell Differentiation

A simple explanation for diminished differentiation of patient monocytes to dendritic cells is that either GM-CSF receptor or IL-4 receptor expression is insufficient on these patients' monocyte surfaces. We have previously published that IL-4 can down-regulate patients' aberrant TNF-α and IL-6 production, suggesting they have adequate IL-4 receptor levels [64]. However, to definitively determine if GM-CSF or IL-4 receptor levels were depressed on these patients' monocytes, patient and normal monocyte IL-4 receptor and GM-CSF receptor levels were compared using flow cytometric analysis. As seen in Figure 4, neither patient monocyte GM-CSF receptor nor their IL-4 receptor levels were reduced as compared to normals.

An additional possible explanation for the failure of patient monocytes to convert to dendritic cells might be early production of IL-10. Although mature dendritic cells are resistant to IL-10 effects, early excessive IL-10 can diminish the

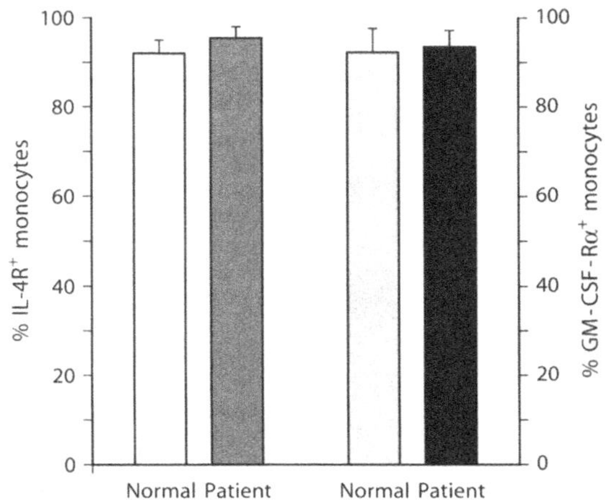

Fig. 4. Expression of IL-4R or GM-CSF-Rα on normal and patient monocytes was assessed by flow cytometry by staining the cells (5×10^5) with α-IL-4R or α-GM-CSF-Rα mAb, respectively, followed by incubation with goat anti-mouse-fluorescein isothyocyanate (FITC)

maturation of dendritic cells by diminishing their endogenous secreted TNF-α production or by inducing TNF receptor shedding, thereby reducing the secreted TNF-α signaling required for dendritic cell maturation [61]. $CD33^+$ monocytes in patients and normals were compared for intracellular IL-10 levels stimulated 8 hours with muramyl dipeptide (MDP). As can be seen in Figure 5, patient monocyte IL-10 levels were depressed, not elevated, at isolation. We then compared patient and normal monocyte IL-10 levels after four days culture with GM-CSF plus IL-4. Similar to the IL-12 results, patient monocyte/dendritic cell IL-10 levels were significantly lower than normal monocyte IL-10 levels (Fig. 6). These data do not support exaggerated monocyte IL-10 production as a mechanism behind decreased monocyte to dendritic cell differentiation in patients with aberrant monocyte function.

Another mechanism which might account for the differences in monocyte to dendritic cell differentiation between normals and patients could be highly increased monocyte apoptosis. Monocytes which partially differentiate toward dendritic cells but fail to receive complete signaling for dendritic cell maturation undergo apoptosis [51, 60]. We assessed the level of apoptosis in IL-4 plus GM-CSF treated (2 days) monocytes using propidium iodide staining. There was a slight increase in apoptosis of patient monocytes. It is possible that the apoptosis levels became progressively greater over time but the slight difference in early apoptosis levels (3.2% vs 6.5%) did not account for the greater than four fold difference between normal and patient dendritic cell differentiation.

It has been shown that activation through the p38 signaling cascade is required for GM-CSF and IL-4-induced differentiation of monocytes to dendritic cells [65]. Consequently, if patient monocytes have a reduction/blockade in p38 cascade signaling components, their dendritic cell differentiation would be depressed. In preliminary experiments, the kinase activity of the p38 substrate mitogen-activated protein kinase activated protein kinase-2 (MAPKAPK-2) was depressed (Fig. 7) in patient monocytes as compared to normal monocytes. These

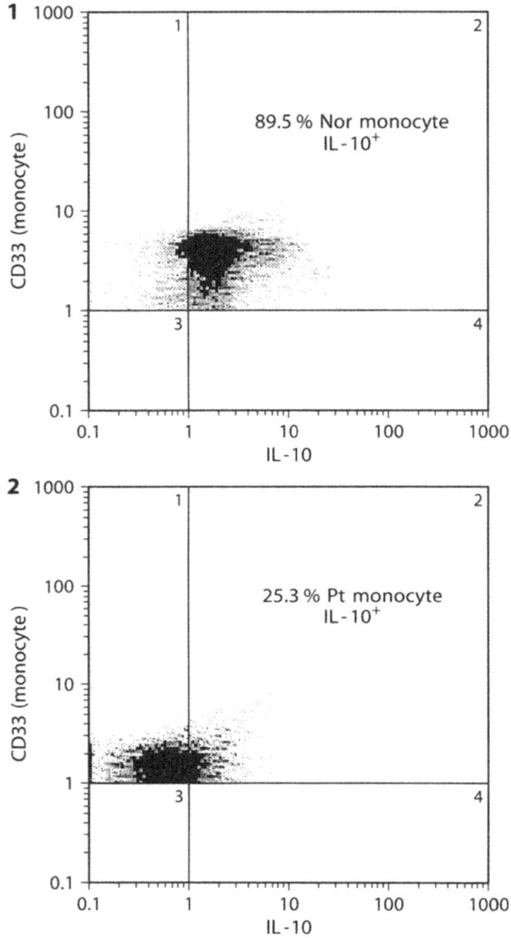

Fig. 5. Flow cytometric analysis of muramyl dipeptide (MDP) stimulated monocytes stained with CD33 prior to fixation and permeablization, followed by intracellular cytokine staining using α-IL-10. Histograms 1 (normal control [nor]) and 2 (patient [pt]) were gated on $CD33^+$ cells. The % dual positive cells for the normal was 89.5% **(Hist. 1)** while patient was 25.3% **(Hist. 2)**

data suggest that monocyte to dendritic cell differentiation is depressed in post-trauma patients while inflammatory macrophage development is favored.

Conclusion

In summary, the three part maturation of peripheral blood monocyte to dendritic cell first requires down-regulation of inflammatory mediator-inducing receptors, like CD14 and FcγRI, by a Th2 type lymphokine, like IL-4 or IL- 13, plus GM-CSF to maintain monocyte viability and differentiation capacity [20–22, 26, 27]. These monocyte-derived dendritic cells then need further stimulation by secreted TNF-α and interaction with antigen to trigger up-regulation of major histo-

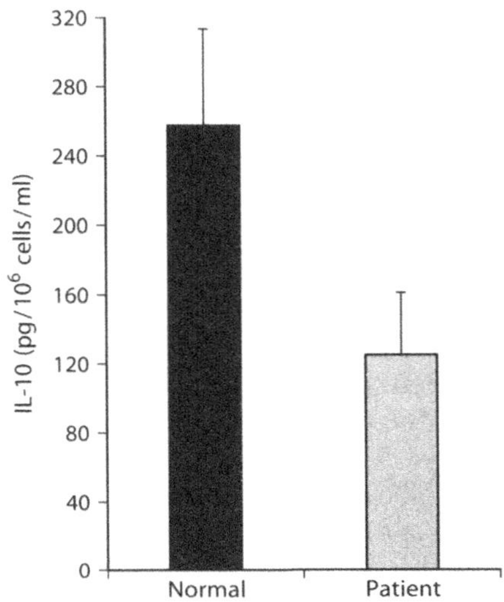

Fig. 6. Normal and patient monocytes were cultured for 4 days in presence of GM-CSF (50 ng/ml) + IL-4 (50 ng/ml) and the culture supernates were assessed for IL-10 by ELISA

compatibility complex (MHC) surface expression and migration to lymphoid organs [21, 66]. If monocytes are induced by LPS and/or complement components like C3b, FcγRI is up-regulated and maturation toward inflammatory macrophages is signaled. Consequently, our data showing retention of FcγRI on patient monocytes which make membrane-associated TNF-α but no secreted TNF-α

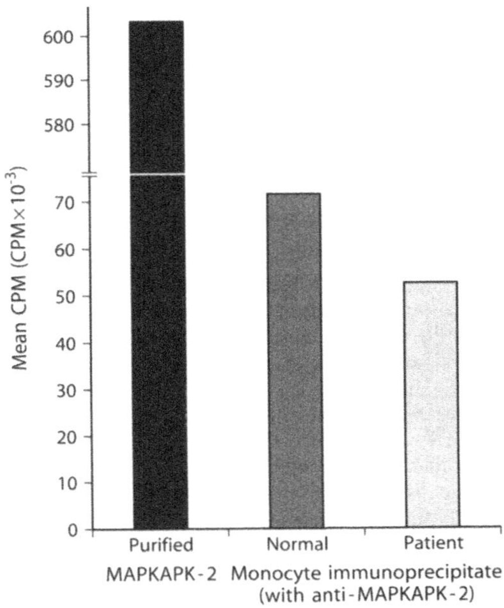

Fig. 7. Normal and patient monocytes (1.5×10^6 cells) were activated for 12 minutes with muramyl dipeptide (MDP, 20 μg/ml) and then lysed with 1% NP-40 lysis buffer. The lysates were immunoprecipitated with anti-mitogen-activated protein kinase activated protein kinase (MAPKAPK)-2 antibody and then the kinase activity of the immunoprecipitate was assessed using a specific substrate and [^{32}P] ATP. The incorporation of [^{32}P] ATP to the substrate was measured by transferring the reaction mixture to phosphocellulose paper and counted by liquid scintillation. CPM: counts per minute

and have a depressed expression of the TNF receptor, indicate a predominance of more macrophage-like differentiation and indicate that these post-trauma monocytes have reduced potential for dendritic cell activity [32, 33]. In addition, we have directly demonstrated that patient monocytes which have exaggerated inflammatory monokine activity have concomitantly depressed conversion to dendritic cells under the influence of IL-4 plus GM-CSF. This diminished capacity of post-trauma monocytes to differentiate to dendritic cells is correlated to post-trauma depressed APC function and decreased IL-12 production. The failure of the post-trauma monocytes to convert to dendritic cells is not a function of monocyte immaturity, since immature monocytes are more easily converted to dendritic cells. Nor is their diminished capacity to differentiate to dendritic cells due to decreased expression of GM-CSF receptor or IL-4 receptor or increased IL-10 production. Our data do not yet discriminate between two other possibilities. The post-trauma inflammatory monocyte population may consist of a disproportionate number of differentiated macrophages which could be converted to dendritic cells if their stimulation with dendritic cell inducing cytokines (GM-CSF/IL-4) was prolonged and their apoptosis prevented. Alternatively, the depression of MAPKAPK-2 activation in these monocytes may represent a block in the p38 signal transduction pathway similar to that seen in anergic T cells, which would require circumvention by alternate cytokine signaling rather than just continued classic cytokine signaling in order to allow activation of these monocytes' dendritic cell gene repertoire. Whatever the underlying mechanism, the depressed APC capacity of post-trauma monocytes concomitant to their increased inflammatory activity and aberrant cytokine regulation is linked to their reduced capacity to differentiate to dendritic cells and an increased potential to become terminally differentiated angry macrophages.

Acknowledgment. This work was supported by Public Health Service Grant #GM36214-13. Its contents are solely the responsibility of the authors and do not necessarily represent the official views of the National Institutes of Health. We thank Laura Orphin for her excellent technical assistance.

References

1. Ayala A, Ertel W, Chaudry IH (1996) Trauma-induced suppression of antigen presentation and expression of major histocompatibility class II antigen complex in leukocytes. Shock 5:79–90
2. Miller-Graziano CL, Szabo G, Takayama T, Wu JY (1989) Alterations of monocyte function following major injury. In: Faist E, Ninnemann JL, Green D (eds) Immune consequences of trauma, shock and sepsis. Springer, Berlin, pp 95–109
3. Waxman K (1996) Shock: Ischemia, reperfusion and inflammation. New Horiz 4:153–160
4. Eigler A, Sinha B, Hartmann G, Endres S (1997) Taming TNF: Strategies to restrain this proinflammatory cytokine. Immunol Today 18:487–492
5. See RH, Chow AW (1992) Role of the adhesion molecule lymphocyte function associated antigen 1 in toxic shock syndrome toxin l-induced tumor necrosis factor alpha and interleukin-1b secretion by human monocytes. Infect Immun 60:4957–4960
6. Pasquale MD, Cipolle MD, Monaco J, Simon N (1996) Early inflammatory response correlates with the severity of injury. Crit Care Med 24:1238–1242

7. Kelly JL, O'Sullivan C, O'Riordain M, et al (1997) Is circulating endotoxin the trigger for the systemic inflammatory response syndrome seen after injury? Ann Surg 225:530–543
8. McBride WT, Armstrong MA, Gilliland H, McMurray TJ (1996) The balance of pro and anti inflammatory cytokines in plasma and bronchoalveolar lavage (BAL) at pediatric cardiac surgery. Cytokine 8:724–729
9. Armstrong L, Millar AB (1997) Relative production of tumor necrosis factor-α and interleukin 10 in adult respiratory distress syndrome. Thorax 52:442–446
10. Saban MR, Saban R, Bjorling D, Haak-Frendscho M (1997) Involvement of leukotrienes, TNF-α, and the LFA-1/ICAM-1 interaction in substance P-induced granulocyte infiltration. J Leukoc Biol 61:445–451
11. Ho WZ, Lai JP, Zhu XH, Uvaydova M, Douglas SD (1997) Human monocytes and macrophages express substance P and neurokinin-1 receptor. J Immunol 159:5654–5660
12. Ayala A, Chaudry IH (1996) Platelet activating factor and its role in trauma, shock, and sepsis. New Horiz 4:265–275
13. Im SY, Han SJ, Ko HM, et al (1997) Involvement of nuclear factor-κB in platelet activating factor-mediated tumor necrosis factor-α expression. Eur J Immunol 27:2800–2804
14. Lo CJ, Cryer HG, Fu MJ, Kim B (1997) Endotoxin-induced macrophage gene expression depends on platelet-activating factor. Arch Surg 132:1342–1347
15. Jeurissen F, Kavelaars A, Korstjens M, et al (1994) Monocytes express a non-neurokinin substance P receptor that is functionally coupled to MAP kinase. J Immunol 152:2987–2994
16. Dries DJ (1996) Activation of the clotting system and complement after trauma. New Horiz 4:276–288
17. Duchemin AM, Anderson CL (1997) Association of non-receptor protein tyrosine kinases with the FcγRI/γ-chain complex in monocytic cells. J Immunol 158:865–871
18. Rose DM, Winston BW, Chan ED, et al (1997) Fcγ receptor cross-linking activates p42, p38, and JNK/SAPK mitogen-activated protein kinases in murine macrophages. Role for $p42^{MAPK}$ in Fcγ receptor stimulated TNF-α synthesis. J Immunol 158:3433–3438
19. Sanghera JS, Weinstein SL, Aluwalia M, Girn J, Pelech SL (1996) Activation of multiple proline-directed kinases by bacterial lipopolysaccharide in murine macrophages. J Immunol 156:4457–4465
20. Palucka KA, Taquet N, Sanchez-Chapuis F, Gluckman JC (1998) Dendritic cells as the terminal stage of monocyte differentiation. J Immunol 160:4587–4595
21. Shortman K, Maraskovsky E (1998) Developmental options. Science 282:424–425
22. Hart DNJ (1997) Dendritic cells: Unique leukocyte populations which control the primary immune response. Blood 90:3245–3287
23. Rescigno M, Winzler C, Delia D, Multini C, Lutz M, Ricciardi-Castagnoli P (1997) Dendritic cell maturation is required for initiation of the immune response. J Leukoc Biol 61:415–421
24. Schuler G, Thurner B, Romani N (1997) Dendritic cells: From ignored cells to major players in T-cell mediated immunity. Int Arch Allergy Immunol 112:317–322
25. Hausser G, Ludewig B, Gelderblom HR, Tsunetsugu-Yokota Y, Akagawa K, Meyerhans A (1997) Monocyte-derived dendritic cells represent a transient stage of differentiation in the myeloid lineage. Immunobiol 197:534–542
26. Morse MA, Zhou LJ, Tedder TF, Lyerly HK, Smith C (1997) Generation of dendritic cells *in vitro* from peripheral blood mononuclear cells with granulocyte/macrophage-colony stimulating factor, interleukin-4 and tumor necrosis factor-α for use in cancer immunotherapy. Ann Surg 226:6–16
27. Chapuis F, Rosenzwajg M, Yagello M, Ekman M, Biberfeld P, Gluckman JC (1997) Differentiation of human dendritic cells from monocytes *in vitro*. Eur J Immunol 27:431 -441
28. Pettit AR, Quinn C, MacDonald KPA, et al (1997) Nuclear localization of RelB is associated with effective antigen-presenting cell function. J Immunol 159:3681–3691
29. Brocker T (1997) Survival of mature CD4 T lymphocytes is dependent on major histocompatibility complex class-II-expressing dendritic cells. J Exp Med 186:1223–1232
30. De Becker G, Moulin V, Van Mechelen M, et al (1997) Dendritic cells and macrophages induce the development of distinct T helper cell populations *in vivo*. Adv Exp Med Biol 417:369–373
31. Gebhard F, Rösch M, Helm M, et al (1997) Is the activity of soluble CD14 enhanced following major trauma? Arch Surg 132:1116–1120

32. Pellegrini JD, Puyana JC, Lapchak P, Kodys K, Miller-Graziano CL (1996) A membrane TNFα/TNFR ratio correlates to MOD score and mortality. Shock 6:389–396
33. Miller-Graziano CL, Szabo G, Kodys K, Griffey K (1990) Aberrations in post-trauma monocyte populations: Role in septic shock syndrome. J Trauma 30 (suppl 12):S86–S97
34. Ziegler-Heitbrock HWL (1996) Heterogeneity of human blood monocytes: the CD14+CD16+ subpopulation. Immunol Today 17:424–428
35. Lugering N, Kucharzik T, Lugering A, et al (1997) Importance of combined treatment with IL-10 and IL-4, but not IL-13, for inhibition of monocyte release of the Ca^{2+} binding protein MRP8/14. Immunology 91:130–134
36. Roth J, Teigelkamp ST, Wilke M, Grun L, Tummler B, Sorg C (1992) Complex pattern of the myelomonocytic differentiation antigens MRP8 and MRP14 during chronic airway inflammation. Immunobiol 186:304–314
37. Grage-Griebenow E, Flad HD, Ernst M (1996) Fcγ receptor 1 (CD64)-negative human monocytes are potent accessory cells in viral antigen-induced T cell activation and exhibit high IFN-γ producing capacity. J Leuk Biol 60:389–396
38. Lentsch AB, Shanley TP, Sarma V, Ward PA (1997) In vivo suppression of NF-κB and preservation of IκBα by interleukin-10 and interleukin-13. J Clin Invest 100:2443–2448
39. Bayon Y, Alonso A, Crespo MS (1997) Stimulation of Fcγ receptor in rat peritoneal macrophages induces the expression of nitric oxide synthase and chemokines by mechanisms showing different sensitivities to antioxidants and nitric oxide donors. J Immunol 159: 887–894
40. Agostini C, Zambello R, Trentin L, et al (1995) Expression of TNF receptors by T cells and membrane TNF-α by alveolar macrophages suggests a role for TNF-α in regulation of the local immune response in the lung of HIV-1 infected patients. J Immunol 154:2928–2938
41. Szabo G, Miller-Graziano CL, Wu JY, Takayama T, Kodys K (1990) Differential tumor necrosis factor production by human monocyte subsets. J Leukoc Biol 47:206–216
42. Ho WZ, Kaufman D, Uvaydova M, Douglas SD (1996) Substance P augments interleukin-10 and tumor necrosis factor-α release by human cord blood monocytes and macrophages. J Neuroimmunol 71:73–80
43. Bost KL (1995) Quantification of macrophage-derived substance P receptor mRNA using competitive polymerase chain reaction. In: Sharp B (ed) The brain: Immune axis and substance abuse. Plenum press, New York, pp 219–223
44. Bozic CR, Lu B, Hopken UE, Gerard C, Gerard N (1996) Neurogenic amplification of immune complex inflammation. Science 272:1722–1724
45. Durden DL, Kim HM, Calore B, Liu Y (1995) The FcγRI receptor signals through the activation of *hck* and MAP kinase. J Immunol 154:4039–4047
46. Blondin C, Dur AL, Cholley B, Caroff M, Haeffner-Cavaillon N (1997) Lipopolysaccharide complexed with soluble CD14 binds to normal human monocytes. Eur J Immunol 156: 430–433
47. Zarewych DM, Kindzelskii AL, Todd RF III, Petty HR (1996) LPS induces CD14 association with complement receptor type 3, which is reversed by neutrophil adhesion. J Immunol 156:430–433
48. Wang B, Fujisawa H, Zhuang L, et al (1997) Depressed Langerhan's cell migration and reduced contact hypersensitivity response in mice lacking TNFG receptor p75. J Immunol 159:6148–6155
49. Peschon JJ, Torrance DS, Stocking KL, et al (1998) TNF receptor-deficient mice reveal divergent roles for p55 and p75 in several models of inflammation. J Immunol 160:943–952
50. Le Hir M, Bluethmann H, Kosco-Vilbois MH, et al (1996) Differentiation of follicular dendritic cells and full antibody responses require tumor necrosis factor receptor-1 signaling. J Exp Med 183:2326–2372
51. Vremec D, Shortman K (1997) Dendritic cell subtypes in mouse lymphoid organs. Cross-correlation of surface markers, changes with incubation, and differences among thymus, spleen and lymph nodes. J Immunol 159:565–573
52. Kronin V, Süss G, Winkel K, Shortman K (1997) The regulation of T cell responses by a subpopulation of $CD8^{+}DEC205^{+}$ murine dendritic cells. Adv Exp Med Biol 417:239–248

53. Triozzi PL, Aldrich W (1997) Phenotypic and functional differences between human dendritic cells derived in vitro from hematopoietic progenitors and from monocytes/macrophages. J Leukoc Biol 61:600-608
54. Salomon B, Cohen JL, Masurier C, Klatzmann D (1998) Three populations of mouse lymph node dendritic cells with different origins and dynamics. J Immunol 160:708-711
55. Winkel KD, Kronin V, Krummel MF, Shortman K (1997) The nature of the signals regulating CD8 T cell proliferative responses to $DC8\alpha^+$ or $CD8\alpha^-$ dendritic cells. Eur J Immunol 27: 3350-3359
56. Josien R, Heslan M, Soulillou JP, Cuturi MC (1997) Rat spleen dendritic cells express natural killer cell receptor protein 1 (NKR-P1) and have cytotoxic activity to select targets via Ca^{2+}-dependent mechanism. J Exp Med 186:467-472
57. Lu L, Qian S, Hershberger P, et al (1997) Blocking of the B7-CD28 pathway increases apoptosis induced in activated T cells by in vitro-generated CD95L (FasL) positive dendritic cells. Transplant Proc 29:1094-1095
58. Sousa CRE, Hieny S, Scharton-Kersten T, et al (1997) In vivo microbial stimulation induces rapid CD40 ligand-independent production of interleukin 12 by dendritic cells and their redistribution to T cell areas. J Exp Med 186:1819-1829
59. McLellan AD, Sorg RV, Fearnley DB, et al (1997) T lymphocyte mediated regulation of costimulator molecule expression on human dendritic cells. Adv Exp Med Biol 417:203-206
60. Bjorck P, Banchereau J, Flores-Romo L (1997) C ligation counteracts Fas-induced apoptosis of human dendritic cells. Int Immunol 9:365-372
61. Schuler G, Romani N (1997) Generation of mature dendritic cells trom human blood - An improved method with special regard to clinical applicability. Adv Exp Med Biol 417:7-13
62. Wong TC, Yant S, Harder BJ, Korte-Sarfaty J, Hirano A (1997) The cytoplasmic domains of complement regulatory protein CD46 interact with multiple kinases in macrophages. J Leukoc Biol 62:892-900
63. Bhardwaj N (1997) Interactions of viruses with dendritic cells: A double-edged sword. J Exp Med 186:795-799
64. Szabo G, Kodys K, Miller-Graziano CL (1991) Elevated monocyte interleukin-6 (IL-6) production in immunsuppressed trauma patients. II. Down regulation by IL-4. J Clin Immunol 11:336-344
65. Arrighi JF, Tropia L, Kindler V, Hausser C (1998) Involvement of p38 MAP kinase in the maturation of human blood-derived dendritic cells. J Interferon Cytokine Res 18:119 (abst)
66. Watts C (1997) Inside the gearbox of the dendritic cell. Nature 388:724-725

Programmed Cell Death (Apoptosis) and the Immunologic Derangements of Critical Illness

R. Taneja, L. Yue, and J. C. Marshall

Introduction

Infection poses a formidable challenge to multicellular organisms. To respond effectively, the host must be able to expand and mobilize a population of effector cells, and accurately direct these to the site of infectious challenge. Here these cells must become activated to contend with the invading pathogen, and further must provide the necessary signals to permit the expansion of antigen-specific immune cells to eliminate the invading organism, and to provide immunity against further challenges in the future. Finally they must regress to a state of resting quiescence, so that normal physiologic homeostasis is restored. Derangements in any component of this complex process can result in disease, rendering the host more vulnerable to the invading pathogen, if the defect involves the activation of a response, or to the injurious effects of the response itself, if the derangement affects its resolution.

Much attention has been focussed on the cellular processes responsible for mobilizing an effective response to an external threat. Until quite recently, those involved in the restoration of normal immune homeostasis have received relatively scant attention. With a heightened recognition that the sequelae of inflammation arise from the response of the host, rather than from the direct cytopathic effects of the invading organism, this situation is changing. Cell populations expand through the controlled division of cells to form two daughter cells. Conversely, they contract under physiologic circumstances through a process of controlled programmed cell death, or apoptosis.

Apoptosis: An Overview

The word 'apoptosis' (pronounced a-puh-*toe*-sis) was first used by Hippocrates more than 2000 years ago in a treatise on the reduction of dislocations (ΜΟΧΛΙΚΟΝ) to describe the structural changes of bone erosion occurring in tissue and cell death [1]. It subsequently found use in a social and political context as a synonym for failure, ruin, decline, and decadence. The term was resurrected in the early 1970s to describe a form of cell death seen primarily during vertebrate ontogeny that was morphologically distinct from necrosis [2, 3]. Over the past decade, appreciation of the fundamental importance of this basic physiologic

Fig. 1. Citations in Index Medicus using the word 'apoptosis', 1990–1997

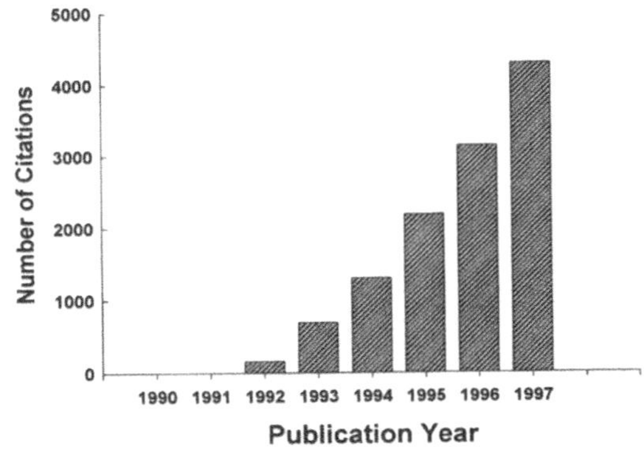

process to normal growth and development has mushroomed, reflected in a massive increase in publications in the scientific literature (Fig. 1). Whereas Index Medicus cited only three publications using the keyword, 'apoptosis' in 1991, by 1997, that number had ballooned to more than 4000.

Apoptosis is the physiologic process through which tissue remodeling occurs during embryogenesis, resulting, for example, in the formation of the interdigital web spaces [4]. In the adult, it is the process underlying the turnover of epithelial cells of the skin and gastrointestinal tracts; apoptosis of the endometrium results in menstruation. Apoptosis is critical to normal immunity. It is the mechanism through which inflammatory cells such as neutrophils are removed from the circulation, and is responsible for the selective deletion of T cells directed against self antigen. Abnormal expression of apoptosis underlies the pathogenesis of a wide variety of disease processes including acquired immunodeficiency syndrome (AIDS) [5], neurodegenerative disorders [6], and autoimmunity [7].

Pathways to Cell Death: Apoptosis and Necrosis

Although each results in the ultimate death of the cell, the processes of necrosis and apoptosis are fundamentally different, both morphologically and biochemically [8]. Pathologic cell death or necrosis is readily evident in tissue sections. It is characterized by cellular swelling, dilatation of mitochondria and injury to other organelles. Disruption of the cell membrane is an early event, while nuclear changes are unremarkable. Loss of membrane integrity results in spillage of cytoplasmic constituents into the local microenvironment, evoking an inflammatory response. Necrosis is a passive process that typically follows direct cellular injury or the inhibition of oxidative phosphorylation.

In contrast, apoptosis is an active process that requires energy to proceed. The apoptotic cell shrinks, and its nuclear chromatin condenses into a characteristic crescent shape; chromatin condensation is followed by nuclear fragmentation into discrete membrane-bound apoptotic bodies (Fig. 2). Key cytostructural and reparative proteins are degraded by the action of pro-apoptotic enzymes, and the

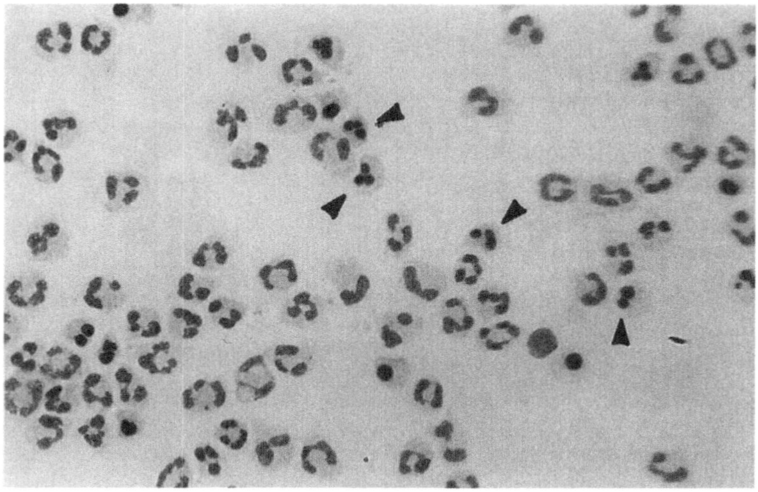

Fig. 2. Morphologic features of apoptosis. The apoptotic neutrophil shows chromatin condensation, and contraction of nuclear contents into discrete membrane bound bodies (arrows)

cytoplasm becomes vacuolated. The cell membrane, however, remains intact with the result that no inflammatory response is elicited. Translocation of phosphatidyl serine residues from the inner to the outer layers of the cell membrane mark the apoptotic cell for phagocytosis by fixed tissue macrophages [9]. The entire sequence of events proceeds rapidly and efficiently, with the result that apoptosis is rarely evident in fixed tissue sections, but instead is more readily identified by the detection of some of its key biochemical events. Nuclear fragmentation, for example, can be seen by DNA gel electrophoresis as a characteristic ladder pattern of DNA fragmentation into fragments that are multiples of 180 base pairs. The nuclear changes of apoptosis can be detected by flow cytometry as the intercalation of the dye, propidium iodide, into the cellular DNA; annexin V binds specifically to phosphatidyl serine permitting the measurement of phosphatidyl serine translocation as a marker of evolving apoptosis.

Necrosis and apoptosis are probably better conceptualized as two extremes of a continuum; the balance between these two forms of cellular death depends on the severity of the triggering injury, and the integrity of cellular adenosine triphosphate (ATP) stores [10].

Biochemical Mechanisms of Apoptosis

Life and Death Genes: The *C. elegans* Connection

A basic template for the biochemical processes involved in apoptosis has been developed through study of the soil nematode, *Caenorhabditis elegans* [11]. During the course of its development to an adult worm comprising 959 cells, the maturing nematode deletes exactly 131 cells, at variable but reproducible times, through the process of apoptosis. Study of the consequences of genetic mutations in *C. elegans* showed that three genes played a central role in the normal involution of these deleted cells. Deletions in genes denoted as *ced-3* and *ced-4* resulted in failure of cellular deletion, suggesting that the products of these genes played a requisite role in the expression of programmed cell death. In contrast, nematodes with defects of *ced-9* showed extensive cell loss, indicating that the product of this gene could block the process of cell death. The coordinated function of these two opposing activities guaranteed normal development.

A search for human genes with homology to the apopototic genes of *C. elegans* revealed a similar, though substantially more complex, situation. The first homolog of *ced-9* to be identified was *bcl-2*, so named because of its isolation from lymphoid cells of a patient with a B cell lymphoma [12]. Subsequent studies have revealed that Bcl-2 is part of a family of proteins that are capable of both inhibiting and inducing apopotosis [13]. Inhibitory members of the Bcl-2 family include Bcl-2 itself, Bcl-x, and Bcl-x_L, while the structurally related genes *bad, bid, bax,* and *bcl-x_S* induce apoptosis [14].

The initial human homolog of *ced-3* to be identified proved to be the same enzyme that converts pro-interleukin-1β to its mature active form, the interleukin-1β (IL-1β) converting enzyme (ICE) [15]. A total of 10 human *ced-3* homologs have been identified [16, 17], and designated caspases, reflecting the fact that they are all cysteine proteases with a distinctive substrate specificity, cleaving their targets at an Asp-X residue [18]. Caspases are formed as inactive precursors with a molecular weight of 30 to 50 kD which are activated by autocatalytic cleavage to form enzymes with molecular weights of 10–20 kD [19].

Analysis of the biologic activities and substrate specificities of the caspases has resulted in their being grouped into three families [20, 21] (Table I). Group I caspases, of which ICE is the prototypical member, probably play a limited role in the expression of apoptosis; indeed cleavage of pro-IL-1β by caspase 1 generates IL-1β, whose activity, at least in hematopoietic cells, is anti-apoptotic [22]. Group

Table 1. Caspases and their intracellular targets

Group	Primary Target Sequence Specificity	Cellular Substrates
Group I: Caspase 1, 4, 5	*WEHD*	Interleukin-1β, interleukin 18
Group II: Caspase 2, 3, 7	*DEVD*	Poly (ADP)-ribose polymerase, sterol regulatory element binding protein, D4-GDI, DNA-dependent protein kinase, 70 kD U1 small ribonucleoprotein
Group III: Caspase 6, 8, 9, 10	*IETD*	Caspases 3, 7; Lamin A

II caspases are the principal effectors of apoptosis, targeting key cytostructural and reparative proteins such as poly (ADP) ribose polymerase, sterol regulatory element-binding proteins, and DNA-dependent protein kinase. Finally, group III caspases serve primarily as activators of the apoptotic cascade. Caspase-8, for example, is activated by engagement of the death receptor Fas, triggering activation of caspase-3, a group II caspase, and activating the death program [23].

A human homolog of *ced-4* has only recently been identified. Apoptosis protease activating factor-1 (APAF-1) bound to cytochrome c from the mitochondria is able to activate the group III caspase, caspase-9, and so to initiate the apoptotic cascade [24, 25].

Mitochondrial Involvement in Cellular Death

The fundamental role played by the mitochondria in the expression of apoptosis has only recently been appreciated. Early studies of Bcl-2 had shown that the protein is localized to the inner leaflet of the mitochondrial membrane [26]. Subsequent investigations demonstrated that apoptosis could be prevented by drugs whose primary pharmacologic action was the inhibition of mitochondrial membrane permeability [27], and that isolated mitochondria can induce chromatin condensation and DNA fragmentation in cell free systems [28]. Two separate groups reported that Bcl-2 exerts its anti-apoptotic effects by inhibiting the release of cytochrome c from the mitochondria [29, 30], and that pro-caspase-3 may have an intramitochondrial distribution [31].

Under normal circumstances, the inner mitochondrial membrane is negatively charged and essentially impermeable to ions. The mitochondrial transmembrane potential ($\Delta\psi m$) results from the asymmetric distribution of charged particles on either side of this inner mitochondrial membrane, a situation that gives rise to an electrochemical gradient. Maintenance of the mitochondrial transmembrane potential is essential for normal function. Loss of the mitochondrial transmembrane potential can be caused by many apoptotic stimuli and has been detected in a variety of cell types undergoing apoptosis. Multiple stimuli including changes in cellular redox state increase inner membrane permeabilty by opening a non-selective large conductance channel known as the mitochondrial permeability transition (MPT), and cause uncoupling of the respiratory chain leading to loss of ATP, depletion of reduced glutathione and NAD(P)H_2, and release of superoxide anions. These changes, in turn, are implicated in the expression of apoptosis. Glutathione protects cells against Fas-induced apoptosis [32], while reactive oxygen species induce apoptosis [33]. Prevention of cell death by Bcl-2 is associated with reduced generation of reactive oxygen species [34]. Indeed there is some evidence that commitment of a cell to an apoptotic or necrotic death is influenced by the intracellular levels of ATP [35].

Thus an alternate model is emerging that posits a central role for the MPT in the initiation of apoptosis. Increased mitochondrial permeability permits the exit from the mitochondria of cytochrome c. Binding of cytochrome c to APAF-1 in the cytosol unmasks a binding site on APAF-1 that in turn recruits and activates caspase-9, initiating the caspase cascade [36]. Apoptosis inducing factor (AIF) is another protein whose release from the mitochondria is permitted by the MPT, and that induces apoptosis within the cytosol [37]. Changes in mitochondrial permeability represent one pathway that initiates apoptotic cellular death; a separate pathway is induced directly through the engagement of death receptors on the cell surface.

The Fas Family of Cell Death Receptors

A family of type 1 membrane protein receptors including Fas (CD95, APO-1), tumor necrosis factor (TNF) receptor p55, CD40, DR3/TRAMP, and the recently-identified receptors for TNF related apoptosis-inducing ligand (TRAIL), TRAIL-R1/DR4 and TRAIL-R2/DR5, transduce signals that activate the apoptotic pathway (Table 2) [38–41]. Each possesses a highly conserved intracellular sequence of 80 amino acids termed the death domain. Engagement of these receptors results in the recruitment of a series of membrane-associated proteins that comprise the death-inducing signalling complex (DISC). Caspase-8 (FLICE/MORT1) is the apical caspase recruited to the DISC [23, 42], and activates a cascade of downstream proteases including caspase-3 (CPP32) [43].

Fas plays an important role in the regulation of immune cell populations. Interactions between Fas and Fas ligand result in the deletion of autoreactive T cells, and are responsible for the elimination of infected or transformed cells [44], and for the maintenance of immune privilege in sites such as the anterior chamber of the eye [45]. It has been hypothesized that autocrine interactions between Fas and its agonistic ligand on the neutrophil membrane may be responsible for spontaneous apoptosis in this cell [46]. Defects in the genes for Fas or its ligand result in autoimmune diseases [47].

The delivery to the interior of the cell of a signal leading to apoptosis is a complex process, involving the association of a family of proteins with the death domain of the receptor, and receptor engagement can, under poorly characterized circumstances, also result in cellular activation (Fig. 3). For example, soluble or

Table 2. The Fas (CD95/APO-1) family of death receptors

Receptor	Ligand
Fas	Fas ligand
TNFR-1 (p55)	Tumor necrosis factor-α
TNFR-2 (p75)	Tumor necrosis factor-α
CD40	CD40 ligand
CD30	CD30 ligand
Nerve Growth Factor Receptor	Nerve growth factor
DR3/TRAMP	
TRAIL R1/DR4	TRAIL (Apo2L)
TRAIL R2/DR5	TRAIL
TRUNDD (Inhibitory)	TRAIL

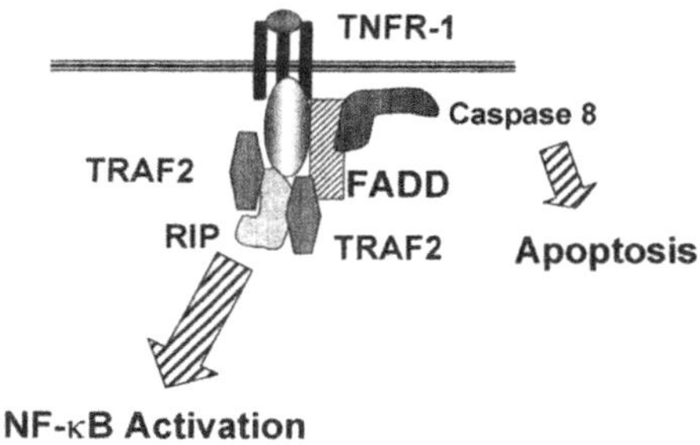

Fig. 3. Trimerization of the receptor for TNF leads to the assembly of a family of membrane-associated proteins that deliver a signal for one of two diametrically opposite cellular responses. Activation of caspase-8 results in apoptosis and cell death, whereas activation of NF-κB leads to the expression of a family of inflammatory genes, and results in the inhibition of apoptosis. See text for details

membrane-associated TNF engages one of two cellular receptors, TNFR1 (p55) or TNFR2 (p75). Trimerization of the TNF receptor causes receptor activation, and recruits a family of membrane-associated proteins to the receptor complex, resulting in transduction of a signal to the interior of the cell [48]. The two TNF receptors share a similar extracellular structure, but different intracellular domains. TNFR1 activation results in recruitment of the TNFR1-associated death domain protein (TRADD), and the TNFR1/TRADD complex then recruits a serine/threonine kinase known as RIP (receptor-interacting protein), the Fas-associated death domain (FADD), and the TNFR-associated protein 2 (TRAF2). FADD induces apoptosis through activation of caspase 8 (FLICE) [23, 42], while TRAF2 and RIP mediate activation of nuclear factor-kappa B (NF-κB), MAPK (mitogen-activated protein kinase), MEKK1 (MAP/ERK kinase kinase 1) and JNK (c-JUN NH_2 terminal kinase) resulting in cellular activation and suppression of apoptosis [49–51]. TNFR2 engagement recruits TRAF1 and TRAF2, as well as the homologs of a group of viral inhibitors of apoptosis, c-IAP1 and c-IAP2 [52], resulting in inhibition of apoptosis and activation of NF-κB.

Inhibitors of Apoptosis

The cellular machinery necessary for the expression of apoptosis is normally present in virtually all mammalian cells. Yet cell death is initiated only under certain circumstances, suggesting that mechanisms must exist in healthy cells to prevent the inadvertent activation of the caspase cascade. Members of the Bcl-2 family (described above) serve as physiologic inhibitors of the expression of apoptosis. Bcl-2 is not expressed in mature neutrophils, however a Bcl-2 homolog, A1 has been identified as a cytoplasmic protein with anti-apoptotic activity [53]. Other families of inhibitory proteins have been identified.

A class of endogenous inhibitory proteins known as the IAP (inhibitors of apoptosis) family was originally identified as viral proteins that blocked apoptosis in cells infected by baculovirus [54]. It has since become evident that IAP are expressed in uninfected mammalian cells [55], and contribute to the normal regulation of the expression of apoptosis [56]. Members of the IAP family possess a common sequence of amino acid repeats termed the BIR (baculovirus IAP repeats) that interact with TRAF2, a component of the TNF receptor complex, to inhibit apoptosis [52]. XIAP (hILP), cIAP1, and cIAP2 may also inhibit apoptosis by preventing the cytochrome c- induced activation of the proximal caspase, procaspase-9, and by directly inhibiting activated caspase-3 [57]. Other cytoplasmic inhibitors of apoptosis include IEX-1L, a transmembrane protein localized to the nuclear membrane and endoplasmic reticulum, that is induced by TNF, and renders cells resistant to TNF-induced apoptosis [58] and survivin, a member of the IAP family [59]. IAP gene expression in response to cytokines is dependent on the activation of the transcription factor NF-κB [60].

A family of membrane-targeted viral proteins, designated FLIPs (FLICE inhibitory proteins), can inhibit TNF or Fas-induced apoptosis by interfering with the receptor-mediated events leading to activation of caspase-8 [61, 62]. Mammalian counterparts of these inhibitory molecules have been identified [63]. Expressed predominantly in lymphoid and muscle cells, these proteins effectively inhibit apoptosis induced by engagement of members of the Fas family of death receptors.

Another biologic process involved in the inhibition of apoptosis has recently been described. Seol and Billiar identified a catalytically inactive variant of caspase-9 in human liver [64]. The protein, termed caspase-9S acts as a dominant negative inhibitor of caspase-9, and blocks the expression of apoptosis induced by TNF, Fas engagement, or the interaction of APF1 and caspase-9.

Modulation of Neutrophil Apoptosis by Inflammatory Mediators

Mature neutrophils are constitutively apoptotic cells. However, the temporal expression of neutrophil apoptosis is exquisitely sensitive to modulation by signals arising from the microenvironment of inflammation. Both the phagocytosis of organisms such as *E. coli* [65] and the engagement of cell surface L-selectin, an adhesion molecule that mediates the initial stages of neutrophil rolling [66] have been shown to accelerate neutrophil apoptosis. In contrast, a large number of inflammatory mediators can inhibit the expression of neutrophil apoptosis (Table 3).

The response to a given mediator may vary with the cell type, the timing of evaluation, and the presence of concomitant modifying signals. Thus a number of cytokines have been shown to either accelerate or inhibit apoptosis, including TNF [49, 67], IL-6 [68, 69], IL-4 [70, 71], and IL-2 [69, 72].

Our own studies have suggested that modulation of the survival of inflammatory neutrophils is a complex process, dependent on both exogenous and endogenous signals (Fig. 4). Inflammatory mediators of either bacterial (lipopolysaccharide, [LPS]) or host (granulocyte/macrophage colony-stimulating factor [GM-CSF]) origin induce significant inhibition of the normal expression of neutrophil apoptosis. This inhibition is an active process, dependent on *de novo* gene expression, and can be prevented by non-specific blockade of tyrosine kinases, prevention of nuclear translocation of NF-κB, or blockade of protein synthesis [22]. Moreover it is associated with increased expression and activity of caspase-1, and results from the preferential processing by caspase-1 of the anti-apoptotic

Table 3. Modulation of neutrophil apoptosis

	Accelerate Apoptosis	Inhibit Apoptosis
Microbial Factors	Ingestion of *E. coli*	LPS fMLP
Physiologic Processes	L-selectin engagement	Endothelial transmigration; β2 integrin engagement
	Thiol depletion	Anti-oxidants
	Inhibition of protein synthesis	NF-κB activation
	Precipitating immune complexes	Soluble immune complexes
Cytokines	FasL, TNF	G-CSF, GM-CSF, IL-1β, TNF, IL-8

cytokine, IL-1β: blockade of the synthesis or cellular binding of IL-1β is largely able to prevent the activation-induced apoptotic delay. However IL-1β-mediated inhibition of apoptosis is also blocked by inhibition of protein synthesis, or of nuclear translocation of NF-κB (Li, unpublished observations), suggesting that the effects of IL-1β do not occur directly through inhibition of the caspase cas-

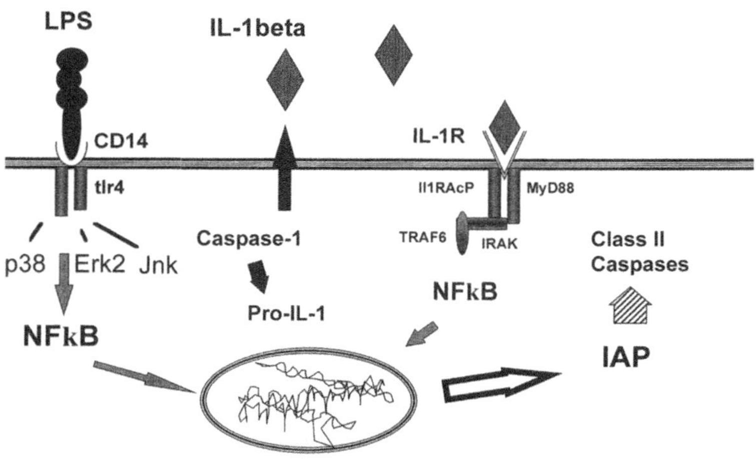

Fig. 4. Modulation of neutrophil programmed cell death appears to be a complex, multi-stage process. Stimuli such as LPS or GM-CSF interact with their cell surface receptors, initiating signal transdustion, NF-κB activation, and transcription of genes for pro-IL-1β and its activating enzyme, caspase-1 (the IL-1β converting enzyme or ICE). Mature IL-1β is secreted by the cell, and initiates a second signaling cascade, again leading to NF-κB activation, and resulting in the expression of one or more as yet unidentified inhibitory genes

cade, but indirectly through the induction of the expression of one or more inhibitory proteins, perhaps members of the IAP family.

Apoptosis plays a critical role in the regulation of cell populations involved in the expression of an immune response. But, just as the expansion of lymphoid cell populations is controlled through the complex interaction of agonist-ligand interactions, modified by the effects of co-stimulatory molecules, regulatory signals from the inflammatory microenvironment influence the expression of innate immunity through the activation of still poorly understood pathways that influence the expression of programmed cell death.

Altered Expression of Apoptosis in Immune Cell Populations

While dysregulation of immune cell populations is the focus of this chapter, it is becoming apparent that altered expression of apoptosis may contribute to the pathogenesis of other forms of organ system dysfunction in the critically ill patient. Pro-inflammatory cytokines up-regulate expression of mRNA for Fas in cultured renal cell lines [73], and renal cell apoptosis can be induced by agonistic anti-Fas antibodies. Similarly, TNF causes apoptosis of renal tubular endothelial cells in mice injected with LPS, suggesting that apoptosis may play a role in the pathogenesis of acute tubular necrosis [74]. Both TNF [75] and Fas [76] induce hepatic failure. Moreover apoptosis of gastrointestinal eptihelial cells can be triggered by toxin A of *C. difficile* [77] or by *Helicobacter pylori* [78]. Indeed the impact of abnormalities in the expression of apoptosis during systemic inflammation appears to be both extensive and complex. Excessive apoptosis results in cellular loss and functional insufficiency, while inadequate execution of the apoptotic program may lead to cell death by necrosis and further inflammatory tissue injury.

Lymphocyte Apoptosis in Critical Illness

The predominant lymphoid cell abnormalities of critical illness include T cell anergy reflected in loss of delayed type hypersensitivity reactivity *in vivo* and impaired mitogen-induced proliferative responses *in vitro*, and altered patterns of immunoglobulin synthesis; increased synthesis of antibody to polysaccharide antigens, but reduced synthesis to protein antigens [79, 80]. Although data from human studies are limited, lymphocyte apoptosis appears to be increased [81], perhaps accounting for the characteristic lymphopenia of critical illness.

Circulating lymphocytes from burned patients show increased rates of apoptosis. Teodorczyk-Injeyan and colleagues evaluated a group of 14 patients with burns to greater than 30% of the total body surface area, and found that the percentage of lymphocytes spontaneously expressing apoptotic features was increased, and further, that mitogenic stimulation with phytohemagglutinin (PHA) induced features of apoptosis [82]. Studies in a rat model of burn injury suggest that augmented thymocyte apoptosis may be a consequence of increased plasma levels of corticosteroids [83].

Oka and co-workers studied apoptosis in peripheral blood mononuclear cells of 18 patients undergoing major elective surgery [84]. They found that numbers of circulating lymphocytes decreased within hours following surgery, and that Fas expression was increased on the surface of these cells. While the number of apoptotic cells evident at the time of harvest did not differ, after 24 hours of *in vitro* culture significantly more lymphocytes from patients who had undergone major surgery showed evidence of apoptosis.

Using a murine model involving the intraperitoneal injection of viable bacteria, Wang and colleagues demonstrated increased thymocyte apoptosis resulting from infection with either Gram-positive or Gram-negative organisms. Apoptosis induced by *E. coli* was TNF-dependent, and could be blocked by inhibition of gene transcription of protein synthesis; in contrast, that induced by *S. pneumoniae* was only partially inhibitable by TNF blockade [85].

The efficiency with which apoptotic cells are phagocytosed and removed by macrophages makes the detection of alterations in the expression of apoptosis difficult. Nonetheless, it would appear that acute stresses commonly encountered in critically ill patients can augment the expression of lymphocyte apoptosis. Whether such changes contribute to altered lymphoid cell function in critical illness is speculative.

Neutrophil Apoptosis in Critical Illness

In contrast to lymphocytes, polymorphonuclear neutrophils harvested from critically ill patients manifest significant delays in the constitutive expression of programmed cell death, and delayed apoptosis is associated with prolonged neutrophil activation.

Chitnis and colleagues studied the expression of neutrophil apoptosis in a cohort of thermally injured patients [86]. They showed that apoptosis was inhibited, and that this inhibition was dependent upon circulating GM-CSF in plasma. Moreover plasma from burn patients induced neutrophil synthesis and release of GM-CSF.

We studied the expression of neutrophil apoptosis in a group of 16 intensive care unit (ICU) patients meeting clinical criteria for systemic inflammatory response syndrome (SIRS), and in a control group of 7 patients who had undergone elective aortic aneurysmectomy [87]. Neutrophil apoptosis was profoundly inhibited in patients with SIRS, and this inhibition persisted throughout the ICU stay (Fig. 5). Conversely, neutrophils from SIRS patients manifested enhanced respiratory burst activity following stimulation with phorbol myristate acetate (PMA), and there was a statistically significant association between the degree of inhibition of apoptosis, and that of augmentation of respiratory burst activity. Western blotting showed a slight increase in pro-caspase-1 protein in comparison to control cells, but no difference in expression of caspase-3.

Keel and co-workers have shown a similar inhibition of neutrophil apoptosis in a cohort of patients with sepsis [88]. Expression of apoptosis could be further inhibited by addition of LPS, and the LPS-induced (but not the sepsis-induced)

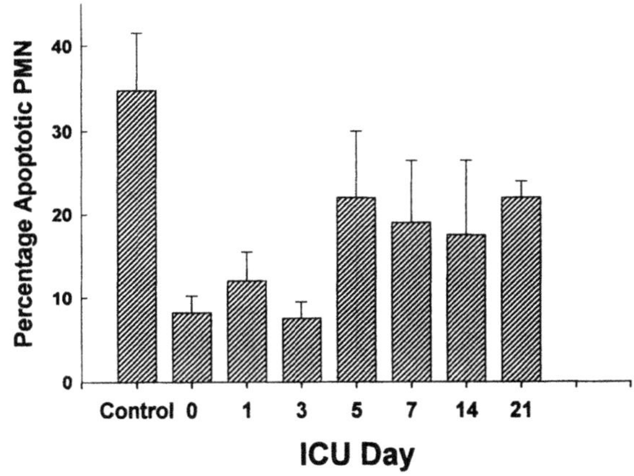

Fig. 5. Critically ill patients with SIRS show marked and prolonged inhibition of the normal expression of neutrophil apoptosis, lasting as long as three weeks after the initiating insult in patients remaining alive in the ICU. (From Jimenez et al [87] with permission)

delay could be completely blocked by IL-10, and partially blocked by anti-TNF antibody. Recent studies from our laboratory also show that the sepsis-induced inhibition is markedly refractory to reversal. Rates of apoptosis in SIRS neutrophils can be restored to about 50% of control levels by incubation with pyrrolidine dithiocarbamate (PDTC), an inhibitor of the nuclear binding of NF-κB, however no intervention yet studied has been able to return rates to those seen in control cells (Taneja, unpublished observations).

The extent to which prolongation of neutrophil survival is a common response to acute homeostatic stress is unknown. We have observed neutrophil apoptosis to be delayed following major elective surgery [87], and in women with pre-eclampsia (von Dadelszen, unpublished observations). Others, however, have shown that normal expression of apoptosis is preserved following multiple trauma, unless infectious complications supervene [89]. Neutrophils harvested from the lungs of critically ill patients with acute respiratory distress syndrome (ARDS) also show inhibition of apoptosis [90], suggesting that prolonged neutrophil functional survival may contribute to the pulmonary injury of ARDS.

Conclusion

Alterations in the expression of the physiologic process of programmed cell death are being implicated in the pathogenesis of an ever-increasing number of disorders; to this list may be added the dysregulated immune response characteristic of critical illness. Excessive apoptosis appears to be a factor in the characteristic lymphopenia of critical illness, while inhibition of a constitutively expressed cell death program contributes to neutrophilia, and likely to neutrophil-mediated tissue injury. In other organ systems, both excessive expression of apoptosis, and preferential activation of necrosis over apoptosis may contribute to tissue injury and physiologic dysfunction.

Dysregulated apoptosis is an attractive therapeutic target. Restoration of the normal expression of neutrophil apoptosis, for example, holds the promise of accelerating the resolution of an inflammatory response, and thereby minimizing neutrophil-mediated tissue injury, without jeopardizing the vital role that neutrophils play in the initial host response to infection or tissue injury. Delineation of the cellular mechanisms that regulate the expression of apoptosis will set the stage for entirely novel immunomodulatory therapies that target the fundamental processes of cellular survival and death.

Acknowledgment. This work was supported in part by the physicians of Ontario through a grant from the Physicians' Services Incorporated Foundation.

References

1. Degli Esposti M (1998) Apoptosis: who was first? Cell Death Diff 5:719–724
2. Kerr JFR (1971) Shrinkage necrosis: a distinct mode of cellular death. J Pathol 105:13–20
3. Kerr JFR, Wyllie AH, Currie AR (1972) Apoptosis: A basic biologcal phenomenon with wide ranging implications in tissue kinetics. Br J Cancer 26:239–257
4. Hammar SP, Mottet NK (1971) Tetrazolium salt and electron microscopic studies of cellular degeneration and necrosis in the interdigital areas of the developing chick limb. J Cell Sci 8: 229–236
5. Meyaard L, Otto SA, Jonker R (1992) Programmed death of T cells in HIV-1 infection. Science 257:217–219
6. Loo DT, Copani A, Pike CJ (1993) Apoptosis is induced by beta-amyloid in cultured central nervous system neurons. Proc Natl Acad Sci USA 90:7951–7955
7. Singer GG, Abbas AK (1994) The Fas antigen is involved in peripheral but not thymic deletion of T lymphocytes in T cell receptor transgenic mice. Immunity 1:365–371
8. Carmody RJ, Cotter TG (1998) Molecular events and mechanisms of apoptosis. Sepsis 2: 9–19
9. Savill JS, Wyllie AH, Henson JE, Henson PM, Haslett C (1989) Macrophage phagocytosis of aging neutrophils in inflammation. J Clin Invest 83:865–875
10. Richter C, Schweizer M, Cossarizza A, Franceschi C (1996) Control of apoptosis by the cellular ATP level. FEBS Lett 378:107–110
11. Ellis RE, Yuan J, Horvitz HR (1991) Mechanisms and function of cell death. Annu Rev Cell Dev Biol 7:663–698
12. Vaux DL, Cory S, Adams JM (1988) Bcl-2 gene promotes haemopoetic cell survival and cooperates with c-myc to immortalise pre-B cells. Nature 335:440–442
13. Yang E, Korsmeyer SJ (1996) Molecular thanatopsis: A discourse on the Bcl-2 family and cell death. Blood 88:386–401
14. Adams JM, Cory S (1998) The bcl-2 protein family: Arbiters of cell survival. Science 281: 1322–1326
15. Yuan J, Shaham S, Ledoux S, Ellis HM, Horvitz HR (1993) The *C. elegans* cell death gene ced-3 encodes a protein similar to mammalian interleukin 1β converting enzyme. Cell 75: 641–652
16. Nagata S (1997) Apoptosis by death factor. Cell 88:355–365
17. Thornberry NA, Lazebnik YA (1998) Caspases: Enemies within. Science 281:1312–1316
18. Alnemri ES, Livingston DJ, Nicholson DW, et al (1996) Human ICE/CED-3 protease nomenclature. Cell 87:171
19. Martin SJ, Green DR (1995) Protease activation during apoptosis: death by a thousand cuts? Cell 82:349–352
20. Thornberry NA, Rano TA, Peterson EP, et al (1997) A combinatorial approach defines specificities of members of the caspase family and granzyme B. J Biol Chem 272:17907–17911
21. Garcia-Calvo M, Peterson EP, Leiting B, Ruel R, Nicholson DW, Thornberry NA (1998) Inhibition of human caspases by peptide-based and macromolecular inhibitors. J Biol Chem 273:32608–32613

22. Watson RWG, Rotstein OD, Parodo J, Bitar R, Marshall JC (1998) The interleukin-1 beta converting enzyme (caspase-1) inhibits apoptosis of inflammatory neutrophils through activation of IL-1β. J Immunol 161:957–962
23. Muzio M, Chinnaiyan AM, Kischkel FC, et al (1996) FLICE, a novel FADD-homologous ICE/CED-3-like protease, is recruited to the CD95 (Fas/APO-1) death-inducing signaling complex. Cell 85:817–827
24. Li P, Nijhawan D, Budihardjo I, et al (1997) Cytochrome c and dATP-dependent formation of Apaf-1/caspase-9 complex initiates an apoptotic protease cascade. Cell 91:479–489
25. Zou H, Henzel WJ, Liu X, Lutschg A, Wang X (1997) Apaf-1, a human protein homologous to C. elegans ced-4, participates in cytochrome c-dependent activation of caspase-3. Cell 90: 405–413
26. Hockenbery D, Nunez G, Milliman C, Schreiber RD, Korsmeyer SJ (1990) Bcl-2 is an inner mitochondrial membrane protein that blocks programmed cell death. Nature 348:334–336
27. Zamzami N, Marchetti P, Castedo M, et al (1995) Sequential reduction of mitochondrial transmembrane potential and generation of reactive oxygen species in early programmed cell death. J Exp Med 182:367–377
28. Zamzami N, Susin SA, Marchetti P (1996) Mitochondrial control of nuclear apoptosis. J Exp Med 183:1533–1544
29. Kluck RM, Bossy-Wetzel E, Green DR, Newmeyer DD (1997) The release of cytochrome c from mitochondria: A primary site for Bcl-2 regulation of apoptosis. Science 275:1132–1136
30. Yang J, Liu XS, Bhalla K, et al (1997) Prevention of apoptosis by Bcl-2: Release of cytochrome c from mitochondria blocked. Science 275:1129–1132
31. Mancini M, Nicholson DW, Roy S (1998) The caspase-3 precursor has a cytosolic and mitochondrial distribution: implications for apoptotic signalling. J Cell Biol 140:1485–1495
32. Watson RWG, Rotstein OD, Jimenez M, Parodo J, Marshall JC (1997) Augmented intracellular glutathione inhibits Fas-triggered apoptosis of activated human neutrophils. Blood 89: 4175–4181
33. Buttke TM, Sandstrom PA (1994) Oxidative stress as a mediator of apoptosis. Immunol Today 15:7–10
34. Kane DJ, Sarafian TA, Anton R, et al (1993) Bcl-2 inhibition of neural death: decreased generation of reactive oxygen species. Science 262:1274–1277
35. Eguchi Y, Shimizu S, Tsujimoto Y (1997) Intracellular ATP levels determine cell death fate by apoptosis or necrosis. Cancer Res 57:1835–1840
36. Slee EA, Harte MT, Martin SJ (1998) A duel to the death: Activated caspases meet their substrates. Sepsis 2:21–29
37. Susin SA, Zamzami N, Custedo M, et al (1996) Bcl-2 inhibits the mitochondrial release of an apoptogenic protease. J Exp Med 184:1331–1341
38. Nagata S, Golstein P (1995) The Fas death factor. Science 267:1449–1456
39. Pan G, Ni J, Wei Y-F, Yu G-L, Gentz R, Dixit VM (1997) An antagonistic decoy receptor and a death domain-containing receptor for TRAIL. Science 277:815–818
40. Pan G, O'Rourke K, Chinnaiyan AM, et al (1997) The receptor for the cytotoxic ligand TRAIL. Science 276:111–113
41. Sheridan JP, Marsters SA, Pitti RM, et al (1997) Control of TRAIL-induced apoptosis by a family of signaling and decoy receptors. Science 277:818–821
42. Boldin MP, Goncharov TM, Goltsev YV, Wallach D (1996) Involvement of MACH, a novel MORT1/FADD-interacting protease, in Fas/APO-1- and TNF receptor-induced cell death. Cell 85:803–815
43. Schlegel J, Peters I, Orrenius S, et al (1996) CPP32/apopain is a key interleukin 1 beta converting enzyme-like protease involved in Fas-mediated apoptosis. J Biol Chem 271:1841–1844
44. Kägi D, Vignaux F, Ledermann B, et al (1994) Fas and perforin pathways as major mechanisms of T cell- mediated cytotoxicity. Science 265:528–530
45. Griffith TS, Brunner T, Fletcher SM, Green DR, Ferguson TA (1995) Fas ligand-induced apoptosis as a mechanism of immune privilege. Science 270:1189–1192
46. Liles WC, Kiener PA, Ledbetter JA, Aruffo A, Klebanoff SJ (1996) Differential expression of Fas (CD95) and Fas ligand on normal human phagocytes: Implications for the regulation of apoptosis in neutrophils. J Exp Med 184:429–440

47. Rieux-Laucat F, Le Deist F, Hivroz C, et al (1995) Mutations in Fas associated with human lymphoproliferative syndrome and autoimmunity. Science 268:1347–1349
48. Wallach D, Boldin M, Varfolomeev E, Beyaert R, Vandenabeele P, Fiers W (1997) Cell death induction by receptors of the TNF family: towards a molecular understanding. FEBS Lett 410:96–106
49. Liu Z, Hsu H, Goeddel DV, Karin M (1996) Dissection of TNF receptor 1 effector functions: JNK activation is not linked to apoptosis while NF-κB activation prevents cell death. Cell 87:565–576
50. Ting AT, Pimentel-Muinos FX, Seed B (1996) RIP mediates tumor necrosis factor receptor 1 activation of NF-kappa B but not Fas/APO-1-initiated apoptosis. EMBO J 15:6189–6196
51. Natoli G, Costanzo A, Ianni A, et al (1997) Activation of SAPK/JNK by TNF receptor 1 through a noncytotoxic TRAF2-dependent pathway. Science 275:200–203
52. Rothe M, Pan M-G, Henzel WJ, Ayres M, Goeddel DV (1995) The TNFR2-TRAF signaling complex contains two novel proteins related to baculoviral inhibitor of apoptosis proteins. Cell 83:1243–1252
53. Chuang PI, Yee E, Karsan A, Winn RK, Harlan JM (1999) A1 is a consitutive and inducible Bcl-2 homologue in mature human neutrophils. Biochem Biophys Res Commun 249: 361–365
54. Hay BA, Wassarman DA, Rubin GM (1995) Drosophila homologs of baculovirus inhibitor of apoptosis proteins function to block cell death. Cell 83:1253–1262
55. Liston P, Roy N, Tamai K, et al (1996) Suppression of apoptosis in mammalian cells by NAIP and a related family of IAP genes. Nature 379:349–353
56. Clem RJ, Duckett CS (1997) The iap genes: unique arbiters of cell death. Trends Cell Biol 7: 337–339
57. Deveraux QL, Roy N, Stennicke HR, et al (1998) IAPs block apoptotic events induced by caspase-8 and cytochrome c by direct inhibition of distinct caspases. EMBO J 17:2215–2223
58. Wu MX, Ao Z, Prasad KVS, Wu R, Schlossman SF (1998) IEX-1L, an apoptosis inhibitor involved in NFκB-mediated cell survival. Science 281:998–1001.
59. Ambrosini G, Adida C, Altieri DC (1997) A novel anti-apoptosis gene, survivin, expressed in cancer and lymphoma. Nature Med 3:917–921
60. Stehlik C, de Martin R, Binder BR, Lipp J (1998) Cytokine induced expression of porcine inhibitor of apoptosis protein (IAP) family member is regulated by NF-kappa B. Biochem Biophys Res Commun 243:827–832
61. Thome M, Schneider P, Hofmann K, et al (1997) Viral FLICE-inhibitory proteins (FLIPs) prevent apoptosis induced by death receptors. Nature 386:517–521
62. Hu S, Vincenz C, Buller M, Dixit VM (1997) A novel family of viral death effector domain-containing molecules that inhibit both CD-95- and tumor necrosis factor receptor-1-induced apoptosis. J Biol Chem 272:9621–9624
63. Irmier M, Thome M, Hahne M, et al (1997) Inhibition of death receptor signals by cellular FLIP. Nature 388:190–195
64. Seol D-W, Billiar TR (1999) A caspase-9 variant missing the catalytic site is an endogenous inhibitor of apoptosis. J Biol Chem 274:2072–2076
65. Watson RWG, Redmond HP, Wang JH, Condron C, Bouchier-Hays D (1996) Neutrophils undergo apoptosis following ingestion of *Escherichia coli*. J Immunol 156:3986–3992
66. Watson RWG, Rotstein OD, Nathens AB, Parodo J, Marshall JC (1997) Neutrophil apoptosis is modulated by endothelial transmigration and adhesion molecule engagement. J Immunol 158:945–953
67. Woods KM, Chapes SK (1993) Three distinct cell phenotypes of induced-TNF cytotoxicity and their relationship to apoptosis. J Leuk Biol 53:37–44
68. Afford SC, Pongracz J, Stockley RA, Crocker J, Burnett D (1992) The induction by human interleukin-6 of apoptosis in the promonocytic cell line U937 and human neutrophils. J Biol Chem 267:21612–21616
69. Armant M, Delespesse G, Sarfati M (1995) IL-2 and IL-7 but not IL-12 protect natural killer cells from death by apoptosis and up-regulate bcl-2 expression. Immunology 85:331–337
70. Mangan EF, Robertson B, Wahl SM (1992) IL-4 enhances programmed cell death (apoptosis) in stimulated human monocytes. J Immunol 148:1812–1816

71. Girard D, Paquin R, Beaulieu AD (1997) Responsiveness of human neutrophils to interleukin-4: induction of cytoskeletal rearrangements, de novo protein synthesis and delay of apoptosis. Biochem J 325:147–153
72. Lenardo MJ (1991) Interleukin-2 programs mouse $\alpha\beta$ T lymphocytes for apoptosis. Nature 353:858–861
73. Ortiz-Arduan A, Danoff TM, Kalluri R, et al (1996) Regulation of Fas and Fas ligand expression in cultured murine renal cells and in the kidney during endotoxemia. Am J Physiol 271:F1193–F1201
74. Faraco PR, Ledgerwood EC, Smith KGC (1998) Apoptosis and renal disease. Sepsis 2:31–37
75. Leist M, Gantner F, Jilg S, Wendel A (1995) Activation of the 55 kDa TNF receptor is necessary and sufficient for TNF-induced liver failure, hepatocyte apoptosis, and nitrite release. J Immunol 154:1307–1316
76. Leist M, Gantner F, Kunstle G, et al (1996) The 55-kD tumor necrosis factor receptor and CD95 independently signal murine hepatocyte apoptosis and subsequent liver failure. Mol Med 2:124
77. Mahida YR, Makh S, Hyde S, Gray T, Borriello SP (1996) Effect of Clostridium difficile toxin A on human intestinal epithelial cells: induction of interleukin 8 production and apoptosis after cell detachment. Gut 38:337–347
78. Moss SF, Calam J, Agarwal B, Wang S, Holt PR (1996) Inductions of gastric epithelial apoptosis by *Helicobacter pylori*. Gut 38:498–501
79. Abraham E, Chang YH (1986) Cellular and humoral bases of hemorrhage-induced depression of lymphocyte function. Crit Care Med 14:81–86
80. Christou NV, Meakins JL, Gordon J, et al (1995) The delayed hypersensitivity response and host resistance in surgical patients. Ann Surg 222:534–548
81. Ayala A, Chung C-S, Chaudry IH (1998) Lymphocyte apoptosis in sepsis. Sepsis 2:55–71
82. Teodorczyk-Injeyan JA, Cembrznska-Nowak M, Lalani S, Peters WJ, Mills GB (1995) Immune deficiency following thermal trauma is associated with apoptotic cell death. J Clin Immunol 15:318–328
83. Nakanishi T, Nishi Y, Sato EF, Ishii M, Hamada T, Inoue M (1998) Thermal injury induces thymocyte apoptosis in the rat. J Trauma 44:148
84. Oka M, Hirazawa K, Yamamoto K, et al (1996) Induction of Fas-mediated apoptosis on circulating lymphocytes by surgical stress. Ann Surg 223:434–440
85. Wang S-D, Huang KJ, Lin YS, Lei HY (1994) Sepsis-induced apoptosis of the thymocytes in mice. J Immunol 5014–5021
86. Chitnis D, Dickerson C, Munster AM, Winchurch RA (1996) Inhibition of apoptosis in polymorphonuclear neutrophils from burn patients. J Leukoc Biol 59:835–839
87. Jimenez MF, Watson RWG, Parodo J, et al (1997) Dysregulated expression of neutrophil apoptosis in the systemic inflammatory response syndrome (SIRS). Arch Surg 132: 1263–1270
88. Keel M, Ungethum U, Steckholzer U, Niederer E, Hartung T, Trentz O (1997) Interleukin-10 counterregulates proinflammatory cytokine-induced inhibition of neutrophil apoptosis during severe sepsis. Blood 90:3356–3363
89. Ertel W, Keel M, Infanger M, Ungethum U, Steckholzer U, Trentz O (1998) Circulating mediators in serum of injured patients with septic complications inhibit neutrophil apoptosis through up-regulation of protein-tyrosine phosphorylation. J Trauma 44:767–775
90. Matute-Bello G, Liles WC (1997) Neutrophil apoptosis in acute respiratory distress syndrome. Am Rev Respir Crit Care Med 156:1969–1977

The Interaction Between the Coagulation System and the Systemic Inflammatory Mediators

S. M. Opal

Introduction

Activation of the coagulation system is commonplace in the presence of severe sepsis. Disseminated intravascular coagulation (DIC) may generate diffuse thrombin formation resulting in tissue necrosis, organ failure [1] and considerable morbidity and mortality [2, 3]. Moreover, consumptive coagulopathy from uncontrolled DIC may precipitate a hemorrhage diathesis as clotting factors are consumed in the process. While clinically overt DIC occurs in the minority of septic patients, sensitive measures of coagulation activation provide evidence that some clotting occurs in almost every patient in septic shock [4–6].

A host of microbial mediators and host-derived pro-inflammatory cytokines are potential inducers of the coagulation system. Human volunteers injected with minute quantities of bacterial endotoxin or tumor necrosis factor (TNF) will activate coagulation cascades within minutes of intravenous challenge [7, 8]. It has been speculated that uncontrolled activation of the coagulation system during generalized inflammation in sepsis contributes to the basic pathophysiology of sepsis. Microthrombi are frequently found in sepsis, and tissue damage, organ dysfunction and circulation failure may ensue as a result of uncontrolled coagulation. The microcirculation in sepsis frequently exhibits evidence of regional hypoperfusion of capillary beds resulting in tissue ischemia and multi-organ dysfunction [9].

Inhibition of the systemic coagulation system has been considered a potential therapeutic strategy for sepsis for several decades [4, 10, 11]. Advances in the understanding of the molecular biology of the endogenous anticoagulants now provides an opportunity to directly test the hypothesis that coagulation activation is detrimental in septic shock. Recent findings clearly demonstrate that the coagulation system is activated by systemic inflammatory mediators [1, 6]. Conversely, systemic inflammation may be induced by activation of the coagulation system. It may be possible to attenuate the generalized host inflammatory response to septic stimuli through careful regulation of the coagulation system. This therapeutic strategy is currently the focus of several controlled clinical trials in human sepsis. The results of these studies should be able to answer a number of questions that remain relating to the role of the coagulation system in sepsis.

Activation of the Coagulation System in Sepsis

It has been convincingly demonstrated that the extrinsic clotting system is primarily responsible for activation of coagulation in the early phases of sepsis [12, 14]. Tissue factor/factor VII complex catalyzes the activation of factor X and drives the common clotting system to generate thrombin and fibrin clots during septic processes [4, 6, 7]. Components of the intrinsic clotting cascade form secondary amplification loops that facilitate the clotting process (Fig. 1).

The intrinsic clotting system consists of the contact factors: Hageman factor (factor XII), factor XI, prekallikrein and high molecular weight kininogen. The contact system may be activated with high doses of endotoxin and may secondarily contribute to the activation of the coagulation system in sepsis. However, administration of a factor XII neutralizing antibody had no effect on the development of intravascular coagulation following an *E. coli* infusion challenge [15]. Despite the apparent inefficiency with which the intrinsic system activates coagulation in sepsis, the contact system does appear to induce many of the hemodynamic alterations observed in sepsis. This may be related to the generation of bradykinin from high molecular weight kininogen or through activation of other pathways such as nitric oxide (NO) or prostacyclin [4, 6]. The contact system also contributes to the activation of the fibrinolytic system (Fig. 2).

The principal inhibitors of the contact system include C1 inhibitor (that inhibits factor XIIa, factor XIIa and kallikrein) and alpha-2 microglobulin (that inhibits kallikrein). While levels of factor XII and prekallikrein are reduced in patients with septic shock, it has recently been observed that factor XII is a negative acute phase reactant and this may also contribute to reduced levels of factor XII observed in severe sepsis [4]. C1 inhibitor may prove to be useful therapeutically as a regulatory element in clotting and as a treatment for severe sepsis [16].

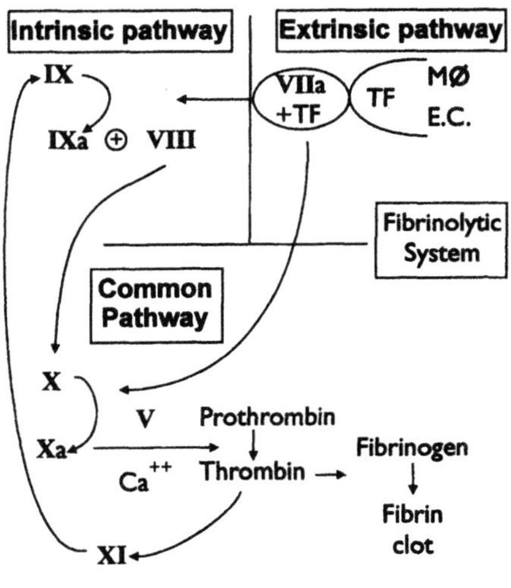

Fig. 1. Activation pathways of the coagulation system in sepsis. The coagulation cascade is primarily activated via the extrinsic clotting cascade with an amplifying role by components of the intrinsic clotting system. TF: tissue factor; MΦ: macrophage; E.C.: endothelial cell

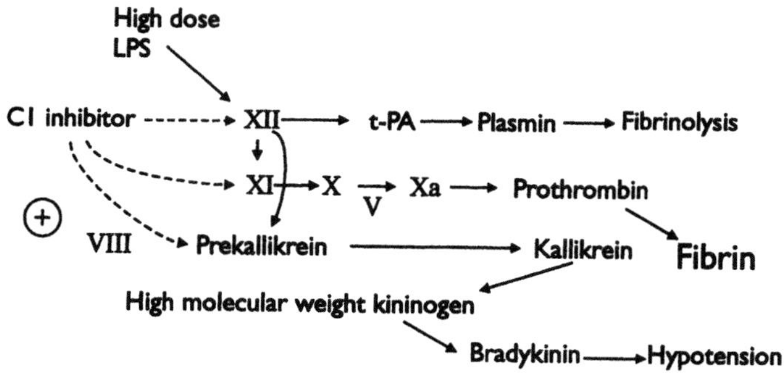

Fig. 2. The contact system (intrinsic clotting system) in sepsis. LPS: lipopolysaccharide; t-PA: tissue plasminogen activator (dotted lines: inhibitory pathways; solid lines: activation pathways)

Endogenous Inhibitors of the Coagulation System

As with other complex biological systems in the human body, the coagulation system has a large number of primary and secondary regulatory elements that control coagulation in health and disease. Consumption of these regulatory components over the course of severe sepsis may result in disordered coagulation, excess thrombin activation, and diffuse fibrin deposition in the microcirculation [1, 4]. There are three major endogenous inhibitors in the coagulation system (Fig. 3). These endogenous anticoagulants work in concert with the fibrinolytic system and hepatic and extra-hepatic clearance mechanisms to prevent unregulated coagulation in the face of a systemic inflammatory response. Degradation of these coagulation inhibitors in septic shock jeopardizes the integrity of this coordinated and complex regulatory network. This may result in vascular compromise in severe sepsis and contribute to the hypoperfusion and tissue sequelae of septic shock.

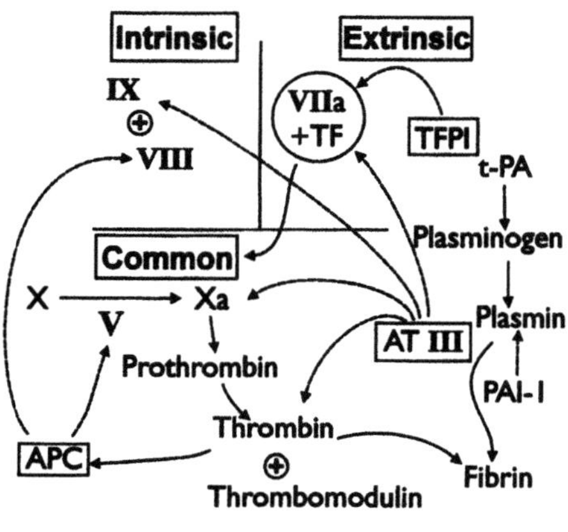

Fig. 3. The endogenous inhibitors of the coagulation system. AT III: antithrombin III; TFPI: tissue factor pathway inhibitor; APC: activated protein C; t-PA: tissue plasminogen activator; TF: tissue factor; PAI-1: plasminogen activator inhibitor-1 (dotted lines: inhibitory pathways; solid lines: activation pathways)

Table 1. The endogenous anticoagulants

Molecule	Site of synthesis	Structural features	Co-factors	Mechanism of action	Inhibitors
Antithrombin III	hepatic	58 Kd glycoprotein	heparin, heparan	inhibits thrombin, tissue factor, factors VII, IX,X,XI,XII	elastase
Activated protein C	hepatic and endothelial cells	heterodimer with internal disulfide bond, post-translational modifications	protein S, thrombomodulin	inhibits factor V, factor VIII	α1-antitrypsin, protein C inhibitor
Tissue factor pathway inhibitor	endothelial cells	42 Kd glycoprotein, 3 Kunitz-type domains	heparin, AT III	inhibits tissue factor/factor VIIa complex, factor Xa	internalized by endothelial cells

The three endogenous anticoagulants include: Antithrombin III (more appropriately referred to as antithrombin); protein C, and tissue factor pathway inhibitor (TFPI). Each of these regulatory elements will be discussed in some detail as important differences exist between these three molecules with regard to the regulation of the coagulation system (Table 1).

Antithrombin III

Antithrombin III is a major inhibitor of the coagulation system affecting the intrinsic, extrinsic and common coagulation pathways. In addition to its function as a specific thrombin inhibitor, antithrombin III is a potent serine protease inhibitor that has the capacity to inhibit the contact factors XIIa and factor XIa in addition to kallikrein. Antithrombin III also inhibits the activity of factor IXa of the intrinsic clotting system, and the final common pathway of clotting at the pivotal position of factor Xa activation. Antithrombin III forms a 1:1 stoichiometric complex with thrombin [17, 18]. Recent evidence confirms that antithrombin III may also function with heparin or in concert with tissue factor pathway inhibitor to inactivate the tissue factor/ factor VII complex of the extrinsic clotting system [19].

Antithrombin III is a classic serine protease inhibitor (SERPIN) and owes its broad spectrum of anticoagulant effects to the fact that most of the activated coagulation components function as serine proteases. Clotting factors are principally zymogens (inactive pro-enzymes) that are converted to active serine protease enzymes through the initiation of the coagulation cascade [4, 6].

Antithrombin III is a hepatically synthesized, single chain, polypeptide protein that is glycosylated and exists in the circulation as a 58 kDa protein [11, 17]. The molecule circulates as a monomer in the plasma and is also found on the cell surfaces of platelets and endothelial cells. This normal plasma concentration is approximately 110–140 mg/liter with a serum half life of 36–48 hours.

Antithrombin III contains a heparin-binding domain and a serine-binding domain at the active site of the molecule. Heparin and other glycosaminoglycans such as heparan sulfate found on endothelial cell surfaces activate antithrombin III via the process of allosteric activation. A pentasaccharide found in heparin and heparan sulfate contains a number of carboxyl and sulfoxyl groups which provide a large concentration of acidic, negative charges. This acidic structure binds to the heparin-binding domain of antithrombin III which contains a large concentration of positively charged lysine and arginine residues. This interaction results in a conformational change in the structure of antithrombin III that potentiates its enzymatic activity as a serine protease by several orders of magnitude [4, 10]. A critical arginine residue at position 393 in the antithrombin III molecule is brought in close proximity to serine at the active site of thrombin or other serine protease molecules of the coagulation system. A covalent bond is generated inactivating thrombin or other serine proteases in the coagulation system. This antithrombin-serine protease complex is then removed by the reticuloendothelial system [17].

Heparin competitively inhibits the binding of antithrombin III to heparan sulfate on endothelial surfaces. In the absence of heparin, antithrombin III will bind the endothelial surfaces and function as an anticoagulant on the cell surface of the microcirculation. In addition to its anticoagulant properties, antithrombin III bound to endothelial surfaces stimulates endothelial cells to increase the synthesis of prostacyclin. Prostacyclin is a potent inhibitor of platelet aggregation. Prostacyclin inhibits the synthesis of the pro-inflammatory cytokines by a prostacyclin-induced, cyclic adenosine monophosphate (cAMP)-mediated process and attenuates neutrophil activation thereby reducing neutrophil degranulation, elastase release and toxic oxygen radical release [20–22].

It should be noted that these anti-inflammatory properties of antithrombin III are only seen in the absence of therapeutic doses of heparin (which interferes with the interaction of antithrombin III with heparan sulfate found on endothelial surfaces). Additionally, the effect is observed primarily at supraphysiologic levels (> 150% normal levels) of antithrombin III [20].

Antithrombin III levels are rapidly depleted as a result of rapid complex formation with multiple activated clotting factors in sepsis-induced DIC [5]. Rapid depletion of antithrombin III is predictive of a fatal outcome in patients with sepsis [23, 24]. Based upon extensive preclinical evaluation of antithrombin III replacement therapy in experimental sepsis models [10, 25], antithrombin III is now in clinical trials in human sepsis [11, 26].

Protein C, Activated Protein C, and Protein S

The second critical regulatory element of the coagulation system is activated protein C. Protein C is synthesized as a zymogen which becomes activated by thrombin in association with another protein found on the cell surface of endothelial cells known as thrombomodulin [27]. The primary mechanism by which activated protein C inhibits the coagulation system is through the enzymatic degradation of activated forms of factor V and factor VIII [2,27,28]. Factor V is an essential component of the common clotting cascade that functions as a pro-thrombin converting complex along with factor Xa, phospholipids and calcium. Factor VIII is part of the intrinsic clotting system and contributes to activation of factor X via the contact system of the coagulation cascade.

Activated protein C is a rather complex molecule that undergoes extensive post-translational modification in order to be physiologically active. Human protein C is initially translated into a 461 amino acid peptide. The first 42 amino acids contain a signal peptide and a pro-peptide that serves as a recognition site for vitamin K-dependent carboxylase reactions [27]. The protein undergoes an internal proteolysis step at position lysine 156-arginine 157. This generates a heterodimer held together by a single di-sulfide bond with a light chain (amino acids 1–155) and a heavy chain (amino acids 157–419). The heavy chain possesses the serine protease domain essential to the inhibitory activity of protein C [4].

The molecule also undergoes extensive glycosylation at several arginine-linked glycosylation sites throughout the molecule. These glycosylation reactions are essential to the biological activity of the molecule. Protein C is a vitamin K-dependent protein which has a series of gamma-carboxyglutamates on the light chain. There is an additional unusual amino acid modification of an aspartate moiety at position 71. This amino acid undergoes a beta-hydroxylation reaction that is essential to generate a fully functional protein C molecule. Circulating protein C exists as zymogen that necessitates activation through the proteolytic cleavage of the first 12 amino acids at the amino terminus of the heavy chain of human protein C. This final proteolytic cleavage gives rise to activated protein C. This activation reaction is generated by thrombin in association with thrombomodulin.

Thrombomodulin expression is regulated by a number of physiologic variables including its synthetic rate, rate of release, and condition of endothelial cells throughout the circulation. Many pro-inflammatory cytokines inhibit the synthesis of thrombomodulin. This impairs the generation of activated protein C and results in a procoagulant state [4, 6]. Thrombomodulin is also inhibited through the action of neutrophil oxidants and elastase release [27]. In this manner, neutrophil-endothelial cell interactions in sepsis may further contribute to the generation of a procoagulant state in the microcirculation.

Protein S is considered a co-factor of protein C activity. Protein S is also a vitamin K-dependent protein and has structural domains and post-translation modifications similar to those found in protein C. Despite these structural similarities, protein S has important differences from protein C. First, protein S lacks a serine protease domain and therefore is inactive as an inhibitor of the coagulation system. Second, protein S will bind to C4b-binding protein. This binding protein is an acute phase reactant, and a regulatory element in the complement cascade [27, 29]. C4b-binding protein will complex with protein S and inactivate protein S as a co-factor for protein C. Free protein S contributes to protein C activity by rendering factor Va more susceptible to the catalytic activity of protein C. Protein S increases the anticoagulant activity of protein C by several fold.

Protein C has other activities in addition to its ability to inhibit the coagulation system. The carbohydrates found on protein S have been shown to attenuate the ability of E selectin to bind to human leukocytes [30]. The selectins are important in the initial interactions between white cells and endothelial cells and initiate the rolling of white cells on endothelial surfaces [31–34]. Prevention of E-selectin-leukocyte interactions may limit the potentially deleterious effects of neutrophil activation and injury to endothelial cells observed in patients with systemic inflammatory states. Through as yet unclear mechanisms, it also appears that protein C limits the generation of pro-inflammatory cytokines in lipopolysaccharide (LPS) challenge models [27]. Therefore, activated protein C, like antithrombin III, may have anti-inflammatory properties, in addition to its anticoagulant properties, that may prove to be therapeutically useful in sepsis.

Protein C and protein S levels fall rapidly at the onset of sepsis, and reduced levels of activated protein C portend a lethal outcome in severe sepsis [2–5, 23, 27, 28]. Protein C is inactivated by α1-antitrypsin, an acute phase protein, and protein C inhibitor (PCI) [4]. Rapid replacement of protein C has been successfully employed in clinical series of septic shock patients [2, 3, 28] and this therapeutic strategy is now the focus of a multicenter trial in severe sepsis.

Tissue Factor Pathway Inhibitor

TFPI is a unique inhibitor of the extrinsic clotting cascade. It is a 42 kDa glycoprotein consisting of 276 amino acids arranged in three Kunitz-type domains [35, 36]. The amino terminus of the molecule is acidic while the carboxy terminus has a series of positively charged, basic amino acid moieties. The first Kunitz domain interacts with surface-associated tissue factor and factor VIIa complex. The second Kunitz-type domain binds and inhibits factor Xa directly. Tissue factor and factor VIIa inhibition are mediated through a quaternary complex consisting of factor Xa-TFPI-factor VIIa-tissue factor [36, 37]. The role of the third Kunitz domain of TFPI is not clearly understood. Positively charged moieties of the third Kunitz domain in addition to the carboxy terminus of the molecule interact with heparin and possibly glycosaminoglycans on the cell surface of endothelial cells. It has recently been demonstrated that antithrombin III and heparin may contribute to the activity of TFPI as a tissue factor/factor VII complex inhibitor [19, 38].

TFPI is primarily synthesized by endothelial cells and is found on the cell surface of endothelial cells and free in the systemic circulation. Plasma levels are low (approximately 2 nanomol) [19]. Most of the circulating TFPI is associated with plasma lipoproteins (particularly low-density lipoprotein [LDL] and high-density lipoprotein [HDL]). Platelets also carry TFPI and this platelet source of TFPI may be released during platelet activation. Heparin increases the circulating levels of TFPI by several fold, an effect that appears to be mediated by release of TFPI from intracellular stores within endothelial cells [38]. Measurement of circulating levels of TFPI during systemic inflammatory states has revealed variable results which may be a reflection of the dynamics of TFPI release, the presence or absence of heparin, and the ability of assays to detect bound versus unbound TFPI in the circulation [4].

Like other endogenous anticoagulants, TFPI may have anti-inflammatory actions in addition to its anticoagulant properties. TFPI appears to interfere with LPS/CD14 interactions by its ability to bind directly to LPS. TFPI-LPS complexes prevent LPS transfer to LPS binding protein [39]. This inhibition blocks transfer of LPS monomer to CD14 on the cell surface of neutrophils and mononuclear cells. The functional significance of this LPS inhibitory property in sepsis is unclear at present and is the focus of current research efforts [40, 41].

Interestingly, TFPI gene disruption in mice is a lethal mutation [37, 42]. Homozygous TFPI (negative/negative) embryos do not survive to gestation. The concepti exhibit marked changes in embryogenesis with extensive hemorrhage and histologic evidence of abnormalities in the circulatory system. TFPI may have physiologic functions in the maintenance of vascular integrity which are unrelated to its anticoagulant properties.

Activation of the Coagulation System by Inflammatory Mediators

It is well known that systemic inflammation is accompanied by activation of the coagulation system [4–6]. The pro-inflammatory cytokines TNF-α, interleukin (IL)-1β, and IL-6 all increase tissue factor expression and inhibit the synthesis of thrombomodulin which is essential for the activation of protein C as a coagulation inhibitor [4]. The pro-inflammatory cytokines also activate the synthesis of plasminogen activator inhibitor (PAI-1) [6]. The fibrinolytic system is rapidly activated in sepsis (primarily via the intrinsic clotting system and through the actions of pro-inflammatory cytokines). However, the rapid activation of plasminogen is subsequently inhibited through the generation of PAI-1. The end result is a disordered state in which the coagulation system is unchecked by the fibrinolytic system resulting in a procoagulant state [4].

Neutrophil activation and degranulation releases elastase and toxic oxygen moieties from activated neutrophils. Neutrophil oxidants and elastase destroy thrombomodulin. Neutrophil elastase also inhibits antithrombin III and C1 inhibitor. C1 inhibitor not only regulates activation of the classic complement pathway but also inhibits a number of the components of the contact system [29, 43], particularly factor XII and prekallikrein [16]. The loss of C1 inhibitor results in a procoagulant state.

The acute phase protein response also results in a procoagulant state. Alpha-1 antitrypsin is a potent inhibitor of activated protein C. C-reactive protein (CRP) promotes the expression of tissue factor by mononuclear cells [4]. Tissue factor is the initial activator of the extrinsic clotting system. CRP has also been shown to activate complement via the classical complement pathway independent of specific antibody interactions [43]. The systemic activation of complement generates the anaphylatoxins (C3a, C5a), activates neutrophils and monocytes, induces cytokine synthesis, and promotes neutrophil/endothelial cell interactions. Complement activation also increases surface exposure of phosphatidylserine on the cell surface of endothelial cells which is a potent procoagulant stimulus [4].

Another acute phase protein is C4b binding protein. This regulatory protein for the complement system also binds to protein S and inactivates protein S. The loss of free protein S interferes with the ability of activated protein C to be fully functional as an inhibitor of factor V and factor VIII [27].

The Role of The Coagulation System in Activation of Inflammatory Mediators

It has been clearly demonstrated that thrombin generation in the systemic circulation is a highly injurious event with numerous pro-inflammatory sequelae [1–6]. Thrombin promotes platelet aggregation throughout the microcirculation. Activated platelets express P-selectin as do endothelial cells exposed to thrombin [32, 34, 44, 45]. P-selectin is the primary initial mediator of leukocyte-endothelial cell rolling and critical for attachment of white cells to endothelial cells. P-selectin glycoprotein ligand type I is expressed on neutrophils and specifically binds to P-selectin on endothelial and platelet surfaces [33, 34]. Thrombin induced P-selectin expression on endothelial surfaces further contributes to diffuse microvascular injury in sepsis as white cells become activated and adhere to capillaries and post-capillary venules.

P-selectin has recently been shown to bind to LPS which may increase local concentrations of LPS in the microcirculation [46]. Release of lytic enzymes from activated neutrophils further contribute to diffuse endothelial injury and vascular compromise in sepsis. Thrombin has also been shown to be an inducer of the potent vasoconstrictor endothelin 1 [29].

Conclusion

It has become increasingly clear that a complex and often synergistic relationship exists between the coagulation system and inflammatory networks observed in the severely septic patient. There is a wealth of preclinical data which supports the contention that inhibitors of the coagulation system may prove to be beneficial in the prevention of the pathophysiologic effects of systemic inflammatory mediators of sepsis. Early clinical trials in septic humans also support the hypothesis that regulation of the coagulation system with endogenous anticoagulants such as antithrombin III, TFPI, and activated protein C may have salutary effects in human sepsis as well. All three of these human anticoagulant regulatory proteins are currently in advanced stages of clinical trials in septic patients to determine their ultimate efficacy.

The levels of antithrombin III, protein C and protein S have all been shown to be reduced in severe sepsis and predict an adverse outcome in septic shock [1, 4, 6]. Therefore, the therapeutic rationale for replacement of these endogenous anticoagulants in human sepsis is quite clear. The major challenge remaining to clinical investigators is to determine the optimal dose, timing, and duration of therapy with these anticoagulants in septic patients. The answers to these questions should be forthcoming within the next few years as these clinical trials are completed.

References

1. Gando S, Kamene T, Nanzaki S, Nakanishi Y (1996) Disseminated intravascular coagulation is a frequent complication of systemic inflammatory response syndrome. Thromb Haemost 75:224–228
2. Smith OP, White B, Vaughan D, et al (1997) Use of protein-C concentrate, heparin, haemodiafiltration in meningococcus-induced purpura fulminans. Lancet 350:1590–1593
3. Rivard GE, David M, Farrell C, Schwarz HP (1995) Treatment of purpura fulminans in meningococcemia with protein C conjugate. J Pediatr 126:646–652
4. Vervloet NG, Thijs LG, Hack CE (1998) Derangements of coagulation and fibrinolysis in critically ill patients with sepsis and septic shock. Semin Thromb Hemost 24:33–34
5. Lorente JA, García-Frade L,J, Landín L, et al (1993) Time course of hemostatic abnormalities in sepsis and its relation to outcome. Chest 103:1536–1542
6. Levi M, ten Cate H, van der Poll T, van Deventer SJH (1993) Pathogenesis of disseminated intravascular coagulation in sepsis. JAMA 270:975–979
7. Van Deventer SJH, Büller HR, ten Cate JW, Aarden LA, Hack CE, Sturk A (1996) Experimental endotoxin in humans: an analysis of cytokine release and coagulation, fibrinolytic and complement pathways. Blood 88:2520–2528
8. van der Poll T, Jansen PW, van Zee KJ, et al (1996) Tumor necrosis factor-α induces activation of coagulation and fibrinolysis in baboons through an exclusive effect on the p55 receptor. Blood 88:922–927
9. Hinshaw LB (1996) Sepsis/septic shock: participation of the microcirculation: an abbreviated review. Crit Care Med 24:1072–1078
10. Dickneite G (1998) Antithrombin III in animal models of sepsis and organ failure. Semin Thromb Haemost 24:61–69
11. Eisele B, Lamy M (1998) Clinical experience with antithrombin III concentrates in critically ill patients with sepsis and multiple organ failure. Semin Thromb Haemost 24:71–80
12. Taylor FB Jr, Chang A, Ruf W, et al (1991) Lethal *E. coli* septic shock is prevented by blocking tissue factor with monoclonal antibody. Circ Shock 33:127–135
13. Gando S, Smanzaki S, Sasaki S, Aoi K, Kemmotsu O (1998) Activation of the extrinsic coagulation pathway in patients with severe sepsis and septic shock. Crit Care Med 26:2005–2009
14. Gray E, Thomas S, Mistry Y, Poole S (1996) Inhibition of tissue factor and cytokine release. Haemostasis 26:92–95
15. Pixley RA, De La Cadena R, Page JD, et al (1993) The contact system contributes to hypotension but not to disseminated intravascular coagulation in lethal bacteremia. J Clin Invest 91:61–70
16. Nuijens JH, Huijbregts C, Erenberg-Belmer AJ, et al (1988) Quantification of plasma factor XIIa C1-inhibitor and kallikrein - CI-inhibitor complexes in sepsis. Blood 72:1841–1848
17. Mammen EF (1998) Antithrombin III: its physiologic importance and role in DIC. Semin Thromb Haemost 24:19–25

18. Eisele B, Lamy N, Thijs LG, et al (1998) Anti-thrombin III in patients with severe sepsis: a randomized, placebo-controlled, double-blind, multicenter trial plus a meta-analysis on all randomized-placebo-controlled, double-blind trials with antithrombin III in severe sepsis. Intensive Care Med 24:663–672
19. Jesty J, Lorenz A, Rodriguez J, Wun TC (1996) Initiation of tissue factor pathway of coagulation in the presence of heparin: control by antithrombin III and tissue factor pathway inhibitor. Blood 15:2301–2307
20. Uchida M, Okajima K, Murakami K (1998) Effects of various doses of antithrombin III and endotoxin-induced endothelial cell injury and coagulation abnormalities in rats. Thromb Res 89:233–241
21. Yamanuchi T, Umeda F, Inoguchi I, Nawata H (1989) Antithrombin III stimulates prostacyclin production by cultured aortic endothelial cells. Biochem Biophys Res Commun 163: 1404–1411
22. Horie S, Ichii H, Kazama M (1990) Heparin-like glycosaminoglycan is a receptor for antithrombin III-dependent but not thrombin-dependent prostacyclin production in human endothelial cells. Thromb Res 59:899–904
23. Fourrier F, Chopin C, Goudemand J, et al (1992) Septic shock, multi-organ failure, and disseminated intravascular coagulation: compared to patterns of antithrombin III-protein C and protein S deficiencies. Chest 101:816–823
24. Mesters RW, Mannucci PW, Coppola R, Keller T, Ostermann H, Kienast J (1996) Factor VII and antithrombin III activity during sepsis and septic shock in neutropenic patients. Blood 88:881–886
25. Uchiba M, Okajima K (1997) Antithrombin III prevents LPS-induced vascular injury: novel biological activity of antithrombin III. Semin Thromb Haemost 23:583–590
26. Inthorn D, Hoffmann JM, Hartl WH, Muhlbayer D, Jochum M (1997) Antithrombin III supplementation in severe sepsis: beneficial effects on organ dysfunction. Shock 8:328–334
27. Yan SB, Grinnell BW (1993) Recombinant human protein C, protein S and thrombomodulin as antithrombotics. Prospectives in Drug Discovery and Design 1:503–520
28. Rintala E, Seppälä O-P, Kotilainen P, Pettilä V, Rasi V (1998) Protein C in the treatment of coagulopathy in meningococcal disease. Crit Care Med 26:965–968
29. Dries DJ (1996) Activation of the clotting system and complement after trauma. New Horiz 4:276–288
30. Grinnell BW, Hermann RB, Yan SB (1994) Human protein C inhibits selectin-mediated cell adhesion: role of unique fucosylated oligosaccharide. Glycobiology 4:221–225
31. Kansas GS (1996) Selectins and their ligands: Current concepts and controversies. Blood 88:3259–3287
32. Coughlan AF, Hau H, Dunlop LC, Berndt MC, Hancock WW (1994) P-selectin and platelet-activating factor mediate initial endotoxin-induced neutropenia. J Exp Med 179:329–334
33. Snapp KR, Ding H, Atkins K, Warnek R, Luscinskas FW, Kansas GS (1998) A novel P selectin glycoprotein ligand-1 monoclonal antibody recognizes and epitope within the tyrosine sulfate motif of human PSGL-1 and blocks recognition of both P- and L-selectin. Blood 91: 154–164
34. Lim YC, Snapp K, Kansas GS, Camphaysen R, Ding H, Luscinskas FW (1998) Important contributions of P-selectin glycoprotein ligand-1-mediated secondary capture of human monocyte adhesin to P-selectin, E-selectin, and TNF-alpha-activated endothelium under flow in vitro. J Immunol 161:2501–2508
35. Bajaj MS, Bajaj SP (1997) Tissue factor pathway inhibitor: potential therapeutic applications. Thrombo Haemost 78:471–477
36. Tieman C, Brinkmann T, Kleesiek K (1997) Detection of Kunitz-single domains in membrane bound tissue factor pathway inhibitor (TFPI) by flow cytometry. Eur J Clin Chem Clin Biochem 35:855–860
37. Huang Z-F, Broze G Jr (1997) Consequences of tissue factor pathway inhibitor gene-disruption in mice. Thromb Haemostas 78:699–704
38. Hamamoto T, Kisiel W (1996) The effect of heparin on the regulation of factor VIIa-tissue factor activity by tissue factor pathway inhibitor. Blood Coagul Fibrinolysis 7:470–476

39. Park CT, Creasey AA, Wright SD (1997) Tissue factor pathway inhibitor blocks cellular effects of endotoxin by binding to endotoxin and interfering with transfer of CD14. Blood 89: 4268–4674
40. Creasey AA, Chang ACK, Feigen L, Wün T-C, Taylor FB, Hinshaw LB (1993) Tissue factor pathway inhibitor reduces mortality in *Escherichia coli* septic shock. J Clin Invest 91: 2850–2860
41. Camerota AJ, Creasey AA, Patla V, Larkin VA, Fink MB (1998) Delayed treatment of recombinant human tissue factor pathway inhibitor improved survival in rabbits with Gram-negative peritonitis. J Infect Dis 177:668–676
42. Broze GJ (1998) Tissue factor pathway inhibitor gene disruption. Blood Coagul Fibrinolysis 9 (suppl 1):S89–S92
43. Wolbink G-J, Bossink AWJ, Groeneveld ABJ, DeGroot MCM, Thijs LG, Hack CE (1998) Complement activation in patients with sepsis is in part mediated by C-reactive protein. J Infect Dis 177:81–87
44. Borges E, Eytner R, Moll T, et al (1997) The P-selectin glycoprotein ligand-1 is important for recruitment of neutrophils into inflamed mouse peritoneum. Blood 90:1934–1942
45. Jung U, Ramos CL, Bullard DC, Lay K (1998) Gene-targeted mice reveal importance of L-selectin-dependent rolling for neutrophil adhesion. Am J Physiol 274:1785–1791
46. Malhotra R, Priest R, Foster MR, Brad MI (1998) P-selectin binds to bacterial lipopolysaccharide. Eur J Immunol 28:985–988

The Endothelium as an Immune Organ: Active Player and Passive Target?

H. Redl

Introduction

The vascular endothelium lines the vascular tree and covers several square meters. One of its characteristics is its heterogeneity, which actually makes it difficult to discuss 'the endothelial cell' and to draw conclusions on results from different types of experiment. Endothelial cells are no longer considered as passive bystanders, but play a central role in the coordination of the inflammatory response. Endothelial cells are dynamic participants in the communication with circulating blood cells, acting as doorkeepers in blood cell margination and extravasation. Endothelial cells are important sites of synthesis of mediators including those providing an adequate vascular tone. Endothelial cells further regulate coagulation and fibrinolysis, maintain selective permeability and at the same time serve as target cells for many substances released during traumatic and septic shock [1]. Endothelial cell regulated vascular growth is beyond the scope of this chapter. Since only a few endothelial cells are circulating [2], it is difficult to monitor their status, and this will be discussed further below.

The response of endothelial cells to mediators differs according to the substance that interacts with the endothelial cell. The different endothelial cell responses can be classified as endothelial stimulation (fast, protein synthesis-independent response) and endothelial activation (slower, protein synthesis-dependent response) analogous to the local inflammatory scenario reviewed by Pober and Cotran [3]. These responses are also referred to as type I and type II endothelial cell activation [4]. Endothelial cell activation leads to a variety of events in the different fields of endothelial investigation (Table 1).

Table 1. Variety of events in endothelial cell activation

Vascular tone	Cellular interaction	Coagulation status
↑ Endothelin	↑ MHC II Expression	↑ Tissue Factor
↑↓Nitric Oxide	↑↓Adhesion	↓ Anti Platelet Activity
↓ Prostacyclin	↑ Cytokine Production	↓ Anti Coagulants
↑ Thromboxane		↓ Fibrinolytic Agents
? Angiotensin		
↑ PAF		

Cellular Interaction

Endothelial cell-leukocyte interactions are dependent largely on adhesion molecules. The endothelial adhesion molecules consist of the selectins (E-selectin, formerly known as endothelial leukocyte adhesion molecules-1 or ELAM-1, P-selectin, formerly known as granule membrane protein 140 or GMP-140) and molecules that belong to the immunoglobulin supergene family (e.g., intercellular adhesion molecule 1 or ICAM-1, vascular cell adhesion molecule-1 or VCAM-1) [5]. In addition, the bulk of available evidence implicates the leukocyte adhesion complex CD11/CD18 and L-selectin as the primary adhesion molecules of neutrophils.

Endothelial Stimulation

In response to agonists, such as thrombin and histamine [6] or oxygen radicals [7] and deposited terminal complement complexes [8], endothelial stimulation occurs. Primary molecules involved in endothelial stimulation are P-selectin [6, 9] and platelet activating factor (PAF) [10] on the endothelial side as well as PSGL-1 (P-selectin glycoprotein ligand receptor) and PAF receptors as their polymorphonuclear leukocyte (PMN) counterparts. P-selectin attaches leukocytes to endothelial cells via o-linked oligosaccharides containing sialyl Lewis^x related structures [11].

P-selectin is located in the Weibel-Palade bodies and is transported to the cell surface upon stimulation [12], where it induces the well known 'rolling' phenomenon of leukocytes. *In vitro* studies have shown that thrombin-stimulated cells, which produce PAF, can augment and prime PMN to produce superoxide, release proteases and enhance their ability to damage endothelial cells [13]. On the other hand, thrombin-stimulated endothelial cells produce prostacyclin [14], which decreases PMN adherence to endothelial cells. Thrombin also stimulates nitric oxide (NO) production which inversely modulates P-selectin expression [15–17]. Beside NO there are further endogenous mediators, such as adenosine, that inhibit the leukocyte-endothelium interaction [18]. In addition to P-selectin, human microvascular endothelial cells contain IL-8 in intracellular granules which co-express with von Willebrand factor. Following exposure of endothelial cells to histamine or thrombin, a dramatic increase in supernatant IL-8 concentration is observed within minutes [19].

Probably the most prominent sign of endothelial-leukocyte activation and interactions is leukostasis demonstrated both in experimental as well as in clinical posttraumatic situations [20]. Similar results have been found in baboon and rat models with hypovolemic shock, showing leukostasis in lung and liver tissues [21, 22]. More direct evidence has been obtained from splanchnic shock experiments in rats, where leukocyte adherence was noted upon reperfusion using intravital fluorescence microscopy. Such effects were attenuated by PAF antagonists [23]. Furthermore, using the intravital microscopic approach, a significant increase in endothelial-leukocyte interactions in liver sinusoids was observed after hemorrhagic shock. Such an early inflammatory reaction in liver sinusoids may reflect an initiation process which probably contributes to the subsequent organ failure [24].

The need for expression of adhesion proteins in neutrophil-dependent acute lung injury (ALI) was shown in rats after vascular injury [25]. Following systemic complement activation, a rapid translocation of P-selectin from cytoplasmic granules to the endothelial cells surface occurred [26]. Adhesion protein expression was demonstrated immunohistochemically and, after treatment with anti-P-selectin antibodies, beneficial effects were demonstrated with evidence of lesser changes in vascular permeability and decreased hemorrhage. This was accompanied by greatly reduced leukostasis and the diminished adherence of neutrophils. Activated complement not only induces P-selectin expression, but contributes to endothelial cell dysfunction after hemorrhage/resuscitation as demonstrated by the use of the complement inhibitor soluble complement receptor-1 (sCR1) [26]. Studies have also shown that ischemia/reperfusion-induced platelet-endothelium interactions are dependent on the expression of P-selectin by endothelial cells [27].

The rolling phenomenon of neutrophils is mediated by members of the selectin family (L-, E- and P-selectin). L-selectin is constitutively present on leukocytes and rapidly shed following neutrophil activation [28]. L-selectin interacts with glycosylation-dependent cell adhesion molecule (GlyCAM)-1, CD34, mucosal addressin cell adhesion molecule (MAdCAM)-1 ligands on the endothelial cells, which contain sulphated, sialylated and fucosylated oligosaccharides [11]. Additionally the cutaneous lymphocyte antigen is an essential component of the L-selectin ligand which is induced on human vascular endothelial cells [29]. L-selectin initiates the interaction of neutrophil adhesion via increasing beta-integrins (CD11/CD18), which are responsible for the strengthening of adhesion and the ensuing migration process with extravasation of neutrophils into the tissue, e.g., lung [28, 30–33]. Ley et al. [34] showed that rolling is initially dependent on P-selectin and later on L-selectin, thus leading them to conclude that L-selectin is prominently involved in rolling and adherence events. Adherence has been proposed to be a two-step process, with rolling as the initial phase, followed by adherence via CD11/CD18–ICAM-1 interactions [32]. In addition to the induction of rolling and adherence, the important role of adhesion molecules for signal transduction should be considered [35].

Endothelial Activation

Direct endotoxin (lipopolysaccharide, LPS)-induced activation of endothelial cells is dependent on the presence of soluble CD14 [36], since endothelial cells do not possess membrane bound CD14, which is necessary for binding the LPS/LPS binding protein (LBP) complex. There is evidence that endothelial activation in the presence of endotoxin is augmented via cytokine release from monocytes which are in turn activated by an LBP/CD14-dependent mechanism [37]. However it remains unknown how the transmembrane signaling occurs. Such signaling might involve toll-like receptors, as currently shown for other cell types [38].

Endothelial cell activation involves nuclear factor-kappa B (NF-κB) [39] and it has been shown that E-selectin expression requires continuous presence of LPS at least *in vitro* [40]. rBPI21, a recombinant N-terminal fragment of human bactericidal/permeability-increasing protein (BPI) acts to reverse LPS-mediated endothelial activation by interrupting the on-going LPS signal. Furthermore E-selectin expression can be down-regulated by interleukin (IL)-4, transforming growth factor (TGF)-β and IFN-γ [41].

De novo expression of adhesion molecules has been shown to occur under septic conditions in subprimate animal models [42], e.g., E-selectin in kidney, liver, lung, heart and skin biopsies. With the use of skin biopsies, it was possible to establish the kinetic expression pattern which was most prominent at 4–6 hours and not detectable 10–24 hours after the induction of sepsis. The above findings are in agreement with septic shock studies in Cynomolgous monkeys [43] where LPS infusion induced a generalized E-selectin expression most pronounced in the vasculature of lung tissue and skin. Again serial skin biopsies showed the onset of E-selectin expression at 2 hours and its maximum expression at 4 hours. Both studies showed that in contrast to earlier findings, E-selectin expression was not restricted to postcapillary venules [42, 43]. However, animals subjected to traumatic/ hypovolemic shock had only minimal expression of E-selectin after 6 hours of shock, which was much less pronounced than observed under septic conditions. This difference could be due to the difference in circulating cytokine/endotoxin concentrations in the two models [42]. Furthermore studies with the use of anti E-selectin antibodies [42] have indicated salutary effects of such an approach on survival following sepsis (Fig. 1).

In contrast to E-selectin, which is not present on normal endothelial cells, ICAM-1 is constitutively expressed on endothelial cells. ICAM-1 can be up-regulated (partly in a thiol-regulated manner [44]) and is responsible for the final

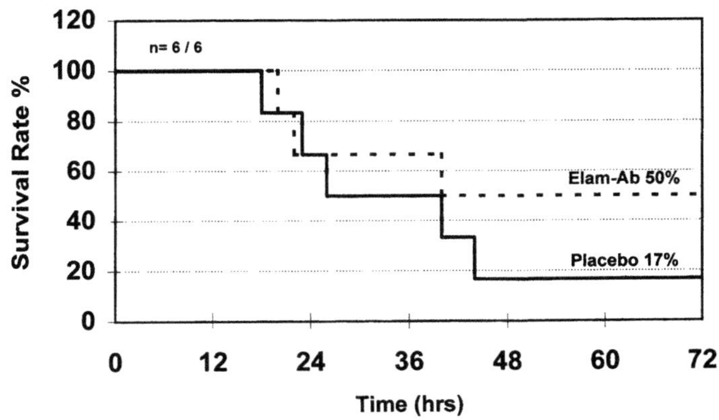

Fig. 1. Survival curves of septic baboons (live *E.coli* 10^9 CFU/kg) with (dashed line) or without (solid line) pretreatment (−2 and 4 hrs) with 5 mg/kg anti E-selectin antibody (in collaboration with M. Robinson, Celltech, Slough, Berkshire, UK)

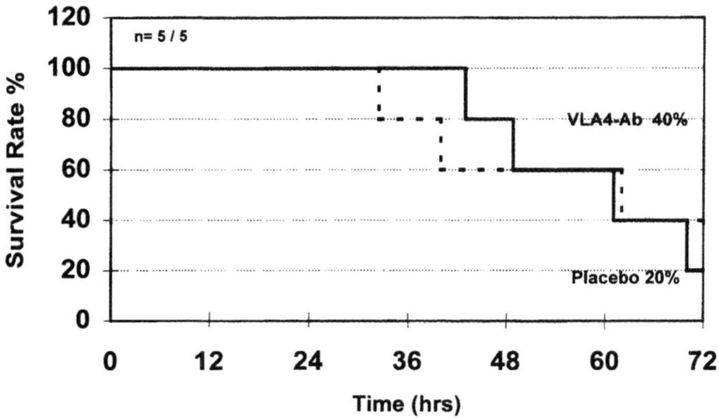

Fig. 2. Survival curves of septic baboons (live *E.coli* 10^9 CFU/kg) with (dashed line) or without (solid line) pretreatment (−1 h) with 1 mg/kg anti VLA4 antibody, potentially interfering with the binding to VCAM-1 on endothelial cells (in collaboration with R. Lobb, Biogen, Cambridge, MA, USA)

attachment, and together with platelet endothelial cell adhesion molecule (PECAM)-1, for transmigration of leukocytes into the surrounding tissue along chemotactic gradients [45]. The exception to this is the liver during endotoxemia [46].

Increased expression of ICAM-1 on cells has been associated with inflammatory disorders known to involve PMNs [47], and ICAM-1 up-regulation is reported to be sufficient to promote cytotoxicity via activated PMNs. ICAM-1 represents a potential target for attenuating PMN-mediated injury to endothelial and other cells [48]. Beside ICAM, VCAM-1 is another member of the immunoglobulin family, which binds to very late antigen (VLA)-4 and seems to be specifically responsible for monocyte adherence. Experimental sepsis studies in a primate model using anti-VLA4 antibodies, however, do not indicate an important role in the septic response. No difference was found between the antibody and placebo group (Fig. 2).

In addition to leukocyte trafficking, endothelial cells have the property of presenting antigen via major histocompatibility antigen (MHC) I present on unstimulated endothelial cells. MHC I up-regulation is seen after TNF exposure, but MHC II expression is found only after IFN-γ stimulation. Furthermore, human endothelial cells also induce and regulate cytolytic T cell differentiation [49].

Anti-Adherence Measures

Since neutrophil adherence to endothelium is mediated by cell surface receptors, experimental studies have been carried out using antibodies and other agents directed against both neutrophil and endothelial cell-surface receptors. Blocking interaction between the CD11/CD18 complex and ICAM with specific monoclonal antibodies has been shown to reduce tissue injury and organ dysfunction following hemorrhagic shock and ischemia/reperfusion in animal models [50, 51]. In addition to CD11/CD18 and ICAM-1, Garcia-Criado et al. [52] demonstrated that early modulation of the interaction between P-selectin and its ligand decreased neutrophil adhesion and migration and consequently diminished damage to the liver.

Using neutralizing monoclonal antibodies that recognize functional epitopes of L-selectin, a reduction in injury following ischemia/reperfusion [53], hemorrhage [54], and sepsis [55] has been found. The results obtained in a recent baboon study demonstrate the protective role of HuDREG-55 (a humanized monoclonal antibody specific for L-selectin) during resuscitation following trauma [56]. Benefit was demonstrated by a significantly higher survival rate after three days (Fig. 3) in a well-established non-human primate model of trauma [57]. To the best of our knowledge, this is the first report of such a salutary effect in a primate model of trauma. In general, these results are in agreement with previous inhibitor studies using anti-L-selectin measures that include not only antibodies [53–55], but also soluble molecules such as low molecular weight carbohydrates, for example sialyl Lewis^x [58]. The microcirculatory protection provided by HuDREG-55, which functionally blocks the L-selectin molecule, may be related to its effect on L-selectin mediated PMN rolling [30] on one hand, and probably to L-selectin as a signal transduction molecule on the other [34, 59, 60]. Alternatively, it could be due to the result of reduced PMN aggregation [61]. All three possibilities could lead to less microcirculatory plugging and less endothelial damage due to activated PMNs.

Despite the positive effects seen in the various studies, blockade of adhesion molecules on the leukocytes carries potential negative side effects [62, 63], including a potential risk of increased infection. Recent studies demonstrate that

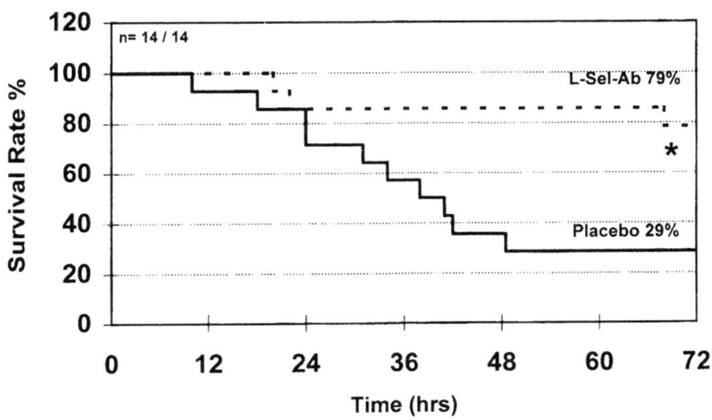

Fig. 3. Improved survival of baboons subjected to hemorrhagic-traumatic shock upon treatment with the anti L-selectin antibody HuDREG55 (2 mg/kg) during the resuscitation period. Data from [56], * $p < 0.05$

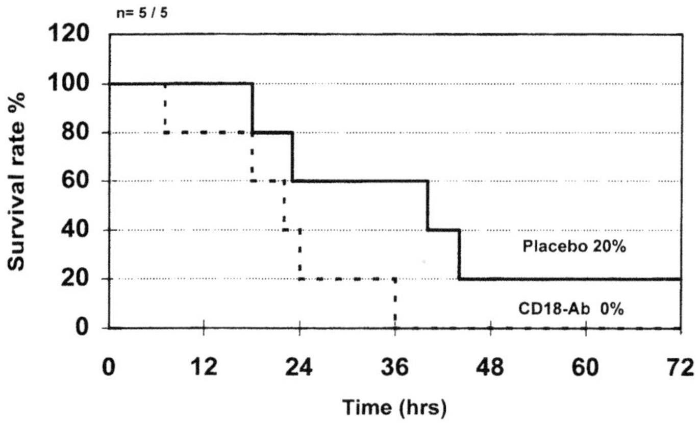

Fig. 4. Unfavorable outcome upon treatment with anti CD18 antibody (−2 hrs, 1 mg/kg) in a baboon sepsis model led to termination of this experimental study

anti-L-selectin antibody-based therapy does not carry such risks [64, 65]. However, an anti-L-selectin therapy approach has not been found to produce any salutary effect in a baboon sepsis model (unpublished observations, in association with Dr. Martin).

The importance of adhesion is further emphasized by studies which utilized monoclonal antibodies (60.3, IB4) against the common CD18 beta-chain. Such antibodies have been shown to produce beneficial effects following hypovolemic shock [50, 66], gut ischemia/reperfusion [67, 68], myocardial infarction [69], LPS-induced leukostasis [70, 71], sepsis induced lung injury [72], or other PMN/monocyte-related tissue injuries [73–75].

Similar to anti-CD18, anti-CD11a and anti-CD11b monoclonal antibodies were found to be tissue-protective. Blockade of ICAM-1 on the endothelial cells has been found to produce a protective effect in isolated lungs [73], and in the mesenteric circulation of rabbits with zymosan-plasma infusion [76]. Pre-treatment with both anti-ICAM-1 and anti-CD11/18 was effective, while only anti-CD11a and anti-CD18 were able to remove the previously adherent leukocytes. Furthermore, antibodies against CD18/ICAM-1 effectively inhibited the development of the local Shwartzman response in rabbit skin [77]. However, anti-CD18 antibody treatment in septic baboons has been shown to produce severe organ damage and failed to improve survival rates [63] (Fig. 4).

Endothelial Cells as a Procoagulant Source

Normally endothelial cells are in an anticoagulant state based on:

i) activation of protein C and S via thrombomodulin/thrombin interaction. Protein C inactivates factors Va and VIII and together with protein S activates plasminogen

ii) endothelial cells expresses surface-bound heparan sulfate which binds antithrombin III (AT III) and catalyses AT III based thrombin inhibition
iii) endothelial cells synthesize tissue factor pathway inhibitor (TFPI) [78]. Endothelial cells also produces tissue plasminogen activator (t-PA), prostacyclin (PGI2) as well as NO, as platelet anti-activation agents. PGI2 induction in endothelial cells is supposed to be one of the protective mechanisms of AT III infusion (Y. Taoko, personal communication). The surface-bound heparan sulfate is not only important for AT III, but also for binding of extracellular superoxide dismutase (ecSOD) [79]. The activated complement fragment C5a can be responsible for the release of heparan sulfate from endothelial cells [80] or activated PMN can degrade heparan sulfate via the release of heparanases [81]. This might also account in part for the fact that heparin or heparin derivatives have beneficial effects on endothelial cell function in sepsis [82].

When the endothelial cell is activated, a shift in favor of procoagulant factors occurs due to down-regulation of anticoagulant, and up-regulation of procoagulant, factors. Of central importance is the tissue factor expression which can be induced by inflammatory mediators as well as hypoxia [83]. In addition, endothelial cell-derived von Willebrand factor and PAF act as cofactors for platelet adhesion. When stimulated, platelets also produce higher amounts of thromboxane A2, which further stimulates platelet aggregation and can lead to microthrombosis. For a recent excellent review on this topic see [84].

Endothelial Cells as Source of Cytokines

Endothelial cells are important producers of IL-1, IL-6 and IL-8 (for a recent review see [85]) as well as colony stimulating factors [86] and chemokines for monocytic cells. In this respect, IL-8 is particularly interesting, since endothelial cells contain pre-stored IL-8 in the Weibel-Palade bodies, from which rapid secretion can occur [19]. The prolonged stimulation of primary human endothelial cells with inflammatory mediators resulted in the accumulation of IL-8 in Weibel-Palade bodies, where it co-localized with von Willebrand factor. These findings suggest that storage of IL-8 in Weibel-Palade bodies may serve as the endothelial cell 'memory' of a preceding inflammatory insult, which then enables the cells to secrete IL-8 immediately without *de novo* protein synthesis [87].

Various factors, especially TNF and IL-1, from inflammatory cell sources can induce endothelial cells to express IL-8 and IL-6 as well as other cytokines. In addition endothelial cells produce IL-1α and IL-1β following stimulation with LPS especially in the presence of soluble CD14 and LBP (natural serum constituents). In the presence of monocytes (co-cultures) the production of cytokines is increased [88]. Agents like histamine, thrombin and endothelium have positive modulatory effects. NO on the other hand decreases cytokine-induced endothelial activation including cytokine synthesis [89].

Like TNF-α and interleukin-1, CD40L on platelets induces endothelial cells to secrete chemokines and to express adhesion molecules, thereby generating signals for the recruitment and extravasation of leukocytes at the site of injury [90].

Endothelial Cell Damage

In general, adhering and activated PMNs are considered crucial in endothelial damage since they create a microenvironment in which mediators are released locally, and damage occurs. This type of damage has been previously attributed to the effect of oxygen radicals, proteases, or both. The endothelium appears to be an early target of oxidant injury as demonstrated by the use of activated adherent neutrophils [91] or acellular systems that produce oxygen radicals. In particular, hydrogen peroxide (H_2O_2) [92], or peroxide-derived products have been shown to induce cell lysis *in vitro* [93] and increased permeability [94, 95] in tissues such as the isolated lungs [96]. Oxygen radical cytotoxicity occurring *in vivo* can, however, be limited by the modulating action of endothelial cells [97], by the protective role of glutathione in the endothelial cell, by intracellular antioxidative enzymes [98], or by the scavenging action of erythrocytes [99].

Studies have also provided *in vivo* visualization of oxidative changes in microvessels during neutrophil activation [100]. In the rat, oxidative changes in the vessel walls of the mesenteric bed were co-localized with neutrophils adhering to the endothelium or migrating to the interstitium. These neutrophil-dependent changes were PAF induced; however, such changes were comparable to the changes induced by hydrogen peroxide without PMNs.

Cell injury is known to cause release of iron [101], thus the conversion of superoxide (O_2^-) and hydrogen peroxide to the aggressive hydroxyl radical ($OH^\cdot$) is likely to occur. Hydroxyl radical is an important oxidant involved in neutrophil-mediated cell injury. Iron chelators or hydroxyl radical scavengers have been shown to significantly attenuate endothelial cell damage [100]. The importance of free radicals and other active oxygen metabolites in trauma and sepsis-induced organ changes, including those induced by the acute respiratory distress syndrome (ARDS), have been reviewed [102, 103]. Studies have also suggested that circulating xanthine oxidase is responsible for lung neutrophil retention after intestinal ischemia and reperfusion [104]. Other sources of O_2^- are endothelial constitutive NO synthase (ecNOS) as well as inducible NOS (iNOS) due to the lack of arginine and supply of oxygen as described below.

NO appears to produce protective effects against hydrogen peroxide induced damage. Pretreatment of cells with different NO donors increased endothelial cGMP content and reduced hydrogen peroxide-related endothelial hyperpermeability. The major cGMP degrading pathway in endothelial cells was phosphodiesterase 2 (PDE2). Simultaneous guanylyl-cyclase activation/PDE2 inhibition may thus be a valuable approach for the treatment of endothelial hyperpermeability [105].

While PMN related endothelial cell damage is crucial in many organs, e.g., lung, plugging of capillaries by leukocytes is not a primary cause for the manifestation of no-reflow in post-ischemic striated muscle. Moreover, *in vivo* studies have shown that thrombus formation and intravascular clotting are not significant and histological examination supports the concept that ischemia/reperfusion induces the disruption of the endothelial integrity with loss of fluid to endothelial cells and the interstitial space. As a consequence, endothelial cell swelling and interstitial edema formation, which contribute to capillary lumenal narrowing, and increase of hydraulic resistance, appears to be important for producing the impairment in perfusion (for review of this topic see [106]).

Endothelial Cells as a Source of Vasoactive Agents

Endothelial cells are both a source of vasoconstrictive agents such as endothelin (for review, see [107]) which is increased in sepsis [108] as well as vasodilatory agents such as NO on which special emphasis is placed in this part of the review.

NO, as both a vasodilator and under certain circumstances cytotoxic molecule, is suggested to be one of the critical mediators of severe inflammation and septic shock [109, 110], even if no infection is involved [111]. There is, however considerable controversy concerning the issue of whether NO is really a critical molecule in sepsis and whether inhibition/scavenging has beneficial or detrimental effects. A vast number of studies exist demonstrating either one or both of these effects, and this topic has been thoroughly reviewed recently [112].

NOS inhibition has been studied in baboons using a well established model of sepsis [113] in which most pitfalls of previous investigations (reviewed in [112]) were avoided. At six days, the survival rate of baboons treated with the non-selective NOS inhibitor N^G-nitro-monomethyl-L-arginine (L-NMMA, 546C88) was significantly improved compared to placebo, thus indicating an overall salutary effect of the therapeutic regimen tested. The beneficial effect was evident despite the fact that treatment was started 12 hours after induction of sepsis. Efficacy of such a delayed treatment in sepsis models is rather unique (except for multiple challenge models [114]) since most experimental studies utilize pre- or early (within 1 hour) post-treatment schedules [115]. Regarding safety issues raised by two recent reviews [112, 116], no negative side effects of 546C88 therapy were found in the experimental setup.

Unfortunately, a clinical study performed in parallel did demonstrate deleterious effects of this drug and the trial had to be stopped. One of the major differences in the treatment regimen used clinically was the dose escalating strategy based on the decrease in arterial pressure drop, versus a fixed dose in the non-human primate study. Another problem might be that non-selective inhibitors of NO synthesis unmask a tonic pressor response of endothelin-1 in human septic shock [117]. It, therefore, appears that new approaches utilizing the so-called selective iNOS inhibitors [118] might prove more successful but might also not be the magic bullet [119].

It is also important to recognize that LPS not only induces iNOS, but also increases the specific activity of ecNOS within the first 10 hours of LPS treatment by a post-translational modification mediated through a protein tyrosine kinase cascade [120]. In contrast to treatment with LPS, Zhou et al. [121] reported that ecNOS is down-regulated during hyperdynamic sepsis as produced by cecal ligation and puncture.

The use of NOS inhibition in hemorrhagic shock is also rather controversial. Both the type and dose of NOS inhibitor are important variables. Of the non-isoform selective inhibitors N^G-nitro-L-arginine methyl ester (L-NAME) worsened injury [122–124], while the use of L-NMMA at an optimized dose of 2 mg/kg used during re-infusion reduced injury and prolonged survival [22]. However, if the dose of L-NMMA was increased to 20 mg/kg, it produced detrimental effects. Beside non-specific inhibitors, selective inhibitors for iNOS have also been tested and found to improve the survival rates of experimental animals [125, 126]. Salutary effects have also been observed by using the NO scavenger NOX-100 (T. Billiar, personal communication). Thus, it appears that the constitutively expressed endothelial enzyme ecNOS (or cNOS), which is activated upon calcium release or influx, is important for the homeostasis of the microcirculation during shock and following reperfusion. It is also known that heat-shock protein 90 associates with ecNOS by agonists that stimulate production of NO, namely vascular endothelial growth factor, histamine, fluid shear stress, and enhances the activation of ecNOS [127]. This reaction could provide the necessary vasorelaxation and most likely the anti-adhesion effects for neutrophils and platelets. In view of this, blocking ecNOS by L-NAME and giving high dose L-NMMA are expected to be detrimental, whereas delayed NOS inhibitor treatment acting partially at neoexpressed iNOS appears to be beneficial [22, 124], similar to iNOS inhibition or scavenging excess NO. However, at least for the local ischemia/reperfusion situation, there is a lack of NO generation, probably due to the limited local substrate of iNOS, arginine. The lack of arginine could provoke the double-faced nature of NOS, being able to use oxygen as a substrate and producing O_2^- [128]. The situation can at least partially be overcome by infusion of arginine [129] or by down-regulation of cNOS by supplying NO donors such as a special S-nitrosated human albumin, which was processed and synthesized to yield a high S-nitroso content (S-nitrosation yield: 85–90 % per mol albumin [130]). Other NO donors have been found to be protective in hemorrhagic-traumatic shock [124, 131] and arginine has also been successfully used as a therapeutic agent in hemorrhagic shock [132–134].

NO has not only vasoactive properties but it also appears to be partly responsible for radical related tissue damage [135, 136], and is an important mediator of immunological responses, e.g., cytokine induction. By using the iNOS inhibitor N6-(iminoethyl)-L-lysine, or iNOS knockout mice, Hierholzer et al. [137] found that the activation of the transcriptional factor, NF-κB, and the signal transducer and activator of transcription 3 (STAT 3) increased IL-6 and granulocyte colony-stimulating factor (G-CSF) messenger RNA levels in the lungs and liver at 4 hours after resuscitation from hemorrhagic shock and these events were iNOS dependent. Furthermore, NO has been found to modulate P-selectin and ICAM-1 mRNA expression [138].

Monitoring of Endothelial Cells

Although it is difficult to directly examine the expression of endothelial-leukocyte cell adhesion molecules in patient organs, the detection of soluble, shed adhesion molecules in serum may provide an indication of the extent of up-regulation during the inflammatory response [139]. According to Law et al., a significant correlation was observed between the absolute levels of soluble ICAM-1 at the time of resuscitation and the severity of subsequent MOF in severely injured trauma patients [140]. Likewise, a subset of major trauma patients manifested elevated levels of circulating shed E-selectin and possibly P-selectin after injury and resuscitation, especially in those with lethal outcomes from infections and organ failure [141]. These data imply that endothelial-leukocyte cell interactions are up-regulated immediately after injury and (based upon successful therapeutic intervention) may be implicated in the systemic inflammatory response that leads to MOF.

Soluble E-selectin was measured in a group of patients undergoing the trauma associated with cardiac surgery and extracorporeal circulation. Some of those patients developed systemic inflammatory response syndrome (SIRS) and had higher, but not significant, levels of soluble E-selectin in association with significantly higher levels of IL-6 [142]. In a study of polytrauma patients, soluble E-selectin and soluble ICAM-1 were found to be different in three outcome groups with lethal, reversible and no organ failure, respectively from day four onwards following trauma [143]. Furthermore, in patients with severe infections, levels of endothelium-derived soluble adhesion molecules and von Willebrand factor antigen were correlated with the severity of illness and may be considered as predictors of survival outcome [144].

In baboons, soluble E-selectin was released *in vivo* after administration of endotoxin and reached a peak level at 24 hours [139]. In contrast to endotoxin, baboons with hemorrhagic shock had much lower levels of soluble E-selectin. Lower soluble E-selectin levels indicate reduced endothelial activation after experimental hemorrhagic shock as compared to endotoxic shock probably due to much lower endotoxin levels, as a result of translocation from the gut, in traumatic shock [139].

It is important to monitor not only endothelial activation but also endothelial damage. One candidate is thrombomodulin, which is a glycoprotein on the endothelial surface that acts as a high-affinity receptor for thrombin and neutralizes thrombin clotting activity [145]. Beside being present on the endothelial surface, a soluble form of thrombomodulin (in reality, several fragments) has also been described in the plasma and urine of normal persons [146, 147]. *In vitro* [148] and *in vivo* [149, 150] studies in rabbits suggest that soluble thrombomodulin is not secreted from the endothelial surface but is the result of cellular damage. Furthermore, several investigators have reported that plasma thrombomodulin levels are elevated in disease states commonly associated with perturbation of the vascular endothelium, such as ARDS [151].

Although no published data on thrombomodulin levels in trauma are available thus far, other results do provide evidence for an *E. coli* dose-related and TNF-dependent thrombomodulin release into the plasma of septic baboons and suggest a possible role of anti-TNF in protection of the endothelium [152]. This suggestion is in line with the studies of Ishii et al. [148] which demonstrate that the release of thrombomodulin from endothelial cells is a marker of endothelial damage induced by activated PMNs. Thus, the concentration of thrombomodulin in plasma might represent a plasma marker for studies of endothelial integrity.

Conclusion

Since the endothelium performs numerous functions, both as an active player and as a passive target, it is only possible to discuss certain selected topics within the field of endothelial responses to activation. Most striking is the induced imbalance in pro- and anti-adhesive forces as well as pro- and anti-coagulation factors. Current emphasis is also on understanding more about the mechanisms behind vascular tone and about the possible therapeutic options to modify the responses. The end result of the different reactions may be hyperpermeability of endothelial cells and edema formation. In view of this, it might be important to place more emphasis in the future on the diagnostic possibilities of evaluating the state of endothelial cell activation and damage so that early therapeutic interventions can be provided.

Acknowledgment. This chapter is dedicated to my mentor, Günther Schlag. I would like to thank the different co-workers and collaborators involved in these studies. Part of the studies were supported by Biogen USA, Celltech UK, Boehringer-Mannheim Germany, and the Lorenz Böhler Funds. The preparation of the manuscript by M. Großauer and the review by I. H. Chaudry were greatly appreciated.

References

1. Schlag G, Redl H (1990) Endothelium as the interface between blood and organ in the evolution of organ failure. In: Schlag G, Redl H, Siegel JH (eds) Shock, Sepsis, and Organ Failure – First Wiggers Bernard Conference. Springer-Verlag, Berlin, pp 210–271
2. Hladovec J (1978) Endothelial injury by nicotine and its prevention. Experientia 34: 1585–1586
3. Pober JS, Cotran RS (1990) The role of endothelial cells in inflammation. Transplantation 50:537–544
4. Hunt BJ, Jurd KM (1998) Endothelial function in inflammatory, sepsis, reperfusion and the vasculitides. In: Halliday A, Hunt BJ, Poston L, Schachter M (eds) An Introduction to Vascular Biology from Physiology to Pathophysiology. Cambridge University Press, Cambridge, pp 225–247
5. Korthuis RJ, Anderson DC, Granger DN (1994) Role of neutrophil-endothelial cell adhesion in inflammatory disorders. J Crit Care 9:47–71
6. Geng JG, Bevilacqua MP, Moore KL, et al (1990) Rapid neutrophil adhesion to activated endothelium mediated by GMP140. Nature 343:757–760
7. Patel KD, Zimmerman GA, Prescott SM, McEver RP, McIntyre TM (1991) Oxygen radicals induce human endothelial cells to express GMP140 and bind neutrophils. J Cell Biol 112: 749–759

8. Hattori R, Hamilton KK, McEver RP, Sims PJ (1989) Complement proteins C5b-9 induce secretion of high molecular weight multimers of endothelial von Willebrand factor and translocation of granule membrane protein GMP140 to the cell surface. J Biol Chem 264: 9053–9060
9. Toothill VJ, vanMourik JA, Niewenhuis HK, Metzelaar MJ, Pearson JD (1990) Characterization of the enhanced adhesion of neutrophil leukocytes to thrombin stimulated endothelial cells. J Immunol 145:283–291
10. Zimmerman GA, McIntyre TM, Mehra M, Prescott SM (1990) Endothelial cell associated platelet activating factor: a novel mechanism for signaling intercellular adhesion. J Cell Biol 110:529–540
11. Rosen SD, Bertozzi CR (1996) Leukocyte adhesion: two selectins converge on sulphate. Curr Biol 6:261–264
12. McEver RP (1991) Selectins: novel receptors that mediate leukocyte adhesion during inflammation. Thromb Haemost 65:223–228
13. Vercellotti GM, Moldow CF, Wickham NWR, Jacobs HS (1990) Endothelial cell platelet activating factor primes neutrophil responses: amplification of endothelial activation by neutrophil products. J Lipid Mediat 2 (suppl):S23–S30
14. Schafer AI, Rodriguez R, Loscalzo J, Gimbrone MA (1989) Inhibition of vascular endothelial cell prostacyclin synthesis by plasmin. Blood 74:1015–1020
15. Eppihimer MJ, Russell J, Anderson DC, Epstein CJ, Laroux S, Granger DN (1997) Modulation of P-selectin expression in the postischemic intestinal microvasculature. Am J Physiol 273: G1326–G1332
16. Armstead VE, Minchenko AG, Schuhl RA, Hayward R, Nossuli TO, Lefer AM (1997) Regulation of P-selectin expression in human endothelial cells by nitric oxide. Am J Physiol 273: H740–H746
17. Horie Y, Wolf R, Anderson DC, Granger DN (1998) Nitric oxide modulates gut ischemia-reperfusion-induced P-selectin expression in murine liver. Am J Physiol 275:H520–H526
18. Perretti M (1997) Endogenous mediators that inhibit the leukocyte-endothelium interaction. Trends Pharmacol Sci 18:418–425
19. Utgaard JO, Jahnsen FL, Bakka A, Brandtzaeg P, Haraldsen G (1998) Rapid secretion of prestored interleukin 8 from Weibel-Palade bodies of microvascular endothelial cells. J Exp Med 188:1751–1756
20. Redl H, Dinges HP, Schlag G (1987) Quantitative estimation of leukostasis in the posttraumatic lung: canine and human autopsy data. Prog Clin Biol Res 236A:43–53
21. Pretorius JP, Schlag G, Redl H, et al (1987) The 'lung in shock' as a result of hypovolemic-traumatic shock in baboons. J Trauma 27:1344–1353
22. Yao Y-M, Bahrami S, Leichtfried G, Redl H, Schlag G (1996) Significance of NO in hemorrhagic-induced hemodynamic alterations, organ injury, and mortality in rats. Am J Physiol 270:H1616–H1623
23. Buehren V, Maier B, Hower R, Holzman A, Redl H, Marzi I (1991) PAF antagonist BN52021 reduces hepatic leukocyte adhesion following intestinal ischemia. Circ Shock 34:537–544
24. Marzi I, Bauer C, Hower R, Buhren V (1993) Leukocyte-endothelial cell interactions in the liver after hemorrhagic shock in the rat. Circ Shock 40:105–114
25. Mulligan MS, Polley MJ, Bayer RJ, Nunn MF, Paulson JC, Ward PA (1992) Neutrophil-dependent acute lung injury. Requirement for P-selectin (GMP-140). J Clin Invest 90:1600–1607
26. Fruchterman TM, Spain DA, Wilson MA, Harris PD, Garrison RN (1998) Complement inhibition prevents gut ischemia and endothelial cell dysfunction after hemorrhage/resuscitation. Surgery 124:782–792
27. Massberg S, Enders G, Leiderer R, et al (1998) Platelet-endothelial cell interactions during ischemia/reperfusion: the role of P-selectin. Blood 92:507–515
28. Kishimoto TK, Jutila MA, Butcher EC (1990) Identification of a human peripheral lymph node homing receptor: a rapidly down-regulated adhesion molecule. Proc Natl Acad Sci USA 87:2244–2248
29. Tu L, Delahunty MD, Ding H, Luscinskas FW, Tedder TF (1999) The cutaneous lymphocyte antigen is an essential component of the L-selectin ligand induced on human vascular endothelial cells. J Exp Med 189:241–252

30. von Andrian UH, Hansell P, Chambers JD, et al (1992) L-selectin function is required for beta2-integrin-mediated neutrophil adhesion at physiological shear rates in vivo. Am J Physiol 263: H1034–H1044
31. Kishimoto TK, Jutila MA, Berg EL, Butcher EC (1989) Neutrophil MAC-1 and MEL-14 adhesion proteins inversely regulated by chemotactic factors. Science 245: 1238–1241
32. von Andrian UH, Chambers JD, McEvoy LM, Bargatze RF, Arfors KE, Butcher EC (1991) Two-step model of leukocyte-endothelial cell interaction in inflammation: distinct roles for LECAM-1 and the leukocyte beta2 integrins in vivo. Proc Natl Acad Sci USA 88: 7538–7542
33. Etzioni A, Frydman M, Pollack S, et al (1992) Brief report: Recurrent severe infections cuased by a novel leukocyte adhesions deficiency. N Engl J Med 327: 1789–1792
34. Ley K, Bullard DC, Arbones ML, et al (1995) Sequential contribution of L and P selectin to leukocyte rolling in vivo. J Exp Med 181: 669–675
35. Aplin AE, Howe A, Alahari SK, Juliano RL (1998) Signal transduction and signal modulation by cell adhesion receptors: the role of integrins, cadherins, immunoglobulin-cell adhesion molecules, and selectins. Pharmacol Rev 50: 197–263
36. Pugin J, Schurer Maly CC, Leturcq D, Moriarty A, Ulevitch RJ, Tobias PS (1993) Lipopolysaccharide activation of human endothelial and epithelial cells is mediated by lipopolysaccharide-binding protein and soluble CD14. Proc Natl Acad Sci USA 90: 2744–2748
37. Pugin J, Ulevitch RJ, Tobias PS (1993) A critical role for monocytes and CD14 in endotoxin-induced endothelial cell activation. J Exp Med 178: 2193–2200
38. Yang RB, Mark MR, Gray A, et al (1998) Toll like receptor 2 mediates lipopolysaccharide induced cellular signalling. Nature 395: 284–288
39. Mantovani A, Bussolino F, Introna M (1997) Cytokine regulation of endothelial cell function: from molecular level to the bedside. Immunol Today 18: 231–240
40. Huang K, Fishwild DM, Wu HM, Dedrick RL (1995) Lipopolysaccharide-induced E-selectin expression requires continuous presence of LPS and is inhibited by bactericidal/permeability-increasing protein. Inflammation 19: 389–404
41. Melrose J, Tsurushita N, Liu G, Berg EL (1998) IFN gamma inhibits activation induced expression of E- and P-selectin on endothelial cells. J Immunol 161: 2457–2464
42. Redl H, Dinges HP, Buurman WA, et al (1991) Expression of endothelial leukocyte adhesion molecule-1 in septic but not traumatic/hypovolemic shock in the baboon. Am J Pathol 139: 461–466
43. Engelberts I, Samyo SK, Leeuwenberg JFM, Van der Linden CJ, Buurman WA (1992) A role for ELAM-1 in the pathogenesis of MOF during septic shock. Ann Surg 53: 136–144
44. Nathens AB, Bitar R, Watson RWG, et al (1998) Thiol-mediated regulation of ICAM-1 expression in endotoxin-induced acute lung injury. J Immunol 160: 2959–2966
45. Christofidou-Solomidou M, Nakada MT, Williams J, Muller WA, DeLisser HM (1997) Neutrophil platelet endothelial cell adhesion molecule-1 participates in neutrophil recruitment at inflammatory sites and is down-regulated after leukocyte extravasation. J Immunol 158: 4872–4878
46. Chosay JG, Fisher MA, Farhood A, Ready KA, Dunn CJ, Jaeschke H (1998) Role of PECAM-1 (CD31) in neutrophil transmigration in murine models of liver and peritoneal inflammation. Am J Physiol 274: G776–G782
47. Burns AR, Takei F, Doerschuk CM (1994) Quantitation of ICAM-1 expression in mouse lung during pneumonia. J Immunol 153: 3189–3198
48. Barnett CC, Moore EE, Moore FA, Biffl WL, Smith MF Jr, Carl VS (1995) Intercellular adhesion molecule-1 promotes neutrophil-mediated cytotoxicity. Surgery 118: 171–175
49. Biedermann BC, Pober JS (1998) Human endothelial cells induce and regulate cytolytic T cell differentiation. J Immunol 161: 4679–4687
50. Vedder NB, Winn RK, Rice CL, Chi EY, Arfors KE, Harlan JM (1988) A monoclonal antibody to the adherence promoting leukocyte glycoprotein CD18, reduces organ injury and improves survival from hemorrhagic shock and resuscitation in rabbits. J Clin Invest 81: 939–944
51. Squadrito F, Altavilla D, Canale P, et al (1994) Contribution of intercellular adhesion molecule 1 (ICAM-1) to the pathogenesis of splanchnic artery occlusion shock in the rat. Br J Pharmacol 113: 912–916

52. Garcia-Criado FJ, Toledo-Pereyra LH, Lopez-Neblina F, Phillips ML, Paez-Rollys A, Misawa K (1995) Role of P-selectin in total hepatic ischemia and reperfusion. J Am Coll Surg 181: 327–334
53. Buerke M, Weyrich AS, Murohara T, et al (1994) Humanized monoclonal antibody DREG-200 directed against L-selectin protects in feline myocardial reperfusion injury. J Pharmacol Exp Ther 271:134–142
54. Ramamoorthy C, Sharar SR, Harlan JM, Tedder TF, Winn RK (1996) Blocking L-selectin function attenuates reperfusion injury following hemorrhagic shock in rabbit. Am J Physiol 271:H1871–H1877
55. Ridings PC, Bloomfield GL, Holloway S, et al (1995) Sepsis-induced acute lung injury is attenuated by selectin blockade following the onset of sepsis. Arch Surg 130:1199–1208
56. Schlag G, Redl H, Till GO, Davies J, Martin U, Dumont L (1999) Anti-L-selectin antibody treatment of traumatic shock in baboons. Crit Care Med (In Press)
57. Schlag G, Redl H, Khakpour Z, Davies J, Pretorius J (1993) Hypovolemic-traumatic shock models in baboons. In: Schlag G, Redl H (eds) Pathophysiology of Shock, Sepsis, and Organ Failure. Springer-Verlag, Berlin, pp 384–402
58. Bertozzi CR, Fukuda S, Rosen SD (1995) Sulfated disaccharide inhibitors in L-selectin: deriving structural leads from a physiological selectin ligand. Biochemistry 34:14271–14278
59. Crockett-Torabi E, Sulenbarger B, Smith CW, Fantone JC (1995) Activation of human neutrophils through L-selectin and MAC-1 molecules. J Immunol 154:2291–2302
60. Simon SI, Burns AR, Taylor AD, et al (1995) L-selectin (CD62L) cross-linking signals neutrophil adhesive functions via the Mac-1 (CD11b/CD18) beta 2 integrin. J Immunol 155: 1502–1514
61. Rochon YP, Simon SI, Lynam EB, Sklar LA (1994) A role for lectin interactions during human neutrophil aggregation. J Immunol 152:1385–1393
62. Eichacker PQ, Hoffman WD, Farese A, et al (1993) Leukocyte CD18 monoclonal antibody worsens endotoxemia and cardiovascular injury in canines with septic shock. J Appl Physiol 74:1885–1892
63. Redl H, Schlag G, Davies J, Robinson M (1993) Detrimental effects of the application of anti-CD18 antibodies in baboon live E. coli sepsis. Circ Shock (Suppl) 2:33 (Abst)
64. Sharar SR, Chapman NN, Flaherty LC, Harlan JM, Tedder TF, Winn RK (1996) L-selectin (CD62L) blockade does not impair peritoneal neutrophil emigration or subcutaneous host defense to bacteria in rabbits. J Immunol 157:2555–2563
65. Garcia NM, Mileski WJ, Sikes P, et al (1994) Effect of inhibiting leukocyte integrin (CD18) and selectin (L-selectin) on susceptibility to infection with Pseudomonas aeruginosa. J Trauma 36:714–719
66. Mileski WJ, Winn RK, Vedder NB, Pohlman TH, Harlan JM, Rice CL (1990) Inhibition of CD18-dependent neutrophil adherence reduces organ injury after hemorrhagic shock in primates. Surgery 108:206–212
67. Schoenberg MH, Poch B, Younes M, et al (1991) Involvement of neutrophils in post-ischaemic damage to the small intestine. Gut 32:905–912
68. Hernandez LA, Grisham MB, Twohig B, Arfors KE, Harlan JM, Granger N (1987) Role of neutrophils in ischemia reperfusion induced microvascular injury. Am J Physiol 253: H699–703
69. Simpson PJ, Tood RF, Fantone JC, Mickelson JK, Griffin JD, Lucchesi BR (1988) Reduction of experimental myocardial reperfusion injury by a monoclonal antibody (anti-Mol, anti-CD11b) that inhibits leukocyte adhesion. J Clin Invest 81:624
70. Cooper JA, Neumann PH, Wright SD, Malik AB (1989) Pulmonary vascular sequestration of neutrophils in endotoxemia: role of CD18 leukocyte surface glycoprotein. Am Rev Respir Dis 139:A301
71. Doerschuk CM, Winn RK, Harlan JM (1990) Mechanisms of neutrophil emigration. In: Springer TA, Anderson DC, Rosenthal AS, Rothlein R (eds) Leukocyte Adhesion Molecules: Structure, Function and Regulation. Springer-Verlag, New York, pp 87–94
72. Walsh CJ, Carey D, Cook DJ, Bechard DE, Fowler AA, Sugerman HJ (1991) Anti CD18 antibody attenuates neutropenia and alveolar capillary membrane injury during gram-negative sepsis. Surgery 110:205–212

73. Barton RW, Rothlein R, Ksiazek J, Kennedy C (1989) The effect of anti-intercellular adhesion molecule MoAb on phorbol ester-induced rabbit lung inflammation. J Immunol 143: 1278–1282
74. Ismail G, Morganroth ML, Todd RF, Boxer LA (1987) Prevention of pulmonary injury in isolated perfused rat lungs by activated human neutrophils preincubated with anti-Mol monoclonal antibody. Blood 69:1167–1177
75. Kaslovsky RA, Horgan MJ, Lum H, et al (1990) Pulmonary edema induced by phagocytosing neutrophils. Protective effect of monoclonal antibody against phagocyte CD18 integrin. Circ Res 67:795–802
76. Argenbright LW, Letts LG, Rothlein R (1991) Monoclonal antibodies to the leukocyte membrane CD18 glycoprotein complex and to intercellular adhesion molecule-1 inhibit leukocyte-endothelial adhesion in rabbits. J Leukocyte Biol 49:253–257
77. Argenbright LW, Barton RW (1991) The Shwartzman response: a model of ICAM-1 dependent vasculitis. Agents Actions 34:208–210
78. Hansen JB, Olsen R, Webster P (1997) Association of tissue factor pathway inhibitor with human umbilical vein endothelial cells. Blood 90:3568–3578
79. Sandström J, Nilsson P, Karlsson K, Marklund SL (1994) 10-fold increase in human plasma extracellular superoxide dismutase content caused by a mutation in heparin binding domain. J Biol Chem 269:19163–19166
80. Platt JL, Dalmasso AP, Lindman BJ, Ihrcke NS, Bach FH (1991) The role of C5a and antibody in the release of heparan sulfate from endothelial cells. Eur J Immunol 21:2887–2890
81. Lucchesi BR (1994) Complement, neutrophils and free radicals: mediators of reperfusion injury. Arzneimittelforschung 44:420–432
82. Morrison AM, Wang P, Chaudry IH (1996) A novel nonanticoagulant heparin prevents vascular endothelial cell dysfunction during hyperdynamic sepsis. Shock 6:46–51
83. Ogawa S, Gerlach H, Esposito C, Pasagian-Macaulay A, Brett J, Stern D (1990) Hypoxia modulates the barrier and coagulant function of cultured bovine endothelium. Increased monolayer permeability and induction of procoagulant properties. J Clin Invest 85:1090–1098
84. Hack CE (1999) Cytokines, coagulation and fibrinolysis. In: Redl H, Schlag G (eds) Cytokines in Severe Sepsis and Septic Shock. Birkhäuser Verlag, Basel, pp 199–212
85. Krishnaswamy G, Kelley J, Yerra L, Smith KJ, Chi DS (1999) Human endothelium as a source of multifunctional cytokines: molecular regulation and possible role in human disease. J Interferon Cytokine Res 19:91–104
86. Rajavashisth TB, Andalibi A, Territo MC, et al (1990) Induction of endothelial cell expression of granulocyte and macrophage colony-stimulating factors by modified low-density lipoproteins. Nature 344:254–257
87. Wolff B, Burns AR, Middleton J, Rot A (1998) Endothelial cell "memory" of inflammatory stimulation: human venular endothelial cells store interleukin-8 in Weibel-Palade bodies. J Exp Med 188:1757–1762
88. Pugin J, Ulevitch RJ, Tobias PS (1994) Human endothelial cell responses to endotoxin are dramatically enhanced by human blood. Agents Actions 41:C183–C184
89. Decaterina R, Libby P, Peng HB, et al (1995) Nitric oxide decrease cytokine induced endothelial activation. Nitric oxide selectively reduces endothelial expression of adhesion molecules and proinflammatory cytokines. J Clin Invest 96:60–68
90. Henn V, Slupsky JR, Gräfe M, et al (1998) CD40 ligand on activated platelets triggers an inflammatory reaction of endothelial cells. Nature 391:591–594
91. Sacks T, Moldow CF, Craddock PR, Bowers TK, Jacobs HS (1978) Oxygen radicals mediate endothelial cell damage by complement-stimulated granulocytes. An in vitro model of immune vascular damage. J Clin Invest 61:1161–1167
92. Martin WJ (1984) Neutrophils kill pulmonary endothelial cells by a hydrogen peroxide dependent pathway. An in vivo model of neutrophil mediated lung injury. Am Rev Respir Dis 130:209–213
93. Weiss SJ, Young J, LoBuglio AF, Slivka A, Nimeh NF (1981) Role of hydrogen peroxide in neutrophil-mediated destruction of cultured endothelial cells. J Clin Invest 68:714–721
94. Shasby DM, Shasby SS, Peach MJ (1983) Granulocytes and phorbol myristate acetate increase permeability to albumin of cultured endothelial monolayers and isolated perfused lungs. Role of oxygen radicals and granulocyte adherence. Am Rev Respir Dis 127:72–76

95. Ward AB (1986) Neutrophil-dependent and independent increases in endothelial permeability. In: Novelli GP, Ursini F (eds) Oxygen Free Radicals in Shock. S. Karger, Basel, pp 83–86
96. Redl H, Schlag G, Schiesser A, Bahrami S, Junger W, Spragg RG (1986) Oxidant-induced alterations in lung adenine nucleotides precede edema formation. In: Novelli GP, Ursini F (eds) Oxygen Free Radicals in Shock. S. Karger, Basel, pp 180–184
97. Fehr J, Moser R, Leppert D, Groscurth P (1985) Antiadhesive properties of biological surfaces are protective against stimulated granulocytes. J Clin Invest 76:535–542
98. Hoover RL, Robinson JM, Karnovsky MJ (1987) Adhesion of polymorphonuclear leukocytes to endothelium enhances the efficiency of detoxification of oxygen-free radicals. Am J Pathol 126:258–268
99. Forsild J, Bjrksten B, Hagersten K, Hed J (1989) Erythrocyte mediated scavenging of reactive oxygen metabolites generated by human polymorphonuclear leukocytes during phagocytosis: comparison between normal and Downs syndrome blood cells. Inflammation 13:543–551
100. Suematsu M, Schmid-Schönbein GW, Chavez-Chavez RH, et al (1993) In vivo visualization of oxidative changes in microvessels during neutrophil activation. Am J Physiol 264: H881–H891
101. Halliwell B, Gutteridge JMC (1986) Oxygen free radicals and iron in relation to biology and medicine: some problems and concepts. Arch Biochem Biophys 246:501–514
102. Bulkley GB (1993) Free radicals and other reactive oxygen metabolites: clinical relevance and the therapeutic efficacy of antioxidant therapy. Surgery 113:479–483
103. Redl H, Gasser H, Schlag G, Marzi I (1993) Involvement of oxygen radicals in shock related cell injury. Br Med Bull 49:556–565
104. Terada LS, Dormish JJ, Shanley PF, Leff JA, Anderson BO, Repine JE (1992) Circulating xanthine oxidase mediates lung neutrophil sequestration after intestinal ischemia-reperfusion. Am J Physiol 263:L394–L401
105. Suttorp N, Hiuppenstiel S, Fuhrmann M, Krüll M, Podzuweit T (1997) Role of NO and phosphodiesterase isoenzyme 2 for reduction of endothelial hyperpermeability. Shock 8:52
106. Menger MD, Rucker M, Vollmar B (1997) Capillary dysfunction in striated muscle ischemia/reperfusion: on the mechanisms of capillary "no-reflow". Shock 8:2–7
107. Webb DJ, Monge JC, Rabelink TJ, Yanagisawa M (1998) Endothelin: new discoveries and rapid progress in the clinic. Trends Pharmacol Sci 19:5–8
108. Redl H, Schlag G, Bahrami S, et al (1994) Big-endothelin release in baboon bacteria is partially TNF dependent. J Lab Clin Med 124:796–801
109. Palmer RMJ, Bridge L, Foxwell NA, Moncada S (1992) The role of nitric oxide in endothelial cell damage and its inhibition by glucocorticoids. Br J Pharmacol 105:11–12
110. Kristof AS, Goldberg P, Laubach V, Hussain SNA (1989) Role of inducible nitric oxide synthase in endotoxin-induced acute lung injury. Am J Respir Crit Care Med 158:1883–1889
111. Cuzzocrea S, Filippelli A, Zingarelli B, Falciani M, Caputi AP, Rossi F (1997) Role of nitric oxide in a nonseptic shock model induced by zymosan in the rat. Shock 7:351–357
112. Kilbourn RG, Szabo C, Traber DL (1997) Beneficial versus detrimental effects of nitric oxide synthase inhibitors in circulatory shock: lessons learned from experimental and clinical studies. Shock 7:235–246
113. Schlag G, Redl H, Davies J, van Vuuren CJJ, Smuts P (1993) Live Escherichia coli sepsis models in baboons. In: Schlag G, Redl H (eds) Pathophysiology of Shock, Sepsis, and Organ Failure. Springer-Verlag, Berlin, pp 1076–1107
114. Schlag G, Redl H, Davies J, Haller I (1994) Anti-tumor necrosis factor antibody treatment of recurrent bacteremia in a baboon model. Shock 2:10–18
115. Redl H, Schlag G, Bahrami S (1999) Endotoxemia in primate models. In: Brade H, Morrison DC, Opal S, Vogel S (eds) Endotoxin in Health and Disease. Marcel Dekker, Inc. New York, pp 795–808
116. Cobb JP, Danner RL (1996) Nitric oxide and septic shock. JAMA 275:1192–1196
117. Avontuur JA, Boomsma F, van den Meiracker AH, de Jong FH, Bruining HA (1999) Endothelin-1 and blood pressure after inhibition of nitric oxide synthesis in human septic shock. Circulation 99:271–275
118. Bahrami S, Strohmaier W, Gasser H, et al (1997) 2,4-Diamino-5,6,7,8-tetrahydro-6-(1-erythro-1, 2-dihydroxypropyl) pteridine (4-ABH4) reduces nitric oxide formation and improves survival rate in experimental endotoxin shock. Shock 8 (Suppl):56 (Abst)

119. Wray GM, Millar CG, Hinds CJ, Thiemermann C (1998) Selective inhibition of the activity of inducible nitric oxide synthase prevents the circulatory failure, but not the organ injury/dysfunction, caused by endotoxin. Shock 9:329–335
120. Huang KT, Kuo L, Liao JC (1998) Lipopolysaccharide activates endothelial nitric oxide synthase through protein tyrosine kinase. Biochem Biophys Res Commun 245:33–37
121. Zhou M, Wang P, Chaudry IH (1997) Endothelial nitric oxide synthase is downregulated during hyperdynamic sepsis. Biochim Biophys Acta 1335:182–190
122. Harbrecht BG, Wu B, Watkins SC, Marshall HPJ, Peitzman AB, Billiar TR (1995) Inhibition of nitric oxide synthase during hemorrhagic shock increases hepatic injury. Shock 4:332–337
123. Adachi T, Hori S, Miyazaki K, et al (1998) Inhibition of nitric oxide synthesis aggravates myocardial ischemia in hemorrhagic shock in constant pressure model. Shock 9:204–209
124. Harbrecht BG, Wu B, Watkins SC, Billiar TR, Peitzman AB (1997) Inhibition of nitric oxide synthesis during severe shock but not after resuscitation increases hepatic injury and neutrophil accumulation in hemorrhaged rats. Shock 8:415–421
125. Thiemermann C, Wu CC, Piper J, Chen SJ, Szabo C, Vane JR (1997) Aminoguanidine attenuates the delayed circulatory failure in endotoxic and haemorrhagic shock in the anaesthetized rat. Can J Physiol Pharmacol 1 (Suppl):471 (Abst)
126. Southan GJ, Zingarelli B, O'Connor M, Salzman AL, Szabo C (1996) Spontaneous rearrangement of aminoalkylguanidines into mercaptoalkyluanidines – a novel class of nitric oxide synthase inhibitors with selectivity towards the inducible isoform. Br J Pharmacol 117: 619–632
127. Garcia-Cardena G, Fan R, Shah V, et al (1998) Dynamic activation of endothelial nitric oxide synthase by Hsp90. Nature 392:821–824
128. Malinski T, Taha Z (1992) Nitric oxide release from a single cell measured in situ by a porphyrinic-based microsensor. Nature 358:676–678
129. Huk I, Nanobashvili J, Neumayer C, et al (1997) L-arginine treatment alters the kinetics of nitric oxide and superoxide release and reduces ischemia/reperfusion injury in skeletal muscle. Circulation 96:667–675
130. Hallström S, Gasser H, Kropik K, et al (1997) Effect of different NO-donors in the isolated rabbit heart perfused with a tyrode-albumin-erythrocyte suspension. Shock 8 (Suppl):53 (Abst)
131. Christopher TA, Ma XL, Lefer AM (1994) Beneficial actions of S-nitroso-N-acetylpenicillamine, a nitric oxide donor, in murine traumatic shock. Shock 1:19–24
132. Angele MK, Smail N, Ayala A, Cioffi WG, Bland KI, Chaudry IH (1999) L-arginine: a unique amino acid for restoring the depressed macrophage functions after trauma-hemorrhage. J Trauma 46:34–41
133. Szabo C, Csaki C, Benyo Z, Reivich M, Kovach AG (1992) Role of the L-arginine-nitric oxide pathway in the changes in cerebrovascular reactivity following hemorrhagic hypotension and retransfusion. Circ Shock 37:307–316
134. Daughters K, Waxman K, Nguyen H (1996) Increasing nitric oxide production improves survival in experimental hemorrhagic shock. Resuscitation 31:141–144
135. Rubbo H, Radi R, Trujillo M, et al (1994) Nitric oxide regulation of superoxide and peroxynitrite-dependent lipid peroxidation. Formation of novel nitrogen-containing oxidized lipid derivatives. J Biol Chem 269:26066–26075
136. Landino LM, Crews BC, Timmons MD, Morrow JD, Marnett LJ (1996) Peroxynitrite, the coupling product of nitric oxide and superoxide, activates prostaglandin biosynthesis. Proc Natl Acad Sci USA 93:15069–15074
137. Hierholzer C, Harbrecht B, Menezes JM, et al (1998) Essential role of induced nitric oxide in the initiation of the inflammatory response after hemorrhagic shock. J Exp Med 187: 917–928
138. Liu P, Xu B, Hock CE, Nagele R, Sun FF, Wong PY (1998) NO modulates P-selectin and ICAM-1 mRNA expression and hemodynamic alterations in hepatic I/R. Am J Physiol 275: H2191–H2198
139. Kneidinger R, Bahrami S, Redl H, Schlag G, Robinson M (1996) Comparison of endothelial activation during endotoxic and posttraumatic conditions by serum analysis of soluble E-selectin in nonhuman primates. J Lab Clin Med 128:515–519

140. Law MM, Cryer HG, Abraham E (1994) Elevated levels of soluble ICAM-1 correlate with the development of multiple organ failure in severely injured trauma patients. J Trauma 37: 100–109
141. Simons RK, Hoyt DB, Winchell RJ, Rose RM, Holbrook T (1996) Elevated selectin levels after severe trauma: a marker for sepsis and organ failure and a potential target for immunomodulatory therapy. J Trauma 41:653–662
142. Kneidinger R, Bahrami S, Redl H, et al (1996) Evaluation of a soluble E-selectin enzyme-linked immunosorbent assay under posttraumatic conditions. J Lab Clin Med 128:520–523
143. Jochum M, Siebeck M, Briegel J, Inthorn D, Waydhas C, Fritz H (1995) Immunological monitoring of new inflammatory parameters in sepsis and trauma patients. Poster at "Kinin '95", September 10–15, Denver, USA
144. Kayal S, Jais JP, Aguini N, Chaudiere J, Labrousse J (1998) Elevated circulating E-selectin, intercellular adhesion molecule 1, and von Willebrand factor in patients with severe infection. Am J Resp Crit Care Med 157:776–784
145. Giddings JC (1990) Cytokines and thrombomodulin. In: Warren JB (ed) The endothelium: an introduction to current research. John Wiley & Sons, New York, pp 141–156
146. Ishii H, Majerus PW (1985) Thrombomodulin is present in human plasma and urine. J Clin Invest 76:2178–2181
147. Ishii H, Nakano M, Tsubouchi J, et al (1990) Establishment of enzyme immunoassay of human thrombomodulin in plasma and urine using monoclonal antibodies. Thromb Haemost 63:157–162
148. Ishii H, Uchiyama H, Kazama M (1991) Soluble thrombomodulin antigen in conditioned medium is increased by damage of endothelial cells. Thromb Haemost 65:618–623
149. Sawada K, Yamamoto H, Matsumoto K, et al (1992) Changes in thrombomodulin level in plasma of endotoxin-infused rabbits. Thromb Res 65:199–209
150. Uchiyama H, Ohtani H, Hiraishi S, Horie S, Ishii H, Kazawa M (1992) Changes in plasma thrombomodulin antigen in rabbits developing endotoxin-induced disseminated intravascular coagulation and the effect of heparin. Thromb Res 65:593–604
151. Takano S, Kimura S, Ohdama S, Aoki N (1990) Plasma thrombomodulin in health and diseases. Blood 10:2024–2029
152. Redl H, Schlag G, Schiesser A, Davies J (1995) Thrombomodulin release in baboon sepsis: its dependence on the dose of Escherichia coli and the presence of tumor necrosis factor. J Infect Dis 171:1522–1527

Immunoregulation in Shock, Trauma, and Sepsis

E. Faist, M. K. Angele, and S. Zedler

Introduction

In the United States, trauma is a leading cause of death during the first three decades of life and ranks as the fourth leading cause of overall mortality with over 100 000 deaths each year [1, 2]. Much of the mortality observed during the first few hours post-trauma is related to irreversible neurological damage or exsanguination [3]. Nonetheless, assuming the patient survives the initial traumatic insult, he or she is still threatened by subsequent infection (sepsis) and multiple organ failure (MOF) [4–7]. It has been reported that upwards of 50% of trauma patients subsequently die due to infection and MOF during the days and week(s) post-trauma [4–7]. In view of this, most scientific and medical research in this area has been directed towards measuring the progression and interrelationship of events which occur following trauma and major surgery. These studies indicate that a causal relationship exists between the traumatic injury and/or shock and the predisposition of these patients to develop septic/infectious complications and/or MOF [8–10]. The excessive inflammatory response together with a dramatic paralysis of cell-mediated immunity following trauma or major surgery [8, 11] appears to be responsible for the increased susceptibility to subsequent sepsis.

In most clinical studies, alterations in immune parameters of patients following trauma or major surgery have been assessed through evaluation of peripheral blood cell function and plasma levels of various mediators. In view of this, it has been advantageous to utilize animal models which simulate the clinical condition. This has allowed us to better define the pathophysiology of the immunoinflammatory response following severe trauma which reduces the trauma victim's capacity to resist subsequent life-threatening infectious complications.

This chapter will focus on the effect of blood loss and injury on cell-mediated immune responses in experimental studies utilizing models of trauma and hemorrhagic shock which have defined effects on the immunoinflammatory response. Subsequently we will discuss how the findings from these experimental studies correlate with data generated from trauma victims and surgical patients. Following this, the effect of trauma and major surgery on the susceptibility to polymicrobial sepsis and infection will be illustrated. Lastly, this chapter will point out a few new results demonstrating the effect of gender and sex hormones on cell-mediated immune responses following trauma and major surgery. These studies might generate new approaches for the treatment of immunodepression following trauma and surgery which might be advantageous for decreasing the susceptibility to infection and for increasing the survival rate of the critically ill surgical patient.

Macrophage Function Following Trauma and Hemorrhage

Macrophage Cytokine Release

Several studies have shown markedly depressed cell-mediated immune function following hemorrhagic shock which was detectable immediately after the hypotensive period [8, 12]. Studies have also demonstrated a significantly depressed capacity of splenic, peritoneal, and alveolar macrophages to release interleukin (IL)-1, IL-6, and tumor necrosis factor (TNF)-α following trauma and hemorrhage *in vitro* [8, 13, 14]. Recent studies indicate that the depression of IL-6 release by splenic and peritoneal macrophages persists for up to seven days following trauma and hemorrhage [15]. However, in animals that are subjected to laparotomy alone (i.e., trauma) or hemorrhage alone, the depression of macrophage cytokine production returned to normal by five days following the initial insult [16]. These findings suggest additive effects of the traumatic injury and the hemorrhagic shock on the depression of immune responses. Moreover, bone fracture in conjunction with soft tissue trauma and hemorrhagic shock produces a more protracted depression of immune function than soft tissue trauma and hemorrhage without bone fracture [17]. Conversely, studies by Nwariaku et al. have shown a depressed capacity of alveolar macrophages to release TNF-α for up to five days following hemorrhage alone in New Zealand White rabbits [14]. The apparent discrepancy between these studies may be due to the anatomical locale of the macrophages studied, or the severity of the hemorrhage model utilized.

In contrast to splenic, peritoneal, and alveolar macrophages, Kupffer cells have been shown to have an enhanced capacity to produce pro-inflammatory cytokines, (i.e., IL-1, IL-6 and TNF-α) during the first 24 hours following hemorrhage [18]. Similarly, an increase in cell-associated TNF-α has been demonstrated on Kupffer cells, but not on splenic macrophages, two hours after hemorrhagic shock and resuscitation [19]. In this regard, studies by Pellegrini et al. [20] in trauma patients indicate that the ratio of cell-associated TNF-α and soluble TNF-α receptor levels correlates with the development of MOF. Thus, the enhanced cell-associated TNF-α appears to play an important role in cellular and immunological alterations following injury.

It should be noted that Kupffer cells, splenic and peritoneal macrophages function in different microenvironments. Thus, the data suggest that trauma and hemorrhagic shock might have potentially different effects on different tissue beds. Alternatively, splenic macrophages are in close contact with T-cells, and mediators released by these cells following hemorrhage might depress the responsiveness of these macrophages as compared to Kupffer cells. Despite the differential cytokine release capacities of macrophages from different microenvironments, a common depression of macrophages to present antigen has been demonstrated following severe blood loss.

Macrophage Antigen Presentation Following Trauma and Hemorrhage

Antigen presentation is defined as the process whereby a cell expresses antigen on its surface in a form capable of being recognized by a T-cell. The proteinacous antigen typically undergoes some form of processing in which it is degraded into small peptides which are capable of associating with major histocompatibility complex (MHC) II for presentation to helper T-lymphocytes or in association with MHC I to become a target for cytotoxic T-lymphocytes [21]. However, for competent antigen presentation to take place the antigen presenting macrophage must provide a second co-stimulatory signal, in the form of a membrane and/or soluble factor.

Several experimental studies demonstrate a marked depression of splenic, peritoneal and liver macrophage (i.e., Kupffer cell) antigen presentation following severe hypotension of one hour [18, 21]. This depression occurs as early as two hours after hemorrhage and persists for up to five days [18, 21]. Regional hypoxia due to decreased organ blood flow appears to be a trigger for depressing macrophage antigen presentation function since studies indicate that chemically induced hypotension [22] and severe hypoxia (unpublished observation) in the absence of any blood loss also produces depression of macrophage antigen presentation. Studies have shown that the depression of antigen presentation capacity of macrophages following trauma-hemorrhage is associated with a decrease of MHC II positive cells as well as with a decreased surface density of MHC II antigen on immune cells [18, 21].

Immune deterioration has also been reported in patients after trauma and surgery. In this respect, studies have shown lack of reactivity of circulating monocytes towards stimulation with bacteria or endotoxin following surgical trauma [23]. This paralysis of monocyte cell function has been reported to persist for three to five days after trauma [24] and appears to be a potential risk factor for postoperative septic complications [23]. Moreover, MacLean et al. [25] and Christou et al. [26] have reported that the outcome of trauma patients is worsened when they exhibit a depressed delayed type hypersensitivity (DTH) reaction. Thus, depressed cell-mediated immunity in patients following injury or major surgery, which is associated with an increased mortality from subsequent sepsis [27, 28], is probably in part due to decreased antigen presenting capacity by macrophages. Additionally, studies following thermal injury have shown that depressed lymphocyte responsiveness due to depressed MHC II expression is associated with depressed antigen presentation [29, 30].

The decrease of monocytic expression of human leukocyte antigen (HLA)-DR represents a very important indicator for the quality of the post-traumatic course of critically ill patients. Polk et al. [31] observes that HLA-DR expression is much more profoundly suppressed in patients with septic complications than in patients with an uneventful post-traumatic course.

These findings collectively suggest that depression of macrophage antigen presentation capacity following injury or major surgery is an important factor contributing to the depression of cell-mediated immunity, that increases subsequent susceptibility to infection. Multiple factors including decreased metabolic activity, anti-inflammatory cytokines, prostaglandins, and nitric oxide (NO) appear to be responsible for the depression of macrophage antigen presenting capacity.

Lymphocyte Function Following Hemorrhagic Shock, Trauma, and Burns

Crucial Parameters of Dysregulation

The central dysregulation of cell-mediated immune responses consists of the dissociation of monocyte T-cell interactions via overrepresentation of suppressor active monocytes and underrepresentation of T-cell help [32]. A disturbance of lymphocyte systems can be observed following any extensive trauma and presents itself frequently within an absolute lymphopenia of $CD3^+$ cells and simultaneously with a monocytosis of $CD14^+$ cells.

Successful and protective immune responses are dependent on the activation of adequate T-lymphocyte subpopulations that exert characteristic effector functions. Within the T-cell subpopulation we observe a shift of the T-helper $CD4^+$/ T-suppressor cytotoxic ($CD8^+$) ratio towards $CD8^+$ cells. This occurs in parallel with a reduction of the proliferative T-cell response, reduced IL-2 production and a disturbance of IL-2 receptor expression.

Both experimental and clinical studies indicate that a wide range of traumatic injuries alter the ability of T-lymphocytes to respond to activation by mitogens such as concanavalin A and phytohemagglutinin [12, 33–37]. These studies demonstrate decreased mitogenic responses of lymphocytes in patients following general surgery, blunt trauma, and thermal injury [34–37]; the degree of lymphocyte depression correlates with the complexity of the surgery. Similarly, following hemorrhagic shock decreased splenocyte proliferative capacity in response to the T cell mitogen, concanavalin A, has been demonstrated extensively in our laboratory [12, 16, 33, 38]. Moreover, the release of Th1 lymphokines, such as IL-2 and interferon (IFN)-γ, by splenocytes has been shown to be significantly depressed as early as two hours following trauma and hemorrhagic shock [12, 16, 33, 38] and this depression persists for up to five days following trauma-hemorrhage [16]. These findings in animal models are supported by several authors in human studies.

Suppressed IL-2 biosynthesis represents the most striking and persistent manifestation of dysregulated cell-mediated immunity. Based on immunomodulatory experiments *in vitro*, the suppression of IL-2 production is a result of the massive release of immunoreactive prostaglandin E_2 (PGE_2) under stressful conditions [39, 40, 41].

In 1988, Faist et al. [42] and Livingston et al. [43] were the first to detect a suppression of IFN-γ release from lymphocytes during traumatic stress. During the post-traumatic course the down-regulation of IL-2 receptor expression plays a crucial role in the disintegration of adequate monocyte/T-cell interactions [44].

In addition to alterations in T-lymphocyte function, changes in B-cell function have also been reported following trauma and shock. The capacity of splenic B-cells to produce antibodies is significantly decreased following hemorrhage [45, 46]. Moreover, a decrease in overall serum levels of immunoglobulin was seen for up to three days after hemorrhagic shock [45, 46]. The decreased IL-2 production by T-lymphocytes has been suggested to be responsible for the down-regulation of antibody production by B-cells following severe injury, since T-cell lymphokines are a prerequisite for adequate B-cell proliferation and immunoglobulin secretion [8]. Whether restoration of T-cell function following severe injury and major surgery, however, restores the depressed B-cell function remains to be determined.

Polarization of Cytokine Release Patterns under Traumatic Stress

We believe that the trauma induced interruption of otherwise integrated cell-mediated immune responses is caused through an overrepresentation of suppressor active monocytes and simultaneous inadequate T-cell help. The trauma induced disturbance of lymphocytic immune function is essentially based on three mechanisms: Deletion (physical destruction, apoptosis); anergy (a lack of immunologic reactivity); and polarization (activation and suppression of partial functions) – a phenomenon that became particularly evident when we analyzed the patterns of cytokine synthesis.

Conventionally, cytokine synthesis of activated peripheral leukocytes is analyzed either at the messenger ribonucleic acid (mRNA) level or via protein release. With these methods it inevitably remains unclear whether the heterogeneity of cytokine expressing cells, for example in peripheral blood mononuclear cell cultures, is responsible for the co-expression of different cytokines, or whether individual cells can co-express different cytokines.

Recent studies have shown that human naive Th0 cells are precursor cells that have the potential to produce the entire spectrum of lymphokines and that respond to certain antigens and cytokines with a polarization into two functionally distinct phenotypes (Table 1). The Th1 subpopulation releases IL-2, IFN-γ and TNF-β and induces the production of immunoglobulin G2a (IgG2a) and cellular immune responses. IL-4, IL-5, IL-6, IL-10 and IL-13 are produced by Th2 cells which stimulate the synthesis of IgG1 and IgE. Both populations represent antagonists for most functions and direct the immune response via a control circuit (Fig. 1). Th1 cells inhibit Th2 differentiation via IFN-γ and IL-12 and promote their own generation, while Th2 cells inhibit the Th1 population via IL-4 and thus enforce their own conversion.

Under most conditions the immune system is able to develop an adequate T-cell response against a specific antigen or pathogen. However, in some cases, the

Table 1. Summary of the changes in Th1 and Th2 lymphokine release by stimulated and non-stimulated T-cells following trauma and shock. The capacity of B-cells to produce antibodies following trauma and shock is also shown

	Non-stimulated	Stimulated
Th1:		
IL-2	↓	↓
IL-2 receptor	↓	↓
IFN-γ	↓	↓
Th2:		
IL-4	?	↑
IL-10	↑	↑
IL-12	?	↑
IL-13	?	↑?
B-cell:		
B-cell antibody production	↓	↓↑

wrong subpopulation will be activated, as, for example, occurs with a Th2 dominant response in tuberculosis, leprosy and leishmaniasis.

The fact that human CD4$^+$ T-cells can be subdivided into various subpopulations depending on their lymphokine profile suggested that similar heterogeneity might exist among CD8$^+$ T-cells. Actually, polarized CD8$^+$ T-cell responses can also be discriminated by analyzing their lymphokine profiles, thus the term T1 and T2 appear to be more appropriate than Th1 and Th2.

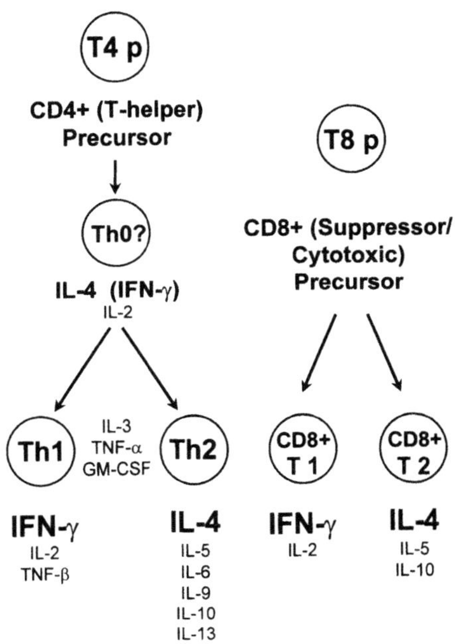

Fig. 1. Differentiation patterns of CD4$^+$ and CD8$^+$ T-cells. CD4$^+$ and CD8$^+$ T-cells differentiate from naive precursors (T4p and T8p, respectively), which do not secrete interleukin (IL)-4 and interferon (IFN)-γ into Th1/Th2 (CD4) or T1/T2 CD8$^+$ cells.
TNF: tumor necrosis factor; GM-CSF, granulocyte/macrophage colony-stimulating factor

The patterns of specific immune responses present themselves more complex than T1 or T2 [47]. Consequently T1 and T2 cells should not be considered as two functional subgroups of $CD4^+$ and perhaps also $CD8^+$ T-cells, but rather as polarized models of the heterogeneous cell-mediated effector response.

The impairment of IL-2 synthesis and gene expression of T-lymphocytes following burn trauma suggested to O'Sullivan and co-workers [48] that a shift within the T-helper cell population towards the direction of a Th2 phenotype occurred, a phenomenon that could play a central role in the pathogenesis of post-traumatic immunodysfunction. The impairment of IFN-γ synthesis in human peripheral blood mononuclear cells following major trauma [42] and a significant increase of IL-4 production compared to healthy controls [48] further suggests a dominant Th2 type cytokine synthesis pattern following major injury. The mechanisms regulating the differentiation of T-helper cells are not completely understood. For example, it is very difficult to decide if an increase in IL-4 production, or the impairment of IL-12 production, represents the decisive event responsible for the shift towards the Th2 direction following massive trauma, although Hseih et al. [49], in a murine leishmaniasis-experiment, found that upregulation of IL-4 is the dominant factor within the process of polarization.

In contrast to Th1 lymphokines, the release of the anti-inflammatory Th2 lymphokine IL-10 has been shown to be increased after trauma-hemorrhage. Neutralization of IL-10 by addition of anti-IL-10 monoclonal antibodies to the culture media, restored the depressed splenocyte proliferative capacity in splenocytes harvested from traumatized animals. These findings suggest that increased release of IL-10 following trauma-hemorrhage contributes to the depressed splenocyte Th1 lymphokine release following trauma-hemorrhage [12].

Diagnostic Approaches to Monitor T-cell Polarization

$CD4^+$ T-cells, some $CD8^+$ T-cells, mast cells and basophilic granulocytes are the most prominent producers of IL-4. However, it remains unclear which cells are the major producers of that cytokine following trauma or burns. The interaction of these cytokines as pro- and anti-inflammatory mediators within the systemic inflammatory reaction, and their potential diagnostic or prognostic importance for the individual patient is poorly understood.

The evaluation of these interactions following major trauma appears to us as most crucial, especially when based on the assumption that we investigate the mechanisms in previously healthy individuals, the clinical picture being solely defined through a specific external damage and the fact that the prognosis will be crucially influenced by the appearance of MOF. We are convinced that adequate bedside monitoring of patients suffering from major trauma will answer one central question: To what degree will pro-and anti-inflammatory mediator release following major injury during the initial post-traumatic phase determine the clinical course towards infection, sepsis and organ failure versus an uneventful clinical course with consecutive healing?

Using flow cytometry, we have studied *de novo* cytokine synthesis at a single cell level. Following *ex vivo* stimulation of mononuclear peripheral leukocytes, flow cytometry allows quantification of the capacity of cytokine synthesis and secretion. We postulated that this diagnostic device would enable us to discriminate patients in respect to their predisposition to develop MOF and sepsis following trauma, based on the capacity of the organism to develop adequate cell biological reactions under stress.

We have been extensively exploring the constitutional phenotype dependent alterations of the signature lymphokine synthesis of the Th1 (IFN-γ) and Th2 (IL-4) subtypes during the post-traumatic course. Ten patients following major burn trauma ($>30\%$ body surface) were studied on four consecutive days following trauma, along with 15 healthy controls. Following density gradient centrifugation over Ficoll-Hypaque, peripheral blood mononuclear cells were separated and incubated (five hours) for cytokine production induced by the accessory cell-independent stimulus of ionomycin and phorbol 12-myristate 13-acetate (PMA) (Fig. 2). After fixation and permeabilization, cell samples were immunofluorescently stained for cell surface antigens (CD4 and CD8) and intracellular IFN-γ and IL-4 synthesis. Results were correlated with corresponding and enzyme-linked immunosorbent assay (ELISA) measurements of the culture supernatants.

The phenotypic analysis of the composition of the helper (CD4) and suppressor (CD8) T-cell subsets demonstrated that patients suffering from major burns and healthy controls express these antigens in similar percentages.

An excessive IL-4 release in the supernatants of the peripheral blood mononuclear cells of burn patients compared to controls (Fig. 3) was noted, while IFN-γ release was elevated only to a small degree compared to healthy controls. Flow cytometric analysis allowed us to identify the $CD8^+$ cell as responsible for the increasing IL-4 and IFN-γ synthesis during the post-traumatic course, while the output capacity for cytokines of the $CD4^+$ subpopulation remained unchanged [50]. The production of IL-4 was up-regulated from 437.8 ± 137.0 pg/ml on day 1 to 1333.8 ± 532.7 pg/ml on day 7 in patients with burns versus 82.3 ± 15.8 pg/ml in controls, while the release of IFN-γ was only slightly increased. As already mentioned, the predominant cell source of IL-4 after burn trauma was a $CD8^+$ cell with a nearly five-fold increase in production on day 5 ($7.2 \pm 2.6\%$) versus $1.5 \pm 0.4\%$ in controls. While $CD8^+$ cells were also capable of enhancing their IFN-γ synthesis under stress by about 50% due to the significant participation of the naive $CD45RA^+$ subset, the $CD4^+$ IFN-γ release remained largely unchanged [51].

With this study, we demonstrated that in non-survivors the number of $CD8^+$ IL-4 producing cells was significantly higher compared with controls (Fig. 4a); the number of IFN-γ releasing memory effector/$CD45R0^+$ was lower compared with survivors (Fig. 4b).

We could confirm with these studies that major burn injury induces a significant shift of cytokine response towards the Th2 direction and we could further demonstrate that the $CD8^+$, rather than the $CD4^+$ phenotype is present. Increased IL-4 synthesis is associated with a Th2 lymphocyte.

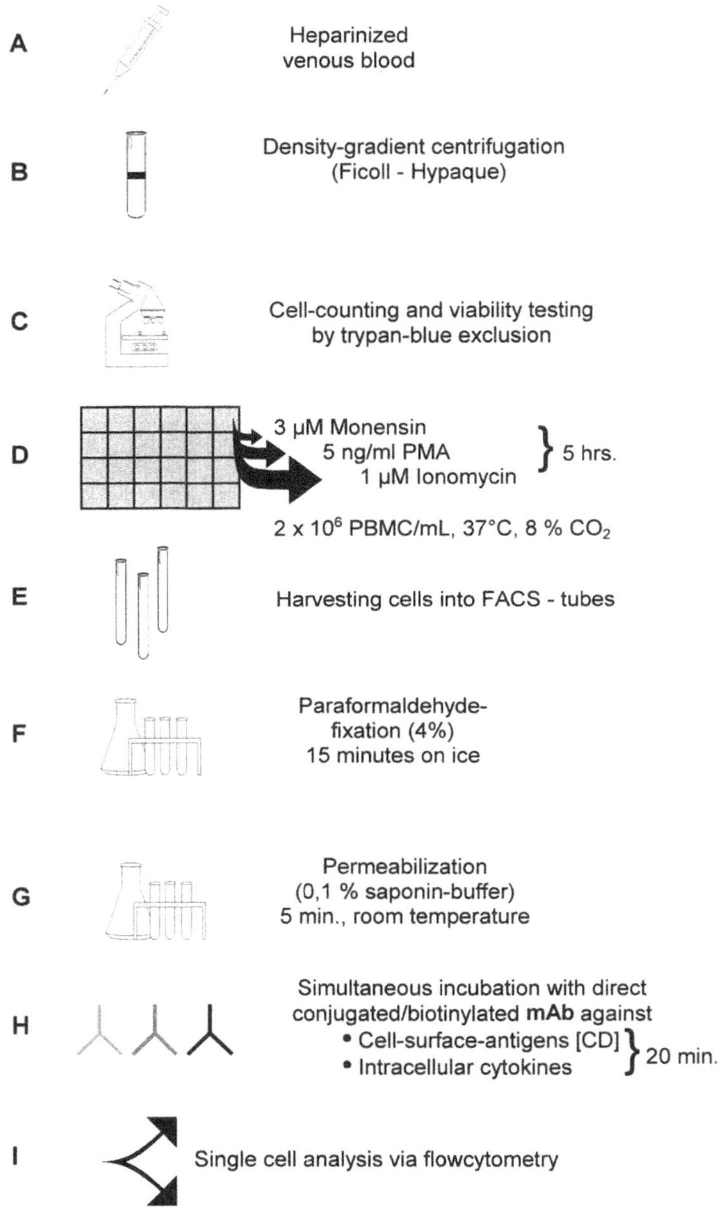

Fig. 2A–I. Schematic of the intracellular cytokine detection technique. Peripheral blood mononuclear cells (PBMC) were activated polyclonally with ionomycin and phorbol 12-myristate 13-acetate (PMA) in the presence of monensin. Initially, fixation of cells in paraformaldehyde is required, followed by permeabilization of cellular membranes with saponin. After staining, the resulting three-color-labeled cells were indicative of protein *de novo* synthesis, allowing classification of individual cytokine-producing cells along with their surface phenotype features

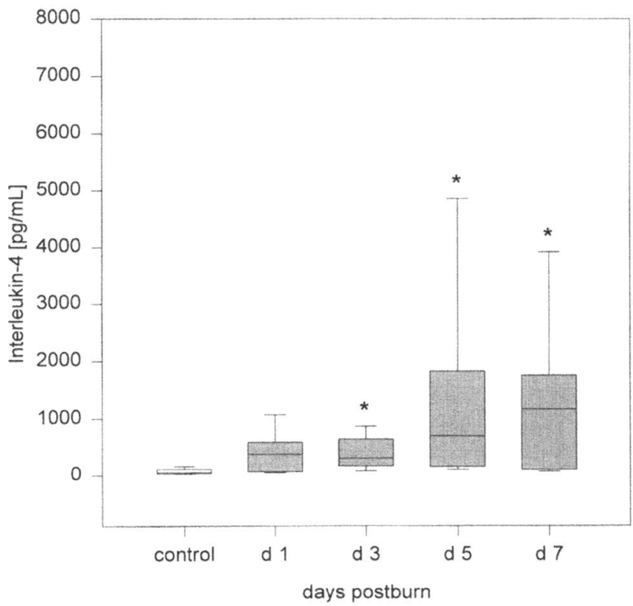

Fig. 3. Changes in the *ex vivo* capacity of peripheral blood mononuclear cells to release interleukin (IL)-4 in response to ionomycin and phorbol 12-myristate 13-acetate (PMA) during a period of 24 hrs after they were harvested on consecutive days after burn injury compared with controls. Peripheral blood mononuclear cells after burn injury enhanced their IL-4 production excessively (*$p < 0.05$ vs. control)

These diagnostic tests may help to differentiate patients with compensatory anti-inflammatory response syndrome and immunosuppression from those patients in the pro-inflammatory state associated with the systemic inflammatory response syndrome.

Circulatory Inflammatory Mediators

The observed immunodeficiency in trauma victims and patients following major surgery has, however, been found to be associated with enhanced concentrations of inflammatory cytokines reflecting activated immunocompetent cells in the same patient [52]. Thus, it appears that the depressed *in vitro* cell-mediated immune responses discussed above reflect hyporesponsiveness to a second stimulus following massive activation *in vivo* [53].

Elevated levels of TNF-α, IL-1 and IL-6 in the plasma have been well described in both animal experiments [8, 54, 55] and patient studies [10, 56–59] following trauma, severe blood loss, and sepsis. The sequence of cytokine release following trauma and hemorrhagic shock includes an increase in plasma TNF-α as early as 30 min after the onset of injury, peak TNF-α levels by two hours post-trauma and

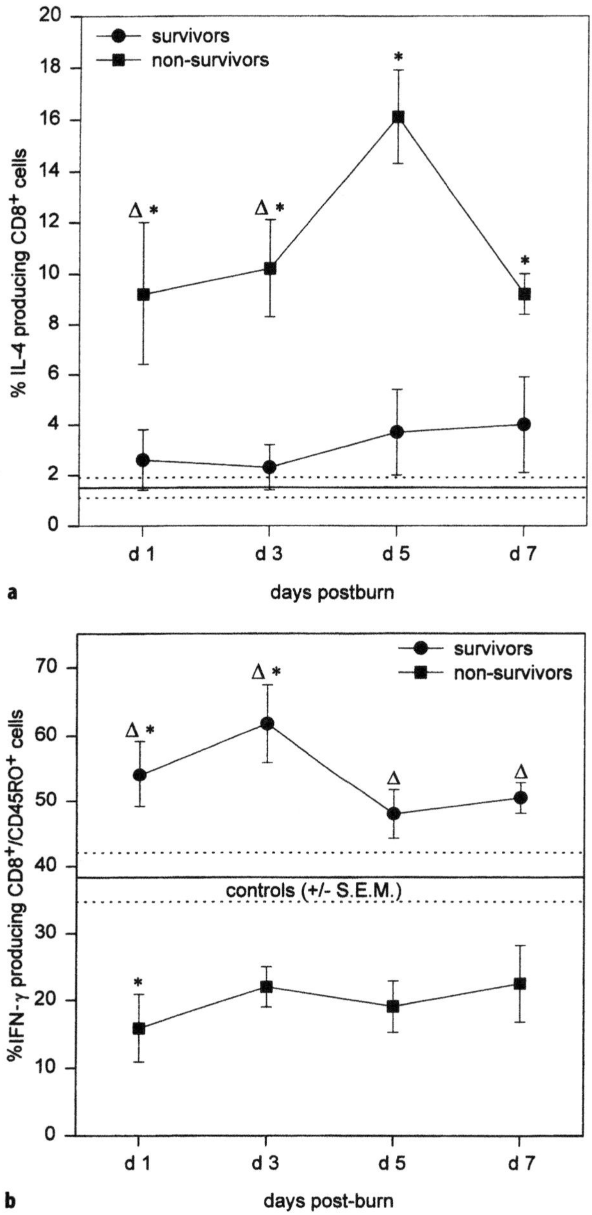

Fig. 4. a Differential interleukin (IL)-4 synthesis in CD8 cells after burns compared with controls. The frequency of $CD8^+$ IL-4 producing cells in nonsurvivors was significantly higher compared with controls, while the response of survivors was within the range of the controls (*p<.05 vs. controls $^{\Delta}$p<.05 vs. survivors). **b** Differential IFN-γ production in the $CD8^+$ memory/effector cell subset ($CD8^+/CD45RO^+$) after burn trauma. The nonsurviving group showed a significant decrease in IFN-γ synthesis compared with survivors ($^{\Delta}$p<.05 vs. survivors), while IFN-γ synthesis in survivors was significantly above control level on days 1 and 3 after burn (*p<.05 vs. control)

hemorrhage and a return towards baseline values at 24 hours [8, 54] (Fig. 5). In contrast to measurements using a bioassay [54], elevated plasma TNF-α levels were detectable at 24 hours post-trauma and blood loss by ELISA (60). This suggests that TNF-α detected 24 hours after injury might not be biologically active. Soluble TNF-α receptors have been isolated from the plasma that might neutralize the biological activity of circulating TNF-α [61]. Unlike TNF-α, plasma IL-6 levels are not significantly elevated until two hours post-hemorrhage, and levels remain elevated up to 24 hours after the induction of hemorrhage [62].

Since *in vivo* administration of IL-1, IL-6, and TNF-α induces a shock-like syndrome similar to that observed following severe blood loss and sepsis [63–66], it has been suggested that these cytokines may play a role in initiating the cascade of events that can lead to the development of multiple organ dysfunction following severe hemorrhagic shock. Furthermore, the increase in the release of pro-inflammatory cytokines by Kupffer cells following the induction of shock is associated with depressed immune function [8]. This suggests that pro-inflammatory cytokines produced by Kupffer cells following hemorrhage act in an autocrine as well as a paracrine fashion to down-regulate Kupffer cell and other macrophage populations. Furthermore, Kupffer cells, which represent the largest pool of macrophages in the body, were found to release increased amounts of IL-1, IL-6, and TNF-α following shock [63], and the selective reduction of this macrophage population by injection of gadolinium chloride significantly reduced plasma IL-6 levels following hemorrhage [67]. This leads to the conclusion that Kupffer cells are a significant source of the increased plasma levels of pro-inflammatory cytokines following trauma and hemorrhage and these cytokines can act to depress macrophage function. Whether or not Kupffer cells are the only contributor to the enhanced pro-inflammatory plasma levels following severe injury and major surgery remains to be determined.

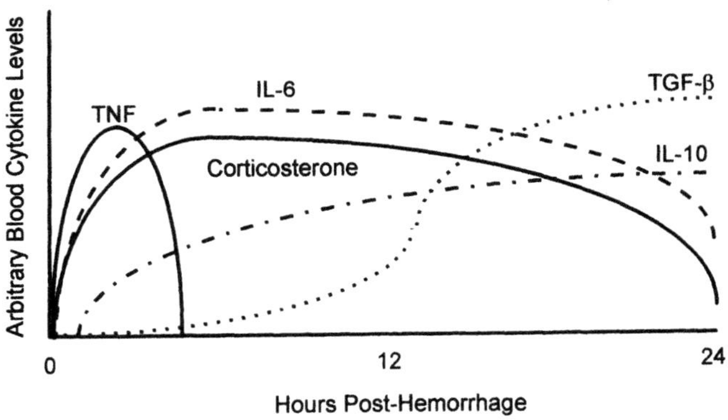

Fig. 5. Arbitrary blood cytokine levels during the first 24 hr following trauma and hemorrhagic shock. Levels of tumor necrosis factor-α (TNF), interleukin-6 (IL-6), and transforming growth factor-β (TGF-β) were determined by specific bioassay. Interleukin-10 (IL-10) was measured by ELISA and corticosterone by radioimmunoassay

In contrast to the early increase in pro-inflammatory cytokines in the plasma following trauma and shock, elevated plasma levels of the anti-inflammatory cytokine, transforming growth factor (TGF)-β, are not detectable until 24 hours after the insult [68]. Furthermore, this elevation in plasma TGF-β persists until 72 hours after trauma and hemorrhage [68]. Neutralization of TGF-β using an anti TGF-β antibody restores depressed antigen presentation to normal levels [68]. These results, along with the studies by Miller-Graziano et al. [69] indicate that the enhanced release of TGF-β is an additional factor responsible for the prolonged suppression of macrophage function following hemorrhagic shock.

In addition to pro- and anti-inflammatory cytokines numerous other mediators in the plasma have been reported to contribute to the depression of cell-mediated immune responses following trauma and shock. Eicosanoids have been extensively studied as agents involved in immunological responses [39, 70, 71]. Early following shock (two hours) an increased release of prostaglandins and leukotrienes by macrophages occurs, leading to elevated plasma levels of eicosanoids [8, 72]. Moreover, PGE_2 has been shown to inhibit cell-mediated immune function [73, 74]. Conversely, administration of ibuprofen, an inhibitor of cyclooxygenase, to animals following severe blood loss, prevents the depression of macrophage function [75]. Ertel et al. [76] have demonstrated that rodents which are pre-fed a fish oil diet high in omega-3-fatty acids, which are known to inhibit the synthesis of PGE_2 through inhibition of arachidonic acid metabolism, have normal macrophage functions following hemorrhage.

Increased levels of circulating cytokines have also been reported following a variety of tissue insults in patients, including trauma, sepsis, thermal injury, and surgery [10, 59, 77, 78]. Increased plasma IL-6 levels in patients have been observed during the first week following trauma [59]. Interestingly, levels of pro-inflammatory cytokines have been shown to be higher in trauma patients with severe blood loss compared to patients with trauma alone [10]. Moreover, in septic patients the increase in the pro-inflammatory cytokines IL-6 and TNF-α has been found to be much higher than in trauma victims without septic complications [59]. These findings suggest additive effects of trauma, blood loss, and septic complications on the immunoinflammatory response. Furthermore, pro-inflammatory cytokine levels, as well as the duration of elevation, appear to correlate with the severity of the insult. Elevated cytokine levels have been shown to persist for five days after gastrectomy compared to three days after mastectomy [78]. Furthermore, several clinical studies have shown an association between elevated plasma levels of pro-inflammatory cytokines and increased infectious complications and higher mortality rates [10, 56, 79–83]. In this respect, Calandra et al. [84] reported a progressive decline in TNF-α levels in survivors of septic shock, whereas TNF-α levels remained persistently elevated after initial diagnosis and attempted treatment in non-survivors from septic shock. Furthermore, studies of patients with meningococcal septic shock demonstrated that serum TNF-α, IL-1β, and IL-6 levels on admission were better prognostic parameters for outcome than leukocyte count, platelet count, or low blood pressure [82].

Therefore, it remains unknown whether increased levels of pro-inflammatory cytokines correlate with the outcome in trauma patients without sepsis. Nonetheless, the above studies suggest the important contribution of pro-inflammatory cytokines to the pathophysiological changes seen in trauma victims. Determination of pro-inflammatory cytokine levels may provide clinicians with an indicator of the intracellular milieu and possible insight into cellular changes taking place. More refinements towards the rapid and online measurements of cytokines are, however, needed before the full benefits of such information can be effectively translated to better management of trauma patients. Although various cytokine therapies in septic patients so far have not yielded satisfactory results, the lack of beneficial effects might be related to the timing and dose of anti-cytokine administration. It is our hypothesis that total blockade/neutralization of cytokines will not be helpful to the host. Instead, modulation of cytokine production/release by immune cells, i.e., macrophages, T-cells, leading to the restoration of cellular homeostasis, might be a better approach for decreasing the susceptibility of trauma victims and patients following major surgery to subsequent sepsis and infection.

Increased Susceptibility to Infection

Increased Susceptibility to Polymicrobial Sepsis

The studies mentioned above indicate depressed immunoresponsiveness after trauma and hemorrhage, which persists despite fluid resuscitation. They do not, however, indicate, whether these observations translate into an actual reduction in the capacity of these traumatized animals to ward off infection of a clinically relevant nature. To determine this, additional studies were conducted by Stephan et al. [33, 85] in which sepsis was induced three days after hemorrhagic shock. The results demonstrate an increased susceptibility of hemorrhaged animals to polymicrobial sepsis as evidenced by an increased mortality rate of hemorrhaged animals following subsequent sepsis (mortality of hemorrhaged animals following subsequent sepsis 100% compared to 50% in sham animals subjected to sepsis). Similarly, Zapata-Sirvent et al. [86] have indicated that the mortality rate in response to a septic challenge was increased in mice. Restoration of the depressed immune responses following trauma and severe blood loss with immunomodulatory agents, specifically flutamide (an androgen receptor blocker) was associated with increased survival rates following subsequent sepsis [85].

Moreover, in patients, an association between the loss of immunocompetence (paralysis of the cell-mediated immunity) following traumatic injury and the development of sepsis and late death has been reported [27, 28] (Fig. 6). Furthermore, alterations in the levels of circulating E-selectin adhesion molecules after trauma and resuscitation have been found to be associated with an increased risk of infectious complications, organ failure and death [87]. In summary, these studies suggest that the immunodepression following injury and major surgery leads to an increased susceptibility to polymicrobial sepsis. Therefore, attempts to modulate the depressed immune responses in trauma victims might decrease the development of septic complications and MOF in those patients.

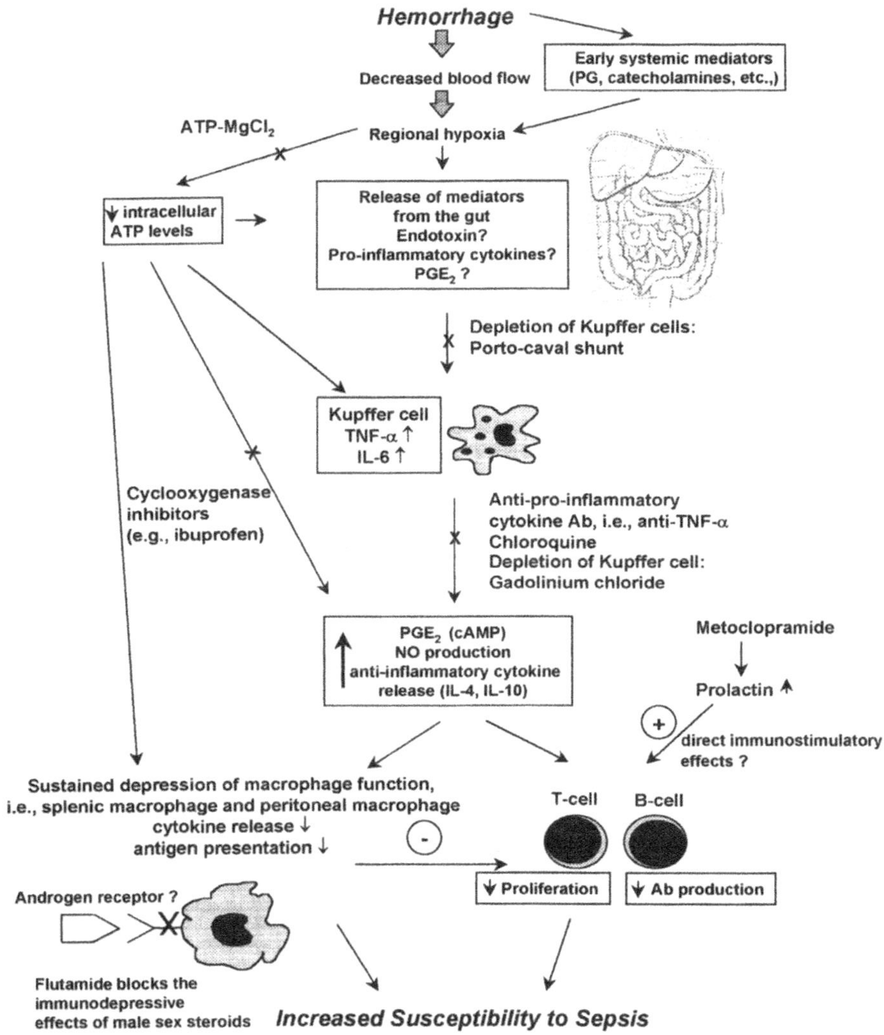

Fig. 6. Hypothesis of the cascade of events following hemorrhagic shock that lead to the development of depressed macrophage function (e.g. decreased cytokine release, antigen presentation capacity), suppression of cell-mediated immunity, and increased susceptibility to sepsis. The cascade inhibitors are marked 'X' and listed in the figure. PG, prostaglandin; Kϕ, Kupffer cells; SMϕ, splenic macrophages; PMϕ, peritoneal macrophages

Increased Rate of Wound Infection

In addition to an increased susceptibility to polymicrobial sepsis, an increased rate of wound infection has been reported in clinical and experimental studies following severe trauma and blood loss [88–91]. In trauma patients, shock and blood loss and the duration of hypotension have been identified as significant risk factors for the development of wound infection [92–93]. Similarly, significantly more wound complications have been documented following surgery for bleeding peptic ulceration compared to non-bleeding ulceration [94]. Livingston et al. [88] noted an increased susceptibility to wound infection following hemorrhagic shock in rats as evidenced by an increased presence of gross purulence at the wound site following *Staphylococcus aureus* injection. Antibiotic prophylaxis failed to reduce the incidence of wound infection [88]. Furthermore, hypovolemic shock or local administration of epinephrine have been shown to increase the virulence of a dermal staphylococcal infection [89]. Recent studies from our laboratory indicate hyporesponsiveness of wound exudate cells to release pro-inflammatory cytokines, i.e., IL-1β and IL-6, following trauma and hemorrhagic shock for up to three days [95]. Furthermore, a depressed phagocytic activity of wound exudate cells has been shown under those conditions [95]. The restored wound exudate cell cytokine release on the fifth post-operative day in these recent studies was associated with an unaltered rate of wound infection in the studies by Livingston et al. [88]. Thus, our recent findings suggest that hyporesponsiveness of wound exudate cells following severe blood loss and trauma might contribute to an increased susceptibility to wound infection. Therefore, attempts to restore immune cell function at the wound site might be helpful for decreasing the incidence of wound infections in trauma victims and in patients following major surgery.

Gender Specific Immune Responses Following Trauma-Hemorrhage

Despite the fact that gender differences in the susceptibility to, and morbidity from, sepsis have been observed in several clinical and epidemiological studies [4, 96–98], little attention has been paid to the influence of gender on immune responses in surgical and trauma patients. Experimental studies investigating alterations in immune function following trauma have largely used male laboratory animals. Recent studies initiated by Zellweger et al. [99], however, examined immune functions in female rodents following the induction of sepsis by cecal ligation and puncture (CLP). The results demonstrated maintenance of splenocyte function in females when they were in the proestrus stage of the estrus cycle as opposed to depression of splenocyte function in males following CLP [99]. Furthermore, the preservation of immune responses in females was also associated with higher survival rates following the induction of sepsis [99]. In light of this, further studies were conducted investigating the effect of gender on cell-mediated immunity following trauma and hemorrhage. In particular, females in the proestrus state of the estrus cycle, showed enhanced IL-1 and IL-6 release by splenic and peritoneal macrophages and enhanced splenocyte IL-2 and IL-3 release, as opposed to depressed macrophage and splenocyte functions in males under such conditions [100]. Higher plasma estradiol and/or higher plasma prolactin levels in proestrus females might contribute to the enhanced immune responses following hemorrhage in proestrus females. Administration of estrogen to castrated male mice supplemented with testosterone improved the depressed immune responses in those animals [101]. Similarly, administration of prolactin to male mice following trauma-hemorrhage prevented the depression of immune responses [102]. These findings suggest immunoprotective properties of female sex hormones following trauma-hemorrhage. The lower levels of male sex steroids in female animals as compared to males might also contribute to the divergent immunoresponsiveness following hemorrhage. Support for the importance of male sex hormones in producing the immune depression in males following hemorrhage comes from recent studies indicating that castration of male mice two weeks prior to hemorrhage prevented the depression of splenic and peritoneal macrophages following the hemorrhagic insult [13, 101]. Moreover, depletion of testosterone by castration prior to hemorrhage normalized the IL-6 release by Kupffer cells following hemorrhage [13, 101]. In attempting to address the issue whether testosterone *per se* is responsible for the depressed macrophage functions following hemorrhage in males, studies were conducted in which castrated male mice were treated with 5α-dihydrotestosterone prior to trauma-hemorrhage [101]. The results demonstrate that castrated male mice treated with testosterone, having elevated plasma testosterone levels (i.e., comparable to intact males), displayed similar immune responses to hemorrhage as males, namely depression of splenic and peritoneal macrophage function [101]. Similarly, treatment of female mice with 5α-dihydrotestosterone also depressed splenic and peritoneal macrophage function as well as splenocyte responses [38, 103]. In addition, gender specific immune responses have also been demonstrated in the thymus, the primary location of T-cell lymphopoiesis [104]. The exact mechanism, however, for the immunomodulatory properties of male and female sex steroids following trauma-hemorrhage remains unknown.

Similar observations have been obtained in clinical trials following sepsis. Bone demonstrated in a retrospective study incorporating four major sepsis studies a preponderance of morbidity and mortality in males as compared to females [4]. McGowan et al. [97] also reported a significantly higher incidence of bacteremic infections in males than in females. A recent prospective study by Schröder et al. [98] confirms gender differences in human sepsis, with a significantly better prognosis for women. The hospital mortality rate in this study was 70% for male, compared to 26% for female patients following sepsis [98].

In summary the above studies suggest that gender, as well as the state of the estrus cycle in females, should be taken into consideration in designing experimental and clinical studies of the immune response following trauma and shock. Moreover, the results of these studies suggest that administration of sex steroids or treatment with their specific blockers may be a useful approach for modulating the immune responses in those patients.

Conclusion

The above studies indicate that injury, trauma, and blood loss produce a marked suppression in cell-mediated immunity and an increased susceptibility to subsequent sepsis and wound infection. Furthermore, both global and local alterations in macrophage function are also evident. Nonetheless, the use of a variety of immunomodulatory agents, e.g., chloroquine, ibuprofen, IFN-γ, prolactin, metclopramide and flutamide (Fig. 6) have been shown to be helpful for the normalization of the altered immune responses following trauma and hemorrhage.

The success in the use of immunomodulatory agents following hemorrhage in rodent models appears to be promising in the development of new therapeutic concepts for the treatment of immunosuppression and for decreasing the mortality from subsequent sepsis in humans. However, careful evaluation of both the benefits and potential adverse effects of therapy is needed before widespread clinical use can be envisioned.

In conclusion, the immunoinflammatory response, and subsequent sepsis, is still one of the major causes of morbidity and mortality following trauma and major surgery. While significant advances have been made, it is important to further define the pathophysiology and identify the precise mechanisms responsible for the depression of cell-mediated immunity using experimental animal models. However, these animal models should take into consideration the various interventions that the patient receives as well as the effect of gender, nutritional status, pre-existing conditions, etc. Only when models of injury begin to consider these factors can effective treatment regimes for patients be developed.

References

1. Shires GT (1985) Principles and management of hemorrhagic shock. In: Shires GT (ed) Principles of Trauma Care, 3rd edn. McGraw-Hill, New York, pp 3–42
2. Trunkey DD (1983) Trauma. Sci Am 249:28–35
3. Akiyoshi T, Koba S, Arinaga S, Miyazaki S, Wada T, Tsuji H (1985) Impaired production of interleukin-2 after surgery. Clin Exp Immunol 59:45–49
4. Bone RC (1992) Toward an epidemiology and natural history of SIRS (systemic inflammatory response syndrome). JAMA 268:3452–3455
5. Baue AE (1990) Multiple organ failure. In: Baue AE (ed) Multiple Organ Failure: Patient Care and Prevention. Mosby Year Book, St. Louis, pp 421–470
6. Deitch EA (1990) Multiple organ failure: pathophysiology and basic concepts of therapy. Thieme Medical Publishers Inc, New York pp 1–299
7. Goris RJA (1993) Sepsis and multiple organ failure: The result of whole body inflammation. In: Faist E, Meakins J, Schildberg FW (eds) Host Defense Dysfunction in Trauma, Shock and Sepsis. Springer-Verlag, Berlin, pp 161–170
8. Chaudry IH, Ayala A (1992) Immunological aspects of hemorrhage. R.G. Landes Company, Austin, pp 1–132
9. Stephan RN, Ayala A, Chaudry IH (1993) Monocyte and lymphocyte responses following trauma. In: Schlag G, Redl H (eds) Pathophysiology of Shock, Sepsis and Organ Failure. Springer-Verlag, Heidelberg, pp 131–144.
10. Roumen RM, Hendriks T, van der Ven-Jongekrijg J, et al (1993) Cytokine patterns in patients after major surgery, hemorrhagic shock, and severe blunt trauma. Ann Surg 6: 769–776

11. Faist E, Baue AE, Dittmer H (1983) Multiple organ failure in polytrauma patients. J Trauma 23:775–787
12. Ayala A, Lehman DL, Herdon CD, Chaudry IH (1994) Mechanism of enhanced susceptibility to sepsis following hemorrhage: Interleukin (IL)-10 suppression of T-cell response is mediated by eicosanoid induced IL-4 release. Arch Surg 129:1172–1178
13. Wichmann MW, Ayala A, Chaudry I (1997) Male sex steroids are responsible for depressing macrophage immune function after trauma-hemorhage. Am J Physiol 273:C1335–C1340
14. Nwariaku FE, McIntyre KL, Sikes PJ, Mileski WJ (1995) Alterations in alveolar macrophage tumor necrosis factor (TNF) response following trauma-hemorrhagic shock. Shock 4: 200–203
15. Xu YX, Ayala A, Chaudry IH (1998) Prolonged immunodepression following trauma and hemorrhagic shock. J Trauma 44:335–341
16. Zellweger R, Ayala A, DeMaso CM, Chaudry IH (1995) Trauma-hemorrhage causes prolonged depression in cellular immunity. Shock 4:149–153
17. Wichmann MW, Zellweger R, Williams C, Ayala A, DeMaso CM, Chaudry IH (1996) Immune function is more compromised following closed bone fracture and hemorrhagic shock than hemorrhage alone. Arch Surg 131:995–1000
18. Ayala A, Perrin MM, Ertel W, Chaudry IH (1992) Differential effects of haemorrhage on Kupffer cells: decreased antigen presentation despite increased inflammatory cytokine (IL-1, IL-6 and TNF) release. Cytokine 4:66–75
19. Ayala A, Perrin MM, Wang P, Ertel W, Chaudry IH (1991) Hemorrhage induces enhanced Kupffer cell cytotoxicity while decreasing peritoneal or splenic macrophage capacity: involvement of cell-associated TNF and reactive nitrogen. J Immunol 147:4147–4154
20. Pellegrini JD, Puyana JC, Lapchak PH, Kodys K, Miller-Graziano CL (1996) A membrane TNF-alpha/TNFR ratio correlates to MODS score and mortality. Shock 6:389–396
21. Ayala A, Ertel W, Chaudry IH (1996) Trauma-induced suppression of antigen presentation and expression of major histocompatibility class II antigen complex in leukocytes. Shock 5:79–90
22. Ertel W, Singh G, Morrison MH, Ayala A, Chaudry IH (1993) Chemically induced hypotension increases PGE_2 release and depresses macrophage antigen presentation. Am J Physiol 264:R655–R660
23. Haupt W, Riese J, Mehler C, Weber K, Zowe M, Hohenberger W (1998) Monocyte function before and after surgical trauma. Dig Surg 15:102–104
24. Faist E, Storck M, Hultner L, et al (1992) Functional analysis of monocyte activity through synthesis patterns of proinflammatory cytokines and neopterin in patients in surgical intensive care. Surgery 112:562–572
25. MacLean LD, Meakins JL, Taguchi K, Duignan J, Dhillon KS, Gordon J (1975) Host resistance in sepsis and trauma. Ann Surg 182:207–211
26. Christou NV, Tellado JM (1993) The impact of preexisting disease conditions for host defense integrity in traumatized and critically ill patients. In: Faist E, Meakins J, Schildberg FW (eds). Host Defense Dysfunction in Trauma, Shock and Sepsis. Springer-Verlag, Berlin, pp 73–82
27. Levy EM, Alharbi SA, Grindlinger G, Black PH (1984) Changes in mitogen responsiveness lymphocyte subsets after traumatic injury: relation to development of sepsis. Clin Immunol Immunopathol 32:224–233
28. Keane RM, Birmingham W, Shatney CM, Winchurch RA, Munster AM (1983) Prediction of sepsis in the multitraumatic patient by assays of lymphocyte responsiveness. Surg Gynecol Obstet 156:163–167
29. Munster AM (1984) Immunologic response of trauma and burns: an overview. Am J Med 76:142–145
30. Antonacci AC, Calvano SE, Reaves LE, et al (1984) Autologous and allogenic mixed-lymphocyte responses following thermal injury in man: the immunomodulatory effects of interleukin-1, interleukin-2 and a prostaglandin inhibitor, WY- 18251. Clin Immunol Immunopathol 30:304–320
31. Polk HC, George CD, Wellhausen SR, et al (1986) A systematic study of host defense processes in badly injured patients. Ann Surg 204:282–299

32. Faist E, Markewitz A, Storck M, Ertel W, Schildberg FW (1992) Der einfluss der ausgedehnten operativen Intervention auf die zellvermittelte Immunantwort. Internist 33:370–378
33. Stephan RN, Kupper TS, Geha AS, Baue AS, Chaudry IH (1987) Hemorrhage without tissue trauma produces immunosuppression and enhances susceptibility to sepsis. Arch Surg 122:62–68
34. Riddle PR, Berenbaum MC (1967) Postoperative depression of the lymphocyte response to phytohaemagglutinin. Lancet i:746–748
35. O'Mahony JB, Palder SB, Wood JJ, et al (1984) Depression of cellular immunity after multiple trauma in the absence of sepsis. J Trauma 24:869–875
36. Daniels JC, Sakai H, Cobb EK, Lewis SR, Larson DL, Ritzmann SE (1971) Evaluation of lymphocyte reactivity studies in patients with thermal burns. J Trauma 11:595–607
37. Sakai H, Daniels JC, Lewis SR, Lynch JB, Watson DL, Ritzmann SE (1972) Reversible alterations of nucleic acid synthesis in lymphocytes after thermal burns. J Reticuloendothelial Soc 11:19–28
38. Angele MK, Ayala A, Cioffi WG, Bland KI, Chaudry IH (1998) Testosterone: The culprit for producing splenocyte depression following trauma-hemorrhage. Am J Physiol 274: C1530–C1536
39. Faist E, Mewes A, Baker CC, et al (1987) Prostaglandin E_2 (PGE_2)-dependent suppression of interleukin-2 (IL-2) production in patients with major trauma. J Trauma 27:837–848
40. Wood JJ, Rodrick ML, O'Mahony JB, et al (1984) Inadequate interleukin-2 production: A fundamental immunological deficiency in patients with major burns. Ann Surg 200: 311–320
41. Abraham E, Chang Y-H (1985) The effects of hemorrhage on mitogen-induced lymphocyte proliferation. Circ Shock 15:141–149
42. Faist E, Mewes A, Strasser T, et al (1988) Alteration of monocyte function following major injury. Arch Surg 123:287–292
43. Livingston DH, Appel SH, Wellhausen SR, et al (1988) Depressed interferon gamma production and monocyte HLA-DR expression after severe injury. Arch Surg 123:1309–1312
44. Ertel W, Faist E, Salmen B, Huber P, Heberer G (1989) Influence of cyclooxygenase inhibition on interleukin-2 receptor (IL-2R) expression after major trauma. Surg Res Comm 5:17–23
45. Abraham E, Freitas AA (1989) Hemorrhage in mice induces alterations in immunoglobulin-secreting B-cells. Crit Care Med 17:1015–1019
46. Abraham E, Freitas AA (1989) Hemorrhage produces abnormalities in lymphocyte function and lymphokine generation. J Immunol 142:899–906
47. Cox FW, Liew FY (1992) T-cell subsets and cytokines in parasitic infections. Immunol Today 13:445–448
48. O'Sullivan ST, Lederer JA, Horgan AF, Chin DH, Mannick JA, Rodrick ML (1995) Major injury leads to predominance of the T helper-2 lymphocyte phenotype and diminished interleukin-12 production associated with decreased resistance to infection. Ann Surg 222:482–490
49. Hseih CS, Macatonia SE, Tripp CS, Wolf SF, O'Garra A, Murphy KM (1993) Development of TH1 CD4+ T cells through IL-12 produced by Listeria-induced macrophages. Science 260: 547–549
50. Zedler S, Faist E, Ostermeier B, et al (1997) Postburn constitutional changes in T-cell reactivity occur in CD8+ rather than in CD4+ cells. J Trauma 42:872–880
51. Zedler S, Bone RC, Baue AE, van Donnersmarck GH, Faist E (1999) T-cell reactivity and its predictive role in immunosuppression after burns. Crit Care Med 27:66–72
52. Fuchs D, Gruber A, Wachter H, Faist E (1996) Activated cell-mediated immunity and immunodeficiency in trauma and sepsis. In: Faist E, Baue AE, Schildberg FW (eds) The immune consequences of trauma, shock and sepsis: Mechanisms and therapeutic approaches. Pabst Science Publishers, Lengerich, pp 235–239
53. Fuchs D, Malkovsky M, Reibnegger G, Werner ER, Forni G, Wachter H (1989) Endogenous release of interferon-gamma and diminished response of peripheral blood mononuclear cells to antigenic stimulation. Immunol Lett 23:103–108
54. Ayala A, Perrin MM, Meldrum DR, Ertel W, Chaudry IH (1990) Hemorrhage induces an increase in serum TNF which is not associated with elevated levels of endotoxin. Cytokine 2: 170–174

55. Ayala A, Wang P, Ba ZF, Perrin MM, Ertel W, Chaudry IH (1991) Differential alterations in plasma IL-6 and TNF levels following trauma and hemorrhage. Am J Physiol 260: R167–R171
56. Damas P, Reuter A, Gysen P, Demonty J, Lamy M, Franchimont P (1989) Tumor necrosis factor and interleukin-1 serum levels during severe sepsis in humans. Crit Care Med 17: 975–978
57. Damas P, Ledoux D, Nys M, et al (1992) Cytokine serum level during severe sepsis in human IL-6 as a marker of severity. Ann Surg 215:356–362
58. Romagnani S (1996) Th1 and Th2 in human diseases. Clin Immunol Immunopathol 80: 225–235
59. Martin C, Boisson C, Haccoun M, Thomachot L, Mege JL (1997) Patterns of cytokine evolution (tumor necrosis factor and interleukin-6) after septic shock, hemorrhagic shock, and severe trauma. Crit Care Med 25:1813–1819
60. Ertel W, Morrison MH, Ayala A, Perrin MM, Chaudry IH (1991) Anti-TNF monoclonal antibodies prevent haemorrhage-induced suppression of Kupffer cell antigen presentation and MHC class II antigen expression. Immunology 74:290–297
61. Porteu F, Nathan C (1990) Shedding of tumor necrosis factor receptors by activated human neutrophils. J Exp Med 172:599–607
62. Ertel W, Morrison MH, Ayala A, Chaudry IH (1991) Chloroquine attenuates hemorrhagic shock induced suppression of Kupffer cell antigen presentation and MHC class II antigen expression through blockade of tumor necrosis factor and prostaglandin release. Blood 78: 1781–1788
63. Wong GC, Clark SC (1988) Multiple actions of interleukin 6 within a cytokine network. Immunol Today 9:137–139
64. Okusawa S, Gelfand JA, Ikejima T, Connolly RJ, Dinarello CA (1988) Interleukin-1 induces a shock like state in rabbits. Synergism with tumor necrosis factor and the effects of cyclooxygenase inhibition. J Clin Invest 81:1162–1172
65. Tracey KJ, Lowry SF, Fahey TJI,et al (1987) Cachectin/tumor necrosis factor induces lethal shock and stress hormone responses in the dog. Surg Gynecol Obstet 164:415–422
66. Lejeune P, Lagadec P, Onier N, Pinnard D, Ohshima H, Jeannin JF (1994) Nitric oxide involvement in tumor-induced immunosuppression. J Immunol 152:5077–5083
67. O'Neill PJ, Ayala A, Wang P, et al (1994) Role of Kupffer cells in interleukin-6 release following trauma-hemorrhage and resuscitation. Shock 1:43–47
68. Ayala A, Meldrum DR, Perrin MM, Chaudry IH (1992) The release of transforming growth factor-β following hemorrhage: Its role as a mediator of host immunosuppression. FASEB J 6:A1604 (Abst)
69. Miller-Graziano CL, Szabo G, Griffey K, Metha B, Kodys K, Catalano D (1991) Role of elevated monocyte transforming growth factor beta (TGF-beta) production in posttrauma immunosuppression. J Clin Immunol 11:95–102
70. Waal Malefyt R, Abrams J, Bennett B, Figdor CG, Vries JE (1991) Interleukin 10 (IL-10) inhibits cytokine synthesis by human monocytes: An autoregulatory role of IL-10 produced by monocytes. J Exp Med 174:1209–1220
71. Knapp W, Baumgartner G (1978) Monocyte-mediated suppression of human B lymphocyte differentiation in vitro. J Immunol 121:1177–1183
72. Johnston PA, Selkurt EE (1976) Effect of hemorrhagic shock on renal release of prostaglandin E. Am J Physiol 230:831–838
73. Bonta IL, Parnham MJ (1982) Immunomodulatory-antiinflammatory functions of E-type prostaglandins. Minireview with emphasis on macrophage mediated effects. Int J Immunopharmacol 4:103–109
74. Plaut M (1979) The role of cyclic AMP in modulating cytotoxic T lymphocytes. I. In vivo-generated cytotoxic lymphocytes, but not in vitro-generated cytotoxic lymphocytes, are inhibited by cyclic AMP- active agents. J Immunol 123:692–701
75. Chaudry IH, Ayala A (1993) Immune consequences of hypovolemic shock and resuscitation. Curr Opin Anaesthesiol 6:385–392
76. Ertel W, Morrison MH, Ayala A, Chaudry IH (1993) Modulation of macrophage membrane phospholipids by n-3 polyunsaturated fatty acids increases interleukin-1 release and prevents suppression of cellular immunity following hemorrhagic shock. Arch Surg 128:15–20

77. Beutler B (1994) Tumor necrosis factor and other cytokines in septic syndrome. In: Vincent JL (ed) Sepsis. Springer-Verlag, Berlin, pp 107–121
78. Shirakawa T, Tokunaga A, Onda M (1998) Release of immunosuppressive substances after gastric resection is more prolonged than after mastectomy in humans. Int Surg 83:210–214
79. Feldbush TL, Hobbs MV, Severson CD, Ballas ZF, Weiler JM (1984) Role of complement in the immune response. Fed Proc 43:2548–2552
80. Marks JD, Marks CB, Luce JM, et al (1990) Plasma tumor necrosis factor in patients with septic shock. Am Rev Respir Dis 141:94–97
81. Marano MA, Fong Y, Moldawer LL, et al (1990) Serum cachectin/tumor necrosis factor in critically ill patients with burns correlates with infection and mortality. Surg Gynecol Obstet 170:32–38
82. Waage A, Halstensen A, Espevik T (1987) Association between tumor necrosis factor in serum and fatal outcome in patients with meningococcal disease. Lancet i:355–357
83. Waage A, Brandtzaeg P, Halstensen A, Kierulf P, Espevik T (1989) The complex pattern of cytokines in serum from patients with meningococcal septic shock. Association between interleukin 6, interleukin 1, and fatal outcome. J Exp Med 169:333–338
84. Calandra T, Baumgartner JD, Gram GE, et al (1990) Prognostic values of tumor necrosis factor/cachectin, interleukin-1, interferon-alpha and interferon-gamma in the serum of patients with septic shock. J Infect Dis 161:982–987
85. Zapata-Sirvent RL, Hansbrough JF, Cox MC, Carter WH (1992) Immunologic alterations in a murine model of hemorrhagic shock. Crit Care Med 20:508–517
86. Angele MK, Wichmann MW, Ayala A, Cioffi WG, Chaudry IH (1997) Testosterone receptor blockade after hemorrhage in males: Restoration of the depressed immune functions and improved survival following subsequent sepsis. Arch Surg 132:1207–1214
87. Simons RK, Hoyt DB, Winchell RJ, Rose RM, Holbrook T (1996) Elevated selectin levels after severe trauma: A marker for sepsis and organ failure and a potential target for immunomodulatory therapy. J Trauma 41:653–662
88. Livingston DH, Malangoni MA (1989) An experimental study of susceptibility to infection after hemorrhagic shock. Surg Gynecol Obstet 168:138–142
89. Miles AA (1956) Nonspecific defense reactions in bacterial infections. Ann N Y Acad Sci 66:356–369
90. O'Keefe GE, Maier RV, Diehr P, Grossman D, Jurkovich GJ, Conrad D (1997) The complications of trauma and their associated costs in a level I trauma center. Arch Surg 132:920–924
91. Nichols RL (1991) Surgical wound infection. Am J Med 91 (suppl 3B):54S-64S
92. Weigelt JA, Haley RW, Seibert B (1987) Factors which influence the risk of wound infection in trauma patients. J Trauma 27:774–781
93. Polk HC Jr (1993) Factors influencing the risk of infection after trauma. Am J Surg 165 (suppl 2A):2S-7S
94. McGinn FP (1976) Effects of hemorrhage upon surgical operations. Br J Surg 63:742–746
95. Angele MK, Knoferl MW, Schwacha MG, et al (1999) Hemorrhage decreases macrophage inflammatory protein-2 (MIP-2) and IL-6 release: A potential mechanism for increased wound infection. Ann Surg 229:651–660
96. Center for Disease Control (1992) Mortality Patterns – United States, 1989. MMWR Morb Mortal Wkly Rep 41:121–125
97. McGowan JE, Barnes MW, Finland N (1975) Bacteremia at Boston City Hospital: occurrence and mortality during 12 selected years (1935–1972) with special reference to hospital-acquired cases. J Infect Dis 132:316–335
98. Schroder J, Kahlke V, Staubach KH, Zabel P, Stuber F (1998) Gender differences in human sepsis. Arch Surg 133:1200–1205
99. Zellweger R, Ayala A, Stein S, DeMaso CM, Chaudry IH (1997) Females in proestrus state tolerate sepsis better than males. Crit Care Med 25:106–110
100. Wichmann MW, Zellweger R, DeMaso CM, Ayala A, Chaudry IH (1996) Enhanced Immune Responses in Females as Opposed to Decreased Responses in Males Following Hemorrhagic Shock. Cytokine 8:853–863
101. Angele MK, Knoferl MW, Ayala A, Cioffi WG, Bland K, Chaudry IH (1999) Male and female sex steroids: do they produce deleterious or beneficial effects on immune responses following trauma-hemorrhage? Surg Forum (in press)

102. Zellweger R, Zhu X-H, Wichmann MW, Ayala A, DeMaso CM, Chaudry IH (1996) Prolactin administration following hemorrhagic shock improves macrophage cytokine release capacity and decreases mortality from subsequent sepsis. J Immunol 157:5748–5754
103. Angele MK, Ayala A, Monfils BA, Cioffi WG, Bland KI, Chaudry IH (1998) Testosterone and/or low estradiol: Normally required but harmful immunologically for males after trauma-hemorrhage. J Trauma 44:78–85
104. Angele MK, Xu YX, Ayala A, et al (1997) Gender differences in immune responses: Increased thymocyte apoptosis occurs only in males but not in females after trauma- hemorrhage. Surg Forum 48:95–97

Endotoxemia in Healthy Subjects as a Human Model of Inflammation

T. van der Poll and S. J. H. van Deventer

Introduction

Endotoxin is a lipopolysaccharide (LPS) that is a major component of the outer membrane of Gram-negative bacteria. Endotoxin has strong pro-inflammatory properties and can activate multiple inflammatory cascades. It is therefore considered to play a key role in the toxic sequelae of Gram-negative sepsis [1,2]. LPS is composed of a lipid moiety, designated lipid A, and a hydrophilic polysaccharide chain. The polysaccharide portion of LPS consists of the O-chain, that protrudes from the bacterial membrane, and a 'core part', connecting the O-chain with lipid A. While the O-chain consists of a series of structurally and antigenically diverse oligosaccharides that determine the many different O-specific serotypes, the core part is identical for many different bacteria. Lipid A is the highly conserved biologically active part of LPS which is completely embedded in the bacterial membrane, shielded by the O-chain. Pro-inflammatory effects of Gram-negative bacteria can, therefore, not be readily explained by the effects of cell-bound LPS. However, LPS can be shed by Gram-negative bacteria via several mechanisms, including destruction of the bacterial cell wall by complement factors.

Reports describing the effects of LPS in humans have been available for at least a century. In the late nineteenth century, the New York surgeon, William B. Coley, injected mixtures of heat-killed *Serratia marcescens* and streptococcus into patients with cancer [3]. These patients developed chills and fever within an hour after the injection. This 'vaccine treatment' with 'Coley's toxin', which had variable success, was based on the observation that certain cancer patients who developed concurrent bacterial infections experienced remissions of their malignant disease. In 1943, it was discovered that LPS was the active substance in Coley's toxin [4]. During the first half of the twentieth century, a number of researchers reported putative beneficial effects of LPS-containing substances in patients with various diseases, including psychiatric disorders, paralysis and neurosyphilis. In a more recently performed series of 'historical' experiments, Greisman and colleagues infused healthy volunteers with increasing doses of LPS by continuous intravenous infusion, and documented the now well recognized phenomenon of endotoxin tolerance [5].

Only in recent years has the injection of endotoxin into humans been employed to study the early inflammatory responses of the host to Gram-negative sepsis. In our opinion, however, human endotoxemia cannot be considered a sepsis model. Rather, intravenous injection of low dose LPS can be used as a model to study mechanisms that contribute to the activation of inflammatory cascades induced by a common bacterial antigen, and to unravel interactions between distinct inflammatory systems (e.g., the cytokine network and the coagulation system). LPS has also been given to humans per aerosol or by bronchoscope, to study its effects within the pulmonary compartment. It is beyond the scope of this chapter to discuss these latter investigations. This chapter will give an overview of investigations in which LPS has been administered to humans intravenously.

Study Design and Clinical Responses

Virtually all studies that have addressed the biological effects of LPS in humans have used the reference standard endotoxin preparation developed by the Office of Biologics of the Food and Drug Administration (FDA) to standardize endotoxin research [6]. This purified LPS, derived from *Escherichia coli* O 113:H 10:K negative (lot EC-5), has been used in most investigations published to date. Recently, the FDA ran out of their stock of lot EC-5, and EC-6 (FDA lot EC-6, USP lot G) has superseded EC-5 as the USP/FDA standard since then, intended to be as similar as possible to EC-5 [7]. Doses of lot EC-5 that have been given to healthy subjects are 2, 3 or 4 ng/kg body weight, inducing largely similar systemic responses. We have used lot G (4 ng/kg) in our studies in healthy human volunteers since 1995, and found that clinical responses are similar to those found after injection of an identical dose of lot EC-5. It should be noted that phase I trials with intravenous LPS in cancer patients have revealed that many of the effects of endotoxin are dose dependent [8, 9]. Unfortunately, direct comparison of doses used in these cancer studies with those administered to healthy humans is hampered by the fact that in the former investigations a different type of LPS, derived from *Salmonella abortus equi*, was given. In all investigations LPS was administered intravenously, either as a bolus or over a few minutes.

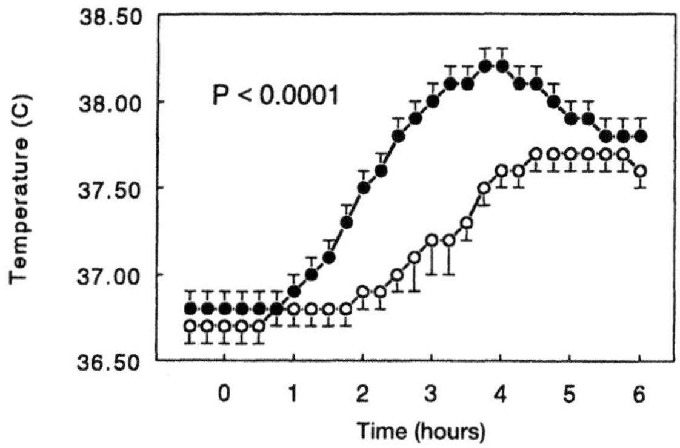

Fig. 1. Febrile response to intravenous administration of LPS to healthy humans, and the effect of neutralization of endogenous TNF activity. LPS induces a monophasic rise in body temperature (closed circles), which is significantly inhibited by infusion of a recombinant dimeric TNF receptor type II fusion protein directly prior to LPS injection (open circles)

The symptoms elicited by intravenous LPS vary considerably between study subjects [10–12]. Although some volunteers experience only mild adverse effects, the majority of subjects complain of headache, generalized malaise and myalgia, sometimes accompanied by nausea and even vomiting. A monophasic fever, preceded by chills, is almost always registered, albeit the rise in body temperature may range from very small to up to 4°C (Fig. 1). All signs and symptoms start to occur one hour to 90 minutes after the injection of LPS, are most prominent after two to three hours, and disappear within one to four hours thereafter, although some degree of fever may last a few hours longer.

Hemodynamic and Pulmonary Effects

The hemodynamic effects of LPS have been carefully documented in normal humans [13–17]. In four studies, all from the same group, hemodynamic responses were monitored by radial artery and pulmonary artery catheters [13–16], while one investigation used M-mode, two-dimensional and Doppler echocardiography [17]. In all studies, LPS was found to induce a hyperdynamic cardiovascular response, characterized by increases in cardiac index and heart rate, and decreases in systemic vascular resistance index and mean arterial pressure. In addition, subjects injected with LPS showed a blunted increase in cardiac index after the preload was increased by intravenous infusion of normal saline, while left ventricular ejection fraction did not increase at all [13]. At higher doses, LPS can cause hypotensive shock, as observed in Phase I trials in patients with malignant disease, and in a man who self-administered a single large dose of LPS [9, 18]. Thus, LPS can qualitatively reproduce the hemodynamic changes found in patients with sepsis, and is, therefore, likely to play an important role in the pathogenesis of cardiovascular collapse in Gram-negative sepsis.

At the doses studied, intravenous LPS influences pulmonary function only moderately. In one study pulmonary gas exchange did not change during the first three hours after injection of LPS [19]. However, a fluid load given thereafter induced a significant decline in PaO_2 and an increase in the alveolar arterial oxygen gradient. In addition, a rise in the clearance rate of inhaled ^{99m}-diethylenetriamine pentacetate, a small marker molecule with a molecular weight of 492, was observed, suggesting an increase in lung permeability to small molecules. The alveolar permeability to protein did not change, as reflected by unaltered IgG/albumin ratios in bronchoalveolar lavage fluids. LPS administration was not associated with influx of neutrophils into the pulmonary compartment, as assessed by unchanged cell counts in bronchoalveolar lavages [19, 20]. A systemic challenge with LPS was associated with priming of alveolar macrophages, reflected in enhanced production of tumor necrosis factor (TNF), interleukin (IL)-1 and prostaglandin E2 (PGE2) on stimulation with LPS '*ex vivo*' 1.5 to six hours after intravenous injection of LPS [20]. Thus, low doses of LPS induce small, clinically unimportant changes in pulmonary function that include alterations in gas exchange, an increase in pulmonary permeability to small molecules, and priming of alveolar macrophages for TNF, IL-1 and PGE2 production.

LPS-Induced Effects on Various Inflammatory Cascades

Effects on Cytokines and Chemokines

Cytokines are small, extremely potent proteins produced and secreted by various cell types in response to a variety of immunologic and infectious stimuli. Although frequently structurally unrelated, individual cytokines have multiple overlapping activities. They closely interact in a highly complex network, in which they influence each other's production and action.

The cytokine network can be arbitrarily divided into three portions [21]:

1) pro-inflammatory cytokines, which facilitate inflammation (e.g., TNF, IL-1, IL-12, interferon [IFN]-γ);
2) anti-inflammatory cytokines (e.g., IL-4, IL-10 and IL-13), which not only inhibit inflammatory responses, but are also capable of inhibiting the production of pro-inflammatory cytokines; and
3) cytokine inhibitors, which can either be soluble (such as the soluble TNF and IL-1 receptors) or cell-bound (such as the 'decoy' type II IL-1 receptor).

Cytokines are involved in immunity and inflammation, and are essential for the orchestration of the host response to local infection. During overwhelming immune activation, however, such as occurs during fulminant sepsis, excessive systemic production of pro-inflammatory cytokines may result in tissue injury.

Chemokines are 8 to 10 kDa chemotactic proteins that play an important role in leukocyte trafficking during inflammation. They can be divided into a number of subgroups, of which CXC and CC chemokines have been studied most thoroughly. This subdivision is based on the relative position of the cysteine residues in the mature protein, whereby in CXC (or α) chemokines the first two cysteine residues are separated by a single amino acid, whereas in the CC (or β) chemokines the first two cysteine residues are adjacent to each other.

Much of the knowledge of the early events leading to the activation of the cytokine network is derived from the human endotoxemia model. The induction of cytokines follows a characteristic pattern after injection of a bolus dose of LPS. TNF is the first cytokine appearing in the circulation, becoming detectable after approximately 45 minutes [10–12]. The release of TNF is transient, with peak levels reached after 90 minutes. As demonstrated by selective hepatic vein catheterization, the splanchnic bed is an important source of TNF produced in response to an intravenous bolus dose of LPS [22]. In human endotoxemia the rise in TNF concentrations is followed by the appearance of IL-6 within 15 to 30 minutes. IL-6 levels peak after approximately three hours. With most assays available, IL-1 is not detected in the circulation after injection of low dose LPS. Interestingly, in one study a clear rise in cell-associated IL-1β, as measured in lysates of peripheral blood leukocytes, was detected following LPS administration [16]. Bioactive IL-12, a heterodimer consisting of a p35 and a p40 subunit, is not released in significant quantities during human endotoxemia. A transient increase in serum IL-12 p40 concentrations can be detected (our own unpublished observations). P40 immunoreactivity represents monomers and dimers of the IL-12 p40 subunit, of which the latter are considered to function as IL-12 inhibitors since they can bind to the IL-12 receptor but cannot induce signal transduction. IFN-γ levels characteristically remain low after LPS injection in humans. Chemotactic and hematopoietic mediators released in response to LPS are the CXC chemokines IL-8 and IFN-inducible protein 10, the CC chemokines monocyte chemoattractant protein 1, macrophage inflammatory protein (MIP)-1α and MIP-1β, and the hematopoietic factor granulocyte-colony stimulating factor (G-CSF)[23–29].

Several endogenous mechanisms exist to protect the host against excessive pro-inflammatory cytokine activity, among which are anti-inflammatory cytokines and soluble cytokine inhibitors. Administration of LPS to normal subjects results in the secretion of soluble inhibitors of TNF and IL-1 [30], factors that are also found in several clinical inflammatory conditions including sepsis. It has become clear that the inducible naturally occurring inhibitors of endogenous TNF are soluble forms of the extracellular domains of the cell-surface TNF receptors. These soluble TNF receptors, of which (as with the transmembrane receptors) two types exist, retain their affinity for free TNF, and, therefore, compete with the cellular TNF receptors for the binding of TNF. Intravenous LPS elicits the release of both types of soluble TNF receptor, and soluble receptors are detectable shortly after the appearance of TNF in the circulation. Levels of soluble TNF receptors remain elevated for several hours [31, 32]. In addition to inhibitors of TNF activity, at least one endogenous inhibitor of IL-1 is detected after administration of LPS to humans, i.e., the IL-1 receptor antagonist (IL-1ra) [33, 34]. This 22–24 kDa cytokine is produced by various cell types including mononuclear cells and neutrophils, and can bind to both known types of IL-1 receptor without exerting any agonistic effect. IL-1ra levels peak after three to four hours, but remain elevated for a considerable time thereafter [33, 34]. The soluble IL-1 receptor type II, which circulates in ng/ml concentrations in healthy humans, does not rise after LPS administration [35].

The activity of the cytokine network can also be regulated at the level of cellular receptors. Administration of LPS to normal subjects results in a transient reduction in TNF receptors on circulating monocytes and granulocytes, as determined by their capacity to bind labeled TNF [36, 37]. This reduced TNF binding is associated with a down-modulation of both the type I and type II TNF receptors. It can be speculated that the reduced expression of cell-surface TNF receptors after LPS injection may represent an attempt by the host to protect itself from excessive TNF activity. LPS also induces a down-regulation of type II IL-1 receptors on circulating monocytes and granulocytes [37].

Among the anti-inflammatory cytokines, IL-10 is the only mediator that is released in detectable quantities during low grade endotoxemia in man. IL-10 release follows that of TNF. LPS injection does not induce a rise in plasma IL-13 levels [35].

Effects on Leukocytes

Leukocytosis is among the most sensitive reactions registered after injection of LPS into humans [9]. Studies in healthy volunteers have invariably documented a characteristic biphasic change in white blood cell count after administration of LPS. Leukocyte counts start to decline 30 minutes post-injection and reach a nadir of less than 2×10^9/l after one hour. This initial leukopenia is followed by a marked leukocytosis. Phase I studies in cancer patients have revealed that the initial leukopenia is dose dependent, and is not found after very low doses of LPS that are still able to induce leukocytosis at later time points [8, 9]. The changes in total leukocyte counts in human endotoxemia largely reflect the changes in the number of circulating neutrophils. The LPS-induced increase in peripheral blood neutrophil counts is associated with the appearance of band forms. LPS administration also provokes a sustained lymphocytopenia of approximately 0.5×10^9/l that lasts at least six hours and involves all lymphocyte subsets, as well as a more transient monocytopenia [38].

Intravenous LPS influences not only leukocyte numbers, but also the activation status of white blood cells. Rises in plasma concentrations of elastase, complexed with its main inhibitor α_1-antitrypsin, lactoferrin, and bactericidal/permeability increasing protein (BPI) occur several hours after injection of endotoxin, indicative of neutrophil degranulation [39–41]. Furthermore, injection of LPS primes neutrophils *in vivo* for respiratory burst activity in response to N-formyl-methionyl-leucine-phenylalanine [42], and induces complement opsonin C3 surface receptors on neutrophils [43]. LPS administration to humans is also associated with a transient reduction in mitogen-induced *ex vivo* peripheral blood mononuclear cell proliferation [28].

The capacity of monocytes to produce pro-inflammatory cytokines in response to stimulation with LPS diminishes after *in vivo* exposure to LPS. This well recognized phenomenon has been designated 'endotoxin tolerance' and can also be found in patients with bacterial sepsis or shortly after surgery. It should be noted that the designation 'tolerance' is not adequate, since LPS is not the only stimulus monocytes are refractory to, and prior exposure to LPS is not a prerequisite for this phenomenon to occur. LPS tolerance can be reproduced by administration of low dose endotoxin to healthy humans [44–46]. Peripheral blood mononuclear cells obtained six hours after *in vivo* injection of LPS produce less TNF, IL-1β, IL-6 and IL-8 upon stimulation with LPS or toxic shock syndrome toxin 1, than cells isolated from blood before LPS injection [44]. These findings have been confirmed in studies in which whole blood was stimulated with LPS [45, 46]. Indeed, three hours after injection of LPS, whole blood obtained from these subjects produced less TNF and IL-1β. Of considerable interest, while the production of pro-inflammatory cytokines is suppressed, blood cells release more IL-1ra on *ex vivo* re-stimulation with LPS [45]. Furthermore, plasma obtained two hours, but not one hour, after *in vivo* administration of LPS inhibited TNF and IL-1ß production by LPS-stimulated whole blood from six other healthy donors not previously exposed to LPS [45]. Together, these data indicate that LPS tolerance represents a purposeful adaptation of the host, rather than a generalized hyporesponsiveness, and is at least partly mediated by soluble factors produced within two hours after previous exposure to LPS.

Effects on Coagulation and Fibrinolysis

The procoagulant response to intravenous injection of LPS has been carefully documented in healthy humans [12, 39, 47–53]. LPS induces a transient activation of the common pathway of the coagulation system, reflected by rises in the plasma concentrations of the prothrombin fragment F1+2 and of thrombin-antithrombin III (TAT) complexes, becoming evident from two hours post-injection. Interestingly, activation of coagulation is preceded by a rapid and transient activation of fibrinolysis (Fig. 2). LPS-induced fibrinolytic activation starts with the release of tissue-type plasminogen activator (tPA) into the circulation, which is followed in time by a brisk rise in plasminogen activator inhibitor type I (PAI-1) levels, indicating that the fibrinolytic response to LPS is highly regulated. The transient generation of active plasmin is confirmed by the detection of elevated plasma concentrations of plasmin-α_2-antiplasmin (PAP) complexes. Three hours after the administration of LPS, fibrinolysis is completely offset, at a time when coagulation activation is still proceeding, resulting in a net procoagulant state.

The contact system can be initiated by autoactivation of factor XII (the Hageman factor) after absorption to negatively charged surfaces such as cell membranes and heparin on endothelial cells. Factor XIIa cleaves factor XI to yield factor XIa, leading to the activation of factor X by the combined action of factor IXa and factor VIIIa in the tenase complex. Yet another substrate for factor XIIa is prekallikrein. Factor XIIa activates this zymogen to kallikrein, which in turn cleaves high molecular weight kininogen to liberate bradykinin. Bradykinin is a major end product of the contact system and one of the most potent vasoactive agents known. Low dose LPS may induce some activation of the contact system,

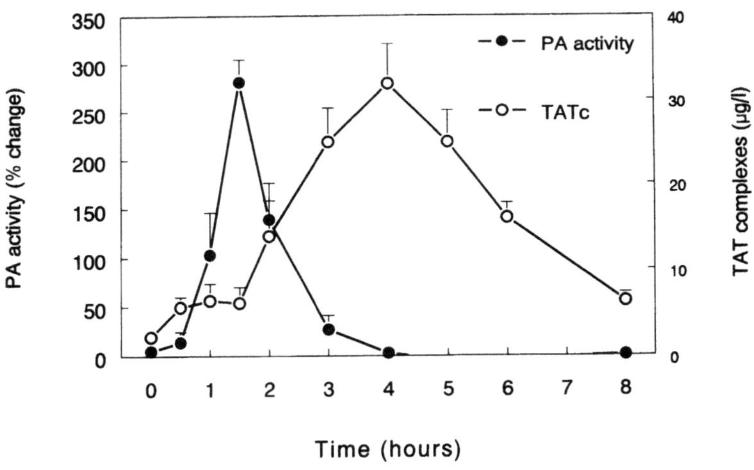

Fig. 2. Activation of fibrinolysis preceeds activation of coagulation during human endotoxemia. LPS induces an early and transient rise in plasma plasminogen activator (PA) activity, followed by a more sustained increase in the plasma concentrations of thrombin-antithrombin III (TAT) complexes

although one study found unchanged levels of factor XIIa-C1-inhibitor and kallikrein-C1-inhibitor complexes after injection of LPS at a dose of 2 ng/kg body weight [12]. Two other studies, both from the same group, did find evidence for contact system activation after administration of 4 ng/kg body weight, demonstrating decreases in functional prekallikrein and factor XI, and an increase in kallikrein-α_2-macroglobulin complexes [53, 54]. Activation of the contact system does not make an important contribution to the activation of the common pathway of the coagulation system in human endotoxemia, since infusion of a specific inhibitor of the extrinsic tissue factor mediated route (i.e., recombinant tissue factor pathway inhibitor) completely prevents LPS-induced coagulation activation in healthy subjects (our own unpublished observations). Hence, intravenous LPS provokes an imbalance between coagulation and fibrinolysis, resulting in a net procoagulant state after several hours. The coagulation system is likely to be activated via the extrinsic route in endotoxemia.

Endocrine and Metabolic Effects

Intravenous injection of LPS elicits a characteristic stress hormone response [11, 55–63]. LPS induces a rise in the plasma concentrations of catecholamines, adrenocorticotrophic hormone (ACTH), cortisol and growth hormone (GH). For most stress hormones, peak levels are reached early, after two to four hours, then rapidly return to baseline values. Plasma cortisol, however, may remain elevated for six hours or longer after LPS injection. LPS does not affect insulin or glucagon concentrations at the doses administered. One study has reported an increase in the peripheral blood concentrations of arginine vasopressin after injection of LPS, while the levels of corticotropin-releasing hormone were unaffected [58]. LPS also influences the GH-insulin-like growth factor (IGF) axis in humans [63]. LPS induced a gradual decrease in total IGF-I concentrations in blood, while IGF-II levels remained unchanged. Concurrently, IGF binding protein-1 (IGFBP-1) and IGFBP-2 increased, whereas IGFBP-3 remained unaltered. Thus, intravenous LPS reproduced the characteristic alterations in the GH-IGF axis found after injury. Another well-described endocrine disturbance in injured patients is the euthyroid sick syndrome. Intravenous administration of low dose LPS to healthy subjects reproduced a number of changes in the plasma concentrations of thyroid hormones and thyrotropin (TSH) commonly seen in this syndrome, including reduced thyroxine (T4), triiodothyronine (T3) and TSH concentrations, and increased reverse T3 (rT3) levels [64, 65].

The effects of LPS on energy and substrate metabolism have been documented thoroughly in humans in a study in which substrate fluxes were monitored by simultaneous measurements in arterial, femoral venous and hepatic venous blood samples [22]. Substrate fluxes were calculated as the product of the arterial-venous difference in substrate concentration and blood flow; the latter was either measured by electrocapacitance plethysmography (extremity blood flow) or estimated by infusion of indocyanine green (splanchnic blood flow). LPS was found to enhance the resting energy expenditure. The rise in total body oxygen consumption was predominantly caused by an increase in extraction of oxygen by the splanchnic bed, i.e., after administration of LPS the estimated splanchnic oxygen consumption increased from 34% of total body oxygen consumption at baseline to 43% of total body oxygen consumption, mimicking the disproportionate increase in splanchnic oxygen consumption compared with total body oxygen consumption seen in clinical sepsis. The production of glucose by the splanchnic bed increased markedly between two and six hours after LPS, presumably a result of a rise in hepatic glucose output. The stimulation of endogenous glucose production was associated with an increase in the splanchnic uptake of lactate and the amino acids glutamine and alanine, all important precursors for gluconeogenesis. A progressive hyperglycemia was observed by two hours, despite an increase in peripheral glucose uptake. It should be noted however, that in this study [22], 5% dextrose was infused during the observation period; without exogenous carbohydrate supplementation, injection of LPS has been associated with a decrease in glucose levels [60]. Arterial free fatty acid (FFA) concentrations increased throughout the six hours after the LPS challenge, in association with a rise in net efflux of FFA from the extremity. In addition, LPS stimulated hepatic uptake of FFA and the efflux of triglycerides from the splanchnic bed. Two studies using stable isotopes to determine protein and glucose kinetics in human endotoxemia have confirmed the presence of increased hepatic glucose production [60, 61]. Furthermore, these investigations demonstrated an increase in whole body protein breakdown in association with an increased splanchnic uptake of amino acids.

Interventions Examined in the Human Endotoxemia Model

The human endotoxemia model is an excellent tool to study mechanisms contributing to inflammatory responses in man *in vivo*. The interventions tested in this model thus far are listed in Table 1.

Interventions Interfering with the Bioavailability of LPS

LPS in serum is bound with high affinity by the acute phase protein LPS binding protein (LBP). Complexing with LBP is essential for LPS to efficiently induce cellular responses. The LPS-LBP complex promotes the binding of LPS to CD14, the cell-surface 'ligand-binding' component of the LPS receptor. By contrast, another host protein, BPI, a constituent of the azurophilic granules of neutrophils, can bind and subsequently inactivate LPS. LPS can also be bound and inactivated by various classes of lipoproteins. Indeed, incubation of LPS with either high density lipoproteins (HDL), low density lipoproteins (LDL), or chylomicrons reduces its activity *in vitro*. In endotoxemia in healthy humans, four different interventions presumably interfering with LPS presentation to cells have been investigated: A recombinant 23 kDa amino terminal fragment of BPI (rBPI23), reconstituted HDL, Intralipid (a triglyceride-rich fat emulsion that resembles chylomicrons

Table 1. Interventions evaluated in the human endotoxemia model

Intervention	Reference
Recombinant amino terminal fragment of bactericidal/permeability increasing protein (rBPI23)	[17, 47, 66]
Reconstituted high density lipoprotein (rHDL)	[49, 67]
Intralipid	[48, 68]
PMX-622 (Polymyxin B)	[69]
Lipid A analog SDZ MRL 953	[70]
Recombinant dimeric tumor necrosis factor receptor type II (TNFR:Fc)	[15, 37, 53, 65, 71]
Recombinant interleukin-1 receptor antagonist (IL-1ra)	[64, 72, 73]
Recombinant soluble interleukin-1 receptor type I	[16]
Recombinant interleukin-10	[26, 50, 74]
Recombinant granulocyte-colony stimulating factor (G-CSF)	[29, 75]
Hydrocortisone	[59, 76–78]
Epinephrine	[51, 79, 80]
Ibuprofen	[14, 11, 23, 40, 56, 60, 82]
Platelet activating factor (PAF) antagonist	[82]
Pentoxifylline	[23, 55]
Metalloproteinase inhibitor GI5402	[83]

with respect to particle size and plasma clearance kinetics), and PMX-622 (an LPS binding agent containing polymyxin B). SDZ MRL 953, a synthetic monosaccharidic lipid A analog, has been evaluated in cancer patients injected with LPS from *Salmonella abortus equi*.

Infusion of rBPI23 (1 mg/kg body weight) directly prior to LPS injection was associated with a significant decrease in LPS activity in plasma, as measured by the Limulus assay. In addition, rBPI23 attenuated major LPS-induced inflammatory responses, including neutrophilic leukocytosis, neutrophil degranulation, cytokine release, and activation of the coagulation and fibrinolytic system [47, 66]. Furthermore, rBPI23 ameliorated the hemodynamic changes elicited by LPS [17]. Remarkably, rBPI23 did not influence clinical symptoms, such as fever, chills and myalgia.

rHDL was administered as a 4-hour infusion at a dose of 40 mg/kg in a study in which LPS was given 3.5 hours after the initiation of the rHDL infusion [49, 67]. During the LPS/rHDL treatment period, LPS levels were higher than during the LPS/placebo treatment period [67]. This seemingly paradoxical finding may reflect the fact that the Limulus assay for LPS activity includes a dilution and heating step during which LPS is recovered from LPS-binding proteins such as rHDL. Therefore, enhanced LPS activity in rHDL-treated volunteers likely reflected successful binding of LPS by rHDL. rHDL reduced LPS-induced symptoms such as chills and myalgia, although the febrile response was not affected. Of considerable interest, rHDL markedly attenuated LPS-induced release of the pro-inflammatory cytokines TNF and IL-8, while modestly inhibiting the secretion of the anti-inflammatory mediators soluble TNF receptors and IL-1ra [67]. In addition, rHDL significantly reduced the activation of the coagulation system (plasma concentrations of F1+2 and TAT complexes) and the fibrinolytic system (plasma tPA concentrations), while not influencing the inhibition of fibrinolysis (release of PAI-1)[49]. The different potencies with which rHDL influenced distinct LPS-induced inflammatory responses may have been related to the fact that some of the LPS administered did not associate with rHDL, and that different responses require different threshold levels of bioactive LPS.

Intralipid is a triglyceride-rich fat emulsion which, in plasma, functions similarly to endogenous lipoproteins. Intralipid inhibited LPS-induced cytokine production in human whole blood *in vitro* in a dose dependent manner; maximal inhibition (up to 70%) was achieved at a concentration of 10 g/l [68]. *In vivo*, LPS was given midway through a 4-hour infusion (125 ml/hour) of either dextrose 5% or Intralipid 20%. Infusion of Intralipid led to an increase in serum triglyceride levels from 95±16 to 818±135 mg/dl prior to LPS administration, i.e., levels that reduced cytokine production in LPS-stimulated whole blood. However, *in vivo* hypertriglyceridemia either did not influence inflammatory responses to LPS (fever, release of TNF, soluble TNF receptors, and leukocytosis), or even potentiated LPS responses (release of IL-6 and IL-8, neutrophil degranulation) [68]. In addition, Intralipid infusion enhanced LPS-induced coagulation activation, while it did not influence the activation of the fibrinolytic system. The LPS-induced appearance of PAI-1 was enhanced by lipid infusion, suggesting that fat emulsion infusion may enhance the tendency towards thrombotic complications in patients with infections [48].

PMX-622 is an agent that contains polymyxin B, a compound known to bind LPS *in vitro*. Infusion of PMX-622 prevented LPS-induced clinical symptoms, as well as cytokine release. In addition, this intervention delayed and attenuated the down-modulation of monocyte TNF receptor expression [69].

The synthetic lipid A analog, SDZ MRL 953, was tested for its LPS neutralizing capacity in a phase I trial in cancer patients injected with LPS from *Salmonella abortus equi* [70]. SDZ MRL 953 itself, i.e., in patients who did not receive LPS, increased granulocyte counts and serum concentrations of G-CSF and IL-6, but not of TNF, IL-1β or IL-8. When given prior to LPS injection, SDZ MRL 953 markedly reduced the release of TNF, IL-1β, IL-6, IL-8 and G-CSF, but augmented the increase in granulocyte counts.

Interventions Directed at the Cytokine Network

Interventions evaluated in the human endotoxemia model aimed at the cytokine network include recombinant TNF receptor proteins, IL-1ra, soluble IL-1 receptor type I, IL-10 and G-CSF.

TNF has long been considered the most important mediator of LPS-induced toxicity. This assumption was primarily based on studies in which neutralization of endogenous TNF resulted in a complete protection of animals treated with lethal doses of live bacteria or LPS. A number of investigations, however, that fo-

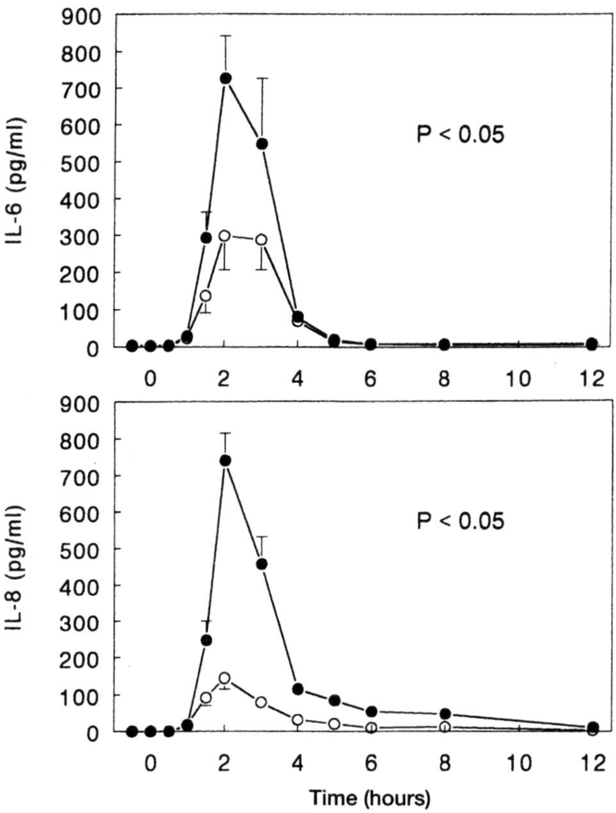

Fig. 3. Release of IL-6 and IL-8 after intravenous injection of LPS, and the effect of neutralization of endogenous TNF activity. LPS induces monophasic increases in the plasma levels of IL-6 and IL-8 (closed circles), which are strongly attenuated by infusion of a recombinant dimeric TNF receptor type II fusion protein directly prior to LPS injection (open circles)

cused on the role of TNF in specific inflammatory responses, have indicated that endogenous TNF is involved only partly in the activation of host mediator systems elicited by LPS. In endotoxemic humans, a recombinant dimeric TNF receptor type II (TNFR:Fc) has been used as a specific TNF inhibitor [15, 37, 53, 65, 71]. One group of investigators infused TNFR:Fc at relatively high doses (10 and 60 mg/m^2) [15, 53], while another group used TNFR:Fc at 6 mg/m^2 [37, 65, 71]. Although all doses provided a large excess of TNF neutralizing capacity in blood, some findings differed between different dosing regiments. When given at high doses TNFR:Fc delayed, but did not reduce, the febrile response to LPS [15], while at the lower dose TNFR:Fc blunted the rise in temperature [71]. TNFR:Fc did not affect the hemodynamic changes induced by intravenous LPS [15]. Elimination of endogenous TNF activity resulted in inhibition of the release of a number of cytokines and chemokines, including IL-6, IL-8 (Fig. 3), G-CSF, growth related protein-α (GRO-α), soluble TNF receptor type I, and IL-1ra. MIP-1α and IL-10 release were not significantly altered [15, 71]. Furthermore, TNFR:Fc inhibited the development of leukocytosis and the extent of neutrophil degranulation. Remarkably, TNFR:Fc exerted a paradoxical effect on cytokine and stress hormone release, i.e. as the dose of TNFR:Fc increased, the degree of inhibition decreased [15], suggesting that TNFR:Fc has a pro-inflammatory effect *per se*. TNFR:Fc did have a consistent inhibitory effect on LPS-induced activation of the fibrinolytic system, completely preventing the increases in tPA, PAI-1 and PAP complexes [53, 71]. Interestingly, TNFR:Fc did not influence the activation of the coagulation system, indicating that endogenous TNF is not required for the procoagulant response to LPS [53, 71]. Indeed, neutralization of TNF may result in a net procoagulant effect due to an unaltered rise in thrombin generation in the presence of a complete elimination of counterregulatory fibrinolytic activation. Endogenous TNF also appeared to be important for endothelial cell activation during endotoxemia, since TNFR:Fc infusion was associated with significant reductions in the plasma levels of von Willebrand factor and soluble E-selectin (Fig. 4) [15, 53]. TNFR:Fc modestly blunted the decrease in monocyte TNF receptors, but did not influence reduced expression of granulocyte TNF receptors or monocyte/granulocyte type II IL-1 receptors. Finally, TNFR:Fc failed to affect the alterations in thyroid hormone and TSH concentrations during endotoxemia [65]. Hence, TNF can be considered a mediator of some of the systemic inflammatory responses found after intravenous injection of LPS. In particular, endogenous TNF is involved in LPS-induced cytokine release, neutrophil degranulation, fibrinolytic changes and endothelial cell activation. An important exception is LPS-induced coagulation activation, which remains unchanged in the absence of detectable TNF activity.

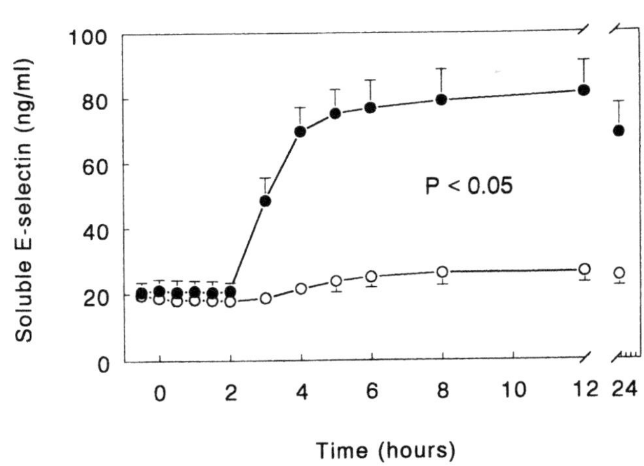

Fig. 4. Endothelial cell activation induced by intravenous injection of LPS, and the effect of neutralization of endogenous TNF activity. LPS induces a marked rise in the plasma levels of soluble E-selectin (closed circles), which is prevented by infusion of a recombinant dimeric TNF receptor type II fusion protein directly prior to LPS injection (open circles)

Attempts to neutralize endogenous IL-1 activity during human endotoxemia include studies in which LPS was administered together with either recombinant IL-1ra [64, 72, 73] or recombinant soluble IL-1 receptor type I [16]. It should be noted in this context that even immunoreactive IL-1 could not be detected in plasma or serum in most investigations in which low dose LPS was given to healthy humans, although this does not exclude expression of IL-1 at tissue level. In one study IL-1ra reduced neutrophilic granulocytosis elicited by LPS given at 3 ng/kg body weight [72], a finding not confirmed in another study in which LPS was injected at a dose of 2 ng/kg [73]. Neither study observed effects of IL-1ra on clinical signs and symptoms, elaboration of stress hormones or acute phase protein response. IL-1ra unexpectedly enhanced TNF release in one study [73], but not in the other [72]. Further, IL-1ra reversed the LPS-induced reduction in *ex vivo* mitogen-triggered peripheral blood mononuclear cell proliferation [72]. IL-1ra treatment did not influence LPS-induced changes in thyroid hormones and TSH concentrations in plasma [64]. Infusion of recombinant soluble type I IL-1 receptor was associated with a marked increase in circulating complexes of soluble type I IL-1 receptor and IL-1ra [16]. This interaction likely resulted in an IL-1 agonistic action, since it is expected to inhibit the anti-inflammatory actions of both exogenous soluble type I IL-1 receptor and endogenous IL-1ra. Thus, high-dose soluble type I IL-1 receptor was associated with increased levels of cell-associated IL-1β, plasma TNF and IL-8, and increased C-reactive protein (CRP) levels compared with subjects injected with LPS only. Other LPS responses were not affected by soluble type I IL-1 receptor, including hemodynamic parameters, leukocyte responses, and release of IL-6 and G-CSF [16].

IL-10 is a 18 kDa polypeptide that can be synthesized by T cells, B cells, monocytes and macrophages. The capacity of IL-10 to inhibit the stimulated production of a number of pro-inflammatory cytokines has received much attention. *In vitro*, IL-10 is a potent inhibitor of the production of TNF, IL-1, IL-6, IL-8, IL-12 and other cytokines. In addition, IL-10 is capable of attenuating the production of other mediators of inflammation, including tissue factor, nitric oxide (NO) and arachidonic acid products. The effect of recombinant human IL-10 on LPS responsiveness in humans *in vivo* has been addressed in an investigation in which IL-10 was given at a dose of 25 μg/kg body weight either two minutes before, or one hour after, LPS injection [26, 50, 74]. IL-10 given prior to LPS reduced the rise in body temperature and in plasma TNF, IL-6, IL-8, MIP-1α, MIP-1β and monocyte chemotactic protein (MCP)-1 concentrations, while post-treatment was without effect [26, 74]. LPS-induced granulocyte accumulation in lungs, as determined by dynamic granulocyte scintigrams, was prevented by IL-10 pretreatment (Fig. 5), while granulocyte degranulation was blunted [74]. Further, IL-10 also inhibited the activation of the fibrinolytic system and the coagulation system [50]. Hence, exogenous IL-10 inhibits inflammation during human endotoxemia, when given directly prior to LPS.

G-CSF is a 18 kDa glycoprotein that increases neutrophil counts in peripheral blood by stimulating proliferation and shortening bone marrow transit time. G-CSF has been advocated as an adjunctive therapy in a number of patient populations, including patients with neutropenia due to chemotherapy and patients

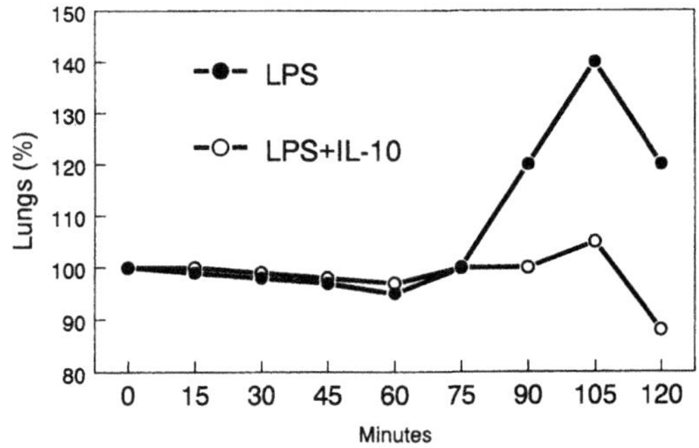

Fig. 5. Accumulation of granulocytes in lungs (expressed as relative radioactivity) after intravenous administration of LPS, and the effect of IL-10 injection given directly prior to LPS. IL-10 prevents granulocyte accumulation in lungs

with severe pneumonia. To determine the effects of G-CSF on inflammatory responses to intravenous LPS, this cytokine has been given in three different treatment regimens to endotoxemic subjects. In one investigation G-CSF was injected subcutaneously at a dose of 300 μg 12 hours prior to administration of LPS derived from *Salmonella abortus equi* (0.8 ng/kg body weight) [75]. In another study G-CSF (5 μg/kg) was given intravenously two hours before, or subcutaneously 24 hours before, injection of LPS from *Escherichia coli* (4 ng/kg)[29]. Interestingly, the effect of G-CSF on LPS-induced cytokine release was dependent on the timing of G-CSF administration. Indeed, G-CSF administered 24 hours before LPS did not influence TNF, IL-6 or IL-1ra levels, diminished IL-8 concentrations, and increased soluble TNF receptor release [29]. When given two or 12 hours before LPS, G-CSF potentiated TNF, IL-6, IL-8, IL-1ra and soluble TNF receptor release [29, 75]. G-CSF administered either two or 24 hours prior to LPS augmented LPS-induced neutrophil responses, including neutrophilia, degranulation and expression of cell surface markers such as CD11b, CD18 and CD67 [29]. Furthermore, these latter two treatment strategies down-modulated neutrophil L-selectin expression and completely prevented the LPS-induced neutrophil accumulation within the pulmonary compartment during the first two hours after LPS challenge, as determined by dynamic granulocyte scintigrams [29]. Together these data suggest that the effects of G-CSF on LPS-induced cytokine release differ when different dosing regimens (two, 12 or 24 hours before LPS injection) are used, while its effects on neutrophil counts and functions are similar.

Influence of Stress Hormones on LPS Effects

The human endotoxemia model has been used to investigate the effects of the stress hormones hydrocortisone and epinephrine on LPS-induced inflammation. A bolus intravenous injection of 100 or 200 mg of hydrocortisone directly before administration of LPS attenuated clinical responses, fever and the increases in TNF, IL-6 and IL-8 [76]. Interestingly, the timing of hypercortisolemia appears to be a major determinant of its effect on LPS responses [59]. Hypercortisolemia, achieved by continuous infusion of hydrocortisone (3 μg/kg body weight/min), resulting in plasma cortisol concentrations up to 800 ng/ml concurrently or six hours before injection of LPS, largely prevented the rise in TNF levels. However, hypercortisolemia 12 hours or six days before injection of LPS, enhanced TNF release. The appearance of IL-6 was not affected by concurrent hypercortisolemia, whereas it was augmented by hypercortisolemia preceding the administration of LPS. Hydrocortisone also influences the production of antagonist members of the cytokine network. Infusion of hydrocortisone directly prior to injection of LPS into normal human beings has been found to inhibit [77], or to have no influence upon release of IL-1ra [76]. The release of soluble TNF receptor type II was influenced by antecedent periods of hypercortisolemia in a similar direction to TNF [77]. In subjects who were infused with hydrocortisone directly prior to LPS administration, IL-10 concentrations were much higher than in those infused with LPS only, while hypercortisolemia six, 12 or 144 hours before LPS injection did not influence LPS-induced IL-10 levels [78]. Taken together, it is likely that antecedent periods of hypercortisolemia participate in the regulation of clinical, hormonal and cytokine responses to LPS. Infusion of hydrocortisone directly before injection of LPS has a net anti-inflammatory effect on the cytokine network by concurrent inhibition of the pro-inflammatory cytokine TNF and enhancement of the anti-inflammatory cytokine IL-10.

Exogenously administered epinephrine influences cytokine production during endotoxemia in a manner similar to hydrocortisone. Epinephrine was given as a continuous infusion at a dose of 30 ng/kg/min, starting either three hours or 24 hours prior to LPS injection [79]. Both epinephrine regimens attenuated LPS-induced TNF release, the infusion started at minus three hours having the more pronounced effect. Epinephrine initiated three hours before LPS, strongly potentiated IL-10 release, which was also associated with a shift of the peak IL-10 response to earlier time points. Epinephrine started 24 hours before LPS injection had no effect on IL-10 release. Epinephrine tended to reduce the appearances of IL-6, IL-8 and IL-1ra during endotoxemia, but these effects did not reach statistical significance. In addition, epinephrine infusion started three hours prior to injection of LPS attenuated the LPS-induced down-regulation of monocyte TNF receptors, an effect that was not observed when epinephrine administration was initiated 24 hours pre-LPS [80]. Hence, epinephrine not only affects the production of TNF, but can also influence the bioavailability of this potent pro-inflammatory cytokine. Interestingly, epinephrine affected hemostatic alterations induced by LPS. Indeed, epinephrine, started either 24 or three hours prior to LPS injection, exerted a strong anticoagulant effect (Fig. 6) [51]. Epinephrine attenuated activation of the coagulation system induced by intravenous LPS, and concurrently enhanced activation of the fibrinolytic system. The anticoagulant properties of epinephrine were further demonstrated by a greater than 50% reduction in the ratio of maximal coagulation activation and maximal fibrinolytic activation [51]. Hence, short term pre-exposure of healthy humans to a constant infusion of epinephrine prior to injection of low dose LPS has strong anti-inflammatory effects, inhibiting the production of the pro-inflammatory cytokine TNF and simultaneously enhancing the synthesis of the anti-inflammatory cytokine IL-10, while also attenuating the procoagulant response.

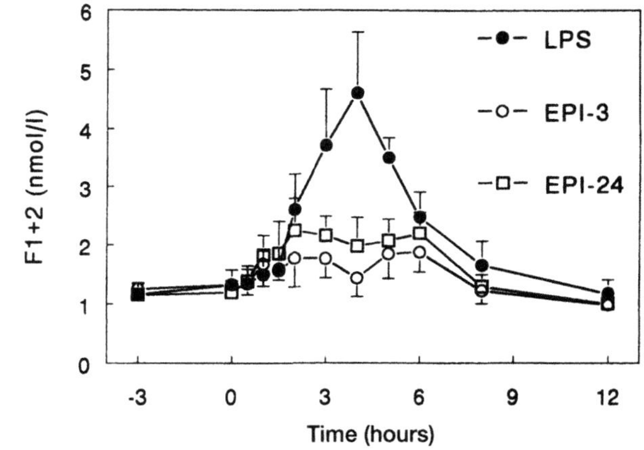

Fig. 6. Epinephrine inhibits LPS-induced coagulation activation (plasma levels of the prothrombin fragment F1 + 2). LPS = subjects injected with LPS only (n = 6); EPI-3 = subjects infused with epinephrine (30 ng/kg/min) from t = −3 h to 6 h (n = 5); EPI-24 = subjects infused with epinephrine (30 ng/kg/min) from t = −24 h to 6 h (n = 6)

Interventions with Various Pharmacological Agents

The cyclooxygenase inhibitor ibuprofen has been used in the human endotoxemia model by a number of investigators. It has become clear that interactions exist between products of the cyclooxygenase pathway and cytokines in endotoxemia. Intravenous administration of LPS induced a transient increase in the plasma concentrations of 6-keto-prostaglandin F1α, the stable metabolite of prostacyclin, indicative of activation of the cyclooxygenase pathway [81]. Inhibition of cyclooxygenase by pre-treatment with ibuprofen blunted the clinical and stress hormone responses to LPS, as well as the increase in the metabolic rate [11, 23, 40, 56, 60, 82]. In two of three studies that reported cytokine levels after pre-treatment with ibuprofen, the induction of the cytokine network by LPS was augmented in ibuprofen treated subjects. Although ibuprofen did not influence the neutrophilic leukocytosis induced by LPS, it augmented the increase in plasma elastase levels, suggesting that cyclooxygenase products inhibit neutrophil degranulation during endotoxemia [40]. In metabolic studies, ibuprofen blunted the effects of LPS on whole body and non-oxidative leucine flux, but enhanced the LPS-induced decrease in plasma glucose levels due to a relative rise in glucose disappearance [60]. Ibuprofen did not alter hemodynamic changes observed during endotoxemia [14]. These data indicate that endogenous cyclooxygenase products mediate some of the biologic effects of LPS, while concurrently inhibiting LPS-induced cytokine production.

Inhibition of platelet activating factor (PAF) has anti-inflammatory effects in rodent models of severe endotoxemia. Oral administration of a PAF antagonist 18 hours before injection of LPS, reduced LPS-induced symptoms such as rigors and myalgia [82]. Further, the PAF antagonist diminished peak cortisol and epinephrine concentrations, but did not influence the febrile response, the release of TNF and IL-6, or the increase in resting energy expenditure.

Pentoxifylline is a compound that is capable of inhibiting TNF synthesis *in vitro*. A four-hour intravenous infusion of pentoxifylline started 30 minutes before

LPS injection prevented the rise in serum TNF concentrations, but had no effect on fever, clinical symptoms, cortisol release and IL-6 secretion [55]. Oral administration of pentoxifylline failed to change leukocyte and cytokine responses or the hemodynamic effects elicited by LPS [23].

TNF is released from the cell surface by cleavage of pro-TNF-α by metalloproteinases. An oral dose of the metalloproteinase inhibitor GI5402 (100 mg) 20 minutes prior to LPS injection strongly reduced LPS-induced TNF release, but did not prevent the increase in monocyte-bound TNF-α. In addition, GI5402 attenuated the rise in plasma soluble TNF-α receptors types I and II after LPS injection, but did not change the LPS-induced decreases in granulocyte and monocyte TNF-α receptor expression [83].

External Factors Influencing LPS Responsiveness

The effects of LPS can be influenced by the route of feeding in the week prior to injection of LPS [52, 62, 84]. Subjects who had received total parenteral nutrition (TPN) for seven days before a single challenge with LPS showed an enhanced response when compared to subjects who received a standardized enteral diet. The augmentation of LPS-induced effects by antecedent TPN involved clinical signs and symptoms, changes in stress hormone levels, peripheral amino acid mobilization, peripheral lactate production and the acute phase protein response [62]. In addition, antecedent TPN potentiated the release of TNF, IL-6 and the type II TNF receptor, as well as the decrease in monocyte TNF receptor expression [84]. Interestingly, TPN was associated with a selectively enhanced activation of the coagulation system during endotoxemia in comparison with enteral feeding. Activation of the fibrinolytic system proceeded similarly in enterally and parenterally fed groups [52]. Although the mechanism underlying this phenomenon remains to be established, its clinical relevance is obvious, demonstrating that the route of feeding and bowel rest may influence the course of disease.

LPS responsiveness is dependent on diurnal variation [85]. Injection of LPS at 9 am or 7 pm resulted in similar increases in the plasma concentrations of TNF and IL-6, but administration in the evening caused about twice the increases in rectal temperature and plasma ACTH and cortisol levels compared to injection in the morning. Considering that endogenous cortisol levels are low in the evening, these data suggest that diurnal variations in the human susceptibility to LPS may be related to a suppression of the biological effects of cytokines by endogenous glucocorticoids.

Conclusion

Intravenous injection of a low dose of LPS induces a number of clinical and laboratory changes that, in a qualitative way, resemble changes found in acute infection. It is important to realize, however, that the human endotoxemia model does not reflect an infectious disease. Indeed, patients with Gram-negative sepsis usually have an infectious focus somewhere in their body, with sepsis originating from pyelonephritis, pneumonia, cholangitis, peritonitis, etc. In such infections, which initially are localized, pro-inflammatory cytokines play an important role in local host defense against bacteria. In models of sterile immune activation such as that produced by intravenous injection of LPS, however, pro-inflammatory cytokines mediate systemic inflammation and are considered harmful. Therefore, we consider this model less suitable to predict which interventions may be useful in clinical infectious disease. Rather, the model can be used to study the early events that lead to activation of different inflammatory cascades in clinical disease, and to evaluate pharmacologic interventions that may attenuate them. Although conclusions drawn from the human endotoxemia model need to be interpreted with caution, the assessment of the biological effects of LPS in healthy humans has contributed significantly to the understanding of the pathophysiology of acute inflammation.

References

1. Manthous CA, Hall JB, Samsel RW (1993) Endotoxin in human disease. Part 1: Biochemistry, assay, and possible role in diverse disease states. Chest 104:1572–1581
2. Hoffmann WD, Natanson C (1993) Endotoxin in septic shock. Anesth Analg 77:613–624
3. Starnes CO (1992) Coley's toxin in perspective. Nature 357:11–12
4. Florman AL, Holzman RS (1975) Nonspecific enhancers of resistance in man. J Pediatr 87: 1094–1102
5. Greisman SE, Woodward WE (1965) Mechanisms of endotoxin tolerance. III. The refractory state during continuous infusions with endotoxin. J Exp Med 121:911–933
6. Hochstein HD, Mills DF, Outschoorn AS, Rastogi SC (1983) The processing and collaborative assay of reference endotoxin. J Biol Stand 11:251–260
7. Poole S, Dawson P, Gaines Das RE (1997) Second international standard for endotoxin: calibration in an international collaborative study. J Endotoxin Res 4:221–231
8. Engelhardt R, Mackensen A, Galanos C, Andreesen R (1990) Biological response to intravenously administered endotoxin in patients with advanced cancer. J Biol Resp Mod 9: 480–491
9. Engelhardt R, Mackensen A, Galanos C (1991) Phase I trial of intravenously administered endotoxin (Salmonella abortus equi) in cancer patients. Cancer Res 51:2524–2530
10. Hesse DG, Tracey KJ, Fong Y, et al (1988) Cytokine appearance in human endotoxemia and primate bacteremia. Surg Gynecol Obstet 166:147–53
11. Michie HR, Manogue KR, Spriggs DR, et al (1988) Detection of circulating tumor necrosis factor after endotoxin administration. N Engl J Med 318:1481–1486
12. Van Deventer SJH, Büller HR, ten Cate JW, Aarden LA, Hack CE, Sturk A (1990) Experimental endotoxemia in humans: analysis of cytokine release and coagulation, fibrinolytic and complement pathways. Blood 76:2520–2526
13. Suffredini AF, Fromm FE, Parker MM, et al (1989) The cardiovascular response of normal humans to the administration of endotoxin. N Engl J Med 321:280–287
14. Martich GD, Parker MM, Cunnion RE, Suffredini AF (1992) Effects of ibuprofen and pentoxifylline on the cardiovascular response of normal humans to endotoxin. J Appl Physiol 73: 925–931
15. Suffredini AF, Reda D, Banks SM, Tropea M, Agosti JM, Miller R (1995) Effects of recombinant dimeric TNF receptor on human inflammatory responses following intravenous endotoxin administration. J Immunol 155:5038–5045
16. Preas II HL, Reda D, Tropea M, et al (1996) Effects of recombinant soluble type I interleukin-1 receptor on human inflammatory responses to endotoxin. Blood 88:2465–2472

17. De Winter RJ, von der Möhlen MAM, van Lieshout H, et al (1995) Recombinant endotoxin-binding protein (rBPI23) attenuates endotoxin-induced circulatory changes in humans. J Inflamm 45:193–206
18. Taveira da Silva AM, Kaulbach HC, Chuidian FS, Lambert DR, Suffredini AF, Danner RL (1993) Brief report: Shock and multiple organ dysfunction after self-administration of Salmonella endotoxin. N Engl J Med 328:1457–1460
19. Suffredini AF, Shelhamer JH, Neumann RD, Brenner M, Baltaro RJ, Parillo JE (1992) Pulmonary and oxygen transport effects of intravenously administered endotoxin in normal humans. Am Rev Respir Dis 145:1398–1403
20. Smith PD, Suffredini AF, Allen JB, Wahl LM, Parillo JE, Wahl SM (1994) Endotoxin administration to humans primes alveolar macrophages for increased production of inflammatory mediators. J Clin Immunol 14:141–148
21. Van der Poll T, van Deventer SJH (1999) Cytokines and anti-cytokines in the pathogenesis of sepsis. Infect Dis Clin North Am 13:413–426
22. Fong Y, Marano MA, Moldawer LL, et al (1990) The acute splanchnic and peripheral tissue metabolic response to endotoxin in humans. J Clin Invest 85:1896–1904
23. Martich GD, Danner RL, Ceska M, Suffredini AF (1991) Detection of interleukin 8 and tumor necrosis factor in normal humans after intravenous endotoxin: the effect of antiinflammatory agents. J Exp Med 173:1021–1024
24. Van Deventer SJH, Hart M, van der Poll T, Hack CE, Aarden LA (1993) Endotoxin and TNF-induced IL-8 release in humans. J Infect Dis 167:461–464
25. Sylvester I, Suffredini AF, Boujoukos AJ, et al (1993) Neutrophil attractant protein-1 and monocyte chemoattractant protein-1 in human serum. J Immunol 151:3292–3298
26. Olszyna DP, Pajkrt D, van Deventer SJH, van der Poll T (1998) Effect of interleukin 10 on CC chemokines during human endotoxemia. 38th Interscience Conference on Antimicrobial Agents and Chemotherapy (ICAAC). September 24–27, 1998. San Diego. Abstract G-2
27. Mackensen A, Galanos C, Engelhardt R (1991) Modulating activity of interferon-gamma on endotoxin-induced cytokine production in cancer patients. Blood 78:3254–3258
28. Granowitz EV, Porat R, Mier JW, et al (1993). Hematologic and immunomodalutory effects of an interleukin-1 receptor antagonist coinfusion during low-dose endotoxemia in healthy humans. Blood 82:2985–2990
29. Pajkrt D, Manten A, van der Poll T, et al (1997) Modulation of cytokine release and neutrophil function by granulocyte colony-stimulating factor during endotoxemia in humans. Blood 90:1415–1424
30. Spinas GA, Bloesch D, Kaufmann MT, Keller U, Dayer JM (1990) Induction of plasma inhibitors of interleukin 1 and TNF-α activity by endotoxin to normal humans. Am J Physiol 259: R993–R997
31. Van Zee KJ, Kohno T, Fischer E, Rock SC, Moldawer LL, Lowry SF (1992) Tumor necrosis factor soluble receptors circulate during experimental and clinical inflammation and can protect against excessive tumor necrosis factor α in vitro and in vivo. Proc Natl Acad Sci USA 89:4845–4849
32. Spinas GA, Keller U, Brockhaus M (1992) Release of soluble receptors for tumor necrosis factor (TNF) in relation to circulating TNF during experimental endotoxinemia. J Clin Invest 90:533–536
33. Granowitz EV, Santos AA, Poutsiaka DD, et al (1991) Production of interleukin-1-receptor antagonist during experimental endotoxaemia. Lancet 338:1423–1424
34. Fischer E, van Zee KJ, Marano MA, et al (1992) Interleukin-1 receptor antagonist circulates in experimental inflammation and in human disease. Blood 79:2196–200
35. Van der Poll T, de Waal Malefyt R, Coyle SM, Lowry SF (1997) Antiinflammatory cytokine responses during clinical sepsis and experimental endotoxemia: sequential measurements of plasma soluble interleukin (IL)-1 receptor type II, IL-10 and IL-13 concentrations. J Infect Dis 175:118–122
36. Van der Poll T, Calvano SE, Kumar A, et al (1995) Endotoxin induces downregulation of tumor necrosis factor receptors on circulating monocytes and granulocytes in humans. Blood 86:2754–2759
37. Van der Poll T, Coyle SM, Kumar A, Barbosa K, Agosti J, Lowry SF (1997) Down-regulation of surface receptors for TNF and IL-1 on circulating monocytes and granulocytes during hu-

man endotoxemia. Effect of neutralization of endotoxin-induced TNF activity by infusion of a recombinant dimeric TNF receptor. J Immunol 158:1490–1497
38. Richardson RP, Rhyne CD, Fong Y, et al (1989) Peripheral blood leukocyte kinetics following in vivo lipopolysaccharide (LPS) administration to normal human subjects. Ann Surg 210: 239–245
39. Suffredini AF, Harpel PC, Parrillo JE (1989) Promotion and subsequent inhibition of plasminogen activation after administration of intravenous endotoxin to normal subjects. N Engl J Med 320:1165–1172
40. Spinas GA, Bloesch D, Keller U, Zimmerli W, Cammisuli S (1991) Pretreatment with ibuprofen augments circulating tumor necrosis factor-α, interleukin-6, and elastase during acute endotoxinemia. J Infect Dis 163:89–95
41. Von der Möhlen MAM, van der Poll T, Jansen J, Levi M, van Deventer SJH (1996) Release of bactericidal/permeability-increasing protein in experimental endotoxemia and clinical sepsis: Role of tumor necrosis factor. J Immunol 156:4969–4973
42. Martich GD, Van Dervort AL, Danner RL, Suffredini AF (1992) Intravenous endotoxin administration to normal humans primes neutrophils for an enhanced respiratory burst. Crit Care Med 20:S100 (abst)
43. Moore FD, Moss NA, Revhaug A, Wilmore DW, Mannick JA, Rodrick ML (1987) A single dose of endotoxin activates neutrophils without activating complement. Surgery 102:200–205
44. Granowitz EV, Porat R, Mier JW, et al (1993) Intravenous endotoxin suppresses the cytokine response of peripheral blood mononuclear cells of healthy humans. J Immunol 151: 1637–1645
45. Van der Poll T, Coyle SM, Moldawer LL, Lowry SF (1996) Changes in endotoxin-induced cytokine production by whole blood after in vivo exposure of normal humans to endotoxin. J Infect Dis 174:1356–1360
46. Kimmings AN, Pajkrt D, Zaaijer K, et al (1996) Factors involved in early in vitro endotoxin hyporesponsiveness in human endotoxemia. J Endotox Res 3:283–289
47. Von der Möhlen MAM, van Deventer SJH, Levi M, et al (1995) Inhibition of endotoxin-induced activation of the coagulation and fibrinolytic pathways using a recombinant endotoxin-binding protein (rBPI23). Blood 85:3437–3443
48. Van der Poll T, Coyle SM, Levi M, et al (1996) Fat emulsion infusion potentiates coagulation activation during human endotoxemia. Thromb Haemostas 75:83–86
49. Pajkrt D, Lerch PG, van der Poll T, et al (1997) Differential effects of reconstituted high-density lipoprotein on coagulation, fibrinolysis and platelet activation during human endotoxemia. Thromb Haemostas 77:303–307
50. Pajkrt D, van der Poll T, Levi M, et al (1997) Interleukin 10 inhibits activation of coagulation and fibrinolysis during human endotoxemia. Blood 89:2701–2705
51. Van der Poll T, Levi M, Dentener M, et al (1997) Epinephrine exerts anticoagulant effects during human endotoxemia. J Exp Med 185:1143–1148
52. Van der Poll T, Levi M, Braxton CC, et al (1998) Parenteral nutrition facilitates activation of coagulation, but not of fibrinolysis, during human endotoxemia. J Infect Dis 177:793–795
53. DeLa Cadena RA, Majluf-Cruz A, Stadnicki A, et al (1998) Recombinant tumor necrosis factor receptor p75 fusion protein (TNFR:Fc) alters endotoxin-induced activation of the kinin, fibrinolytic, and coagulation systems in normal humans. Thromb Haemostas 80:114–118
54. DeLa Cadena RA, Suffredini AF, Page JD, et al (1993) Activation of the kallikrein-kinin system after endotoxin administration to normal human volunteers. Blood 81:3313–3317
55. Zabel P, Wolter DT, Schönharting MM, Schade UF (1989) Oxpentifylline in endotoxaemia. Lancet ii:1474–1477
56. Revhaug A, Michie HR, Manson JM, et al (1988) Inhibition of cyclo-oxygenase attenuates the metabolic response to endotoxin in humans. Arch Surg 123:162–170
57. Michie HR, Spriggs DR, Manogue KR, et al (1988) Tumor necrosis factor and endotoxin induce similar metabolic responses in human beings. Surgery 104:280–286
58. Michie HR, Majzoub JA, O'Dwyer ST, Revhaug A, Wilmore DW (1990) Both cyclooxygenase-dependent and cyclooxygenase-independent pathways mediate the neuroendocrine response in humans. Surgery 108:254–261
59. Barber AE, Coyle SM, Marano MA, et al (1993) Glucocorticoid therapy alters hormonal and cytokine responses to endotoxin in man. J Immunol 150:1999–2006

60. Bloesch D, Keller U, Spinas GA, Kury D, Girard J, Stauffacher W (1993). Effects of endotoxin on leucine and glucose kinetics in man: contribution of prostaglandin E_2 assessed by a cyclooxygenase inhibitor. J Clin Endocrinol Metab 77:1156–1163
61. Fong Y, Matthews DE, He W, Marano M, Moldawer LL, Lowry SF (1994) Whole body and splanchnic leucine, phenylalanine, and glucose kinetics during endotoxemia in man. Am J Physiol 266:R419–R425
62. Fong Y, Marano MA, Barber A, et al (1989) Total parenteral nutrition and bowel rest modify the metabolic response to endotoxin in humans. Ann Surg 210:449–456
63. Lang CH, Pollard V, Fan J, et al (1997) Acute alterations in growth hormone-insulin-like growth factor axis in humans injected with endotoxin. Am J Physiol 273:R371–R378
64. Van der Poll T, van Zee KJ, Endert E, et al (1995) Interleukin-1 receptor blockade does not affect endotoxin-induced changes in plasma thyroid hormone and thyrotropin concentrations in man. J Clin Endocrinol Metab 80:1341–1346
65. Van der Poll T, Endert E, Coyle SM, Agosti JM, Lowry SF (1999) Neutralization of tumor necrosis factor does not influence endotoxin-induced changes in thyroid hormone metabolism in man. Am J Physiol 276:R357–R362
66. Von der Möhlen MAM, Kimmings AN, Wedel NI, et al (1995) Inhibition of endotoxin-induced cytokine release and neutrophil activation in humans by use of recombinant bactericidal/permeability-increasing protein. J Infect Dis 172:144–151
67. Pajkrt D, Doran JE, Koster F, et al (1996) Antiinflammatory effects of reconstituted high-density lipoprotein during human endotoxemia. J Exp Med 184:1601–1608
68. Van der Poll T, Braxton CC, Coyle SM, et al (1995) Effect of hypertriglyceridemia on endotoxin responsiveness in man. Infect Immun 63:3396–3400
69. Lin E, Coyle SM, Randhawa S, et al (1998) PMX-622 prevents endotoxin-induced inflammation in humans. Surg Forum 49:6–8
70. Kiani A, Tschiersch A, Gaboriau E, et al (1997) Downregulation of the proinflammatory cytokine response to endotoxin by pretreatment with the nontoxic lipid A analog SDZ MRL 953 in cancer patients. Blood 90:1673–1683
71. Van der Poll T, Coyle SM, Levi M, et al (1997) Effect of a recombinant dimeric tumor necrosis factor receptor on inflammatory responses to intravenous endotoxin in normal humans. Blood 89:3727–3734
72. Granowitz EV, Porat R, Mier JW, et al (1993) Hematologic and immunomodulatory effects of an interleukin-1 receptor antagonist coinfusion during low-dose endotoxemia in healthy humans. Blood 82:2985–2990
73. Van Zee KJ, Coyle SM, Calvano SE, et al (1995) Influence of interleukin-1 receptor blockade on the human response to endotoxemia. J Immunol 154:1499–1507
74. Pajkrt D, Camoglio L, Tiel-van Buul MCM, et al (1997) Attenuation of proinflammatory response by recombinant human IL-10 in human endotoxemia; the effect of timing of rhIL-10 administration. J Immunol 158:3971–3977
75. Pollmächer T, Korth C, Mullington J, et al (1996) Effects of granulocyte colony-stimulating factor on plasma cytokine receptor levels and on the in vivo host response to endotoxin in healthy men. Blood 87:900–905
76. Santos AA, Scheltinga MR, Lynch E, et al (1993) Elaboration of interleukin 1-receptor antagonist is not attenuated by glucocorticoids after endotoxemia. Arch Surg 128:138–144
77. Barber AE, Coyle SM, Fischer E, et al (1995) Influence of hypercortisolemia on soluble TNF receptor II and interleukin-1 receptor antagonist responses to endotoxin in human beings. Surgery 118:406–411
78. Van der Poll T, Barber AE, Coyle SM, Lowry SF (1996) Hypercortisolemia increases plasma interleukin 10 concentrations during human endotoxemia. J Clin Endocrin Metab 81:3604–3606
79. Van der Poll T, Coyle SM, Barbosa K, Braxton CC, Lowry SF (1996) Epinephrine inhibits tumor necrosis factor α and potentiates interleukin 10 production during human endotoxemia. J Clin Invest 97:713–719
80. Van der Poll T, Calvano SE, Kumar A, Coyle SM, Lowry SF (1997) Epinephrine attenuates downregulation of monocyte tumor necrosis factor receptors during human endotoxemia. J Leukoc Biol 61:156–160

81. Van der Poll T, van Deventer SJH, Büller HR, Sturk A, ten Cate JW (1991) Comparison of the early dynamics of systematic prostacyclin release after administration of tumor necrosis factor and endotoxin to healthy humans. J Infect Dis 164:599–601
82. Thompson WA, Coyle SM, van Zee K, et al (1994) The metabolic effects of platelet-activating factor antagonism in endotoxemic man. Arch Surg 129:72–79
83. Dekkers PEP, Lauw FN, ten Hove T, et al (1998) Effect of a metalloproteinase inhibitor (GI4502) in endotoxemia in healthy subjects. 38th Interscience Conference on Antimicrobial Agents and Chemotherapy (ICAAC). September 24–27, 1998. San Diego. Abstract G-4
84. Braxton CC, Coyle SM, Montegut WJ, et al (1995) Parenteral nutrition alters monocyte TNF receptor activity. J Surg Res 59:23–28
85. Pollmächer T, Mullington J, Korth C, et al (1996) Diurnal variations in the human host response to endotoxin. J Infect Dis 174:1040–1045

Monitoring Immune Status in Critically Ill Patients

M. R. Pinsky and A. J. Rosenbloom

Introduction

Although the systemic inflammatory response syndrome (SIRS) has been well described [1, 2] in gross clinical terms, its actual cellular components and their interactions have only just recently come into focus. The overall inflammatory state and subsequent organ injury occurs as a result of inflammatory mechanisms. Many of the organ-system injury pathways are linked through immune effector cell activation and cytotoxic cell injury. The understanding of the processes that lead to immune injury and external modulation of the endogenous control of these immune effector cells during SIRS has proven to be complex. No simple cascade of initiating sequences followed by activation of intracellular inflammatory responses and subsequent cell and organ injury explains the process seen clinically, although such a cascade does describe the initial aspects of isolated cell culture experiments. Clinically, multiple pro- and anti-inflammatory mediators appear in the blood of patients with SIRS. Most of the time when one measures the levels of inflammatory mediators in the blood of patients with SIRS, the concentration of anti-inflammatory mediators vastly outweighs that of pro-inflammatory mediators [3]. Furthermore, it has been difficult to demonstrate bioactivity of the pro-inflammatory substances in the plasma of patients with SIRS [4]. Potentially, bursts of inflammatory mediator release are very brief or pro-inflammatory mediator molecules are bound to cell surfaces and are presented locally at high concentrations, cell to cell [5]. However, based on measures of circulating pro- or anti-inflammatory mediators in the serum, it is unclear under what circumstances biologically relevant inflammation exists in the vascular compartment. This reality has led investigators to explore alternative methods of assessing the balance between pro- and anti-inflammatory mediators on a functional level. One of the means of assessing these complex interactions is to measure immune responsiveness of circulating immune effector cells.

CD11b as a Marker of PMN Activation

One important potential consequence of pro-inflammatory activity in the blood is the activation of circulating polymorphonuclear neutrophil leukocytes (PMN). Activated PMN can bind to already injured endothelial surface cells. They have increased oxidative burst activity and are limited in natural apoptosis, thus insuring that their inflammatory activity will be prolonged. In this regard, PMN have been implicated in the organ dysfunction of SIRS. We [6] and others [7] have shown that circulating PMN from patients with SIRS appear partially activated with a higher than normal display of CD11b, a β2-integrin adhesion molecule that is increased in density on the cell surface upon PMN activation. CD11b combines with CD18 to form the integrin adhesion molecule necessary for firm adhesion of PMN to activated endothelial cells. As shown in previous studies using both *in vivo* and *in vitro* models, the display of adhesion molecules on circulating PMN can be used to identify a potentially activated phenotype. With pro-inflammatory stimulation, PMN display increased CD11b and diminished L-selectin.

CD11b is a good marker of PMN activation because it is a functional molecule that is involved in many of the potent inflammatory mechanisms of the PMN. CD11b is up-regulated within minutes of exposure to pro-inflammatory substances such as tumor necrosis factor-alpha (TNF-α), interleukin-8 (IL-8), formyl-methionyl-leucyl-phenylalanine, C5a, leukotriene B4, and platelet activating factor (PAF). However, like other integrins, CD11b must not only increase in density on the cell to work, but it must undergo a qualitative change as well. When PMN activate, intracellular signals alter the conformation of CD11b to a new 3-dimensional structure that can bind its target receptors. Activated CD11b can be recognized by antibodies that bind to 'activation neoepitopes' present only on active CD11b. Specific antibodies can be made which bind only to this neoepitope allowing one to assess the degree to which CD11b expression reflects actual PMN activation. The antibody CBRM1/5, for example, recognizes a subset of CD11b molecules (10–50%) on activated PMN, but does not recognize any CD11b on cells in the resting state [8]. Binding of CBRM1/5 to CD11b blocks adhesion to counter-receptors. Only activated CD11b binds to the vascular endothelium via intracellular adhesion molecule-1 (ICAM-1) and to complement component iC3b, clotting factor X, fibrinogen and collagen type I. Furthermore, engagement of active CD11b with counter-receptors sends a signal into the cell markedly enhancing the respiratory burst [9]. Thus, the activation of CD11b plays a role in attachment to endothelium, phagocytosis of bacteria, enhancing the respiratory burst, bacterial killing, interaction with clotting components and migration of PMN within tissues. Many of the potent inflammatory functions of the PMN require the activation of CD11b, and active CD11b defines PMN engagement in inflammatory behavior.

The circulating PMN of patients with SIRS are constantly exposed to a complex mix of inflammatory mediators. They have a higher density of CD11b at rest than do PMN from normal controls. We hypothesized that these PMN are partially activated. The level of activation, however, cannot be assessed by merely measuring the PMN expression of CD11b or its activated epitope CBRM1/5, because these markers only denote what has happened, not what can subsequently occur in response to an immunological challenge. If these PMN from patients with SIRS have a greater potential for further activation of CD11b this would lead to greater PMN adhesiveness and a more vigorous respiratory burst. These events may increase endothelial and tissue injury. Thus, assessing the ability of these cells to increase further their expression of CD11b would characterize the relative balance between pro- and anti-inflammatory stimuli as they interact in a complex fashion with circulating PMN. If these partially activated PMN could be demonstrated to further activate their phenotype in response to pro-inflammatory stimuli, then this situation would provide a rationale for the use of anti-inflammatory therapies, including the use of monoclonal antibodies against CD11b in SIRS. However, if these PMN had a blunted activation response to pro-inflammatory stimuli, as compared to normal controls, then these data would demonstrate a relative immuno-suppression of circulating PMN, arguing more for immunostimulating therapies, if any form of immunomodulation were to be undertaken at all.

Accordingly, we measured the quantitative and qualitative changes in CD11b that occur during PMN activation *in vitro*. We stimulated freshly isolated whole blood PMN by adding increasing doses of TNF-α (from 0 to 200 U/mL) for 15 minutes prior to fixation for flow cytometry.

We selected 36 patients who fulfilled the SIRS criteria [10] and also had a known source of serious infection, including peritonitis, intra-abdominal or intra-thoracic abscess, pneumonia, upper urinary tract infection with obstruction and perforated abdominal viscus [23]. Thirty-one had positive cultures either at the site of suspected infection or in the blood. Twenty-one SIRS patients (58%) survived and 15 (42%) died of causes attributable to their SIRS. Twenty-three healthy volunteers served as controls. All subjects had leukocyte adhesion molecule studies performed by flow cytometry, as well as serum assays for TNF-α, IL-6, IL-8, IL-10, and soluble TNF-α receptors I and II.

The essence of our study was to describe both the *in vitro* expression of CD11b and its active form on circulating PMN and their subsequent immediate response to varying levels of TNF-α. Thus, we used the immediate *in vitro* expression of CD11b as a measure of the *in vivo* responsiveness or immune competence of our subjects. The goal of this assay is to document immune competence by the immediate response of circulating PMN to a pro-inflammatory stimulant in terms of their basal and subsequent response to TNF-α.

Conventional flow cytometry is not sensitive enough to detect cell surface markers of low density. Even fully activated PMN display only 10–50% of total CD11b with the CBRM1/5 epitope. Thus, high sensitivity flow cytometry [13] was used to assess CBRM1/5 (+) CD11b on PMN. Thus, the quantitative and qualitative changes of CD11b in our subjects associated with activation of PMN with TNF-α were assessed by reactivity with anti-CD11b and CBRM1/5, respectively. The resting surface density of leukocyte adhesion molecules was estimated by relative fluorescence index (RFI), obtained by subtracting the mean log fluorescence of the control cells (unstained) from the mean log fluorescence of the positive cells (stained with the monoclonal antibody of interest).

Not surprisingly, the patients with SIRS had elevated levels of pro-inflammatory cytokines IL-6, IL-8 and TNF-α compared to normal controls. However, as previously shown, there was no correlation between serum cytokine levels and either organ failure or outcome. Importantly, both patients with SIRS and control subjects had antagonists of inflammation in the blood. However, the levels of antagonists of inflammation were much higher in patients with SIRS. Soluble TNF-RII but not soluble TNF-RI correlated inversely to organ failure in the patients, while neither correlated with mortality or severity of illness scores. Similarly, the patients with SIRS had higher CD11b levels and lower L-selectin levels than controls.

The normal response of CD11b on PMN upon exposure to TNF-α appears to be a rapid up-regulation of the density of total CD11b, with a simultaneous increase of the density of CBRM1/5 staining. These changes indicate a conformational change in CD11b, which is associated with activation and receptor binding capability. We compared the RFI at increasing doses of TNF-α between patients and normal controls (Fig. 1). Although SIRS patients start out with a slightly higher average CD11b display, as PMN are exposed to TNF-α *in vitro*, the density of CD11b on healthy PMN challenged with TNF-α surpasses that on the patients' cells as the amount of TNF-α used is increased. The amount of CD11b displaying the activation epitope reactive with CBRM1/5 followed a similar pattern.

Although most patients with SIRS had diminished responsiveness of total CD11b and its conformational change as detected by CBRM1/5, a small number of very ill patients had preserved up-regulation of total CD11b but had virtually no conformational change as measured by the appearance of the CBRM1/5 epitope. No cytokine level measured in the blood correlated significantly with the diminished responsiveness of CD11b.

Since patients with SIRS have increased levels of soluble TNF-α receptors in the blood, these soluble receptors can bind endogenous or exogenous TNF-α and hence interfere with the TNF-α induced responses we measured in our assay. However, plasma concentrations of TNF-α receptors did not correlate with either the reactivity of total CD11b to TNF-α nor the switch to the active form. Thus, diminished TNF-α sensitivity was not due to soluble TNF-α receptors alone. It is

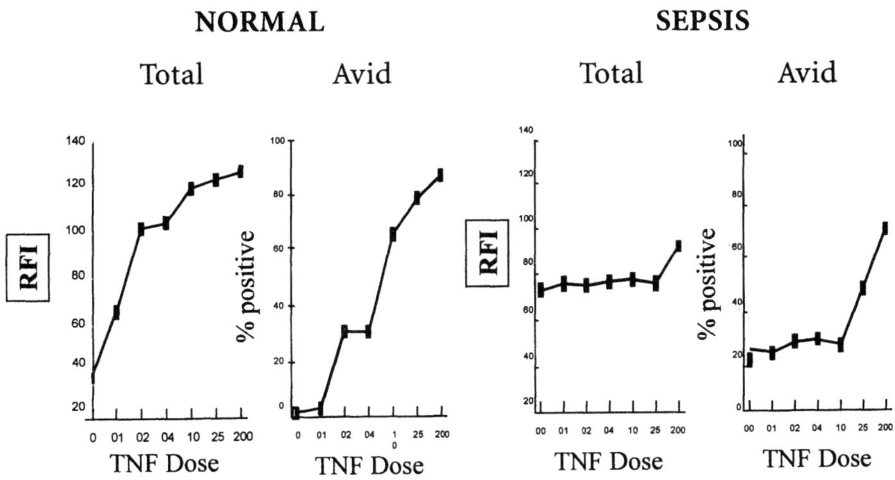

Fig. 1. Dose response of total CD11b density and CBRM1/5 generation on PMN to TNF-α *in vitro* in normal controls (n = 23) and patients with SIRS (n = 36)

also known that a variety of inflammatory stimuli down-regulate responsiveness to TNF-α by causing the shedding of its receptors from the cell surface. Such a loss of TNF-α receptors on circulating PMN would have the effect of decreasing their responsiveness to exogenous TNF-α exposure even if their intracellular processes were not affected by the initial SIRS process. However, there was no significant difference in the density of cellular TNF-α type I receptors between healthy controls and the patients with SIRS. If anything, the septic patients had a significantly higher density of TNF-α type II receptors than controls. Thus, diminished TNF-α sensitivity was not due to TNF-α receptor loss from PMN. Finally, PMN hypo-responsiveness could be due to an increased number of immature PMN in the circulation. Many patients with SIRS have an increased number of band forms. However, there was no correlation between the degree of PMN desensitization to TNF-α and the immature PMN (band) count.

The activation state of PMN exposed to this milieu is important since activated PMN can be auto-destructive. The inflammatory phenotype of circulating PMN from patients with SIRS appears to be partially activated. However, based on the above preliminary findings, the cells display a higher density than normal of the β2 integrin CD11b. However, the quantitative and qualitative changes associated with CD11b activation in response to increasing concentrations of TNF-α are depressed as compared to normal controls.

The suppression of CD11b responsiveness to TNF-α on PMN is most likely of multi-factorial etiology. The functional defect appears to be within the cells themselves, since there was no correlation with levels of soluble TNF receptors and no relationship to TNF receptor loss from the PMN. Also, CD11b dysfunction did not appear to be due to cell immaturity. There was no correlation with the number of circulating immature forms. Potentially, exhaustion of intracellular stores of CD11b [14] or senescence of PMN due to inhibition of apoptosis [15] could induce these phenomena. Whatever the causes of diminished CD11b responsiveness, this dysfunction appears to affect all circulating PMN.

The magnitude of CD11b unresponsiveness in the patients with SIRS that we studied correlated with the degree of organ failure. However, SIRS is a grossly non-specific criteria and up to two thirds of all hospitalized patients fulfill the SIRS criteria. This implies that diminished CD11b function is widespread in critically ill patients, and may be a non-specific effect of critical illness. In support of this hypothesis, a diminished quantitative CD11b up-regulation in response to mediators of inflammation has also been shown in burn patients [16]. In fact, these phenomena probably reflect the broader immune response referred to as inflammatory-stimuli-induced-anergy as proposed by Cavaillion.

Conclusion

Does immune responsiveness reflect process or outcome from acute illness? More than likely, outcome from SIRS is a complex endpoint. In our population, there was no relationship between the magnitude of CD11b dysfunction and mortality. We favor the hypothesis that immune suppression is the natural process of inflammation activation. The diminished immune responsiveness of circulating PMN in infected, critically ill patients probably reflects the natural down-regulation of the inflammatory response which initially induces a pro-inflammatory response, including migration of PMN to the site of inflammation, followed by a down-regulation of this response as repair occurs. This is an analogous process to thrombolysis following thrombus formation. Thus, immune suppression may be the method by which localized inflammation balances the risks of PMN over-stimulation and remote tissue injury versus under-stimulation and diminished clearance of infection. In support of this hypothesis, the relationship between CD11b function and both inflammation and infection are closely linked in a reciprocal fashion. Blockade of CD11b with monoclonal antibodies diminishes inflammatory injury in animal models [17]. The oxicam class of anti-inflammatory drugs antagonizes the appearance of the CBRM1/5 neoepitope and this is thought to be one of the mechanisms of action. Conversely, CD11b blockade [18] or congenital absence of CD11b [19] increases the severity of infection.

We did not measure the adhesiveness of PMN, but rather the up-regulation of CD11b density and the appearance of the 'activation epitope', CBRM1/5. Thus, the TNF-α titration assay cannot be equated to an analysis of *in vivo* adhesion, but rather to immune responsiveness. Antibodies that block this site antagonize PMN adhesion. However, some drugs block adhesion without diminishing CBRM1/5 display. For example, the anti-inflammatory leumedins block cytokine-mediated CD11b adhesion but the CBRM1/5 epitope still appears [21]. Thus, adhesiveness can be abrogated at other control points and patients with normal CBRM1/5 kinetics may still have impaired PMN adhesion. Nonetheless, the observation of widespread suppression ofthe CBRM1/5 epitope is strong evidence that cytokine-driven cell adhesion and CD11b signaling is diminished on circulating PMN in patients with SIRS.

References

1. Sands KE, Bates DW, Lanken PN, et al (1997) Epidemiology of sepsis syndrome in 8 academic medical centers. JAMA 278:234–240
2. Rangel-Frausto MS, Pittet D, Costigan M, Hwang T, Davis CS, Wenzel RP (1995) The natural history of the systemic inflammatory response syndrome (SIRS). A prospective study. JAMA 273:117–123
3. Goldie AS, Fearon KC, Ross JA, et al (1995) Natural cytokine antagonists and endogenous antiendotoxin core antibodies in sepsis syndrome. JAMA 274:172–177
4. Brandtzaeg P, Osnes L, Ovstebo R, Joo GB, Westvik AB, Kierulf P (1996) Net inflammatory capacity of human septic shock plasma evaluated by a monocyte-based target cell assay: identification of interleukin-10 as a major functional deactivator of human monocytes. J Exp Med 184:51–60
5. Dayer JM, Isler P, Nicod LP (1993) Adhesion molecules and cytokine production. Am Rev Respir Dis 148:S70–S74
6. Rosenbloom AJ, Pinsky MR, Bryant JL, Shin A, Tran T, Whiteside T (1995) Leukocyte activation in the peripheral blood of patients with cirrhosis of the liver and SIRS. Correlation with serum interleukin-6 levels and organ dysfunction. JAMA 274:58–65
7. Lin RY, Astiz ME, Saxon JC, Rackow EC (1993) Altered leukocyte immunophenotypes in septic shock. Studies of HLA-DR, CD11b, CD14, and IL-2R expression. Chest 104:847–853

8. Diamond MS, Springer TA (1993) A subpopulation of Mac-1 (CD11b/CD18) molecules mediates neutrophil adhesion to ICAM-1 and fibrinogen. J Cell Biol 120:545–556
9. Shappell SB, Toman C, Anderson DC, Taylor AA, Entman ML, Smith CW (1990) Mac-1 (CD11b/CD18) mediates adherence-dependent hydrogen peroxide production by human and canine neutrophils. J Immunol 144:2702–2711
10. Bone RC, Balk RA, Cerra FB, et al (1992) Definitions for sepsis and organ failure and guidelines for the use of innovative therapies in sepsis. The ACCP/SCCM Consensus Conference Committee. Chest 101:1644–1655
11. Knaus WA, Harrell FE, Fisher CJ, et al (1993) The clinical evaluation of new drugs for sepsis. A prospective study design based on survival analysis. JAMA 270:1233–1241
12. Goris RJ, Tee BT, Nuytinck JK, Gimbrere JS (1985) Multiple-organ failure. Generalized autodestructive inflammation? Arch Surg 120:1109–1115
13. Zola H, Flego L, Sheldon A (1992) Detection of cytokine receptors by high-sensitivity immunofluorescence/flow cytometry. Immunobiol 185:350–365
14. Singer II, Scott S, Kawka DW, Kazazis DM (1989) Adhesomes: specific granules containing receptors for laminin, C3bi/fibrinogen, fibronectin, and vitronectin in human polymorphonuclear leukocytes and monocytes. J Cell Biol 109:3169–3182
15. Colotta F, Re F, Polentarutti N, Sozzani S, Mantovani A (1992) Modulation of granulocyte survival and programmed cell death by cytokines and bacterial products. Blood 80:2012–2020
16. Rodeberg DA, Bass RC, Alexander JW, Warden GD, Babcock GF (1997) Neutrophils from burn patients are unable to increase the expression of CD11b/CD18 in response to inflammatory stimuli. J Leukocyte Biol 61:575–582
17. Mulligan MS, Vaporciyan AA, Warner RL, et al (1995) Compartmentalized roles for leukocytic adhesion molecules in lung inflammatory injury. J Immunol 154:1350–1363
18. Conlan JW, North RJ (1992) Monoclonal antibody NIMP-R10 directed against the CD11b chain of the type 3 complement receptor can substitute for monoclonal antibody 5C6 to exacerbate listeriosis by preventing the focusing of myelomonocytic cells at infectious foci in the liver. J Leukocyte Biol 52:130–132
19. Etzioni A (1994) Adhesion molecule deficiencies and their clinical significance. Cell Adhes Commun 2:257–260
20. Macey MG, Jiang XP, Veys P, McCarthy D, Newland AC (1992) Expression of functional antigens on neutrophils. Effects of preparation. J Immunol Methods 149:37–42
21. Endemann G, Feng Y, Bryant CM, et al (1996) Novel anti-inflammatory compounds prevent CD11b/CD18, alpha M beta 2 (Mac-1)-dependent neutrophil adhesion without blocking activation-induced changes in Mac-1. J Pharmacol Exp Ther 276:5–12
22. Overton WR (1988) Modified histogram subtraction technique for analysis of flow cytometry data. Cytometry 9:619–626
23. Rosenbloom AJ, Pinsky MR, Napolitano C, et al (1999) Suppression of cytokine mediated β2-integrin activation on circulating neutrophils in critically ill patients. J Leukoc Biol (in press)

Tumor Necrosis Factor Receptors in Systemic Inflammation

E. Lin, S. E. Calvano, and S. F. Lowry

Introduction

The systemic inflammatory response arising from severe injury or sepsis continues to pose a significant challenge in the management of critically ill patients. Clinical trials employing antagonists of pro-inflammatory mediators produced by activated immunocytes have, thus far, only shown modest efficacy in reducing the incidence of multiple organ failure (MOF) and mortality in these patients [1-3]. There is a recognized need for identifying endogenous markers that can serve as early predictors of outcome so that those patients who might benefit from novel, resource-intensive therapies can be identified. In addition, the expression of such biological markers may offer critical insights into the function of activated immunocytes responsible for inflammatory cytokine production.

Acute systemic inflammation, such as that induced by lipopolysaccharide (LPS) administration, causes the release of pro-inflammatory cytokines, of which tumor necrosis factor-α (TNF-α) is the first to appear in the circulation [2]. While TNF-α may be an essential element in host defense, it is clear that excessive production of TNF-α can precipitate detrimental systemic effects including circulatory shock and death. TNF-α exerts its biologic effects by binding to specific cellular receptors, TNFR1 (55 kD) and TNFR2 (75 kD) [3]. Optimal TNF-α activity only occurs with trimerized ligands interacting simultaneously with dimerized or trimerized receptors [4]. Although TNFR1 and TNFR2 share the same ligand, they possess multiple highly regulated intracellular signaling pathways that potentially influence the inflammatory response. Hence, characterization of the expression and function of transmembrane TNF receptors during systemic inflammation may enhance insight into the pleiotropic effects of TNF-α.

This chapter will first discuss what is known about TNF receptor function and signal transduction as they relate to inflammatory processes. Due to similarities in receptor structure and signaling pathways, the function of related TNF receptor family members during systemic inflammation will also be highlighted. The remainder of the discussion will then focus on clinically-derived data, beginning with immunocyte TNF receptor alterations exhibited during acute systemic inflammation and culminating in potential clinical implications stemming from such changes.

Tumor Necrosis Factor Receptors 1 and 2

TNFR1 and TNFR2 share a 28% extracellular sequence homology, a characteristic of several other TNF receptor-like cell surface proteins collectively referred to as the 'TNF receptor-superfamily' [5]. However, TNFR1 and TNFR2 possess dissimilar intracellular domains that suggest distinct signaling mechanisms. Under physiologic conditions, TNFR1 mediates most known biologic effects of soluble TNF-α (17 kDa), including inflammatory responses, nuclear factor-kappa B (NF-κB) activation, and apoptosis [6]. Activation of TNFR2 by soluble TNF-α promotes proliferation of T-cells, fibroblasts, and natural killer (NK) cells. Recent evidence has further demonstrated that TNFR2 function can be significantly enhanced if the ligand is membrane-associated TNF-α (26 to 29 kDa) [7]. In this regard, it is important to note that most *in vitro* studies of TNF-α-mediated toxicity refer to the soluble, 17 kDa, form.

Early data had suggested receptor cooperativity where TNFR2 transfers TNF-α to adjacent TNFR1 and thereby enhances TNFR1 function [8]. However, recent data have demonstrated that TNFR1 and TNFR2 functional cooperation is attributed to shared intracellular signaling molecules and pathways (ie., 'cross talk') [9, 10]. While it may be conceptually convenient to ascribe distinct roles for each of the TNF receptors, available data indicate compellingly that despite non-overlapping cytoplasmic domains, both TNFR1 and TNFR2 can exhibit signaling pathway overlap resulting in similar end-points, as well as divergent signaling pathways leading to disparate end-points [11–13]. The conditions that determine which signals predominate remain unclear.

TNF Receptor-Mediated Inflammation

Discerning the individual functions of TNFR1 and TNFR2 in acute injury and systemic inflammation has been an ongoing challenge. Much of the original information on TNF receptor signal transduction was derived from stable or tumor cell lines, rather than the primary immunocytes that mediate the systemic inflammatory response. Extensive *in vivo* autocrine and paracrine influences upon inflammatory cells further compound the complexity of TNF receptor biology.

Technical advances in the pre-clinical arena have afforded investigators the ability to systematically characterize the relative contributions of TNFR1 and TNFR2 in the inflammatory response. Such advances include the employment of receptor-specific monoclonal and polyclonal antibodies. More recently, the advent of murine transgenic and knockout models, and the availability of chimeric receptor constructs have provided invaluable models for systematic *in vivo* receptor function studies.

Blocking monoclonal antibodies against TNFR1, but not against TNFR2 can protect mice from TNF-α-mediated toxicity [12]. Mice genetically altered to lack TNFR1 exhibited a similar lack of responsiveness to TNF-α [13]. However, while mice lacking only TNFR2 exhibited a lethal response to TNF-α, this response was reduced when compared to wild-type mice [14]. In murine fibroblasts expressing only TNFR1, TNF-α is capable of inducing adhesion molecule expression, interleukin (IL)-6 and granulocyte/macrophage colony-stimulating factor (GM-CSF) release, cell proliferation, and NF-κB activation. In contrast, fibroblasts expressing only TNFR2 did not exhibit such responses to TNF-α activation [15]. Taken together, these data suggest that the bulk of the TNF-α inflammatory signaling is mediated by TNFR1, and that TNFR2 functions in an accessory role. Two additional observations have also been made in TNFR1-deficient mice [16]. First, while these mice exhibit an attenuated inflammatory response when sensitized with D-galactosamine followed by low-dose LPS challenge, they are normally sensitive to high-dose LPS administration. This further supports the concept that TNF-α release may not be solely responsible for the toxicity associated with Gram-negative endotoxemia. Second, TNFR1-deficient mice that do not respond to TNF-α challenge have increased susceptibility to infection with *Listeria monocytogenes* but maintain normal immune response against vaccinia or lymphocytic choriomeningitis virus infections. This may suggest a specific role for TNFR1-mediated signaling in eradicating selected bacterial pathogens. There is also evidence that both TNF receptors can independently mediate antiviral activity [17].

Studies in non-human primates also suggest a dominant role for TNFR1 in TNF-α-mediated toxicity. The administration of mutant TNF-α with exclusive TNFR1 binding-capacity precipitated circulatory shock reminiscent of severe sepsis [18]. However, the administration of mutant TNF-α binding exclusively to TNFR2 failed to induce any inflammatory responses or shock [19].

Another set of experiments used TNFR1 knockout, TNFR2 knockout, or double TNFR1 and TNFR2 knockout mice to characterize the response to localized pulmonary infections [20]. Compared to wild-type mice, *Micropolyspora faeni*-induced neutrophil accumulation within the lung was significantly reduced in TNFR1 knockout and double knockout mice, but was markedly enhanced in TNFR2 knockout mice. This appears to suggest a role for TNFR2 in attenuating pulmonary inflammation in response to *M. faeni* antigens. This dependence on TNF receptor expression also appears to be organism-specific because LPS administration into the lungs of all TNF receptor-deficient mouse strains resulted in no differences in leukocyte accumulation compared to wild-type mice.

In TNF receptor knockout mice, there also appears to be a difference in the magnitude of inflammatory response as measured by TNF-α release following high-dose LPS challenge. Mice lacking either TNFR1 or TNFR2 exhibited a 5-fold increase in serum TNF-α release over wild-type mice. Double knockout mice exhibited a 15- to 20-fold elevation in TNF-α [24].

Soluble TNF Receptors in Systemic Inflammation

Both human and non-human studies demonstrate that activation of immunocytes and other cell types is associated with rapid shedding of membrane-bound TNF receptors, resulting in soluble forms of TNFR1 and TNFR2 (sTNFR1 and sTNFR2). This shedding is facilitated by metalloproteinase-mediated cleavage of the extracellular domain of the transmembrane receptors into 30 kDa and 40 kDa components, respectively [21, 22]. Soluble TNF receptors shed during systemic inflammation are postulated to serve as endogenous inhibitors of TNF-α activity by two mechanisms [23, 24]. TNF-α can be sequestered by soluble TNF receptors, thereby attenuating further ligand activity [25]. Furthermore, the shedding of surface TNF receptors reduces the availability of functional receptors on the immunocyte surface, thereby down-modulating intracellular signaling [26].

Animal studies using type-2 TNFR: Fc demonstrated no reversal in lung injury or mortality from sepsis [27]. Human studies using the type-1 TNFR: Fc [28] and type-2 TNFR: Fc [29] demonstrated effective neutralization of circulating TNF-α but failed to improve outcome from severe sepsis.

Moreover, treatment with higher doses of type-2 TNFR: Fc was associated with a loss of anti-inflammatory activity in endotoxemia [30], and in one study, greater mortality in patients with septic shock. This may suggest greater *in vivo* affinity of TNFR1 for TNF-α, and that the type-2 TNFR: Fc paradoxically serves as a 'carrier' of TNF-α for later release [31, 32].

The evolving clinical evidence underscores the frustrations of selective neutralization of inflammatory mediators in the management of sepsis despite demonstrable efficacy in several less severe inflammatory conditions [33].

TNFR-Mediated Signal Transduction

Apoptosis and Inflammation

Members of the TNF receptor-superfamily (more than 20) regulate cell proliferation or cell death (apoptosis) through highly regulated signaling mechanisms [34, 35].

Apoptosis is the principal mechanism by which senescent or dysfunctional cells, including macrophages and polymorphonuclear cells (neutrophils, PMNs), are systematically eliminated [36]. The inflammatory milieu is recognized to alter the normal apoptotic machinery, delaying the disposal of activated macrophages and PMNs [37–40]. The prolonged survival of these inflammatory immunocytes is hypothesized to perpetuate the inflammatory response, and thereby participate in the evolution of MOF. Therefore, key signaling mechanisms that govern programmed cell death may serve as potential sites for regulating the life span of inflammatory cells during systemic inflammation [38].

CD95 Pathway

Several members of the TNF receptor-superfamily (e.g., CD95/Fas, TNFR1, death receptor (DR) 3/TNF receptor-related apoptosis-mediated protein [TRAMP], DR4/TNF-related apoptosis-inducing ligand [TRAIL]R-1, DR5/TRAILR-2, DR6, p75-nerve growth factor receptor [NGFR]) exhibit similar intracellular sequence motifs referred to as the 'death domain' [39]. Of these receptors, CD95 and TNFR1 intracellular signaling have been most extensively investigated. Similar to TNF-α,

CD95-ligand (CD95L) also trimerizes in order to activate a trimerized receptor aggregate [40]. The fact that a significant component of the TNFR1 signaling pathway is common with CD95 signaling, makes it necessary to highlight the functional dynamics of both receptor types when discussing TNF receptor response in acute systemic inflammation.

The only known function for CD95 is to induce apoptosis. Upon CD95 activation, an adapter protein, FADD (Fas-associated death domain), is recruited to the receptor death domain region (Fig. 1]. FADD also contains an N-terminus region known as the 'death effector domain' (DED) that associates with and activates caspase-8 (also referred to as FLICE, for Fas-like interleukin-1β converting enzyme) [41]. The simultaneous clustering of the CD95 death domain, FADD, and FLICE is commonly referred to as the death-inducing signaling complex (DISC) and is an obligatory process in CD95 signal transduction [42]. Caspase-8 possesses pro-apoptotic enzymatic activity which further activates other downstream caspases [43].

The caspase cascade mediates intracellular apoptotic pathways. Recent experiments have demonstrated that CD95-mediated caspase cascade activation can progress by two pathways: A mitochondria-independent pathway associated with caspase-8 recruitment at the DISC, or a mitochondria-dependent pathway associated with reduced caspase-8 activation [44, 45]. While these two pathways are not mutually exclusive, progression via the mitochondria-independent pathway

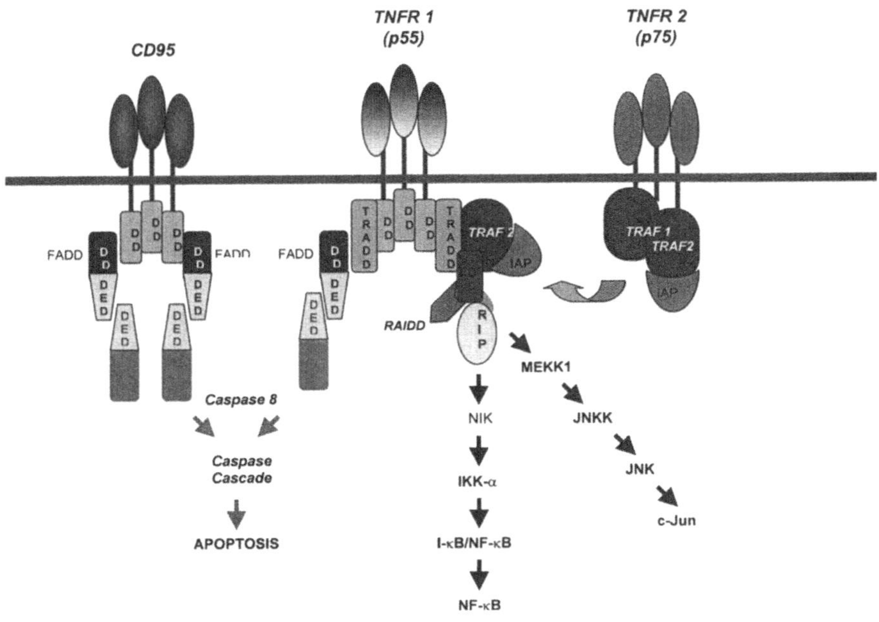

Fig. 1. Signaling pathway for CD95, TNFR1 (p55) and TNFR2 (p75). (Adapted from [7] with permission)

occurs more rapidly (minutes), as determined by cleavage of a terminal caspase (caspase-3), than the dependent pathway (hours). It is presently unclear whether CD95-mediated apoptosis in immune cells such as macrophages and PMNs is mitochondria-dependent, independent or neither.

Distal caspase activation, with mitochondrial membrane disruption usually indicates a critical point of 'no-return' in the apoptotic pathway. An important link between caspase activation and endonuclease activity leading to desoxyribonucleic acid (DNA) fragmentation, a hallmark of programmed cell death, has been identified [46, 47]. Downstream activation of caspase-3 cleaves the inhibiting component of ICAD (inhibitor of caspase-activated DNAse), facilitating internucleosomal DNA degradation. Terminal caspases functioning in the manner of caspase-3 are loosely dubbed 'executioners', as opposed to middle-level caspases that are often dubbed 'effectors' [48].

CD95-mediated apoptosis can be inhibited by a host of proteins (e.g., FLICE inhibitory protein [FLIP], E1B 19K) that interferes directly and indirectly with DISC formation [49, 50]. It should also be noted that in certain tumor cell lines, an alternative CD95 pathway is present where the intracellular adapter protein Daxx induces apoptosis by associating with the death domain portion of CD95 and, in turn triggering ASK1 (apoptosis signal-regulating kinase 1) activation [51].

TNFR1 Pathway

TNFR1 activation may direct several responses that are either pro-inflammatory or anti-inflammatory. TNFR1 mediates most of the pro-inflammatory effects of TNF-α and it has been demonstrated that the early activation of c-Jun N-terminal kinase (JNK) and p38 kinase prevents TNFR1-mediated apoptosis [52].

Analogous to signaling through CD95, TNFR1 activation recruits the adapter molecule, TRADD (TNF receptor-associated death domain) to the receptor death domain. Recently, it has been proposed that SODD (silencer of death domains), constitutively found on the death domain of TNFR1, serves as a mechanism that prevents spontaneous signaling of the receptor during rest [53]. TNFR1 can recruit TRADD and TNF receptor-associated factor 2 (TRAF2) only when SODD is released from the death domains.

Unlike FADD, TRADD lacks a DED. However, TRADD can recruit FADD via interaction between their respective death domains. Hence, TNFR1 can mediate apoptosis upon receptor ligation through the CD95 pathway [54]. Alternatively, TNFR1 can mediate apoptosis through the recruitment of RIP (receptor interacting protein) to TRADD. RIP has a death domain component that interacts with TRADD and may share part of the CD95 apoptotic pathway [55]. However, more recent evidence suggests that RIP directly activates the caspase cascade through an adapter molecule called CRADD (caspase and RIP adapter with death domain or RAIDD) that recruits caspase-2 to the TNFR1 complex [56]. RAIDD-to-caspase or caspase-to-caspase interaction occurs specifically at sequences referred to as CARDs (caspase recruitment domains) [57]. RIP also carries a kinase component that, when activated by TRAF2, leads to NF-κB and JNK activation [58]. At least six known TRAF proteins interact with the death domains of various TNF receptor-superfamily members [59].

TRAF2 interaction with RIP promotes activation of NIK (NF-κB-inducing kinase), which precipitates a sequence of enzymatic events culminating in NF-κB activation [60]. TRAF2 activation of RIP also induces an enzymatic cascade that leads to activation of MEKK1 (mitogen-activated protein/ERK kinase kinase-1), a proximal mediator of the JNK pathway [61]. The activation of NF-κB and JNK is believed to be the major anti-apoptotic, and therefore pro-inflammatory, signal induced by TNFR1 and TNFR2 [62, 63]. It is well-known that TNF-α-induced NF-κB-activation delays cell death [64–66], and is associated with the activation of diverse genes that include pro-inflammatory mediators. Inhibiting NF-κB activation in endothelial cells has been shown to reduce the expression of E-selectins, P-selectins, tissue factor and IL-8 [65]. Exaggerated peripheral blood monocyte NF-κB activation has been associated with mortality in septic shock [66].

Overexpression of endogenous regulators that interact with TRAF2 (I-TRAF) potently inhibited TRAF2-mediated NF-κB activation initiated by TNFR1, TNFR2 and CD40 [67].

Finally, the duality of TNFR1 as a pro-apoptotic mediator and as an anti-apoptotic receptor has been demonstrated in cells transfected with dominant negative-FADD (FADD-DN). FADD-DN expressing cells inhibited both TNFR1- and Fas-mediated apoptosis, but did not alter NF-κB or JNK activity [68].

TNFR1 and CD95 appear to activate the sphingomyelin pathway as a second messenger mediating cell death through the activation of stress-activated protein kinase (SAPK)/JNK cascade to apoptosis [69, 70]. While ceramide induces apoptosis in acute inflammation [71], the involved pathways appear to be independent of TNFR1 and CD95 signal transduction [72, 73].

In summary, the regulation of TNFR1-mediated apoptosis or cell survival occurs early following TNF-α induction, and is dependent on whether TRADD interacts with FADD or with TRAF2 [61]. Almost immediately downstream of TRADD is an apparent signaling trifurcation where RIP-TRAF2 activates NF-κB via the NIK pathway, where RIP-TRAF2 also activates MEKK1 in the JNK pathway, and where RIP facilitates apoptosis through recruitment of caspases [74]. The precise extracellular factors that determine which pathways prevail are uncertain.

TNFR2 Pathway

Unlike TNFR1, information on TNFR2-signaling during systemic inflammation is comparatively scarce. TNFR2 does not have a death domain, and hence, is not known to induce TRADD signaling pathways [14]. TNFR2 is capable of recruiting a heterocomplex of TRAF2/TRAF1, which in turn, mediates the recruitment of mammalian cellular inhibitors of apoptosis proteins (c-IAP1 and c-IAP2) to the TNFR2 signaling complex [75]. Several investigators have now identified IAPs in human cells (h-IAP1, h-IAP2, x-IAP, NAIP) [76]. IAP can be shuttled to TRADD on TNFR1 via its interaction with TRAF2, which then promotes NF-κB activation [Fig. 1]. TRAF2 activation of NF-κB can be inhibited by the endogenous intracellular regulator TRIP (TRAF-interacting protein) [77].

Although TRAF2 promotes NF-κB activation and cell survival, the simultaneous stimulation of TNFR1 and TNFR2 in a cell may down-modulate TRAF2 activity, and thereby promote apoptosis [78]. This effect, seen in HeLa cell lines, occurs independently of the CD95-FADD pathway, and suggests that TNFR1-mediated cytotoxicity can be enhanced through TNFR2-mediated degradation of TRAF2 and TRAF2-induced antiapoptotic proteins.

Additional Considerations in TNF Receptor Signal Transduction

Death Receptor 3

DR3 (TRAMP) is similar in structure and function to TNFR1, and is capable of recruiting TRADD, RIP, FADD and activating the caspase cascade [79]. DR3 is activated by the Apo3-ligand (Apo3L or TWEAK), which is structurally similar to TNF-α. However, there is no evidence that Apo3L and TNF-α have cross-reactivity. Unlike TNFR1, which is expressed on most cell surfaces, DR3 is mostly present on cells of lymphoid origin and on activated T cells [80]. Therefore, Apo3L-DR3 interaction in activated monocytes and neutrophils is presently unclear.

DR4, DR5, Decoy Receptor 1, DcR2

This group of receptors are hypothesized to be cell mechanisms for evading immune surveillance. The ligand for these receptors is TRAIL or Apo2L, which closely resembles the CD95L [81]. DR4 (TRAILR-1) and DR5 (TRAILR-2) both possess a death domain. However, they are only able to induce apoptosis when overexpressed on cell surfaces. Furthermore, it is unclear whether their apoptotic machinery involves that of CD95 or TNFR1.

The decoy receptors DcR1 (TRAILR-3), DcR2 (TRAILR-4) express similar extracellular domains to DR4 and DR5, but lack functional cytoplasmic domains [82, 83]. They appear to compete with DR4 and DR5 for TRAIL, but are unable to induce a post-receptor response.

Bcl-2 Family and Mitochondria

The oncogene product Bcl-2 and its homologs are found on the outer mitochondrial membrane, and exert an important regulatory role in TNFR1 mediated apoptosis (Table 1). A central event in Bcl-2 regulation of cell survival is its ability to heterodimerize with its family members [84]. The Bcl-2 family members include both pro-apoptotic and anti-apoptotic homologs, and their relative concentrations may determine the fate of the cell [85].

Table 1. The known Bcl-2 homolog family (unless indicated, these homologs are mammalian)

Sub-family	Name	
Bcl-2	Bcl-2	
(Anti-apoptotic)	Bcl-X_L	
	Bcl-w	
	mcl-1	
	A1/Bfl-1	
	NR-13	(chicken)
	BHRF1	(viral)
	LMW5-HL	(viral)
	ORF16	(viral)
	KS-Bcl-2	(viral)
	E1B 19K	(viral)
	CED-9	(nematode)
Bax	Bax	
(Pro-apoptotic)	Bak	
	Bok	
BH3	Bik	
(Pro-apoptotic)	Blk	
	Hrk	
	BNIP3	
	Bim_L	
	Bad	
	Bid	
	EGL-1 (nematode)	

Disruption of the highly selective mitochondrial membrane and its energy gradient known as the transmembrane potential ($\Delta\Psi m$) is another hallmark of apoptosis. The disrupted mitochondrial membrane subsequently loses its inner membrane selectivity, permitting free passage of ions and molecules across the membrane in a process referred to as permeability transition [86]. Bcl-2 and its antiapoptotic homologs appear to have a significant role in preventing apoptosis by stabilizing the transmembrane potential, inhibiting permeability transition, and blocking the release of apoptosis-inducing factor and cytochrome-C. It has been suggested, based on three-dimensional analysis, that the Bcl-2 homologs stabilize or destabilize mitochondrial membranes by forming porous channels. Conformational changes of these proteins will permit the influx or efflux of ions [87].

There is increasing evidence demonstrating the roles of human Bcl-2 homologs in regulating human immunocyte survival in systemic inflammation. The expression of Bfl-1, the human homolog of the proapoptotic murine A1, is directly dependent upon NF-κB activity and capable of suppressing TNF-α-induced apoptosis [88]. Bfl-1 messenger ribonucleic acid (mRNA) is inducible in neutrophils stimulated with agonists such as G-CSF, GM-CSF, and LPS [89]. Inflammatory cytokines can also enhance neutrophil Mcl-1 expression, another antiapoptotic Bcl-2 homolog, suggesting one mechanism by which inflammatory states prolong neutrophil survival [90]. Monocytes activated by inflammatory stimuli such as TNF-α can also have prolonged survival as a result of up-regulated Bfl-1 gene expression [91].

TNF Receptors In Human Systemic Inflammation

Systemic inflammation is associated with diverse biological alterations in the host that may influence the clinical course. The alterations in human immune cell TNF-α receptor expression, as several have observed during systemic inflammation, is one such response. As the receptor for one of the earliest and most potent inflammatory mediators, alterations in TNF receptor expression may not be merely a manifestation of host injury but a marker of important functional changes.

Soluble TNF Receptor

Soluble TNFR is released into the circulation early following injury or sepsis. In trauma patients, both sTNFR1 and sTNFR2 were elevated within 1 hour of injury and the elevations lasted more than 7 days. sTNFR2 release was significantly higher than sTNFR1, and levels of both receptors were higher in non-survivors [92]. TNF receptor shedding has also been observed in critically ill patients and in experimental endotoxemia. Among critically ill patients, non-survivors also released higher levels of soluble TNF receptor than survivors [93]. It was further demonstrated using *in vitro* cytotoxicity assays that the release of physiologic levels of soluble TNF receptor was sufficient to attenuate endogenous TNF-α activity during endotoxemia, but was insufficient for neutralizing TNF-α toxicity in severe sepsis [94]. In experimental human endotoxemia models, the administration of low dose (6 mg/m^2) soluble recombinant human dimeric type-2 TNFR:Fc attenuated the febrile response, completely neutralized fibrinolysis activation and endothelial activation, and partially neutralized neutrophil responses [95]. There was no attenuation in LPS-induced activation of coagulation, phospholipase A_2 or LPS binding protein (LBP) release. Lower doses of TNFR:Fc administered during experimental endotoxemia were paradoxically more effective than higher doses in abrogating the pro-inflammatory response [34].

Surface TNF Receptors

Cell surface TNF receptors on monocytes and neutrophils also exhibit changes during systemic inflammation. In experimental endotoxemia, TNFR1 and TNFR2 expression on both circulating monocytes and granulocytes is significantly down-regulated 2 hours following LPS administration, in association with a transient decrease in TNF-α binding capacity. The down-regulation was more pronounced in monocytes ($>90\%$ reduction), with receptor recovery by 6 hours [96]. However, 24 hours following LPS administration, monocyte-TNF receptor expression was increased and only returned to baseline expression after 48 hours (Fig. 2). Receptor recovery in granulocytes appeared to progress over a longer course. It was also apparent that higher doses of LPS led to greater changes in surface receptor expression and soluble receptor release.

Monocyte-TNF receptor down-regulation following LPS administration was attenuated by the infusion of recombinant dimeric TNFR:Fc construct [97]. Importantly, using mutant TNF-α with specifity for only TNFR1 or only TNFR2, it was demonstrated *ex vivo* that TNFR1 activation was responsible for the down-regulation of both types of receptors, and TNFR2 activation did not affect the expression of either receptor.

Cell surface TNF receptors are down-regulated in response to most inflammatory stimuli. LPS induces sTNFR2 release from monocytes, but not the release of sTNFR1 [98]. This particular response was abrogated with antibodies that block CD14, as well as with bactericidal/permeability-increasing (BPI) protein, but the addition of LBP enhanced sTNFR2 release. *In vitro*, the expression of monocyte surface TNF receptors was reduced in a dose-dependent fashion in response to high doses of LPS, an effect that was blunted by BPI.

In vivo administration of a conjugated polymyxin, an agent which binds and neutralizes the lipid A moiety of LPS, effectively inhibited clinical symptoms in experimental human endotoxemia. Furthermore, LPS neutralization by the conjugated polymyxin markedly attenuated the typical LPS-induced down-regulation in monocyte TNF receptor expression [99] (Fig. 3].

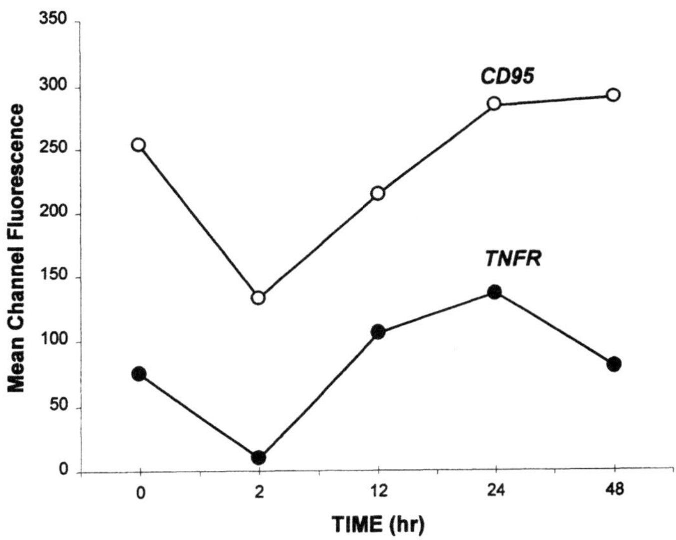

Fig. 2. Average monocyte surface CD95 and TNF receptor (TNFR) expression following 2 ng/kg intravenous bolus of endotoxin given at 0 hours. Receptor density measured sequentially by fluorochrome-ligand staining of the receptors. (Adapted from [4] with permission)

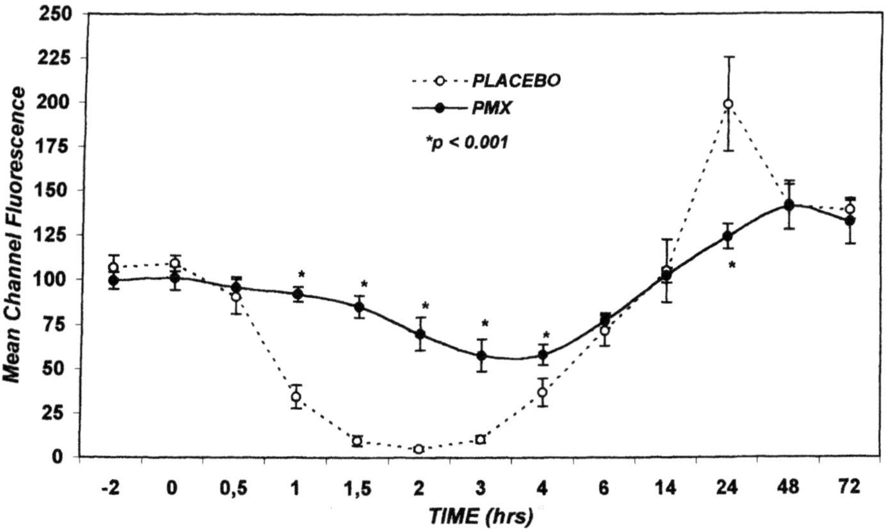

Fig. 3. Monocyte TNF receptor expression following intravenous administration of 2 ng/kg of endotoxin, given at 0 hours. 5 subjects were also treated with a conjugated polymyxin (PMX, filled circles) beginning at −2 hours. 5 subjects received no polymyxin (placebo, open circles). Note the supranormal recovery at 24 hours in the placebo group. (Adapted from [108] with permission)

Another series of experiments using U-937 cells demonstrated that the down-regulation of surface TNF receptors is mediated through TNFR1 activation [100]. Activation of TNFR2 only, and TNF-α stimulation of cell lines that only express TNFR2 did not induce receptor down-regulation. Moreover, TNFR1 down-regulation was the result of internalization as demonstrated by receptor labeling with ^{125}I-TNF-α. The experimental and clinical data collectively suggest that monocyte TNF receptor expression is altered during inflammation, and that the alterations are the combined results of specific receptor shedding and internalization.

Monocyte receptor expression is down-regulated in severely septic patients [101]. Survivors of sepsis had monocyte receptor levels equal to those of normal healthy subjects at the onset of illness. Non-survivors, in contrast, had significantly lower receptor expression at the onset, and expression remained unchanged throughout the course of illness (Fig. 4). Multivariate analysis suggests that the degree of monocyte-TNF receptor expression on the first day of sepsis may be predictive of subsequent outcome [102].

CD95 Response

Alterations in CD95 expression on monocytes and neutrophils during experimental endotoxemia reflect those of monocyte and neutrophil TNF receptors, although the magnitude of the changes is smaller [103]. Following LPS administra-

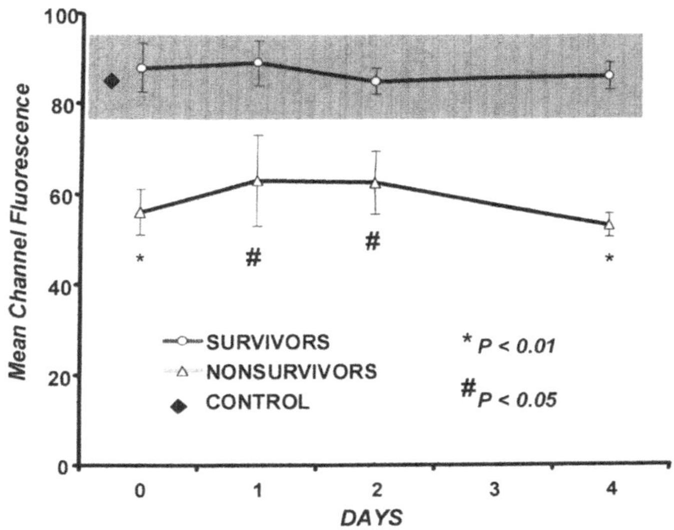

Fig. 4. Monocyte TNF receptor expression in healthy subjects, and in surviving and non-surviving sepsis patients on Days 0 to 4. Gray box encompasses range of monocyte TNF receptor expression in surviving patients and healthy subjects. (Adapted from [110] with permission)

tion, an acute reduction in receptor expression is observed at two hours, followed by recovery over 48 hours. This receptor down-regulation is probably the result of combined internalization and shedding [104]. In certain cell types, CD95 can be stored intracellularly and transported to the cell surface upon stimulation [105]. Preliminary reports have also documented elevated soluble Fas release in critically ill pediatric sepsis patients [106].

Hormonal Regulation

In addition to changes in the response to inflammatory mediators, TNF receptor expression on monocytes is also subject to external hormonal influences. Catecholamines up-regulate total monocyte-TNF receptor expression following LPS stimulation through a β_2- and adenylate cyclase-dependent mechanism [107]. Similar results have been reported from *in vivo* human studies where short-term (3 hours) epinephrine infusion attenuated the down-regulation of monocyte-TNF receptors following LPS administration [108]. However, longer periods of epinephrine infusion (24 hours) failed to attenuate LPS-induced receptor down-regulation, perhaps due to tachyphylaxis to catecholamines. Continuous epinephrine administration, without LPS, did not alter monocyte-TNF receptor expression. The effects of endogenous or exogenous hormones on TNF receptor or CD95 expression remain to be fully elucidated.

Programmed Cell Death

It is hypothesized that changes in TNF receptor and CD95 expression on inflammatory immune cells will impact the apoptotic machinery via the TNF receptor pathway. Indeed, there is strong evidence that the inflammatory environment following injury or in sepsis delays normal immune cell apoptosis [109, 110]. The ability to regulate activated immune cells is therefore important for the resolution of local and systemic inflammation.

While not all apoptotic mechanisms involve the TNF receptor pathways, these pathways are important in many human cell types involved in the inflammatory response. For example, human neutrophils co-express both CD95 and CD95L and normally undergo autocrine-induced cell death. This pathway can be modulated by a vast array of mediators [111, 112]. Furthermore, optimum induction of neutrophil apoptosis appears to require activation of both TNF receptors [113]. Mutant TNF-α with specificity for only TNFR1 is capable of inducing apoptosis, but with significant decrease in potency compared to wild type TNF-α. Mutant TNF-α with specificity for only TNFR2 was unable to induce apoptosis. Therefore, reduction in monocyte or neutrophil TNF receptor expression following LPS challenge or in sepsis (e.g., internalized TNFR1 and shed TNFR2) can potentially delay the deletion of these activated cells, thereby prolonging their contribution to the inflammatory process.

Finally a distinction must be made between parenchymal (tissue) apoptosis and leukocyte apoptosis. During systemic inflammation, parenchymal cell apoptosis is increased [114], as is the case in hepatic failure. It is hypothesized that tissue injury is directly induced by activated immunocytes or their inflammatory mediators, and timely termination of these inflammatory cells can attenuate further organ injury.

Conclusion

Acute systemic inflammation observed in critically ill patients is associated with diverse alterations in the immune response. Specific alterations in the expression of immunocyte-associated and soluble TNF-α receptors have been documented experimentally and clinically. Furthermore, similar alterations have been observed in other members of the TNF receptor-superfamily. These receptor alterations may serve as biomarkers of systemic inflammation and potentially predict subsequent outcome.

Alterations in receptor expression, such as in TNF receptor and CD95, during systemic inflammation, also have important functional implications. Although mechanistically complex, the intracellular signals emanating from these receptors are critical determinants of the response of activated immunocytes following host injury. While inflammation is necessary to restore the injured host to homeostasis, prolonged inflammatory activity by immunocytes can perpetuate tissue and vital organ injury. Hence, the ability to regulate signals emanating from these receptors can potentially modulate the immune response during systemic inflammation.

Acknowledgment. This work was supported in part by National Institutes of Health Grant GM34695. Dr. Lin is also supported by a Surgical Infection Society Fellowship Award

References

1. Baue AE (1997) Multiple organ failure, multiple organ dysfunction syndrome, and systemic inflammatory response syndrome. Why no magic bullets? Arch Surg 132:703–707
2. Lin E, Lowry SF (1999) The human response to endotoxin. Sepsis (in press)
3. Tartaglia LA, Goeddel DV (1992) Two TNF receptors. Immunol Today 13:151–153.
4. Van der Poll T, Lowry SF (1995) Tumor necrosis factor in sepsis: Mediator of multiple organ failure or essential part of host defense? Shock 3:1–12
5. Lin E, Calvano SE, Lowry SF (1997) The biologic control of systemic inflammatory response. Curr Opin Crit Care 3:299–307
6. Hsu H, Xiong J Goeddel DV (1995) The TNF receptor 1-associated protein TRADD signals cell death and NF-kappa B activation. Cell 81:495–504
7. Grell M, Douni E, Wajant H, et al (1995) The transmembrane form of tumor necrosis factor is the prime activating ligand of the 80 kDa tumor necrosis factor receptor. Cell 83:793–802
8. Tartaglia LA, Pennica D, Goeddel DV (1993) Ligand passing: the 75-kDa tumor necrosis factor (TNF) receptor recruits TNF for signaling by the 55-kDa TNF receptor. J Biol Chem 268:18542–18548
9. Vandenabeele P, Declercq W, Vanhaesbroeck B, Grooten J, Fiers W (1995) Both TNF receptors are required for TNF-mediated induction of apoptosis in PC60 cells. J Immunol 154: 2904–2913
10. Weiss T, Grell B, Hessabi S, et al (1997) Enhancement of TNF receptor p60-mediated cytotoxicity by TNF receptor p80. J Immunol 158:2398–2404
11. Bazzoni F, Beutler B (1996) The tumor necrosis factor ligand and receptor families. N Engl J Med 334:1717–1725
12. Sheehan KC, Pinckard JK, Arthur CD, Dehner LP, Goeddel DV, Schreiber RD (1995) Monoclonal antibodies specific for murine p55 and p75 tumor necrosis factor receptors: Identification of a novel in vivo role for p75. J Exp Med 181:607–617
13. Rothe J, Lesslauer W, Lotscher H, et al (1993) Mice lacking the tumour necrosis factor receptor 1 are resistant to TNF-mediated toxicity but highly susceptible to infection by Listeria monocytogenes. Nature 364:798–802
14. Erickson SL, de Sauvage FJ, Kikly K, et al (1994) Decreased sensitivity to tumour-necrosis factor but normal T-cell development in TNF receptor-2-deficient mice. Nature 372: 560–563
15. Mackay F, Rothe J, Bluethmann H, Loetscher H, Lesslauer W (1994) Differential responses of fibroblasts from wild-type and TNF-R55-deficient mice to mouse and human TNF-alpha activation. J Immunol 153:5274–5284
16. Rothe J, Mackay F, Bluethmann H, Zinkernagel R, Lesslauer W (1994) Phenotypic analysis of TNFR1-deficient mice and characterization of TNFR1-deficient fibroblasts in vitro. Circ Shock 44:51–56
17. Ruby J, Bluethmann H, Peschon JJ (1997) Antiviral activity of tumor necrosis factor (TNF) is mediated via p55 and p75 TNF receptors. J Exp Med 186:1591–1596
18. Van Zee KJ, Stackpole SA, Montegut WJ, et al (1994) A human tumor necrosis factor (TNF) α mutant that binds exclusively to the p55 TNF receptor produces toxicity in the baboon. J Exp Med 179:1185–1191
19. Welborn MB, Van Zee K, Edwards PD, et al (1996) A human tumor necrosis factor p75 receptor agonist stimulates in vitro T cell proliferation but does not produce inflammation or shock in the baboon. J Exp Med 184:165–171
20. Peschon JJ, Torrance DS, Stocking KL, et al (1998) TNF receptor-deficient mice reveal divergent roles for p55 and p75 in several models of inflammation. J Immunol 160:943–952
21. Aderka D, Engelmann H, Maor Y, Brakebusch C, Wallach D (1992) Stabilization of the bioactivity of tumor necrosis factor by its soluble receptors. J Exp Med 175:323–329

22. Bemelmans MHA, Gouma DJ, Buurman WA (1993) LPS-induced sTNF-receptor release in vivo in a murine model: Investigation of the role of TNF, IL-1, leukemia inhibiting factor, and IFN-γ. J Immunol 151:5554–5562
23. Van der Poll T, Jansen J, van Leenen D, et al (1993) Release of soluble receptors for tumor necrosis factor in clinical sepsis and experimental endotoxemia. J Infect Dis 168:955–960
24. Rogy MA, Coyle SM, Oldenburg HSA, et al (1994) Persistently elevated soluble tumor necrosis factor receptor and interleukin-1 receptor antagonist levels in critically ill patients. J Am Coll Surg 178:132–138
25. Van Zee KJ, Kohno T, Fischer E, Rock SC, Moldawer LL, Lowry SF (1992) Tumor necrosis factor soluble receptors circulate during experimental and clinical inflammation and can protect against excessive tumor necrosis factor-α in vitro and in vivo. Proc Natl Acad Sci USA 89:4845–4849
26. Leeuwenberg JFM, Jeunhomme TMAA, Buurman WA (1994) Slow release of soluble TNF receptors by monocytes in vitro. J Immunol 152:4036–4040
27. Lechner AJ, Johanns CA, Matuschak GM (1997) A recombinant tumor necrosis factor-α p80 receptor: Fc fusion protein decreases circulating bioactive tumor necrosis factor-α but not lung injury or mortality during immunosuppression-related gram-negative bacteremia. J Crit Care 12:28–38
28. Abraham E, Glauser MP, Butler T, et al (1997) p55 tumor necrosis factor receptor fusion protein in the treatment of patients with severe sepsis and septic shock. A randomized controlled multicenter trial. JAMA 277:1531–1538
29. Fisher CJ, Agosti JM, Opal SM, et al (1996) Treatment of septic shock with the tumor necrosis factor receptor: Fc fusion protein. N Engl J Med 334:1697–1702
30. Suffredini AF, Reda D, Banks SM, Tropea M, Agosti JM, Miller R (1995) Effects of recombinant dimeric TNF receptor on human inflammatory responses following intravenous endotoxin administration. J Immunol 155:5038–5045
31. Mohler KM, Torrance DS, Smith CA, et al (1993) Soluble tumor necrosis factor (TNF) receptors are effective therapeutic agents in lethal endotoxemia and function simultaneously as both TNF carriers and TNF antagonists. J Immunol 151:1548–1561
32. Evans TJ, Moyes D, Carpenter A, et al (1994) Protective effect of 55- but not 75-kDa soluble tumor necrosis factor receptor-immunoglobulin G fusion proteins in an animal model of gram-negative sepsis. J Exp Med 180:2173–2179
33. Grau GE, Maennel DN (1997) TNF inhibition and sepsis—sounding a cautionary note. Nature Med 3:1193–1195
34. Ware CF, van Arsdale S, van Arsdale TL (1996) Apoptosis mediated by the TNF-related cytokine and receptor families. J Cell Biochem 60:47–55
35. Baker SJ, Reddy EP (1998) Modulation of life and death by the TNF receptor superfamily. Oncogene 17:3261–3270
36. Squier MKT, Sehnert AJ, Cohen J (1995) Apoptosis in leukocytes. J Leukocyte Biol 57:2–10
37. Mangan DF, Wahl SM (1991) Differential regulation of human monocyte programmed cell death (apoptosis) by chemotactic factors and proinflammatory cytokines. J Immunol 147: 3408–3412
38. Marshall JC, Watson RWG (1997) Apoptosis in the resolution of systemic inflammation. In: Vincent JL (ed) Yearbook of Intensive Care and Emergency Medicine. Springer-Verlag, Berlin, pp 100–108
39. Tartaglia LA, Ayres TM, Wong GH, Goeddel DV (1993) A novel domain within the 55 kd TNF receptor signals cell death. Cell 74:845–853
40. Huang B, Eberstadt M, Olejniczak ET, Meadows RP, Fesik SW (1996) NMR structure and mutagenesis of the Fas (APO-1/CD95) death domain. Nature 384:638–641
41. Medema JP, Scaffidi C, Kischkel FC, et al (1997) FLICE is activated by association with the CD95 death-inducing signaling complex (DISC). EMBO J 16:2794–2804
42. Kischkel FC, Hellbardt S, Behrmann I, et al (1995) Cytotoxicity-dependent APO-1 (Fas/CD95)-associated proteins form a death-inducing signaling complex (DISC) with the receptor. EMBO J 14:5579–5588
43. Nagata S (1997) Apoptosis by death factor. Cell 88:355–365

44. Scaffidi C, Fulda S, Srinivasan A, et al (1998) Two CD95 (APO-1/Fas) signaling pathways. EMBO J 17:1675–1687
45. Kuwana T, Smith JJ, Muzio M, Dixit V, Newmeyer DD, Kornbluth S (1998) Apoptosis induction by caspase-8 is amplified through the mitochondrial release of cytochrome C. J Biol Chem 273:16589–16594
46. Sakahira H, Enari M, Nagata S (1998) Cleavage of CAD inhibitor in CAD activation and DNA degradation during apoptosis. Nature 391:96–99
47. Liu X, Zou H, Slaughter C, Wang X (1997) DFF, a heterodimeric protein that functions downstream of caspase-3 to trigger DNA fragmentation during apoptosis. Cell 89:175–184
48. Thornberry NA, Lazebnik Y (1998) Caspases: enemies within. Science 281:1312–1316
49. Thome M, Schneider P, Hofmann K, et al (1997) Viral FLICE-inhibitory proteins (FLIPs) prevent apoptosis induced by death receptors. Nature 386:517–521
50. Perez D, White E (1998) E1B 19K inhibits Fas-mediated apoptosis through FADD-dependent sequestration of FLICE. J Cell Biol 141:1255–1266
51. Chang HY, Nishitoh H, Yang X, Ichijo H, Baltimore D (1998) Activation of apoptosis signal-regulating kinase 1 (ASK1) by the adapter protein Daxx. Science 281:1860–1863
52. Roulston A, Reinhard C, Amiri P, Williams LT (1998) Early activation of c-Jun N-terminal kinase and p38 kinase regulate cell survival in response to tumor necrosis factor-α. J Biol Chem 273:10232–10239
53. Jiang Y, Woronicz JD, Liu W, Goeddel DV (1999) Prevention of constitutive TNF receptor 1 signaling by silencer of death domains. Science 283:543–546
54. Hsu HL, Shu HB, Pan MG, Goeddel DV (1996) TRADD-TRAF2 and TRADD-FADD interactions define two distinct TNF receptor 1 signal transduction pathways. Cell 84:299–308
55. Stanger BZ, Leder P, Lee TH, Kim E, Seed B (1995) RIP: a novel protein containing a death domain that interacts with Fas/APO-1 (CD95) in yeast and causes cell death. Cell 81:513–523
56. Yuan H, Dixit VM (1997) RAIDD is a new death adaptor molecule. Nature 385:86–89
57. Chou JJ, Matsuo H, Duan H, Wagner G (1998) Solution structure of the RAIDD CARD and model for CARD/CARD interaction in caspase-2 and caspase-9 recruitment. Cell 94:171–180
58. Ting AT, Pimentel-Muinos FX, Seed B (1996) RIP mediates tumor necrosis factor receptor 1 activation of NF-B but not Fas/APO-1-initiated apoptosis. EMBO J 15:6189–6196
59. Chaudhuri A, Orme S, Eilam S, Cherayil BJ (1997) CD40-mediated signals inhibit the binding of TNF receptor-associated factor 2 to the CD40 cytoplasmic domain. J Immunol 159: 4244–4251
60. Ling L, Cao Z, Goeddel DV (1998) NF-κB-inducing kinase activates IKK-α by phosphorylation of Ser-176. Proc Natl Acad Sci USA 95:3792–3797
61. Lee FS, Hagler J, Chen ZJ, Maniatis T (1997) Activation of the IκBα kinase complex by MEKK1, a kinase of the JNK pathway. Cell 88:213–222
62. Liu ZG, Hsu HL, Goeddel DV, Karin M (1996) Dissection of TNF receptor 1 effector functions: JNK activation is not linked to apoptosis, while NF-κB activation prevents cell death. Cell 87:565–576
63. Yujiri T, Sather S, Fanger GR, Johnson GL (1998) Role of MEKK1 in cell survival and activation of JNK and ERK pathways defined by targeted gene disruption. Science 282:1911–1914
64. Beg AA, Baltimore D (1996) An essential role for NF-κB in preventing TNFα-induced cell death. Science 274:782–784
65. Anrather J, Csizmadia V, Brostjan C, Soares JP, Bach FH, Winkler H (1997) Inhibition of bovine endothelial cell activation in vitro by regulated expression of a transdominant inhibitor of NF-κB. J Clin Invest 99:763–772
66. Böhrer H, Qiu F, Zimmermann T, et al (1997) The role of NF-κB in the mortality of sepsis. J Clin Invest 100:972–985
67. Rothe M, Xion J, Shu HB, Williamson K, Goddard A, Goeddel DV (1996) I-TRAF is a novel TRAF-interacting protein that regulates TRAF-mediated signal transduction. Proc Natl Acad Sci USA 93:8241–8246
68. Wajant H, Johannes FJ, Haas E, et al (1998) Dominant-negative FADD inhibits TNFR60-, Fas/Apo1- and TRAIL-R/Apo2-mediated cell death but not gene induction. Curr Biol 8: 113–116

69. Gamard CJ, Dbaibo Gs, Liu B, Obeid LM, Hannun YA (1997) Selective involvement of ceramide in cytokine-induced apoptosis. Ceramide inhibits phorbol ester activation of nuclear factor-κB. J Biol Chem 272:16474–16481
70. Basu S, Kolesnick R (1998) Stress signals for apoptosis: ceramide and c-Jun kinase. Oncogene 17:3277–3285
71. Haimovitz-Friedman A, Cordon-Cardo C, Bayoumy S, et al (1997) Lipopolysaccharide induces disseminated endothelial apoptosis requiring ceramide generation. J Exp Med 186: 1831–1841
72. Adam D, Ruff A, Strelow A, Wiegmann K, Kronke M (1998) Induction of stress-activated protein kinases/c-Jun N-terminal kinases by the p55 tumour necrosis factor receptor does not require sphingomyelinases. Biochem J 333:343–350
73. Hsu SC, Wu CC, Luh TY, Chou CK, Han SH, Lai MZ (1998) Apoptotic signal of Fas is not mediated by ceramide. Blood 91:2658–2663
74. Song HY, Regnier CH, Kirschning CJ, Goeddel DV, Rothe M (1997) Tumor necrosis factor (TNF)-mediated kinase cascades: bifurcation of nuclear factor-κB and c-jun N-terminal kinase (JNK/SAPK) pathways at TNF receptor-associated factor 2. Proc Natl Acad Sci USA 94:9792–9796
75. Rothe M, Pan MG, Henzel WJ, Ayres TM, Goeddel DV (1995) The TNFR2-TRAF signaling complex contains two novel proteins related to baculoviral inhibitor of apoptosis proteins. Cell 83:1243–1252
76. Rajcan-Separovic E, Liston P, Lefebvre C, Korneluk RG (1996) Assignment of human inhibitor of apoptosis protein (IAP) genes xiap, hiap-1, and hiap-2 to chromosomes Xq25 and 11q22q23 by fluorescence in situ hybridization. Genomics 37:404–406
77. Lee SY, Lee SY, Choi Y (1997) TRAF-interacting protein (TRIP): a novel component of the tumor necrosis factor receptor (TNFR)- and CD30-TRAF signaling complexes that inhibits TRAF2-mediated NF-κB activation. J Exp Med 185:1275–1285
78. Weiss T, Grell M, Siemienski K, et al (1998) TNFR80-dependent enhancement of TNFR60-induced cell death is mediated by TNFR-assoicated factor 2 and is specific for TNFR60. J Immunol 161:3136–3142
79. Chinnaiyan AM, O'Rourke K, Yu GL, et al (1996) Signal transduction by DR3, a death domain-containing receptor related to TNFR1 and CD95. Science 274:990–992
80. Kitson J, Raven T, Jiang YP, et al (1996) A death-domain-containing receptor that mediates apoptosis. Nature 384:372–375
81. MacFarlane M, Ahmad M, Srinivasula SM, Fernandes-Alnemri T, Cohen GM, Alnemri ES (1997) Identification and molecular cloning of two novel receptors for the cytotoxic ligand TRAIL. J Biol Chem 272:25417–25420
82. Sheridan JP, Marsters SA, Pitti RM, et al (1997) Control of TRAIL-induced apoptosis by a family of signaling and decoy receptors. Science 277:818–821
83. Marsters SA, Sheridan JP, Pitti RM, et al (1997) A novel receptor for Apo2L/TRAIL contains a truncated death domain. Curr Biol 7:1003–1006
84. Yang E, Korsmeyer SJ (1996) Molecular thanatopsis: a discourse on the BCL2 family and cell death. Blood 88:386–401
85. Zha J, Harada H, Osipov K, Jockel J, Waksman G, Korsmeyer SJ (1997) BH3 domain of BAD is required for heterodimerization with BCL-XL and pro-apoptotic activity. J Biol Chem 272:24101–24104
86. Kroemer G, Zamzami N, Susin SA (1997) Mitochondrial control of apoptosis. Immunol Today 18:44–51
87. Schlesinger PH, Gross A, Yin XM, et al (1997) Comparison of the ion channel characteristics of proapoptotic BAX and antiapoptotic BCL-2. Proc Natl Acad Sci USA 94:11357–11362
88. Zong WX, Edelstein LC, Chen C, Bash J, Gelinas C (1999) The prosurvival Bcl-2 homolog Bfl-1/A1 is a direct transcriptional target of NF-κB that blocks TNF-α-induced apoptosis. Genes Dev 13:382–387
89. Chuang PI, Yee E, Karsan A, Winn RK, Harlan JM (1998) A1 is a constitutive and inducible Bcl-2 homologue in mature human neutrophils. Biochem Biophys Res Commun 249: 361–365

90. Moulding DA, Quayle JA, Hart CA, Edwards SW (1998) Mcl-1 expression in human neutrophils: Regulation by cytokines and correlation with cell survival. Blood 92:2495–2502
91. Perera LP, Waldmann TA (1998) Activation of human monocytes induces differential resistance to apoptosis with rapid down regulation of caspase-8/FLICE. Proc Natl Acad Sci USA 95:14308–14313
92. Cinat M, Waxman K, Vaziri ND, et al (1995) Soluble cytokine receptors and receptor antagonists are sequentially released after trauma. J Trauma 39:112–120
93. Rogy MA, Coyle SM, Oldenburg HAS, et al (1994) Persistently elevated soluble tumor necrosis factor receptor and interleukin-1 receptor antagonist levels in critically ill patients. J Am Coll Surg 178:132–138
94. Van Zee KJ, Kohno T, Fischer E, Rock CS, Moldawer LL, Lowry SF (1992) Proc Natl Acad Sci USA 89:4845–4849
95. Van der Poll T, Coyle SM, Levi M, et al (1997) Effect of a recombinant dimeric tumor necrosis factor receptor on inflammatory responses to intravenous endotoxin in normal humans. Blood 89:3727–3734
96. Van der Poll T, Calvano SE, Kumar A, et al (1995) Endotoxin induces downregulation of tumor necrosis factor receptors on circulating monocytes and granulocytes in humans. Blood 86:2754–2759
97. Van der Poll T, Coyle SM, Kumar A, Barbosa K, Agosti JM, Lowry SF (1997) Down-regulation of surface receptors for TNF and IL-1 on circulating monocytes and granulocytes during human endotoxemia. J Immunol 158:1490–1497
98. Leeuwenberg JFM, Dentener MA, Buurman WA (1994) Lipopolysaccharide LPS-mediated soluble TNF receptor release and TNF receptor expression by monocytes. J Immunol 152:5070–5076
99. Lin E, Calvano SE, Coyle SM, et al (1999) PMX-622 abrogates the inflammatory response in human endotoxemia. J Immunol (in press)
100. Higuchi M, Aggarwal BB (1994) TNF induces internalization of the p60 receptor and shedding of the p80 receptor. J Immunol 152:3550–3558
101. Calvano SE, van der Poll T, Coyle SM, Barie PS, Moldawer LL, Lowry SF (1996) Monocyte tumor necrosis factor receptor levels as a predictor of risk in human sepsis. Arch Surg 131:434–437
102. Calvano SE, Coyle SM, Barbosa KS, Barie PS, Lowry SF (1998) Multivariate analysis of 9 disease-associated variables for outcome prediction in patients with sepsis. Arch Surg 133:1347–1350
103. Lin E, Katz J, Calvano SE, et al (1998) The influence of human endotoxemia on CD95-induced apoptosis. Arch Surg 133:1322–1327
104. Tanaka M, Itai T, Adachi M, Nagata S (1998) Downregulation of Fas ligand by shedding. Nature Med 4:31–36
105. Bennett M, Macdonald K, Chan S-W, Luzio JP, Simari R, Weissberg P (1998) Cell surface trafficking of Fas: a rapid mechanism of p53-mediated apoptosis. Science 282:290–293
106. Doughty L, Clark R, Carcillo J (1998) Soluble Fas receptor (sFasR) in pediatric sepsis-induced MOF. Crit Care Med 26 (suppl): A79 (abst)
107. Guirao X, Kumar A, Katz J, et al (1997) Catecholamines increase monocyte TNF receptors and inhibit TNF through β_2-adrenoreceptor activation. Am J Physiol 273:E1203–1208
108. Van der Poll T, Calvano SE, Kumar A, Coyle SM, Lowry SF (1997) Epinephrine attenuates down-regulation of monocyte tumor necrosis factor receptors during human endotoxemia. J Leukoc Biol 61:156–160
109. Jimenez MF, Watson WG, Parodo J, et al (1997) Dysregulated expression of neutrophil apoptosis in the systemic inflammatory response syndrome. Arch Surg 132:1263–1270
110. Ertel W, Keel M, Infanger M, Ungethum U, Steckholzer U, Trentz O (1998) Circulating mediators in serum of injured patients with septic complications inhibit neutrophil apoptosis through up-regulation of protein-tyrosine phosporylation. J Trauma 44:767–776
111. Liles WC, Kiener PA, Ledbetter JA, Aruffo A, Klebanoff SJ (1996) Differential expression of Fas (CD95) and Fas ligand on normal human phagocytes: implications for the regulation of apoptosis in neutrophils. J Exp Med 184:429–440

112. Leuenroth S, Lee C, Grutkoski P, Keeping H, Simms H (1998) Interleukin-8-induced suppression of polymorphonuclear leukocyte apoptosis is mediated by suppressing CD95 (Fas/Apo-1) Fas-1 interactions. Surgery 124:409–417
113. Murray J, Barbara JA, Dunkley SA, et al (1997) Regulation of neutrophil apoptosis by tumor necrosis factor-α: requirement for TNFR55 and TNFR75 for induction of apoptosis in vitro. Blood 90:2772–2783
114. Riadh K, Colagiovanni DB, Josephs MD, et al (1998) Disparate roles for TNF-α and Fasl ligand in concanavalin A-induced hepatitis. J Immunol 160:4082–4089

Cytokine Neutralization: An Overview

E. Abraham

Introduction

An excessive inflammatory response accompanies the initial stages of severe infection and appears to contribute to organ system failure and death in this setting [1–3]. A number of immunomodulatory therapies aimed at decreasing the dysregulated inflammatory response have been examined in patients with sepsis (Table 1). Despite initially encouraging results with many of these approaches in Phase II clinical trials, larger Phase III studies have not demonstrated benefit. In contrast to the lack of effect of immunomodulatory agents in sepsis, therapies directed against specific pro-inflammatory cytokines, such as tumor necrosis factor (TNF)-α or interleukin (IL)-1, have produced remarkable clinical response in diseases such as rheumatoid arthritis and Crohn's disease [4–6].

The fact that agents such as anti-TNF-α antibodies are clinically effective in the setting of rheumatoid arthritis and Crohn's disease, but not sepsis, provokes

Table 1. Some immunomodulatory therapies examined in sepsis

Agent	Number of trials completed with results reported through 1998	Total number of patients enrolled in trials of the agent
Corticosteroids	9	1298
Antiendotoxin antibodies		
HA-1A	2	2742
E5	2	1335
IL-1ra	3	1688
Bradykinin antagonist	2	755
Anti-TNF-α monoclonal antibodies		
Murine anti-TNF	3	3414
Murine anti-TNF-α Fab'_2 fragments	3	607
TNF receptor fusion proteins		
p75 TNF receptor fusion protein	1	141
p55 TNF receptor fusion protein	2	1838
Platelet activating factor (PAF) antagonists	2	930
Ibuprofen (cyclooxygenase inhibitor)	3	514

questions about the clinical heterogeneity of patients with sepsis as compared to those with rheumatoid arthritis or Crohn's disease. Overly broad clinical definitions for sepsis may have diluted out any effect that such therapies had in more limited patient populations. In particular, whereas rheumatoid arthritis or Crohn's disease are well described entities with specific immunologic, radiologic, and pathophysiologic criteria, the diagnosis of sepsis is less well defined and based on organ system dysfunctions in the appropriate clinical setting.

Definitions and Entry Criteria

Entry criteria for sepsis trials have primarily been designed to include patients with clinical evidence of infection associated with the recent development of organ system dysfunction believed to be due to this infectious process [7, 8]. Because of the perceived need to enroll patients early in their clinical course, positive cultures have not been required. In recent studies, only a minority of patients had positive cultures, with bacteremia present in about a third of the patients [9–13].

The definitions of sepsis and septic shock used in most of the clinical trials did not include consideration of the length of time that the infectious process had been present or of the anatomic source of infection. Such classification may be particularly important since animal studies have shown different patterns of response to anti-cytokine therapy, such as anti-TNF-α monoclonal antibodies, for intraabdominal infections compared to bacteremias, and for rapidly initiated infectious processes, such as acute bacteremia, compared to more slowly developing infections, such as peritonitis [14]. No microbiologic classifications were used prospectively in the clinical trials of immunomodulatory agents even though responses to anti-inflammatory therapies may differ between Gram-positive and Gram-negative infections, and also may be more marked in patients with documented infections [11, 15].

Even though recent clinical trials have targeted specific mediators, such as endotoxin, IL-1, or TNF-α, which were postulated to have a pivotal role in the inflammatory cascade leading to organ system failure and death in sepsis, the actual presence of excessive levels of these mediators was not required for entry into the study. Rather, clinical criteria, such as the presence of one or more organ failures, with or without shock, were used for patient inclusion in these studies. Although elevation of the mediator of interest was postulated to accompany organ system dysfunction in septic patients, data gathered from the IL-1 receptor antagonist (IL-1ra) and anti-TNF clinical trials suggested that such correlation occurred in only a minority of cases. For example, in the NORASEPT II trial of a murine monoclonal antibody for septic shock, fewer than 25% of patients had detectable circulating TNF-α levels at the time of enrollment [13].

The lack of a requirement to recruit demonstrably infected patients with elevation of the mediator of interest may have adversely affected outcome in trials examining immunomodulatory agents in sepsis. For example, improved efficacy of therapies, such as monoclonal anti-TNF-α antibodies, was found when blinded data-safety monitoring committees eliminated patients without clear evidence of infection [16]. In the NORASEPT II trial of murine monoclonal anti-TNF-α antibodies, there was an 18% relative reduction in day 28 mortality compared to placebo in patients with detectable circulating TNF-α levels at the time of enrollment [13]. In contrast, no effect of such anti-TNF therapy was seen in patients without elevation of circulating TNF-α concentrations.

IL-1ra

IL-1ra is a naturally occurring inhibitor of IL-1, which competitively binds to the IL-1 receptor [17, 18]. In pre-clinical studies, primarily involving rabbits and mice, infusion of IL-1ra, starting before or shortly after endotoxemia or bacteremia, improved survival [17, 18]. Interestingly, in baboon studies [19, 20], IL-1ra therapy appears to have minimal effect in blunting endotoxemia-induced increases in IL-6, TNF-α, or circulating levels of soluble TNF receptors, suggesting that IL-1 may not have a central role in sepsis-induced inflammatory responses in primates.

Although a small, dose ranging, unblinded Phase II trial in 99 septic patients [21] suggested that IL-1ra could improve survival, two large subsequent Phase III studies [12, 22] were unable to demonstrate similar efficacy. In part, the inability of IL-1ra to provide benefit may be because IL-1 does not occupy a central, pivotal role in perpetuating the inflammatory response and producing organ system dysfunction in human sepsis, as suggested by the baboon endotoxemia studies [19, 20] reviewed above. Additionally, the failure of IL-1ra to reduce mortality may reflect a timing issue, generic in sepsis studies. In particular, even if IL-1 is important in initiating a pro-inflammatory response, its role may be minimal by the time the patients are recognized and entered into a clinical trial. Of note, very few septic patients have elevations in circulating IL-1, so the number of patients who truly had increased IL-1 tissue expression at the time of enrollment into the IL-1ra studies is unknown. Such information is of obvious importance because therapies inhibiting IL-1 would be expected to have effect only in patients with increased expression of this cytokine.

Anti-TNF Therapies

The two major approaches taken to neutralizing TNF have involved either monoclonal murine or chimeric anti-TNF antibodies or fusion protein constructs in which the extramembrane portion of the p55 (Type I) or p75 (Type II) TNF receptor is joined to the Fc fragment of a human IgG1 antibody. Pre-treatment of endotoxemic or bacteremic animals with anti-TNF-α antibodies or TNF receptor fusion protein constructs, results in improvement in survival and amelioration of organ system dysfunction [23–26]. In some models of Gram-negative or Gram-positive bacteremia, administration of anti-TNF-α antibodies at the time of initiation of the bacteremic insult or even shortly thereafter (i.e., within the first hour) still is associated with significant survival benefit [27]. However, the use of such antibodies at later time points in endotoxemia or bacteremia models does not appear to be associated with any clear benefits.

Although several small studies [28, 29] suggested that anti-TNF-α antibody therapy improved physiologic parameters, such as cardiac output, in septic patients, these studies were too small to detect any effect on survival. The NORASEPT I trial examined a murine IgG1 monoclonal antibody in 994 patients with severe sepsis and septic shock [9]. There was no statistically significant benefit associated with anti-TNF therapy in the overall patient group enrolled in NORASEPT I. However, in the prospectively defined subgroup of patients with septic shock, a statistically significant reduction in mortality compared to placebo was present during the first two weeks following therapy with monoclonal anti-TNF-α antibody. At day 28 after anti-TNF-α therapy, the reduction in mortality among septic shock patients was 17% compared to those receiving placebo (p = not significant).

In the NORASEPT I shock patients, the beneficial effect of anti-TNF-α antibodies on survival appeared within the first 24 hours after enrollment, with the greatest separation between the survival curves for placebo and anti-TNF antibody treated patients occurring within this time window. Approximately 60% of the placebo deaths occurred within the first three days of the study. Treatment with 7.5 mg/kg monoclonal anti-TNF-α antibodies was associated with a 49% reduction in mortality versus placebo at day three after study enrollment.

A second study (INTERSEPT) with the same murine monoclonal anti-TNF-α antibody used in the NORASEPT I study was undertaken in 14 countries, primarily in Europe [10]. Although the INTERSEPT study initially enrolled septic patients with and without shock, after the results of NORASEPT I were available, only shock patients were entered into INTERSEPT. A total of 564 patients, of whom 420 were in septic shock, were enrolled in the INTERSEPT study. Day 28 mortality was reduced by 14.5% in patients who received 3 mg/kg monoclonal anti-TNF-α antibody (p = not significant), with no reduction in mortality found in the patients given 15 mg/kg. There was no evidence in the INTERSEPT trial of early survival benefit (i.e., within the first three days after anti-TNF antibody infusion) as had been seen in NORASEPT I. Additionally, whereas 60% of the placebo deaths among patients in shock occurred within the first three study days in the NORASEPT I trial, less than 45% of placebo deaths occurred within this period in the INTERSEPT study.

A recently completed study (NORASEPT II) enrolled 1900 patients with septic shock and examined the potential utility of 7.5 mg/kg of the murine monoclonal anti-TNF-α antibody [13]. No improvement in survival was found in septic shock patients treated with the monoclonal anti-TNF-α antibody compared to those who received placebo. All-cause mortality at day 28 was 40.3% in monoclonal anti-TNF-α antibody treated patients compared to 42.8% in placebo-treated patients. Even though the APACHE II scores, day 28 mortality rates, sex ratio, and percentage of patients with one or more organ failures present at baseline were similar in NORASEPT I and NORASEPT II, there did appear to be substantial differences in patient survival patterns. Whereas more than 60% of the deaths in the placebo arm of NORASEPT I occurred in the first three days after study entry, the mean time to death in the placebo group of NORASEPT II was more delayed, averaging 6.8 days. These differences in survival may reflect interval improvement in the supportive care provided to patients with septic shock resulting in better survival from the initial hypotensive episode and associated immediate complications, a period where pro-inflammatory cytokine release, including TNF-α, may be greatest. If advances in management have permitted critically ill septic patients to better survive the initial state of accelerated pro-inflammatory cytokine expression, then this would diminish the efficacy of therapies, such as anti-TNF-α antibodies, aimed at modulating these early responses.

The utility of administration of $F(ab')_2$ fragments of a murine IgG3 monoclonal antibody to TNF-α has been examined in patients with severe sepsis or septic shock [30]. There were 122 patients entered in the clinical trial, and no increase in survival from sepsis for the patients receiving anti-TNF treatment was present in the overall study population. However, a retrospective stratification of patients by IL-6 concentration suggested beneficial effects for the drug in patients ($n=37$) with baseline circulating IL-6 concentrations greater than 1000 pg/ml. In patients with IL-6 levels greater than 1000 pg/ml, mortality decreased from 80% in the placebo group to 35% in patients who received the highest dose (1 mg/kg) of the anti-TNF-α therapy. However, a larger subsequent study was unable to substantiate the hypothesis that a beneficial response to anti-TNF-α therapy could be predicted by IL-6 levels at the time of enrollment. These results were consistent with those found in NORASEPT II [13], INTERSEPT [10], and the p55 TNF receptor fusion protein [11] studies which found no relationship between IL-6 levels and response to anti-TNF therapy. There is, however, another study ongoing in Canada and the U.S.A which is examining the predictive value of IL-6 levels in defining patients who may respond to anti-TNF therapy.

Three clinical studies have reported results using soluble TNF receptor constructs as anti-TNF agents. In the first of these studies, the molecule used consisted of the extramembrane components of the human type II (p75) receptor joined to the Fc portion of a human IgG1 antibody molecule [15]. Patients ($n = 141$) with septic shock, with or without associated organ system dysfunction, were entered into the study. A statistically significant ($p=0.014$), dose dependent increase in mortality occurred in patients treated with this p75 soluble TNF receptor construct, with mortality rising from 30% in the placebo group to 53% in the patients treated with the highest dose (1.5 mg/kg) of the anti-TNF compound.

The enhanced mortality associated with treatment with the p75 TNF receptor molecule may be related to the high doses used in the study. Soluble TNF receptor fusion proteins appear to inactivate TNF-α more than fifty times as well as monoclonal antibodies [11]. Therapy with a dose of 1.5 mg/kg of the p75 TNF receptor fusion protein would therefore be expected to neutralize TNF-α for a prolonged period, especially given the long half life of the compound (>60 hours). TNF-α is an essential component of the normal inflammatory responses, and prolonged neutralization of its activity may have potent immunosuppressive effects leading to increased mortality.

Two clinical trials have examined the role of a p55 TNF receptor fusion protein construct in septic patients. In the initial 498 patient study, separate randomization lists were used for patients with severe sepsis with or without early shock and for patients with refractory septic shock [11]. The doses of the p55 TNF receptor complex used in this study (0.008 mg/kg, 0.042 mg/kg, and 0.08 mg/kg) were substantially lower than those administered in the p75 TNF receptor complex clinical trial. Therapy with 0.08 mg/kg of the p55 TNF receptor fusion protein complex, but not other doses, was associated with a 36% reduction ($p = 0.07$) in day 28 mortality in the prospectively defined patient group with severe sepsis with or without early septic shock. In contrast, no apparent beneficial effects were seen with any dose of the p55 receptor complex in patients with refractory septic shock.

Because of the apparent benefit of the p55 TNF receptor fusion protein in severe sepsis with or without early septic shock, a 1340 patient, Phase III study was undertaken in this patient population (unpublished data). No improvement in 28-day all cause mortality or in surrogate endpoints, such as organ failure scores, was found in patients treated with the p55 TNF receptor construct compared to placebo. Of note, the p55 TNF receptor fusion protein used in this Phase III study was from a different lot than the Phase II study, with differences in glycosylation, and had slightly lower TNF neutralizing ability, so that higher doses (approximately 0.125 mg/kg) were used. It is unknown what role, if any, these alterations in molecular structure or binding potency of the p55 TNF receptor fusion protein played in the different outcomes between the Phase II and Phase III clinical trials.

Future Directions

As noted above, almost all of the clinical trials of immunomodulatory therapies have enrolled patients with clinical evidence of infection associated with organ system dysfunction, without requiring any evidence that the immunologic abnormality of interest is present. Such inclusion criteria may allow entry of excessively heterogeneous patient populations into clinical trials and may prevent detection of beneficial effects that could be present in more homogeneous subgroups with organ system failures due to the mediator of interest. Positive results associated with endotoxin blockade for meningococcemia [31] suggest that there are specific groups of infected patients that do respond to immunomodulatory agents.

Classification of infected patients based on demonstrable abnormalities in immunologic or biochemical pathways may permit inclusion into therapeutic studies at earlier points in their clinical course, before organ dysfunction develops and becomes irreversible. In this case, patients with clinical evidence of infection and alteration of the mediator of interest, such as TNF-α, would be eligible for study enrollment. Such a classification scheme, in addition to allowing appropriate targeting of patient populations who may benefit from a specific therapeutic agent, would also mean that the development of clinically relevant organ system dysfunction could be used as an endpoint, rather than as an entry criterion for clinical trials.

There are substantial differences in the intracellular signaling cascades initiated by Gram-negative and Gram-positive infections [32], as well as by the site of infection [14]. It would therefore appear reasonable to limit the nature and site of the infection in future trials of immunomodulatory agents. For example, an immunomodulatory therapy would initially be investigated only in patients with evidence of meningococcemia or pneumococcal pneumonia.

Conclusion

Although large clinical trials of anti-inflammatory therapies in sepsis have been disappointing, it is unclear if such results are due to inefficacy of this approach or to problems in study design. All sepsis trials have used entry criteria based on the patients' clinical characteristics, and did not demonstrate or require elevation of the mediator of interest. Administration of effective therapies to patients with documented presence of endotoxemia or hypercytokinemia may demonstrate an impact of such treatment on the development of infection-induced organ dysfunction or death. Using more stringent definitions in clinical trials would, of course, restrict the numbers of patients eligible for a specific therapy until subsequent studies examine larger at risk populations. However, unless benefit can first be shown in a rigorously defined patient population in which there is specific evidence of mediator activation, there is little reason to anticipate that efficacy will be achieved in larger, more heterogeneous patient groups.

References

1. Abraham E (1997) Therapies for sepsis. Emerging therapies for sepsis and septic shock. West J Med 166:195–200
2. Parrillo JE, Parker MM, Natanson C, et al (1990) Septic shock in humans. Ann Intern Med 113:227–242
3. Zeni F, Freeman B, Natanson C (1997) Anti-inflammatory therapies to treat sepsis and septic shock: a reassessment. Crit Care Med 25:1095–1100
4. Targan SR, Hanauer SB, van Deventer SJ, et al (1997) A short-term study of chimeric monoclonal antibody cA2 to tumor necrosis factor alpha for Crohn's disease. New Engl J Med 337:1029–1035
5. Lorenz HM, Antoni C, Valerius T, et al (1996) In vivo blockade of TNF-alpha by intravenous infusion of a chimeric monoclonal TNF-alpha antibody in patients with rheumatoid arthritis. Short term cellular and molecular effects. J Immunol 156:1646–1653
6. Elliott MJ, Maini RN, Feldmann M, et al (1994) Repeated therapy with monoclonal antibody to tumor necrosis factor alpha (cA2) in patients with rheumatoid arthritis. Lancet 344:1125–1127
7. Bone RC, Balk RA, Cerra FB, et al (1992) ACCP/SCCM consensus conference: Definitions for sepsis and organ failure and guidelines for the use of innovative therapies in sepsis. Chest 101:1644–1655
8. Bone RC, Fisher Jr. CJ, Clemmer TP, et al (1989) Sepsis syndrome: A valid clinical entity. Crit Care Med 17:389–393
9. Abraham E, Wunderink R, Silverman H, et al (1995) Monoclonal antibody to human tumor necrosis factor alpha (TNF MAb): Efficacy and safety in patients with the sepsis syndrome. JAMA 273:934–941
10. Cohen J, Carlet J (1996) INTERSEPT: An international, multicenter, placebo-controlled trial of monoclonal antibody to human tumor necrosis factor-α in patients with sepsis. Crit Care Med 24:1431–1440
11. Abraham E, Glauser MP, Butler T, et al (1997) p55 tumor necrosis factor receptor fusion protein in the treatment of patients with severe sepsis and septic shock. JAMA 277:1531–1534

12. Opal SM, Fisher CJ, Pribble JP, et al (1997) The confirmatory interleukin-1 receptor antagonist trial in severe sepsis: a phase III randomized, double-blind, placebo-controlled, multicenter trial. Crit Care Med 25:1115–1124
13. Abraham E, Anzueto A, Gutierrez G, et al (1998) Monoclonal antibody to human tumor necrosis factor alpha (TNF Mab) in the treatment of patients with septic shock: A multi-center, placebo controlled, randomized, double-blind clinical trial. Lancet 351:929–933
14. Zanetti G, Heumann D, Gerain J, et al (1992) Cytokine production after intravenous or peritoneal gram-negative bacterial challenge in mice. J Immunol 148:1890–1897
15. Fisher CJ Jr., Agosti JM, Opal SM, et al (1996) Treatment of septic shock with the tumor necrosis factor receptor Fc fusion protein. N Engl J Med 334:1697–1702
16. Sprung CL, Finch RG, Thijs LG, Glauser MP (1996) International sepsis trial (INTERSEPT): role and impact of a clinical evaluation committee. Crit Care Med 24:1441–1447
17. Ohlsson K, Bjork P, Bergenfeldt M, Hageman R, Thompson RC (1990) Interleukin-1 receptor antagonist reduces mortality from endotoxin shock. Nature 348:550–552
18. Wakabayashi G, Gelfand JA, Burke JF, Thompson RC, Dinarello CA (1991) A specific receptor antagonist for interleukin-1 prevents Escherichia coli-induced shock. FASEB J 5:338–343
19. Hawes AS, Fischer E, Marano MA, et al (1993) Comparison of peripheral blood leukocyte kinetics after live Escherichia coli, endotoxin, or interleukin-1 alpha administration. Studies using a novel interleukin-1 receptor antagonist. Ann Surg 218:79–90
20. Fischer E, Marano MA, Van Zee KJ, et al (1992) Interleukin-1 receptor blockade improves survival and hemodynamic performance in Escherichia coli septic shock, but fails to alter host responses to sublethal endotoxemia. J Clin Invest 89:1551–1557
21. Fisher CJ Jr., Slotman GJ, Opal SM, et al (1994) Initial evaluation of human recombinant interleukin-1 receptor antagonist in the treatment of sepsis syndrome: a randomized, open-label, placebo-controlled multicenter trial. The IL-1RA Sepsis Syndrome Study Group. Crit Care Med 22:12–21
22. Fisher CJ Jr, Dhainaut JF, Opal SM, et al (1994) Recombinant human interleukin 1 receptor antagonist in the treatment of patients with sepsis syndrome. Results from a randomized, double-blind, placebo-controlled trial. Phase III rhIL-1ra Sepsis Syndrome Study Group. JAMA 271:1836–1843
23. Tracey KJ, Fong Y, Hesse DG, et al (1987) Anti-cachectin/TNF monoclonal antibodies prevent septic shock during lethal bacteremia. Nature 330:662–664
24. Fong Y, Tracey KJ, Moldawer LL, et al (1989) Antibodies to cachectin/TNF reduce interleukin-1 and interleukin-6 appearance during lethal bacteremia. J Exp Med 170:1627–1633
25. Hinshaw LB, Tekamp-Olson P, Chang AC, et al (1990) Survival of primates in LD_{100} septic shock following therapy with antibody to tumor necrosis factor (TNF). Circ Shock 30: 279–292
26. Van Zee KJ, Moldawer LL, Oldenburg HAS, et al (1996) Protection against lethal *Escherichia coli* bacteremia in baboons (Papio anubis) by pretreatment with a 55-kDa TNF receptor (CD120a)-Ig fusion protein, Ro 45-2081. J Immunol 156:2221–2230
27. Hinshaw LB, Emerson TE Jr., Taylor FB Jr., et al (1992) Lethal *S. aureus* shock in primates: prevention of death with anti-TNF antibody. J Trauma 33:568–573
28. Vincent JL, Bakker J, Marecaux G, Schandene L, Kahn RJ, Dupont E (1992) Administration of anti-TNF antibody improves left ventricular function in septic shock patients. Results of a pilot study. Chest 101:810–815
29. Dhainaut JF, Vincent JL, Richard C, et al (1995) CDP571, a humanized antibody to human tumor necrosis factor-α: Safety, pharmacokinetics, immune response, and influence of the antibody on cytokine concentrations in patients with septic shock. Crit Care Med 23:1461–1469
30. Reinhart K, Wiegand-Lohnert C, Grimminger F, et al (1996) Assessment of the safety and efficacy of the monoclonal anti-tumor necrosis factor antibody-fragment, MAK 195F, in patients with sepsis and septic shock: A multicenter, randomized, placebo-controlled, dose-ranging study. Crit Care Med 24:733–742
31. Giroir BP, Quint PA, Barton P, et al (1997) Preliminary evaluation of recombinant amino-terminal fragment of human bactericidal/permeability-increasing protein in children with severe meningococcal sepsis. Lancet 350:1439–1443
32. Bone RC (1994) Gram-positive organisms and sepsis. Arch Intern Med 154:26–34

Immunostimulation with Cytokines in Patients with 'Immunoparalysis'

H. D. Volk, P. Reinke, and W. D. Döcke

Introduction

The main function of the immune system is the protection of the body's integrity, and antimicrobial defense against pathogens is an important component. The increased risk of developing infective complications in patients with exogenous immunosuppression (transplant patients) and following major surgery and trauma is well established. For optimal immunological management of such patients we require an immune monitoring program which is easy to perform and has a good cost-benefit ratio.

In the case of transplant patients it would be helpful to find parameters which help to individualize immunosuppressive therapy in order to prevent both inadequate immunosuppression leading to rejection and over-immunosuppression resulting in increased infections. Clinical parameters are not very useful as transplant patients show diminished clinical signs of inflammation in response to infection. Moreover, it would be good to detect the infectious risk before manifestations of infection become clinically apparent.

Infections are one of the main complications in non-transplant intensive care unit (ICU) patients, and can develop into sepsis associated with a very high mortality. Over the last two decades our understanding of the pathophysiology of sepsis has progressed considerably. After realizing that an overwhelming inflammatory response to microbial invasion may be involved in the pathogenesis of the systemic inflammatory response syndrome (SIRS), sepsis and multiple organ failure (MOF), and that tumor necrosis factor (TNF) and interleukin-1 (IL-1) may mimic sepsis and septic shock in preclinical models, several clinical trials focused on neutralization of the production or action of these inflammatory mediators, but the results were very disappointing.

Several reasons have been proposed for the failure of the anti-inflammatory approach in sepsis [1–3]. From the immunological point of view, we have had to learn that our model of sepsis pathogenesis (invasion of bacteria and/or toxins → systemic release of pro-inflammatory cytokines → shock → MOF) was oversimplified [4].

The Inflammatory Response may be of Benefit in Severe Infection

As a result of the emphasis on TNF/IL-1 as the 'bad guys' during the 90s, many overlooked important experimental and clinical data contradicting this approach. For example, it was shown that anti-TNF therapy was successful in preventing shock following a single intravenous/intraperitoneal challenge of lipopolysaccharide (LPS) or bacteria, but was of no benefit, or even harmful, in the cecal ligation and puncture (CLP)-peritonitis models which are closer to the clinical situation [5]. Moreover, mice which are genetically deficient in their ability to produce or respond to TNF (knock-out mice), are relatively resistant to LPS mediated injury but fail to control infection with living bacteria [6]. Despite delayed elimination, more or less harmless laboratory *Escherichia coli* strains do not induce severe sepsis in these knock-out mice, whereas infection with more pathogenic germs (e.g., *Salmonella thyphimurium*, listeria species) results in septic death of the TNF-deficient mice. Similar observations have been made with LPS binding protein (LBP) knock-out mice [7]. We have had to learn that a bolus injection of LPS or bacteria does not completely reflect the complex host-pathogen interaction that takes place during sepsis. On the other hand, mice deficient in anti-inflammatory cytokines, like transforming growth factor-β (TGF-β) or IL-10, are very sensitive to LPS or bacteria-induced shock due to an uncontrolled inflammatory response. These data suggest that well balanced inflammation is important to control bacterial infections; obviously, we can die from both too much inflammation in response to infection (hyperinflammation) and too little inflammation (uncontrolled infection) (Fig. 1). Further studies should address the mechanisms of death by infection in the latter group.

Clinical data have also challenged the simple concept of septic death 'by too much inflammation'. Pro-inflammatory and anti-inflammatory cytokines have been detected in the serum and body fluids of septic patients [8]. However, the complex network and the short half-life of cytokines complicate the interpretation of these data. In addition, the concentration of a mediator in the serum does not automatically reflect its availability in the tissue, particularly at the site of infection. So it is not surprising that some studies found an association between

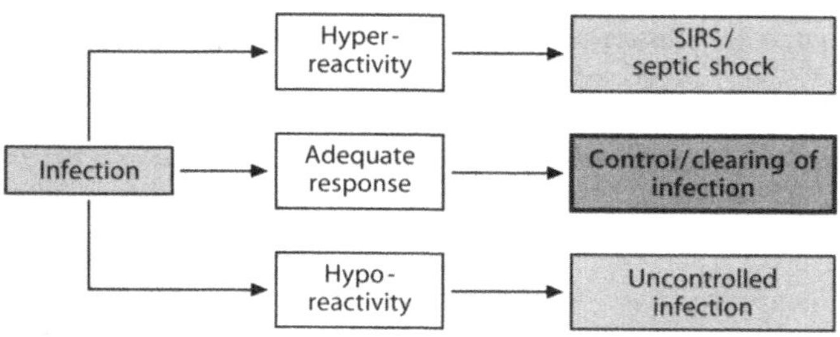

Fig. 1. The quality of the immune response determines the clinical outcome of severe infections

sepsis outcome and the serum levels of pro-inflammatory cytokines, and others described a relation to anti-inflammatory cytokine serum levels (reviewed in [9]).

Several groups have described deactivation of monocytes and granulocytes in septic patients, particularly during the later stages of disease [4] (reviewed in [8, 9]). In contrast to the unstable phenotype of cytokine plasma levels (half-life of minutes), after leaving the bone-marrow, monocytes and granulocytes have a half-life of about 24 hrs in the peripheral blood. Whereas monocytes migrate into the tissues where they differentiate into different subtypes of macrophages, granulocytes are short-lived and can only go into inflammatory tissues. These properties make analysis of monocyte and granulocyte function suitable for daily monitoring.

In contradiction to the assumption of persistent hyperinflammation, we demonstrated a state of the inflammatory system in prolonged sepsis in which monocytic TNF secretion capacity, as well as human leukocyte antigen (HLA)-DR expression and antigen-presenting capacity, are severely depressed whereas the capacity for IL-1 receptor antagonist (IL-1ra) and, at least temporarily, also for IL-10 production, is largely preserved. This switch to predominant anti-inflammatory mediator release was associated with a high risk of fatal outcome from persistent, in part opportunistic, infection and MOF. In our experience, no septic patient ever survived without substantial recovery of monocytic pro-inflammatory function and major histocompatibility complex (MHC)-class II expression. We first observed this phenomenon in septic transplant patients. If immunosuppression was rapidly reduced then, commonly, the patient survived without any signs of acute rejection, despite a reduction in the immunosuppression. In contrast, septic transplant patients with normal monocytic phenotype and function rapidly rejected their graft if immunosuppression was reduced. Obviously, monocytic deactivation reflects the *in vivo* situation of the cell-mediated immune system. Therefore, we called this phenomenon 'immunoparalysis' [10, 11].

Mechanisms of Developing 'Immunoparalysis'

Monocytes are a crucial component of resistance to infection. They phagocytose and kill pathogenic microorganisms, mediate an inflammatory response to endotoxins and exotoxins originating from pathogens, and as antigen-presenting cells they are an important link between the innate resistance system and the highly specialized adoptive immune response. All functions are disturbed in monocytes from patients with immunoparalysis.

What are the possible mechanisms? In the search for factors which trigger this phenomenon we noticed that the occurrence of immunoparalysis was not dependent on certain pathogens or toxins. It was striking, however, that almost every case of Candida sepsis (mostly appearing in combination with bacterial sepsis) was associated with immunoparalysis but not *vice versa*. Candida sepsis is, therefore, to be regarded as a result, rather than the cause, of the immunodepression (opportunistic infection). Another indication that immunoparalysis is not the direct result of pathogenic action is the fact that we, and others, found monocyte deactivation in some patients after a primarily sterile injury (burns, trauma, major surgery) or following high-dose immunosuppression (induction or anti-rejection therapy) (reviewed in [8, 9, 11]).

Immunoparalysis can be the result of different factors (Fig. 2). Monocyte phenotype and function is closely associated with the 'net'-immunosuppression of cell-mediated immunity, particularly the type 1 T-cell response. The pro-inflammatory capacity of monocytes (secretion of TNF, IL-1, IL-12, etc.), as well as their antigen-presenting capacity (expression of surface HLA-DR, HLA-DP, HLA-DQ, CD80/86) is positively regulated by immunostimulatory cytokines (e.g., interferon-gamma [IFN-γ], granulocyte/macrophage colony-stimulating factor [GM-CSF]) and negatively influenced by several factors (IL-10, TGF-β, prostaglandins, catecholamines, apoptotic material, etc.).

Following high dose immunosuppression (steroid bolus, OKT 3 mAb, antithymocyte globulin [ATG]) we have seen a temporary decrease in monocytic HLA-DR expression (and *ex vivo* TNF secretion capacity) [11]. The reason for this phenomenon may be the lack of stimulatory cytokines (e.g., IFN-γ which is strongly down-regulated by immunosuppression) as well as the induction of inhibitory factors (e.g., steroids block cytokine action on monocytes and other cells, cyclosporin up-regulates TGF-β secretion). In some patients the monocyte deactivation reached the critical level we defined as immunoparalysis ($HLA\text{-}DR^+CD14^+$ monocytes: $<30\%$, *ex vivo* TNF secretion in response to 500 pg/ml LPS: <300 pg/ml). This phenomenon was associated with an increased risk of developing infectious complications within the next few weeks (after two days immunoparalysis bacterial/fungal infections were seen in about 30% of patients vs. 4% in patients without immunoparalysis following high-dose immunosuppression, $p<0.01$; the longer the immunoparalysis persists, the higher the incidence of infections) [11]. In general, the immunocompetence rapidly recovers following reduction of immunosuppression. Moreover, if clinical signs of infection appeared in transplant patients with immunoparalysis, the patients had a poor outcome if the immunosuppression was not immediately tapered [10, 11].

But what are the mechanisms of immunoparalysis in non-transplanted ICU patients? Following *in vitro* LPS stimulation of murine or human blood leukocytes, TNF secretion peaks as early as two hrs after LPS administration, whereas IL-10 peak secretion is delayed by more than 14 hrs. TNF by itself could induce IL-10 mRNA (but not protein) and, in combination with other stimuli (e.g., low-dose LPS, prostaglandins), also IL-10 protein. Moreover, blocking of TNF by neutralizing antibodies inhibits the IL-10 secretion suggesting a negative feedback regulation (high TNF level = hyperinflammation = high IL-10 level = strong down-regulation). In fact, *in vitro* IL-10 could mimic monocyte deactivation, and neutralization of IL-10 prevented the low-dose LPS-induced deactivation of monocytes (LPS desensitization) [4, 12]. These data suggest that inflammation by itself may induce its own down-regulation via the nuclear factor kappa-B (NF-κB), TNF and cAMP (prostaglandin) dependent pathways (Fig. 2). The monocyte deactivation frequently observed in patients surviving septic shock (late sepsis) may be related to this phenomenon.

However, this phenomenon appears not to be the only mechanism. Up-take of apoptotic material by monocytes also down-regulates TNF secretion capacity and up-regulates IL-10 secretion (Fig. 2). The molecular mechanism is not fully understood but the CD36 receptor seems to be involved. So a massive induction of apoptosis in organ failure (e.g., liver failure) may contribute to the phenomenon of immunoparalysis in septic and trauma patients.

Loss of monocytic HLA-DR expression and diminished *ex vivo* TNF secretion capacity have also been observed in many primarily non-infected patients after trauma, burn injury, or major surgery. How can this be explained? In fact, the activation of the stress axis following local or systemic inflammation plays an important role in down-regulation of the systemic immune response. Whereas the regulatory role of activation of the hypothalamo-pituitary-adrenal axis which results in corticosteroid release is long established, we recently showed that activation of the catecholamine axis is also strongly involved in monocyte deactivation following stress. cAMP dependent up-regulation of IL-10 plays a key role in this process (Fig. 2) [13]. Experimental studies in rats confirmed the hypothesis based on clinical observations. Local injury in rat brains (increase of intracranial pressure by an intraventricular balloon or intraventricular infusion of pro-inflammatory cytokines simulating head trauma and neurosurgical procedures) which was not associated with systemic release of pro-inflammatory cytokines (TNF, IL-1, IFN-γ, IL-6) induced a rapid systemic release of IL-10 which was preventable by parallel intravenous administration of β-adrenergic receptor blockers (e.g., propranolol) (Fig. 3) [13].

Moreover, this axis also seems to be involved in the regulation of IL-10 released during systemic inflammation. In contrast to the *in vitro* situation, *in vivo* TNF and IL-10 are secreted in parallel within one hour following LPS challenge (in both humans and mice) suggesting involvement of TNF-independent mechanisms for IL-10 regulation. Using reverse transcription polymerase chain reaction (RT-PCR) analyses we found a very high TNF and IL-10 mRNA expression in

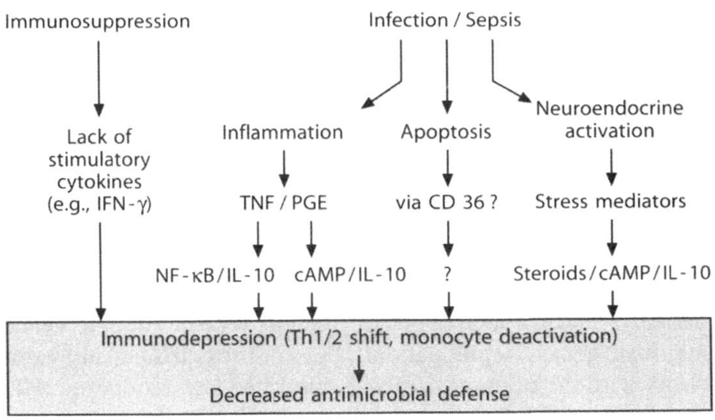

Fig. 2. Mechanisms of immunodepression

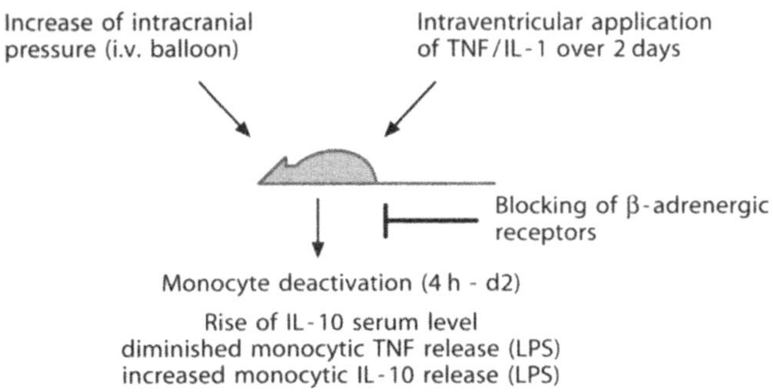

Fig. 3. Triggering of the neuroendocrine axis deactivates the peripheral monocytic system

mouse or rat livers one hour alter LPS injection, while peripheral blood leukocytes expressed only TNF. Eight hours later, IL-10 mRNA was also detectable in blood leukocytes and the protein was, in contrast to TNF, still detectable in the plasma. Both late IL-10 mRNA and IL-10 protein expression were inhibited by the use of a neutralizing anti-TNF antibody in parallel with LPS. By contrast, early IL-10 was not influenced, or even increased, following TNF blockade. However, parallel administration of β-adrenergic receptor blockers strongly inhibited early IL-10 release and further increased early TNF release following LPS application (Volk et al., unpublished data).

In addition to the different regulatory factors, the patient's predisposition has a major impact on the balance between inflammation and anti-inflammation. Thus, we and others have shown that patients with advanced tumors already reveal a diminished inflammatory response pre-operatively, which is further exacerbated by the trauma. Moreover, it has been observed that the capacity to produce cytokines in response to a trigger differs between individuals. Interestingly, recent data suggest that the capacity to produce pro-inflammatory or anti-inflammatory cytokines is genetically determined. Allelic polymorphisms have been described which are associated with low or high IL-10 and TNF production, respectively [14, 15]. Recently, it was reported that in febrile patients, usually due to bacterial infection, a high IL-10/TNF production rate on admission was associated with increased mortality [16].

As suggested above, IL-10 seems to play a key role in down-regulation of the inflammatory system. In fact, septic patients with immunoparalysis express low levels of TNF mRNA but high levels of IL-10 mRNA while septic patients without immunoparalysis (and better outcome) show the opposite picture (Syrbe et al., unpublished data). Is IL-10 the only mediator of monocyte deactivation in ICU patients? Plasma samples from patients with monocyte deactivation following major surgery or septic patients, but not those from healthy donors or septic patients without immunoparalysis, inhibited the monocytic HLA-DR expression and *ex vivo* TNF secretion of indicator cells from healthy donors. This inhibitory activity is heat labile and not dialyzable. Moreover, in most samples, elevated IL-

10 levels were detectable. However, neutralizing IL-10 mAb showed variable effects; it abolished the inhibitory activity of the plasma samples by 20 to 100% suggesting that, at least in some samples, additional immunosuppressive factors are present (Syrbe et al., unpublished data). Moreover, we recently performed a clinical trial in psoriasis, in which patients received up to 12 μg/kg/day IL-10 subcutaneously for up to six weeks, resulting in plasma IL-10 levels comparable with those seen in many ICU patients (20–100 pg/ml). As expected, monocytic HLA-DR expression, antigen-presenting activity, *ex vivo* TNF/IL-12 secretion capacity, and the Th1-/Th2-cytokine ratio were significantly inhibited ([12], Döcke et al., unpublished data). However, we never observed such a strong down-regulation of the monocytic system as in ICU patients, suggesting that IL-10 is an important player in monocyte deactivation but not the only one.

How Can We Explain the High IL-6 Plasma Levels in Septic Patients With Immunoparalysis?

Despite the monocyte deactivation (including deficient TNF-α/IL-6 secretion), many septic patients with immunoparalysis express moderately increased TNF and highly elevated IL-6 plasma levels – how can this be explained?

First, monocyte deactivation is not automatically tissue macrophage deactivation. However, the monocytes' half-life in the blood is about 24 hours and the longer immunoparalysis is detectable in the blood, the more tissue macrophages are replaced by 'deactivated' monocytes. In fact, the duration of the immunoparalysis is inversely related to the outcome. Secondly, even in cases of monocyte deactivation we never observed complete blocking of TNF/IL-6 secretion explaining low-level cytokine levels in patients with persistent infection. Thirdly, and most importantly, IL-6 is not only produced by immune cells. It is also secreted by non-immune cells (endothelial cells, fibroblasts, keratinocytes, etc.), in response to inflammatory cytokines secreted by macrophages, but also directly following contact with LPS (via sCD14) or hypoxia. In other words, IL-6 is a marker of tissue injury independent of the situation in the monocyte/macrophage system (Fig. 4).

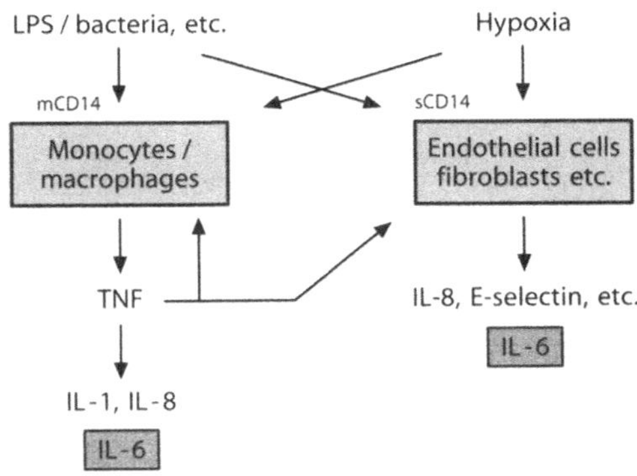

Fig. 4. Cellular sources of systemic IL-6 plasma levels

How Can We Restore the Immune Responsiveness?

If immunoparalysis is not only an epiphenomenon which is associated with an increased incidence of infectious complications in different patient populations and a poor outcome in septic patients, but in fact a causal relationship exists, recovery from immunodeficiency should be a novel therapeutic approach. The first evidence that this concept may be valid was obtained from the transplant population. In transplant patients, we monitor monocyte function (HLA-DR expression by flow cytometry, *ex vivo* TNF secretion by semiautomatic enzyme-linked immunosorbent assay [ELISA]) of patients with high-dose immunosuppression (induction therapy, anti-rejection therapy) two to three times per week. The development of signs of 'over-immunosuppression' (critical level: $<30\%$ HLA-DR^{+} monocytes and/or <300 pg/ml TNF secretion) is associated with a 7.5 times increased risk of developing infectious complications within the next two to three weeks [11]. Therefore, we then reduce the immunosuppression carefully and start to monitor procalcitonin and IL-6 plasma levels in order to detect ongoing systemic infection very early. If immunoparalysis is observed in transplant patients with established infections, immunosuppression is immediately tapered in order to prevent death by sepsis. With two exceptions in more than 100 cases during the last 10 years, we have never seen acute graft rejection as a result of tapering immunosuppression in patients with immunoparalysis which demonstrates the general immunodeficiency in these patients. In contrast, reduction of immunosuppression in infected transplant patients without immunoparalysis is frequently followed by acute rejection [10, 11].

In summary, the transplant data suggest that recovery of the inflammatory response is important for the control of bacterial/fungal infections and not harmful even in septic patients. These observations were the rationale for similar approaches in non-transplant septic patients (Fig. 5). *In vitro*, *ex vivo* and in experimental models, we could show that the monocytic activators IFN-γ and GM-CSF were able to restore the deactivation state [18, 19]. Moreover, we demonstrated in a pilot trial that IFN-γ can also reverse immunoparalysis in septic patients [4]. This was the first therapeutic approach in sepsis using immune monitoring parameters as a guideline for treatment. Nine septic patients with immunoparalysis

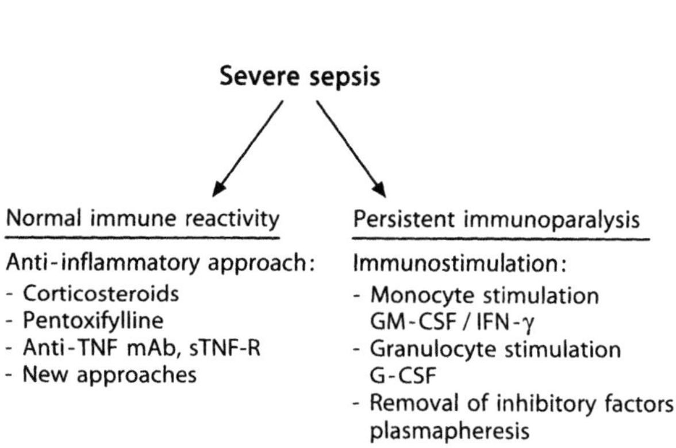

Fig. 5. Immune competence should determine the therapeutic approach in septic patients

for at least two days (HLA-DR$^+$ monocytes <30%) were treated every day with 100 μg/d IFN-γ subcutaneously. Treatment was continued until more than 50% of monocytes were HLA-DR$^+$ for three consecutive days (duration of treatment: Mean 6 days, range 4 to 11 days). Although IFN-γ dramatically increases LPS related mortality in experimental sepsis models, it was well tolerated by the patients with immunoparalysis, supporting our concept. Although kinetics and the level of the response was varied, monocyte recovery was observed in all nine patients. The slightly up-regulated TNF plasma levels (23 pg/ml peak level on day 4, vs. 4 pg/ml before therapy measured by the Quantikine™ ELISA [recognizing bioactive TNF]) reflected the restoration of monocyte function *in vivo* and indicated recovery of antimicrobial response. Eight of nine patients recovered from sepsis shortly after treatment; however, two of them relapsed at a later stage at a time when IFN-γ treatment was discontinued. In parallel, the MOF score improved significantly. This pilot trial was not designed to prove effects on mortality but the results were promising.

We are aware of at least two other groups (Paris, Mannheim) who have also treated septic patients with IFN-γ using similar inclusion criteria (immunoparalysis), with comparable promising results.

Several groups have reported on diminished granulocyte function in sepsis. Moreover, monocytes from patients with immunoparalysis also show a diminished G-CSF secretion (Zuckermann et al., unpublished data). As G-CSF is not only important for granulocytopoesis but also for the antimicrobial function and the survival time of mature granulocytes (Fig. 6), we wondered whether G-CSF application would be a therapeutic alternative in sepsis (Fig. 7). Twelve septic patients (abdominal/thoracic sepsis; three with acute respiratory distress syndrome [ARDS]) with immunoparalysis for at least two days were treated with G-CSF (3 × 300 μg) despite leukocytosis (mean 13000 cells/μl). No significant side effects were observed. Leukocyte counts increased up to 75000 cells/μl (mean 35000) in 10/12 patients. Nine of the patients recovered from sepsis. This was associated with a decrease in procalcitonin plasma levels (Zuckermann et al., unpublished data).

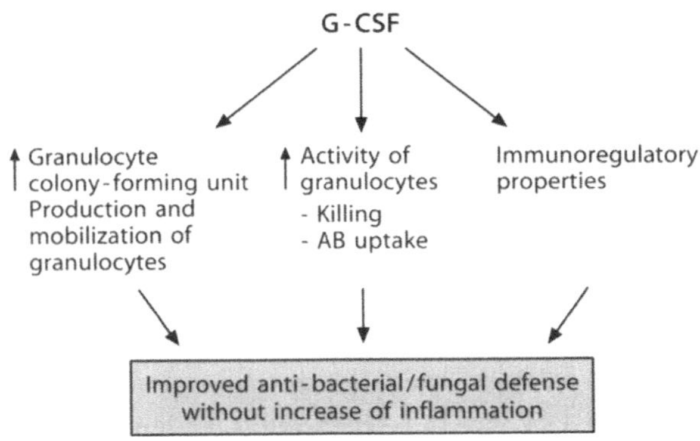

Fig. 6. Biological effects of granulocyte-colony stimulating factor (G-CSF)

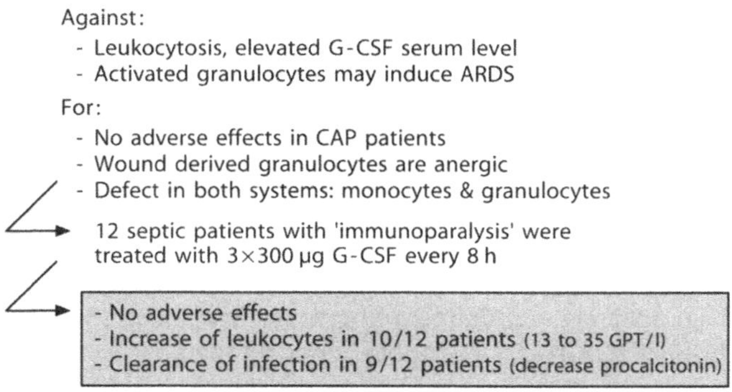

Fig. 7. Rationale for the administration of G-CSF in non-neutropenic septic patients

In another approach we tested the feasibility of plasmapheresis in septic patients with immunoparalysis. The rationale for this therapy is the removal of inhibitory factors from the plasma as dialysis seems to be insufficient for this approach. In this pilot trial, 76 septic patients (mostly with peritonitis as focus) with immunoparalysis for more than four days were included: 35 of them underwent plasmapheresis (3 × 4–5 l). Stable recovery of monocyte function was observed in 18/35 patients, 17 of them survived but none of the 17 non-responders. Overall mortality in this open label trial was 52% vs. 80% in the untreated group ($p<0.01$) [11, 20].

Conclusion

As our understanding of the pathogenesis of sepsis has advanced, we have come to realize that, like other organs, the immune system can also fail. Whereas the monitoring of other organ systems (kidney, liver, blood pressure, lung, coagulation, etc.), is well established on ICUs, monitoring of the immune system is still poorly developed. However, the immune response is essential for the control of infection. Moreover, the introduction of immunotherapeutic approaches in sepsis without immune monitoring has resulted in disappointing results.

Our data from several pilot trials suggest that immunostimulation in septic patients with defined 'immunoparalysis' may be a novel approach. However, controlled multicenter trials are necessary to confirm the hypothesis. In the past this aim was limited due to poor standardization of immune monitoring making multicenter trials very difficult, but recently a panel of immune parameters with high-quality standardization has been developed (Fig. 8). Immune competence can be measured by a standardized HLA-DR flow cytometric measurement (read-out: molecules/cell) and the semi-automatic *ex vivo* whole blood TNF secretion assay. Inflammation and tissue injury can be detected by measurement of plasma TNF and IL-6 levels using semiautomatic systems. Moreover, it has been

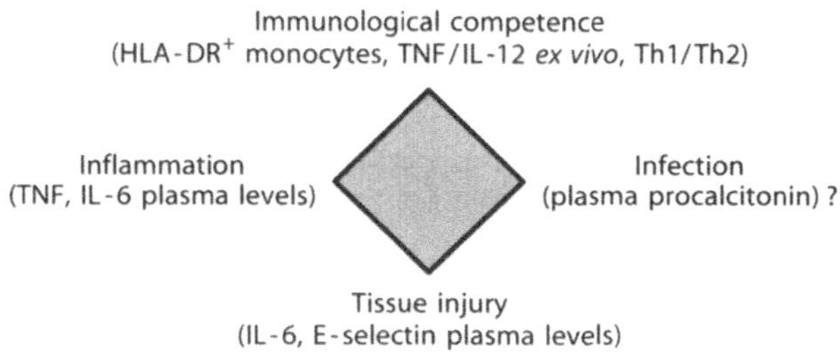

Fig. 8. Immune monitoring of ICU patients

shown in some studies that measurement of procalcitonin plasma levels is helpful for early detection of invasive bacterial/fungal infections [21].

In our opinion, preemptive therapy of high-risk patients would be an even better approach than treatment of established sepsis. Using measurement of immunocompetence (e.g., monocytic HLA-DR expression, whole blood TNF/IL-12 release) it is possible to detect patients who are at high risk of developing infective complications after major surgery and trauma as early as two to three days postoperatively. After initial down-regulation of the monocytic system which is seen in almost all patients after major surgery and trauma, immune function recovers in most patients. We believe that this early down-regulation of the inflammatory system, particularly via the stress axis, is of important biological significance in order to prevent over-reaction to injury and infection. In general, the patients recover from immune deactivation after trauma or major surgery within a few days. However, persistence of the immune deactivation for several days is associated with an increased risk of developing infective complications. For example, in neurosurgical patients on day two the predictive value is already >90% [13]. Therefore, it may be useless or even dangerous (over-reaction, autoimmunity) to prophylactically treat all patients with a putative risk of developing infective complications (e.g., after major surgery) with immunostimulatory approaches immediately after or even before the trauma. Using immune monitoring it should be possible to select high risk patients on day two or three who may benefit from preemptive immunostimulatory therapy. With the availability of standardized immune monitoring it should now be possible to design prospective clinical trials.

Acknowledgment. We would like to acknowledge the invaluable contribution of Dr. H. Zuckerman and Dr. W. Kox to the clinical work described in this chapter.

References

1. Natanson C, Hoffman WD, Suffredini AF, Eichacker PQ, Danner RL (1994) Selected treatment strategies for septic shock based on proposed mechanisms of pathogenesis. Ann Intern Med 120:771–783
2. Abraham E (1999) Cytokine neutralization: An overview. In: Marshall JC, Cohen J (eds) Immune response in the critically ill. Springer, Heidelberg, pp 385–392

3. Zeni F, Freeman B, Natanson C (1997) Anti-inflammatory therapies to treat sepsis and septic shock: a reassessment. Crit Care Med 25:1095-1100
4. Döcke WD, Randow F, Syrbe U, et al (1997) Monocyte deactivation in septic patients: restoration by IFN-γ treatment. Nature Med 3:678-681
5. Echtenacher B, Falk W, Mannel DN, Krammer PH (1990) Requirement of endogenous tumor necrosis factor/cachectin for recovery from experimental peritonitis. J Immunol 145: 3762-3766
6. Pfeffer K (1993) Mice deficient for the p55 kD tumor necrosis factor receptor are resistant to endotoxic shock, yet succumb to L. monocytogenes infection. Cell 73:457-467
7. Jack RS, Fan X, Bernbein M, et al (1997) Lipopolysaccaride binding protein is required to combat a murine gram-negative bacterial infection. Nature 389:742-745
8. Faist E, Angele MK, Zedler S (1999) Immunoregulation in shock, trauma and sepsis. In: Marshall JC, Cohen J (eds) Immune response in the critically ill. Springer, Heidelberg, pp 312-334
9. Calandra T, Heumann D (1999) Inhibitory cytokines. In: Marshall JC, Cohen J (eds) Immune response in the critically ill. Springer, Heidelberg, pp 67-83
10. Volk HD, Reinke P, Falck P, et al (1989) Diagnostic value of an immune monitoring program for the clinical management of immunosuppressed patients with septic complications. Clin Transplant 3:246-252
11. Döcke WD, Reinke P, Syrbe U, et al (1997) Immunoparalysis in sepsis - from phenomenon to treatment strategies. Tex Med 9:55-65
12. Randow F, Syrbe U, Meisel C, et al (1995) Mechanism of endotoxin desensitization - involvement of IL-10 and TGFβ. J Exp Med 5:1887-1892
13. Woiciechowsky Ch, Asadullah K, Nestler D, et al (1998) Sympathetic activation triggers systemic IL-10 release in immunodepression induced by brain injury. Nature Med 4:808-813
14. van Deventer SJH, Stokkers P (1999) Genomics of the sepsis syndrome. In: Marshall JC, Cohen J (eds) Immune response in the critically ill. Springer, Heidelberg, pp 22-36
15. Eskdale J, Gallagher G, Verweij CL, et al (1998) Interleukin 10 secretion in relation to human IL-10 locus haplotypes. Proc Natl Acad Sci USA 95:9465-9470
16. van Dissel J, van Langevelde P, Westendorp RG, Kwappenberg K, Frolich M (1998) Anti-inflammatory cytokine profile and mortality in febrile patients. Lancet 351:950-953
17. Asadulah K, Sterry W, Stephanek K, et al (1998) IL-10 is a key cytokine in psoriasis. Proof of principle by IL-10 therapy: a new therapeutic approach. J Clin Invest 101:1-12
18. Randow F, Döcke WD, Bundschuh D, et al (1997) In vitro prevention and reversal of LPS desensitization by IFN-γ, IL-12, and GM-CSF. J Immunol 158:2911-2918
19. Bundschuh D, Barsig J, Hartung T, et al (1997) GM-CSF and interferon-gamma restore the systemic TNF-alpha response to endotoxin in lipopolysaccaride-desensitized mice. J Immunol 158:2862-2871
20. Reinke P (1996) Plasmapheresis in the therapy of septic disease. Int J Artif Organs 19: 127-128
21. de Werra I, Jaccard C, Corradin SB, et al (1997) Cytokines, nitrite/nitrate, soluble TNF receptors, and procalcitonin concentrations: comparison in patients with septic shock, cardiogenic shock, and bacterial pneumonia. Crit Care Med 25:607-613

Prospects for a Vaccine to Prevent Bacterial Sepsis

S. M. Opal

Introduction

The development of vaccines against common bacterial diseases has been the ultimate goal of medical researchers since the first recognition of microbial pathogens as a cause of human disease in the late 19th century. Some vaccines against bacterial exotoxins have been remarkably successful (e.g., the tetanus toxoid vaccine and diphtheria toxoid vaccine). Tetanus and diphtheria have been virtually eliminated from developed countries largely as the result of universal immunization policies. Other bacterial vaccines directed against specific microbial pathogens (e.g., *Vibrio cholerae, M. tuberculosis, S. pneumoniae*) have been less successful; nonetheless, they have made a significant impact on the morbidity and mortality related to these bacterial pathogens worldwide [1].

Unfortunately, bacterial vaccines that protect patients from the adverse sequelae of systemic microbial infections complicated by septic shock have not yet been developed. Considerable time and effort continues to be expended in an attempt to develop such vaccines. The challenges presented in the successful development of an anti-sepsis vaccine are daunting but not insurmountable. There are a relatively limited number of microbial mediators that are thought to play a major role in the pathophysiology of septic shock. It may be feasible to develop a vaccine against these principal microbial mediators and disrupt the molecular pathogenesis of the septic process [2].

This chapter examines the current status of active immunization strategies in the prevention and treatment of bacterial sepsis. Progress is being made on several fronts of vaccine development, and it is anticipated that clinical trials with active immunization protocols against bacterial sepsis will be initiated within the next few years. Despite recent disappointments with immunotherapies in the treatment of septic shock [3], immunoprophylaxis with active vaccine strategies continues to hold promise as a means of prevention and treatment of the early phases of bacterial sepsis. The therapeutic rationale of bacterial vaccines and sequence of developmental milestones that must be attained in the successful clinical development of a vaccine against sepsis will be the focus of this chapter.

Prerequisites for an Effective Anti-Sepsis Vaccine

Many critical questions must be addressed before a candidate vaccine strategy against the bacterial pathogens responsible for sepsis can be seriously contemplated. The fact that bacterial sepsis is caused by a multitude of different microbial pathogens complicates, but does not eliminate, the possibility that an anti-sepsis vaccine could be developed. Answers to the following sequence of essential questions must be found before an anti-sepsis vaccine becomes a viable candidate for clinical testing in humans.

1) Basic Immunobiology Questions:
   What are the common microbial mediators that are central to the pathogenesis of septic shock? What are the relevant epitopes that could serve as potential vaccine components from these microbial mediators? Does the naturally-acquired disease process itself (septic shock) provide survivors with long lasting, natural immunity (i.e., does a protective immune response develop in animals [or humans] after an episode of bacterial sepsis)? What is the nature of the cellular and humoral immune response to the microbial pathogens that induce sepsis?
2) Basic Clinical Immunology Questions:
   Some additional fundamental vaccine research questions need to be answered before endeavoring to develop a vaccine approach to bacterial pathogens. Does the passive transfer of serum or cells from animals that have survived a septic challenge protect naive animals from an otherwise lethal challenge of the microbial pathogen (i.e., is it possible to provide protection through passive immunization)? Is it possible to develop a vaccine that retains its immunogenicity yet is rendered non-reactogenic (i.e., generation of protective antibody response without causing disease or toxicity in vaccine recipients)?
3) Clinical Immunology and Trial Design Questions:
   Even after a basic understanding of the immune response to sepsis has been formulated, and potential vaccines for sepsis have been developed, major hurdles would remain before a potential vaccine could be put to clinical use. Further pre-clinical and clinical evaluations must be undertaken to answer questions relating to vaccine efficacy and safety in a clinical setting. These are critical milestones to reach before large scale vaccine trials are undertaken. Is it possible to immunize naive animals (or patients) with a vaccine and generate high titers of protective antibodies against microbial mediators of sepsis? Is it possible to protect vaccine recipients (both animal models and human volunteers) from a subsequent septic challenge? Is it possible to define a patient population that has a sufficiently high frequency of sepsis to perform an adequately controlled clinical trial? Is it possible to demonstrate efficacy and confirm safety in human volunteers of a candidate vaccine? What would be the duration, relative efficacy, and limitations of an anti-sepsis vaccine strategy in actual clinical medicine?

The Overall Vaccine Strategy

The intrinsic complexities of human sepsis make it inevitable that a vaccine strategy against bacterial sepsis will not be a simple, single component vaccine. It is quite likely that a multi-component vaccine will be necessary in order to achieve efficacy against a wide variety of invasive microbial pathogens and potent microbial mediators. Despite all the obstacles inherent in the process of vaccine development for such an unpredictable and heterogeneous disorder as sepsis, an active immunization strategy continues to be an active preventative and therapeutic approach to sepsis. The ever increasing incidence of sepsis [4], progressive development of antimicrobial resistance among common bacterial pathogens [5], and limited therapeutic options currently available to treat sepsis [3, 6] provides the impetus for current anti-sepsis vaccine approaches.

Microbial mediators that have been identified as inducers of human bacterial sepsis are all potential targets for vaccine development. Candidate vaccine targets

Table 1. Microbial mediators of bacterial sepsis as vaccine targets

Mediators	Advantages	Disadvantages
Core glycolipid endotoxin structure [3, 6, 8, 14, 16]	Major mediator, advanced vaccine development	Not highly immunogenic, not effective in Gram-positive sepsis
O Antigens of bacterial endotoxin [7, 12, 15]	Highly immunogenic, limited number of serotypes respon-sible for sepsis	Polyvalent vaccine approach, opsonic but not anti-toxic, not effective in Gram-positive sepsis
Bacterial superantigens [19–22]	Highly protective immune response	Serotype specific, only effective in a sub-group of septic patients
Peptidoglycan [23–25]	Common to both Gram-negative and Gram-positive bacteria	Relevant epitopes not yet defined, protective efficacy unproven
Lipoteichoic acid [24, 26]	Immunogenic, structure is well defined	Only effective in a sub-group of septic patients, protective efficacy unproven
Unmethylated CpG motifs of bacterial DNA [27, 28]	Highly inflammatory to human immune system	Immunogenicity not yet demonstrated, cross reactions with human DNA
Bacterial exotoxins (alpha toxin, Pseudomonas exotoxin A, phospholipase, etc.) [3, 6, 8]	Highly immunogenic, virulence factors for specific pathogens	Only effective in a small sub-group of septic patients
Polysaccharide capsular antigens, outer membrane proteins [6]	Immunogenic, important virulence factors	Multiple serotypes, lack of cross protection

for an active immunization program against sepsis include endotoxin [3, 6–18], bacterial superantigens [19–22], peptidoglycan [23–25], lipoteichoic acid [24, 26], bacterial desoxyribonucleic acid (DNA) [27, 28] and other microbial mediators [3, 6, 8, 24] (Table 1). The summary of the potential advantages and disadvantages of a vaccine approach to bacterial sepsis are listed in Table 2.

In addition to all the potential problems with vaccine development listed above, it is clear that a preventive vaccine for sepsis will need to have an excellent safety profile. If such a vaccine is to be of practical clinical utility, it must be well tolerated and readily administered to a wide variety of compromised patients.

The risk/benefit ratio with a vaccine of uncertain benefit for a low frequency event (sepsis) that may occur some time in the future dictates that the vaccine possess little or no risk to the recipient. A poorly tolerated vaccine with frequent side effects will clearly not be acceptable. The most highly developed vaccines under current clinical development are anti-endotoxin vaccines and vaccines against bacterial superantigens. Both of these vaccine programs are considered separately in the sections that follow.

The Anti-Endotoxin Vaccine Approach

Most of the pathophysiologic consequences of Gram-negative sepsis can be reproduced by administration of purified lipopolysaccharide (LPS) or cell wall fragments for the outer membrane of non-viable Gram-negative bacteria [11, 14, 18]. The widely held belief that endotoxin is the principal mediator of bacterial sepsis remains a likely, yet unproved, hypothesis at the present time [29, 30]. It will be necessary to demonstrate that specific anti-endotoxin agents actually improve the outcome in patients with Gram-negative bacterial sepsis to prove that endotoxin is a key mediator in human sepsis. There are a number of agents currently under development that should be able to conclusively demonstrate the central role of endotoxin in the pathophysiology of human sepsis [14].

There has been an explosion of new information over the last several years regarding the interactions of LPS with proteins and immune effector cells [18,

Table 2. Vaccines against bacterial sepsis

Advantages	Disadvantages
1. Specifically targets microbial pathogens	1. Wide variety of microbial pathogens
2. Avoids inherent risk of immunomodulation of the human immune response	2. Target population for vaccine is difficult to identify
3. May be effective as a preventative strategy	3. Level of protection and duration of immunity not defined
4. Antibodies present in the early phases of sepsis when intervention most effective	4. May not be effective in immuno-compromised patients
5. Complements antibiotic therapy against bacterial pathogens	5. May not be effective in un-immunized trauma patients

30–33]. Blocking sepsis at the bacterial toxin level is appealing because it is a precipitating upstream event, so that the deleterious secondary host-derived inflammatory networks of sepsis will not be activated. A variety of anti-endotoxin strategies have been proposed. A vaccine strategy is only one of a number of novel anti-sepsis agents under consideration at the present time [14].

The Structure and Function of Endotoxin

The biochemistry of bacterial endotoxin reveals that it is a complex, polar macromolecule consisting of three basic components:

1) a highly conserved lipid A structure that is principally responsible for its endotoxic properties;
2) a relatively conserved yet variable core oligosaccharide region covalently linked to lipid A;
3) repeating units of distinct polysaccharide molecules (the O side chain).

The lipid A portion of the molecule is a highly conserved structure that consists of a diphosphorylated β1–6 linked diglucosamine backbone structure with six acyl groups linked by ester or amide bonds. Most pathogenic Gram-negative organisms have 12–14 carbon atom fatty acids (lauric or myristic acid) linked to the diglucosamine nucleus [13, 18, 29].

The Immunology and Biochemistry of Lipid A: Lipid A biosynthesis is a highly complex synthetic process performed by Gram-negative bacteria. Lipid A is an essential component of outer membrane structure and physiology. Inhibition of lipid A biosynthesis is lethal to Gram-negative bacteria [18]. Lipid A is an amphophilic molecule that forms supramolecular aggregates in aqueous solution. Recent evidence suggests that a unique 3-dimensional 'endotoxic conformation' needs to be maintained in order to fully express endotoxin activity of the lipid A component of bacterial endotoxin [13, 18]. Monomeric, diphosphorylated lipid A has a hexagonal three dimensional structure and is the most biologically active. Monophosphorylated or membrane bound lipid A is often found in a lamellar three dimensional structure that is intrinsically less biologically active.

While lipid A is the toxic moiety of bacterial endotoxin, it is immunorecessive with respect to the immunogenicity of bacterial endotoxin. Lipid A is buried deep into the substance of the outer membrane and is not surface exposed and available to circulating antibodies. This has proven to be a major impediment to vaccine development against this common, highly conserved, and toxic portion of the LPS molecule [9, 10, 29, 30].

Two anti-lipid A monoclonal antibodies have undergone extensive clinical testing over the past decade [34–37]. Neither antibody possessed high affinity binding to endotoxin and neither proved to be effective in large, multi-center Phase 3 trials. One antibody appeared to bind to autoantigens on red blood cells and B cells [38] and actually worsened the mortality rate in a canine sepsis model [39]. Lipid A is not the focus of current vaccine efforts.

The Immunology and Biochemistry of the Core Oligosaccharide: Lipid A is covalently linked to a oligosaccharide core structure which consists of both inner and outer core components. This oligosaccharide component combined with lipid A is known as the core glycolipid structure[18]. The oligosaccharides found in this region of the molecule are the major focus of vaccine development. This region is highly immunogenic, reasonably well preserved, and common among many Gram-negative bacterial species [3, 30, 40]. The inner core region consists of ketodeoxyoctonate (KDO) linked to a small series of unique heptose sugars. The inner core is attached to a more variable group of hexose sugars (the outer core structure). There is microheterogeneity of these outer core hexose molecules. There are five different core types among *E. coli* strains and one major core type in *Salmonella* species [18]. Monoclonal antibodies have been derived which bind to unique core types among Gram-negative bacteria [9–11, 18].

Since the initial discovery of common antigenic components among endotoxin structures from different Gram-negative bacterial species, it was hypothesized that antibodies generated in response to this common antigen could protect against endotoxin-mediated pathophysiologic events [41–45]. This seemingly simple and testable hypothesis has proven to be rather difficult to confirm or refute [9, 29, 30, 46]. Evidence that such antibodies could be exploited to prevent septic shock and other deleterious effects of systemic endotoxin release comes from a number of laboratory and clinical studies. Anti-core antibodies have been shown to prevent endotoxin-mediated lethality in a number of animal studies [9]. Elevated serum antibody titers against the core glycolipid of endotoxin has been associated with a lower incidence of mortality from *P. aeruginosa* sepsis [47], and morbidity following major surgery [48, 49].

Despite these findings, the protective efficacy of core glycolipid antibodies as a prevention or treatment of sepsis remains unproved [29, 30]. Earlier clinical studies with polyclonal antisera directed against the common core structures of endotoxin have been mired in controversy [30, 50, 51]. Monoclonal antibodies have recently been discovered which will cross react with multiple different species and genera of Gram-negative bacteria. These monoclonal antibodies support the hypothesis that core glycolipid structures among Gram-negative bacteria may serve as a potential vaccine to generate a cross protective antibody response [14, 18, 40].

The best known core glycolipid structure is expressed by the galactose epimerase mutant of *E. coli* 0111:B4. This mutant, known as *E. coli* J5 is unique among the LPS as its inner core structure and lipid A molecule are highly exposed and immunogenic [9, 17, 50]. This mutant expresses a core glycolipid structure that is functionally a Rc mutant form of rough LPS. The core structure consists only of three unusual heptose molecules and a terminal alpha 1–7 linked D-glucosamine and an alpha 1–3 linked glucose moiety on the second heptose molecule [16, 18].

Another commonly used core structure is the Re mutant of *Salmonella minnesota* [44, 45]. This molecule consists only of lipid A and KDO (the Re mutant). Unfortunately, most of the antibodies that are raised in response to the core glycolipid structure are directed against the KDO molecule [18]. This molecule is not available for antibody binding with smooth LPS structures that contain complete core structure and O specific side chains. Since most invasive Gram-negative bacteria express smooth LPS, such antibodies will not bind to pathogenic Gram-negative bacteria and predictably would not be effective in actual septic states [18, 29].

However, other monoclonal antibodies have been defined (mAb SDZ 219-800) that bind to the core oligosaccharide structure of bacterial endotoxin of multiple species and genera of Gram-negative bacteria [40]. This IgG antibody is able to bind to smooth LPS with O side chains in place. This indicates that the O side chains do not sterically inhibit the binding of this antibody. This allows the antibody to bind to native LPS structures found in most pathogenic microorganisms. This antibody binds to the lateral segment of the core region at the junction of the inner and outer core. The minimal structure that this antibody will bind is the core structure presented by *E. coli* J5 (Rc) [18, 40].

Additional support for the potential efficacy of the protective anti-core glycolipid hypothesis comes from a recent series of studies using purified LPS from the rough mutant bacteria, *E. coli* J5. Bhattacharjee and colleagues prepared affinity purified, J5 LPS specific IgG from antisera raised to *E. coli* J5 using a solid phase matrix to which J5 LPS had been coupled. This IgG preparation (as well as the parent antisera preparations) protected neutropenic rats against a lethal infection with *P. aeruginosa* [52]. It appears that there are critical conformational epitopes at the core region of the glycolipid structure of LPS which may cross react with other LPS serotypes of other enteric bacteria. The major challenge in vaccine development is to present these conformational epitopes in a fashion which will generate the production of these protective anti-core glycolipid antibodies [3, 11, 16, 53].

The Immunology and Biochemistry of the Polysaccharide Structure of Endotoxin: The O polysaccharide of bacterial endotoxin consists of repeating units of distinct high molecular weight polymers formed by multiple repeating oligosaccharide structures. These are serotype-specific polysaccharide structures that define the serotype of the somatic O antigens of Gram-negative bacteria. Antibodies to these polysaccharide structures generate highly protective immune responses to subsequent challenge in experimental animals [9, 54]. Unfortunately, these are serotype-specific antibody responses and no cross protection is generated against other serotypes. Since there are several hundred serotypes of pathogenic Gram-negative bacteria, this has limited the use of polysaccharide antigens as a vaccine approach.

However, careful analyses by Cross and colleagues have demonstrated that a relatively limited number of serotypes are primarily responsible for Gram-negative bacteremia in humans [7, 14, 15]. This situation is somewhat analogous to the limited number of polysaccharide capsular antigens found in bacteremic isolates of *Streptococcus pneumoniae* and forms the basis of the pneumococcal vaccine [55]. As a result of these investigations, an attempt has been made to develop a polyclonal anti-O-specific antibody approach to bacterial sepsis. These O specific antibodies are opsonophagocytic, but not anti-endotoxic. They promote rapid phagocytosis and clearance of Gram-negative bacterial pathogens but do not intrinsically inhibit the ability of endotoxin to activate host-derived immune mediators [54].

A hyperimmune serum consisting of the 23 most common capsular polysaccharides in clinical isolates of *Klebsiella*, eight O serotypes of *Pseudomonas aeruginosa* and 12 O serotypes of *E. coli* has been tested in humans. A large Veteran's Administration cooperative study [7] was undertaken to analyze the protective activity of this passive immunotherapeutic strategy. While the study failed to demonstrate an overall improvement in survival from bacterial sepsis, it did demonstrate that there appeared to be a reduction in the incidence of serotype-specific Gram-negative infections.

Interestingly, it was observed that active immunization of a vaccine which contained 24 capsular antigens of *Klebsiella* and 8 O polysaccharide antigens of *Pseudomonas aeruginosa* in victims of severe trauma resulted in high level antibody responses. It was observed that antibody responses were similar to those observed in normal volunteers [15]. While antigen processing by macrophages may be adversely affected by trauma, Th2-type cytokine responses induced by trauma (i.e., interleukin [IL]-4, IL-10, and IL-13) promote a humoral antibody response [15]. Trauma patients may yet be candidates for active immunization with an anti-endotoxin vaccine. The sepsis-related mortality observed in severe trauma may occur weeks to months after the initial injury [2, 3, 6]. This time course should provide a 'window of opportunity' in which to initiate an active immunization strategy against endotoxin in trauma patients.

The Anti-Core Glycolipid Vaccine Strategy

Careful analysis of the immunologic response to the core glycolipid structure of bacterial endotoxin has allowed for the development of a candidate anti-core glycolipid vaccine. Once the target epitope of the core structure was defined, it was apparent that a candidate vaccine would need to be safe and well tolerated. It was mandatory to first detoxify the endotoxic properties of bacterial endotoxin. Severe vaccine reactions related to the endotoxin components of the vaccine would be clearly unacceptable as a preventative vaccine approach.

The endotoxin molecule was first de-O-acylated by mild alkali hydrolysis to cleave off ester linked C-12 and C-14 fatty acids. This detoxification step removes the endotoxicity of the macromolecule yet preserves the essential immunogenic epitopes of the core region of the molecule. The detoxified LPS structure was then complexed with the outer membrane protein (OMP) of group B *Neisseria meningitidis*. This step was taken to increase the immune response to the critical conformational epitopes of the core region of detoxified LPS [3, 16].

Our group has previously demonstrated that a vaccine consisting of detoxified J5 LPS alone, or conjugated with a protein carrier, elicited only a 2–10 fold rise in anti-core glycolipid antibody responses and failed to provide significant protection in animal sepsis models [3]. Linkage of the detoxified J5 LPS with the OMP of *N. meningitidis* resulted in a 100–1000 fold greater antibody response in the core glycolipid structure [53]. This non-covalent complex with the OMP and detoxified J5 LPS was highly soluble and stable in aqueous solutions. The complex expresses a critical conformational epitope of the core oligosaccharide of J5 LPS

Table 3. Binding of dLPS J5-OMP vaccine-induced antibodies to whole bacterial (% binding by fluoresence-activated cell sorting analysis)*

Bacterial Strain	Pre-Immune IgG	Post-Immune IgG
E. coli	0	18.4
Pseudomonas aeruginosa	3.4	35.0
Enterobacter cloacae	2.2	55.0
Enterobacter aerogenes	3.4	41.7
Klebsiella pneumoniae	37.4	95.3
Staphylococcus aureus	6.7	1.4

* Bacteria were exposed to an antibiotic (imipenem) and then treated with rabbit sera prior to (pre-immune) or following (post-immune) vaccination and then coated with FITC-labeled goat anti-rabbit IgG. (See reference [53] for details of assay).

that remains cryptic and unavailable for antibody binding with covalent linker protein constructs. The vaccine induces the formation of anti-core glycolipid antibodies that cross react with a wide variety of pathogenic Gram-negative bacteria and provides protection from lethal Gram-negative sepsis in animal models [17]. This vaccine predictably fails to induce antibodies that can recognize cell wall antigens found on Gram-positive bacterial pathogens (Table 3) [53]. This vaccine material is now undergoing phase I testing in human volunteers.

Vaccine Approaches to Bacterial Superantigens

The pyrogenic exotoxins of Group A streptococci (SPEs) and the enterotoxins of *Staphylococcus aureus* are a family of structurally related bacterial exotoxins that share similar immunologic properties [56, 57]. They have the capacity to stimulate CD4, CD8 and γδ T cells by an unusual mechanism (Fig. 1). They bind to the variable region of specific β chains (Vβ) of the T cell receptor (TCR) adjacent to the usual epitope recognition site. They simultaneously bind to the lateral surface of the class II major histocompatibility complex (MHC) of antigen presenting cells. This binding site is adjacent to the specific antigenic groove that makes up the normal antigen presenting motif of the MHC class II structure. This results in aberrant activation and proliferation of an unusually large subset of T-cells [56].

Activation of the monocyte/macrophage cell lines by superantigens results in the concomitant release of pro-inflammatory cytokines from both the T lymphocyte and monocyte populations. The crosslinking of TCR and MHC-II molecules by superantigens leads to profound blastogenesis of lymphocytes and antigen presenting cells. The resulting stimulation of leukocytes leads to a significant increase in cytokine production [56–60].

Inflammatory cells stimulated with bacterial superantigens produce the Th1 cytokines IL-2 and interferon (IFN)-γ along with the anti-inflammatory cytokine IL-10 [59, 61], while monocytes activated by superantigen stimulation produce IL-12 [62]. Mixed cultures of peripheral blood mononuclear cells containing lym-

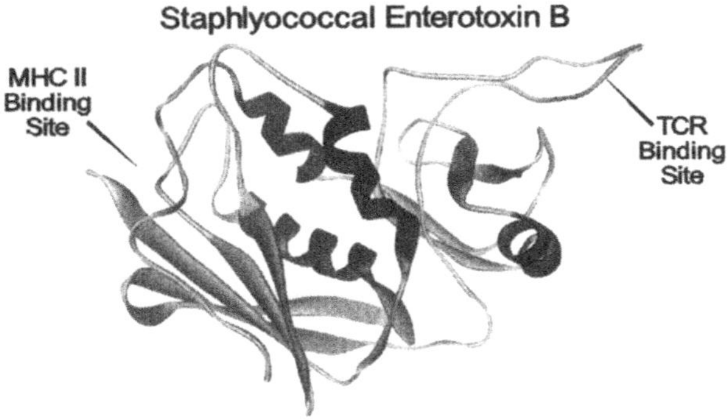

Fig. 1. The three dimensional structure of a bacterial superantigen: Staphylococcal enterotoxin B (obtained from the Brookhaven National laboratory datafiles). Note the compact structure with a central helical core region. The MHC II binding site is located on the amino terminal region of the toxin while the Vβ binding region of the T cell receptor is located on the C-terminal side of the molecule

phocytes and antigen presenting cells generate a wide range of inflammatory cytokines in significant amounts. Monocyte cytokines IL-1, IL-6, and tumor necrosis factor (TNF)-α were dependent on the presence of T cells [63].

Co-stimulatory molecules that participate in conventional immune responses play a significant role in the response of immune cells to superantigens as well (Fig. 2). The co-stimulatory T-cell antigen, CD28, and its corresponding ligand on MHC-II bearing cells, B7, contribute to superantigen mitogenicity [64, 65]. Other co-stimulatory molecules, such as LFA-1/ICAM-1 (lymphocyte function associated-1/intercellular adhesion molecule-1) and VLA-4/VCAM-1 (very late antigen-4/vascular cell adhesion molecule-1) also contribute to the activation of im-

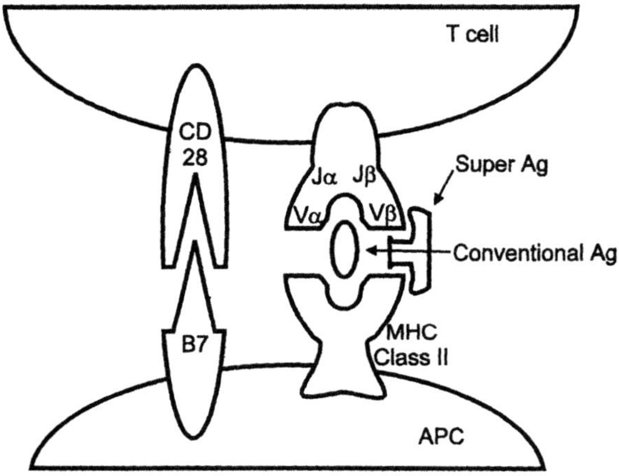

Fig. 2. A schematic representation of the interactions between the T cell receptor (TCR), antigen presenting cell (APC) and bacterial superantigen. Accessory signals provided by B7 antigens on APCs are essential for the full expression of superantigen-induced pro-inflammatory cytokine generation. The superantigen binds to a region adjacent to the epitope presenting groove for conventional antigens and activates T cells via the Vβ region of the TCR complex

mune cells by superantigens [66]. These immunostimulatory activities of superantigens are central to their pathophysiologic effects in humans. This excessive activation of the immune system may culminate in such severe consequences that septic shock may result [56, 59, 60].

The physiologic response to superantigens is similar to septic shock induced by bacterial endotoxin produced by Gram-negative organisms. In fact, LPS and superantigens can work synergistically to produce lethal toxic shock [67, 68]. Toxic shock syndrome can be exacerbated by the synergistic effects of toxic shock syndrome toxin-1 (TSST-1) with the staphylococcal enterotoxin (SE)/ streptococcal pyrogenic exotoxin (SPE) family of toxins [58, 69].

Structure-Function Relationships of the Superantigens

Staphylococcal exotoxins that function as superantigens cause a variety of syndromes in humans. These exotoxins were first recognized in staphylococcal food poisoning [56, 57]. It was subsequently shown that the same toxins induced proinflammatory cytokines and produced toxic shock-like syndromes [59, 60]. The gene sequences and corresponding primary amino acid sequences of at least seven staphylococcal enterotoxins have been described: SEA-SEE and SEH [56, 70].

The SPEs are responsible for the pathogenesis of scarlet fever and streptococcal toxic shock-like syndrome (i.e., toxic strep syndrome) [59, 60]. The sequences of the SPEs have many structural similarities to the staphylococcal enterotoxins [71–73].

TSST-1 from *Staph. aureus* is a potent superantigen; however, amino acid sequences of this toxin differ significantly from those of SEs and SPEs [74]. Despite the differences in primary amino acid sequence, the overall topology of TSST-1 and the SE/SPE family of exotoxins is similar [19, 20, 75]. All the bacterial superantigens are soluble proteins of approximately 230 amino acids and have a central disulfide loop, except for TSST-1 which has only 194 amino acids and lacks a disulfide bridge [76] (Fig. 1).

Mutational analysis reveals that mutations at various positions throughout the SPEA and SEB molecules are sufficient to inactivate biological activity [77, 78]. Mutations at various points have different effects, indicating that functional activities are not attributable to any one region of the toxins [79]. A functional tertiary structure must be maintained. Chemical modifications of highly conserved histidine residues inactivated biologic activity [80].

The central disulfide loop is required for mitogenic activity of staphylococcal enterotoxins SEA and SEB. Reduction of the disulfide loop inactivated T cell stimulatory activity, but did not affect MHC-II binding and stimulation of monocytes [22, 81]. Peptide cleavages within the loop had no effect on T-cell mitogenicity; however cleavage of conserved sequences outside the loop of SEA resulted in loss of mitogenic activity [81].

The loop and conserved adjacent sequences bind to the TCR, and do not contribute to the specificity of toxins for a particular Vβ type [77]. Residues determining TCR Vβ specificity appear to be located within the carboxyl-terminus of the SE/SPE toxins [22, 82], while residues critical for MHC-II binding are located in the amino-terminal region, and the central portion of the molecule near the disulfide loop [22, 83]. The disulfide loop and adjacent highly conserved sequences contribute to the structural integrity of the toxins, and serve to bring the TCR and MHC binding regions in functional proximity to each other [20, 76]. The variable sequences in the TCR binding region and the MHC-II binding regions account for different specificities for specific Vβ molecules and MHC-II types for each unique superantigen [84].

The Immune Response to Common Antigenic Components in Superantigens

Two distinct regions of the SE/SPE toxins have been identified which share highly conserved amino acid homology. The first consensus region begins immediately after the carboxyl side of the cysteine loop. Sequence homology in this region has been identified in all of the staphylococcal enterotoxins and streptococcal pyrogenic exotoxins, but not in TSST-1 [85].

The second consensus region sequence (K-x(2)-(LIV)-x(4)-(LIV)-D-x(3)-R-x(2)-L-x(5)-(LIV)-Y) has been identified in all of the staphylococcal enterotoxins, streptococcal pyrogenic exotoxins, and TSST-1. The conserved regions are separated by roughly thirty residues. The second consensus region has been shown to be functionally important for the activity of at least two SEs [85, 86]. The high degree of sequence homology in these regions contributes to the immunologic cross reactivity shared by many members of the SE/SPE family [87, 88]. These highly conserved regions may serve as a substrate for the development of therapeutic measures against these superantigens [85, 89].

Recent laboratory investigations suggest that specific immunoglobulins directed against the conserved regions of the SE/SPE toxins might prove an effective therapeutic approach [85]. Peptides constructed of the combined consensus regions of the toxins have been used to raise antibodies in mice. These antibodies inhibited blastogenesis of human mononuclear cells to various superantigens. Passive protection of immune serum in rabbits to SEB and SPEA challenge was also demonstrated.

Experimental evidence for the beneficial effects of intravenous immunoglobulin (IVIG) in superantigenic shock appears promising [90–92]. There is considerable experimental evidence that the adverse cytokine response stimulated by superantigens can be down-regulated by the use of IVIG. Human plasma from patients treated with IVIG can inactivate the mitogenic effects of SE/SPEs [93, 94]. There are anecdotal reports of the beneficial effects of this therapy in human patients. The practical value of IVIG therapy in human sepsis and superantigen-induced toxic shock patients is still debated [95]. Well controlled, multicenter clinical studies are needed to fully evaluate the efficacy of this therapy.

The use of peptide derived vaccines to develop anti-toxin antibodies against critical epitopes found within superantigen structures is the focus of current research efforts. Whether such a strategy will prove to be beneficial in the clinical setting remains to be seen. It is worth pointing out that in an experimental model of fasciitis, an active vaccine against one streptococcal superantigen (SPEA) actually worsened outcome. It is possible that the administration of a superantigen as a vaccine strategy may lead to clonal deletion of relevant Vβ specific T cells and this can result in T cell anergy to subsequent microbial challenge with a SPEA-producing strain of *S. pyogenes* [96]. Potential immune-mediated toxicity of candidate anti-sepsis vaccines will need to be fully investigated before clinical trials can begin.

Conclusion

Septic shock is the result of a deleterious, generalized host immune response to microbial mediators. Viewed in this context, septic shock is essentially a toxigenic illness. Antibody strategies designed to inhibit the toxin properties of microbial toxins remain a viable therapeutic approach in the prevention and treatment of sepsis. While a formidable number of challenges persist in the development of an anti-sepsis vaccine, recent advances in the molecular structure and basic immunology of bacterial toxins have provided new insights into vaccine development against sepsis.

Critical epitopes that are essential to the action of microbial toxins have been identified that may serve as vaccine targets. Clinical investigations employing an active immunization approach to sepsis are anticipated in the near future. The goal of this research is to prevent the deleterious consequences of uncontrolled immune activation in susceptible patients at greatest risk of sepsis.

References

1. Hayden GF, Sato PA, Wright PF, et al (1989) Progress in worldwide control and elimination of disease through immunization. J Pediatrics 114:520–527
2. Zeni F, Freeman B, Natanson C (1997) Anti-inflammatory therapies to treat sepsis and septic shock: a reassessment. Crit Care Med 25:1059–1100
3. Bhattacharjee AK, Cross AS (1999) Vaccines and antibodies in the prevention and treatment of sepsis. Infect Dis Clin North Am 13:285–297
4. Brun-Buisson C, Doyon F, Carlet J, et al (1995) Incidence, risk factors, and outcome of severe sepsis and septic shock in adults: a multicenter, prospective study in intensive care units. JAMA 274:968–974
5. Flaherty JP, Weinstein RA (1996) Nosocomial infections caused by antibiotic-resistant organisms in the intensive care unit. Infect Control Hosp Epidemiol 17:236–248
6. Opal SM (1998) Sepsis. Sci Am Med 30:1–17
7. Donta ST, Paduzzi P, Cross AS, et al (1996) Immunoprophylaxis against *Klebsiella* and *Pseudomonas aeruginosa* infections. J Infect Dis 174:537–543
8. Goldie AS, Fearon KCH, Ross JA, et al (1995) Natural cytokine antagonists and endogenous antiendotoxin core antibodies in sepsis syndrome. JAMA 274:172–177
9. Hustinx WNM, Kraaijeveld K, Hoepelman AIM, et al (1997) Cross protection by anti-core glycolipid antibodies: evidence from animal experiments. J Antimicrob Chemother 40:475–486
10. Lugowski C, Niedziela TN, Jachymek W (1996) Anti-endotoxin antibodies directed against *Escherichia coli* R1 oligosaccharide core-tetanus toxoid conjugate bind to smooth, live bacteria and smooth lipopolysaccharides and attenuate their tumor necrosis factor stimulating activity. FEMS Immunol Med Microbiol 16:31–39

11. Muller-Loennies S, Holst O, Brade H (1994) Chemical structure of the core region of *Escherichia coli* J5 lipopolysaccharide. Eur J Biochem 224:751–759
12. Bailat S, Heummann D, LeRoy D, et al (1997) Similarities and disparities between core-specific and O-side chain-specific antilipopolysaccharide monoclonal antibodies in models of endotoxemia and bacteremia in mice. Infect Immun 65:811–814
13. Rietschel ET, Schletter J, Weidemann B, et al (1998) Lipopolysaccaride and peptidoglycan: CD14-dependent bacterial inducers of inflammation. Microb Drug Resist 1:37–44
14. Opal SM, Yu RL Jr. (1998) Antiendotoxin strategies for the prevention and treatment of septic shock. Drugs 55: 497–508
15. Campbell WN, Hendrix, E, Cryz S Jr, Cross AS (1996) Immunogenicity of a 24-valent Klebsiella capsular polysaccharide vaccine and an eight-valent Pseudomonas O-polysaccharide conjugate vaccine administered to victims of severe trauma. Clin Infect Dis 23; 179–181
16. Bhattacharjee AK, Cross AS Opal, et al (1996) New trends in *Escherichia coli* O111: B4 J5 mutant (Rc chemotype) vaccine development for use in Gram-negative bacillary sepsis. In: Morrison DC, Ryan JL (eds) Novel therapeutic strategies in the treatment of sepsis. Marcel Dekker, Inc, New York, pp 31–41
17. Opal SM, Cross AS, Bhattacharjee A, et al (1996) Active immunization with an *E. coli* J5 LPS vaccine in an experimental model of Gram-negative sepsis. Program abstracts of the 36th ICAAC Meeting (abstract G-1)
18. Rietschel ET, Brade H, Holst O, et al (1996) Bacterial endotoxin; chemical composition, biological recognition, host response, and immunological detoxification. Curr Top Microbiol Immunol 216:39–81
19. Swaminathan S, Furey W, Pletcher, et al (1992) Crystal structure of staphylococcal enterotoxin B, a superantigen. Nature 359:801–805
20. Jardetzky TS, Brown JH, Gorga JC, et al (1994) Three-dimensional structure of a human class II histocompatibility molecule complexed with superantigen. Nature 368:711–718
21. Wahlsten JL, Ramakrishman S (1998) Separation of function between the domains of toxic shock syndrome-1. J Immunol 160:854–859
22. Woody MA, Krakauer T, Ulrich RG, Stiles BJ (1998) Differential immune responses to Staphylococcal enterotoxin B mutation in a hydrophobic loop dominating the interface with major histocompatibility complex class II receptors. J Infect Dis 177:1013–1022
23. Kusunoki T, Wright SD (1996) Chemical characteristics of *Staphylococcus aureus* molecules that have CD14-dependent cell-stimulating activity. J Immunol 157:5112–5118
24. Weidemann B, Schletter J, Dziarski R, et al (1997) Specific binding of soluble peptidoglycan and muramyl dipeptide to CD14 on human monocytes. Infect Immun 65:858–863
25. Dziarski R, Tapping RI, Tobias PS (1998) Binding of bacterial peptidoglycan to CD14. J Biol Chem 273:8680–8686
26. van Langevelde P, van Dissel JT, Ravensbergen E, et al (1998) Antibiotic-induced release of lipoteichoic acid and peptidoglycan from *Staphylococcus aureus*: quantitative measurements and biological reactivities. Antimicrob Agents Chemother 3073–3078
27. Krieg AM, Love-Homan L, Ae-Kyung Y, et al (1998) CpG DNA induces sustained IL-12 expression in vivo and resistance to *Listeria monocytogenes* challenge. J Immunol 161: 2428–2434
28. Krieg AM, Wu T, Weeratna R, et al (1998) Sequence motifs in adenoviral DNA block immune activation by stimulatory CpG motifs. Proc Natl Acad Sci USA 95:12631–12636
29. Baumgartner JD (1991) Immunotherapy with antibodies to core lipopolysaccharide: A critical appraisal. Infect Dis Clin North Am 5:753–764
30. Cross AS (1994) Antiendotoxin antibodies: A dead end? Ann Intern Med 121:58–60
31. Ge Y, Ezzell RM, Tompkins RG, et al (1994) Cellular distribution of endotoxin after injection of chemically purified lipopolysaccharide differs from that after injection of live bacteria. J Infect Dis 169:95–104
32. Wurfel MM, Hailman E, Wright SD (1995) Soluble CD14 acts as a shuttle in the neutralization of lipopolysaccharide (LPS) by LPS-binding protein and reconstituted high density lipoprotein. J Exp Med 181:1743–1754
33. Yang R-B, Mark MR, Gray A, et al (1998) Toll-like receptor-2 mediates lipopolysaccharide-induced cellular signaling. Nature 395:284–286

34. Bone RC, Balk RA, Fein AM, et al (1995) A second large controlled clinical study of E5, a monoclonal antibody to endotoxin: Results of a prospective, multicenter, randomized, controlled trial. Crit Care Med 23:994–1005
35. Greenman RL, Schein RMH, Martin MA, et al (1991) A controlled clinical trial of E5 murine monoclonal IgM antibody to endotoxin in the treatment of Gram-negative sepsis. JAMA 266:1097–1102
36. McCloskey RV, Straube RC, Sanders C, et al (1994) Treatment of septic shock with human monoclonal antibody HA-1A. A randomized, double-blind, placebo-controlled trial. Ann Intern Med 121:1–5
37. Ziegler EJ, Fisher CJ, Jr., Sprung CL, et al (1991) Treatment of Gram-negative bacteremia and septic shock with HA-1A human monoclonal antibody against endotoxin: a randomized, double-blind, placebo-controlled trial. N Engl J Med 324:429–436
38. Bhat NM, Bieber MM, Chapman CJ, et al (1993) Human anti-lipid A monoclonal antibodies bind to human B cells and the i antigen on cord red blood cells. J Immunol 151:5011–5021
39. Quezado ZMN, Natanson C, Alling DW, et al (1993) A controlled trial of HA-1A in a canine model of Gram-negative septic shock. JAMA 269:2221–2227
40. Di Padova F, Brade H, Barclay GR, et al (1993) A broadly cross-protective monoclonal antibody binding to *Escherichia coli* and *Salmonella* lipopolysaccharides. Infect Immun 61: 3863–3872
41. Braude AI, Douglas H, Davis CE (1973) Treatment and prevention of intravascular coagulation with antiserum to endotoxin. J Infect Dis 128:S157–164
42. Chedid L, Parant M, Boyer F (1968) A proposed mechanism for natural immunity to enterobacterial pathogens. J Immunol 100:292–306
43. Greisman SE, Young EJ, DuBuy JB (1973) Mechanisms of endotoxin tolerance. VIII. Specificity of serum transfer. J Immunol 111:1349–1355
44. McCabe WR, Kreger BE, Johns M (1972) Type-specific and cross-reactive antibodies in Gram-negative bacteremia. N Engl J Med 287:261–267
45. McCabe WR, DeMaria A, Berberich H, et al (1998) Immunization with rough mutants of *Salmonella minnesota*: protective activity of IgM and IgG antibody to the R595 (Re Chemotype) mutant. J Infect Dis 158:291–300
46. Warren HS, Amato SF, Fitting C, et al (1993) Assessment of ability of murine and human anti-lipid A monoclonal antibodies to bind and neutralize lipopolysaccharide. J Exp Med 177: 89–97
47. Pollack M, Huang AI, Prescott RW, et al (1983) Enhanced survival in *Pseudomonas aeruginosa* septicemia associated with high levels of circulating antibody to *Escherichia coli* endotoxin core. J Clin Invest 72:1874–1881
48. Nys M, Darnas P, Joassin L, et al (1993) Sequential anti-core glycolipid immunoglobulin antibody activities in patients with and without septic shock and their relation to outcome. Ann Surg 217:300–306
49. Bennett-Guerrero E, Ayuso L, Hamilton-Davies C, et al (1997) Relationship of pre- operative anti-endotoxin core antibodies and adverse outcomes following cardiac surgery. JAMA 277: 646–650.
50. Ziegler EJ, McCutchan JA, Fierer J, et al (1982) Treatment of Gram-negative bacteremia and shock with human antiserum to a mutant *Escherichia coli*. N Engl J Med 307:1225–1230
51. Hellman J, Zanzot EM, Loiselle PM, et al (1997) Antiserum against *Escherichia coli* J5 contains antibodies reactive with outer membrane proteins of heterologous Gram-negative bacteria. J Infect Dis 176:1260–1268
52. Bhattacharjee AK, Opal SM, Palardy JE, et al (1994) Affinity-purified *Escherichia coli* J5 lipopolysaccharide-specific IgG protects neutropenic rats against gram-negative bacterial sepsis. J Infect Dis 170:622–629
53. Bhattacharjee AK, Opal SM, Taylor R, et al (1996) A noncovalent complex vaccine prepared with detoxified *Escherichia coli* J5 (Rc chemotype) lipopolysaccharide and *Neisseria meningitidis* Group B outer membrane protein produces protective antibodies against gram-negative bacteremia. J Infect Dis 173:1157–1162
54. Kim KS, Kang JH, Cross AS, et al (1988) Functional activities of monoclonal antibodies to the O side chain of *Escherichia coli* lipopolysaccharides in vitro and in vivo. J Infect Dis 157:47–53

55. Shapiro ED, Berg AT, Austrian R, et al (1991) The protective efficacy of polyvalent pneumococcal polysaccharide vaccine. N Engl J Med 352: 1453–1458
56. Marrack P, Kappler J (1990) The staphylococcal enterotoxins and their relatives. Science 248:705–711
57. Schleivert PM (1993) Role of superantigens in human disease. J Infect Dis 167:997– 1002
58. Hensler T, Köller M, Geoffroy C, et al (1993) *Staphylococcus aureus* toxic shock syndrome toxin 1 and *Streptococcus pyogenes* erythrogenic toxin A modulate inflammatory mediator release from human neutrophils. Infect Immun 61:1055–1061
59. Kotzin BL, Leung DY, Kappler J, et al (1993) Superantigens and their potential role in human disease. Adv Immunol 54:99–166
60. Stevens DL, Tanner MH, Winship J, et al (1989) Severe group A streptococcal infections associated with a toxic shock-like syndrome and scarlet fever toxin A. N Engl J Med 321:1–7
61. Astiz M, Saha D, Lustbader D, et al (1996) Monocyte response to bacterial toxins, expression of cell surface receptors, and release of anti-inflammatory cytokines during sepsis. J Lab Clin Med 128:594–600
62. Leung DY, Travers JB, Giorno R, et al (1995) Evidence for a streptococcal superantigen-driven process in acute guttate psoriasis. J Clin Invest 96:2106–2112
63. Muller-Alouf H, Alouf JE, Gerlach D, et al (1994) Comparative study of cytokine release by human peripheral blood mononuclear cells stimulated with *Streptococcus pyogenes* superantigenic erythrogenic toxins, heat killed streptococci, and lipopolysaccharide. Infect Immun 62:4915–4921
64. Goldbach-Mansky R, King PD, Taylor AP, et al (1992) A co-stimulatory role for CD28 in the activation of CD4+ T lymphocytes by staphylococcal enterotoxin B. Int Immunol 4: 1351–1360
65. Blankson JN, Morse SS (1994) The CD28/B7 pathway costimulates the response of primary murine T cells to superantigens as well as to conventional antigens. Cell Immunol 157:306–312
66. Krakauer T (1994) Cell adhesion molecules are co-receptors for staphylococcal enterotoxin B-induced T-cell activation and cytokine production. Immunol Lett 39:121–125
67. Leonard BA, Schlievert PM (1992) Immune cell lethality induced by streptococcal pyrogenic exotoxin A and endotoxin. Infect Immun 60:3747–3755
68. Blank C, Luz A, Bendigs S, et al (1997) Superantigens and endotoxin synergize in the induction of lethal shock. Eur J Immunol 27:825–833
69. Smith RJ, Schlievert PM, Himelright IM, et al (1994) Dual infections with *Staphylococcus aureus* and *Streptococcus pyogenes* causing toxic shock syndrome. Possible synergistic effects of toxic shock syndrome toxin-1 and streptococcal pyrogenic exotoxin C. Diag Micro Infect Dis 19:245–247
70. Ren K, Bannan JD, Pancholi V, et al (1994) Characterization and biological properties of a new staphylococcal exotoxin. J Exp Med 180:1675–1683
71. Reda KB, Kapur V, Mollick JA, et al (1994) Molecular characterization and phylogenetic distribution of the streptococcal superantigen gene (ssa) from *Streptococcus pyogenes.* Infect Immun 62:1867–1874
72. Weeks CR, Ferretti JJ (1986) Nucleotide sequence of the type A streptococcal exotoxin (erythrogenic toxin) gene from *Streptococcus pyogenes* bacteriophage T12. Infect Immun 52:144–150
73. Goshorn SC, Schlievert PM (1988) Nucleotide sequence of streptococcal exotoxin type C. Infect Immun 56:2518–2520
74. Blomster-Hautama DA, Kreiswirth BN, Kornblum JS, et al (1986) The nucleotide and partial amino acid sequence of toxic shock syndrome toxin-1. J Biol Chem 261:15783–15786
75. Acharya KR, Passalacqua EF, Jones EY, et al (1994) Structural basis of superantigen action inferred from crystal structure of toxic-shock syndrome toxin-1. Nature 367:94–97
76. Warren JR, Spero L, Metzger JF (1974) Stabilization of native structure by the closed disulfide loop of staphylococcal enterotoxin B. Biochem Biophys Acta 359:351–363
77. Grossman D, Van M, Mollick JA, et al (1991) Mutation of the disulfide loop in staphylococcal enterotoxin A. Consequences for T cell recognition. J Immunol 147:3274–3281

78. Kappler JW, Herman A, Clements J, et al (1992) Mutations defining functional regions of the superantigen staphylococcal enterotoxin B. J Exp Med 175:387–396
79. Hartwig UF, Fleisher B (1993) Mutations affecting MHC class II binding of the superantigen streptococcal erythrogenic toxin A. Int Immunol 5:869–875
80. Stelma GN, Jr, Bergdoll MS (1982) Inactivation of staphylococcal enterotoxin A by chemical modification. Biochem Biophys Res Comm 105:121–126
81. Grossman D, Cook RG, Sparrow JT, et al (1990) Dissociation of the stimulatory activities of staphylococcal enterotoxins for T cells and monocytes. J Exp Med 172:1831–1841
82. Mollick JA, McMasters RL, Grossman D, et al (1993) Localization of a site on bacterial superantigens that determines T cell receptor beta chain specificity. J Exp Med 177:283–293
83. Griggs ND, Pontzer CH, Jarpe MA, et al (1992) Mapping of multiple binding domains of the superantigen staphylococcal enterotoxin A for HLA. J Immunol 148:2516–2521
84. Soos JM, Johnson HM (1994) Multiple binding sites on the superantigen, staphylococcal enterotoxin B, imparts versatility in binding to MHC class II molecules. Biochem Biophys Res Comm 201:596–602
85. Bannan JD, Mingo F, Viteri A, et al (1997) Neutralization of streptococcal pyrogenic exotoxins and staphylococcal enterotoxins by antisera to synthetic peptides representing conserved amino acid motifs. Adv Exp Med Biol 418:903–907
86. Jett M, Neill R, Welch C, et al (1994) Identification of staphylococcal enterotoxin B sequences important for induction of lymphocyte proliferation by using synthetic peptide fragments of the toxin. Infect Immun 62:3408–3415
87. Bohach GA, Hovde CJ, Handley JP, et al (1988) Cross-neutralization of staphylococcal and streptococcal pyrogenic toxins by monoclonal and polyclonal antibodies. Infect Immun 56: 400–404
88. Spero L, Morlock B, Metzger J (1978) On the cross-reactivity of staphylococcal enterotoxins A, B, and C. J Immunol 120:86–89
89. Pontzer CH, Griggs ND, Johnson HM (1993) Agonist properties of a microbial superantigen peptide. Biochem Biophys Res Commun 193:1191–1197
90. Andersson J, Skansén-Saphir U, Björk L, et al (1994) Lymphokine production induced by streptococcal pyrogenic exotoxin-A is selectively down-regulated by pooled human IgG. Eur J Immunol 24:916–922
91. Björk L, Andersson U, Chauvet J-M, et al (1994) Quantification of superantigen induced IFN-γ production by computerised image analysis-inhibition of cytokine production and blast transformation by pooled human IgG. J Immunol Method 175:201–213
92. Kaul R, McGeer A, Norrby-Teglund, et al (1999) Intravenous immunoglobulin therapy for streptococcal toxic shock syndrome – a comparative observational study. Clin Infect Dis 28:800–807
93. Norrby-Teglund A, Basma H, Andersson J, et al (1998) Varying titers of neutralizing antibodies to streptococcal superantigens in diferdent preparations of normal polyspecific immunoglobulin G: Implications for therapeutic efficacy. Clin Infect Dis 26:631–638
94. Norrby-Teglund A, Kaul R, Low DE, et al (1996) Plasma from patients with severe invasive group A strepcococcal infections treated with normal polyspecific IgG inhibits streptococcal superantigen-induced T cell proliferation and cytokine production. J Immunol 156: 3057–3064
95. Werdan K, Pilz G (1996) Supplemental immune globulins in sepsis: a critical appraisal. Clin Exp Immunol 104 (suppl 1):83–90
96. Sriskandan S, Moyes D, Buttery LK, et al (1996) Streptococcal pyrogenic exotoxin A release, distribution, and role in a murine model of fasciitis and multiorgan failure due to *Streptococcus pyrogenes.* J Infect Dis 173: 1399–1407

Subject Index

Printing: Mercedes-Druck, Berlin
Binding: Buchbinderei Lüderitz & Bauer, Berlin

GPSR Compliance

The European Union's (EU) General Product Safety Regulation (GPSR) is a set of rules that requires consumer products to be safe and our obligations to ensure this.

If you have any concerns about our products, you can contact us on ProductSafety@springernature.com

In case Publisher is established outside the EU, the EU authorized representative is:

Springer Nature Customer Service Center GmbH
Europaplatz 3
69115 Heidelberg, Germany

Batch number: 10583998

Printed by Printforce, the Netherlands